International Trauma Life Support
for Emergency Care Providers

seventh edition

International Trauma Life Support
for Emergency Care Providers

John Campbell, MD, FACEP
and Alabama Chapter, American College of Emergency Physicians

PEARSON

Boston Columbus Indianapolis New York San Francisco Upper Saddle River Amsterdam
Cape Town Dubai London Madrid Milan Munich Paris Montreal Toronto Delhi
Mexico City São Paulo Sydney Hong Kong Seoul Singapore Taipei Tokyo

Publisher: Julie Levin Alexander
Publisher's Assistant: Regina Bruno
Editor-in-Chief: Marlene McHugh Pratt
Senior Acquisitions Editor: Stephen Smith
Associate Editor: Monica Moosang
Senior Managing Editor for Development: Lois Berlowitz
Development Editor: Jo Cepeda
Editorial Assistant: Samantha Sheehan
Director of Marketing: David Gesell
Marketing Manager: Brian Hoehl
Marketing Specialist: Michael Sirinides
Marketing Assistant: Crystal Gonzalez
Managing Production Editor: Patrick Walsh
Production Liaison: Julie Boddorf
Production Editor: Peggy Kellar
Senior Media Editor: Amy Peltier
Media Project Manager: Lorena Cerisano
Manufacturing Manager: Alan Fischer, Lisa McDowell
Senior Art Director: Maria Guglielmo
Art Director: Chris Weigand
Interior Designer: Kevin Kall
Cover Designer: Jodi Notowitz/Wicked Design
Composition: Aptara®, Inc.
Printing and Binding: Quad/Graphics
Cover Printer: Lehigh-Phoenix Color/Hagerstown

Notice on Care Procedures

It is the intent of the authors and publisher that this textbook be used as part of an education program taught by qualified instructors and supervised by a licensed physician. The procedures described in this textbook are based upon consultation with paramedics, nurses, and physicians. The authors and publisher have taken care to make certain that these procedures reflect currently accepted clinical practice; however, they cannot be considered absolute recommendations.

The material in this textbook contains the most current information available at the time of publication. However, federal, state, and local guidelines concerning clinical practices, including, without limitation, those governing infection control and universal precautions, change rapidly. The reader should note, therefore, that new regulations may require changes in some procedures.

It is the responsibility of the reader to familiarize himself or herself with the policies and procedures set by federal, state, and local agencies as well as the institution or agency where the reader is employed. The authors and the publisher of this textbook and the supplements written to accompany it disclaim any liability, loss, or risk resulting directly or indirectly from the suggested procedures and theory, from any undetected errors, or from the reader's misunderstanding of the text. It is the reader's responsibility to stay informed of any new changes or recommendations made by any federal, state, and local agency as well as by his or her employing institution or agency.

Notice on Gender Usage

The English language has historically given preference to the male gender. Among many words, the pronouns, he and his are commonly used to describe both genders. Society evolves faster than language, and the male pronouns still predominate our speech. The authors have made great effort to treat the two genders equally, recognizing that a significant percentage of EMS providers are female. However, in some instances, male pronouns may be used to describe both males and females solely for the purpose of brevity. This is not intended to offend any readers of the female gender.

If you purchased this book within the United States or Canada you should be aware that it has been imported without the approval of the Publisher or the Author.

Credits and acknowledgments for content borrowed from other sources and reproduced, with permission, in this textbook appear on appropriate page within text.

PEARSON

10 9 8 7 6 5 4 3 2 1
PIE ISBN-10: 0-13-276666-3
PIE ISBN-13: 978-0-13-276666-1

Dedication

"Individual commitment to a group effort—that is what makes a team work, a company work, a society work, a civilization work."—Vince Lombardi

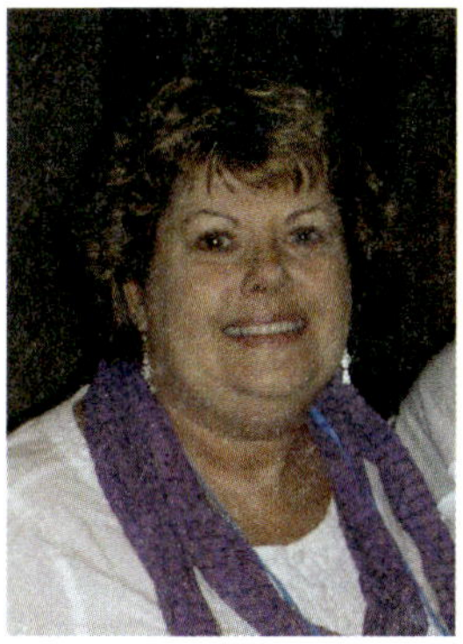

The Seventh Edition of ITLS is dedicated to Ginny Kennedy Palys.

Ginny Kennedy Palys became our Executive Director over 17 years ago and has served admirably as the anchor for our Board, Editorial Board, and the entire organization. Ginny's individual commitment to our group effort has facilitated the growth of ITLS products, services, and availability worldwide. Thank you for your loyalty and leadership.

In gratitude from the Board of Directors and the Editorial Board of International Trauma Life Support, Inc.

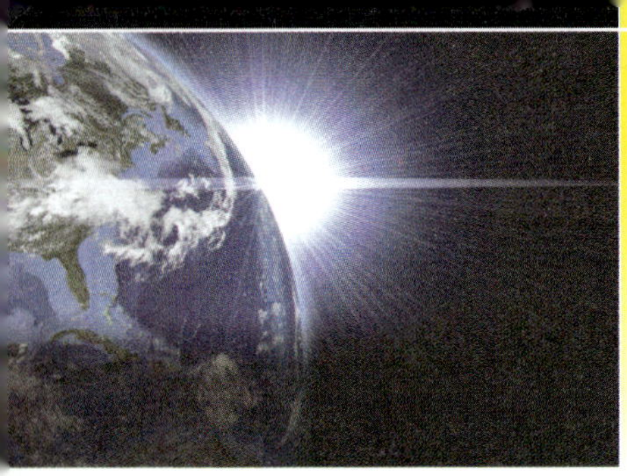

Brief Contents

Contents

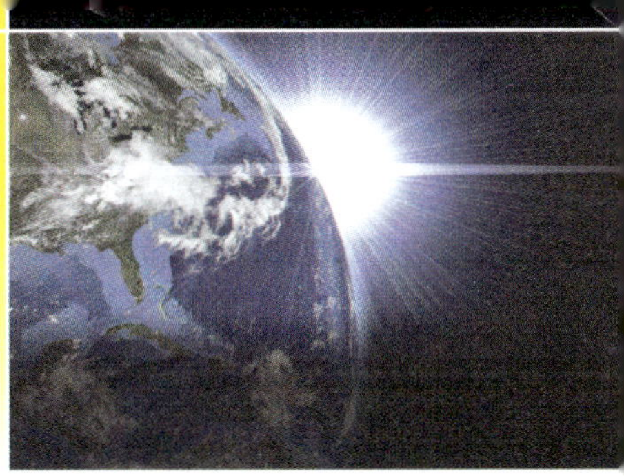

Chapter 7
Thoracic Trauma Skills 131

Chapter 8
Shock 140

Chapter 9
Vascular Access Skills 162

Chapter 10
Head Trauma 172

Chapter 11
Spinal Trauma 193

Chapter 12
Spine Management Skills 219

Chapter 13
Abdominal Trauma 236

Chapter 14
Extremity Trauma 245

Chapter 15
Extremity Trauma Skills 271

Chapter 16
Burns 285

Chapter 17
Pediatric Trauma 308

Chapter 18
Geriatric Trauma 332

Chapter 19
Trauma in Pregnancy 342

Chapter 20
The Impaired Patient 352

Chapter 21
Trauma Arrest 359

About the Editor

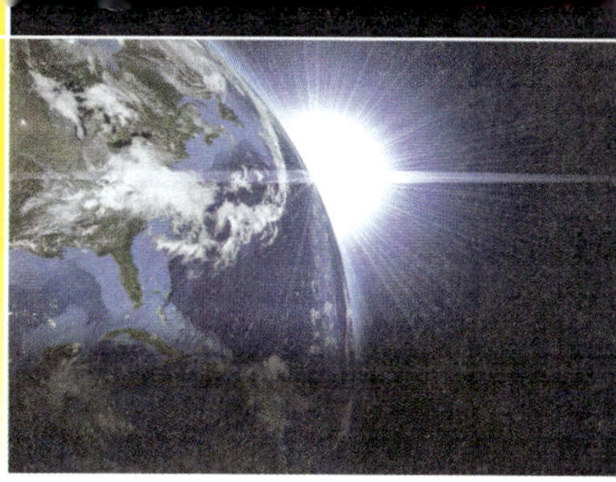

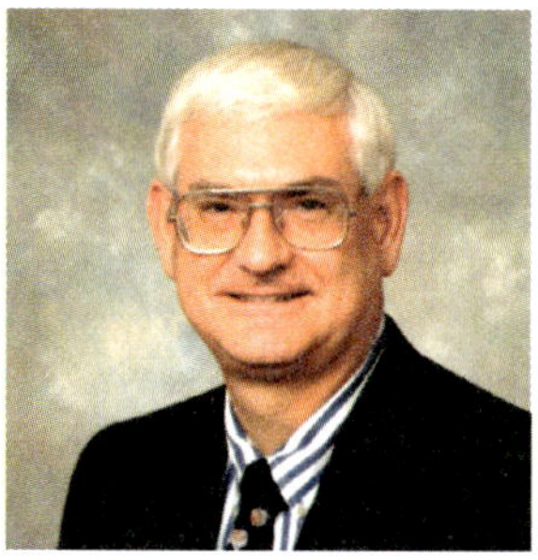

JOHN E. CAMPBELL, *MD, FACEP*

Dr. Campbell received his BS degree in pharmacy from Auburn University in 1966 and his medical degree from the University of Alabama at Birmingham in 1970. He has been in the practice of Emergency Medicine for 40 years, practicing in Alabama, Georgia, New Mexico, and Texas. He became interested in prehospital care in 1972 when he was asked to teach a basic EMT course to members of the Clay County Rescue Squad. He is still an honorary member of that outstanding group. Since then, he has served as medical director of many EMT and paramedic training programs. He recently retired as the Medical Director for EMS and Trauma for the State of Alabama.

From the original basic trauma life support course developed an international organization of teachers of trauma care called "International Trauma Life Support, Inc.," or ITLS. Dr. Campbell has served as its president since the inception of the organization.

Dr. Campbell is the author of the first edition of the *Basic Trauma Life Support* textbook and has continued to be the editor through to this new edition, now entitled *International Trauma Life Support for Emergency Care Providers.* He also is the coauthor of *Homeland Security and Emergency Medical Response* and *Tactical Emergency Medical Essentials.*

He was a member of the first faculty of Emergency Medicine at the School of Medicine, University of Alabama at Birmingham. In 1991 he was the first recipient of the American College of Emergency Medicine's EMS Award for outstanding achievement of national significance in the area of EMS. In 2001 he received the Ronald D. Stewart Lifetime Achievement Award from the National Association of EMS Physicians. He is currently retired from clinical practice and resides on his farm in Camp Hill, Alabama.

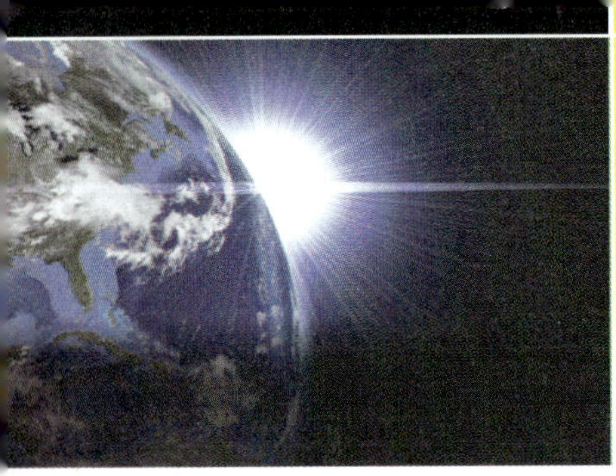

Authors

ITLS for Emergency Care Providers

Roy L. Alson, PhD, MD, FACEP, FAAEM
Associate Professor of Emergency Medicine and Director, Office of Prehospital and Disaster Medicine, Wake Forest University School of Medicine, Winston-Salem, NC
Medical Director, Forsyth County EMS, Winston-Salem, NC
Medical Advisor, Disaster Services, NC Office of EMS, Raleigh, NC

James J. Augustine, MD
Director of Clinical Operations, EMP Ltd, Canton, OH
Assistant Clinical Professor, Department of Emergency Medicine, Wright State University, Dayton, OH
Chair, ASTM Task Group E54.02.01, Standards for Hospital Preparedness Under Committee E54 on Homeland Security Applications
Former Medical Director, Atlanta Fire Rescue Department and the District of Columbia Fire and EMS Department

Jere Baldwin, MD, FACEP, FAAFP
Chief, Department of Emergency Medicine and Ambulatory Services, Mercy Hospital, Port Huron, MI

Graciela M. Bauza, MD
Assistant Professor of Surgery, University of Pittsburgh

Russell Bieniek, MD, FACEP
Director of Emergency Preparedness, UPMC Hamot, Erie, PA

William Bozeman, MD, FACEP, FAAEM
Associate Professor, Department of Emergency Medicine, and Associate Research Director, Wake Forest University School of Medicine, Winston-Salem, NC

Walter J. Bradley, MD, MBA, FACEP
Medical Director, Illinois State Police
SWAT Team Physician, Moline Police Department
Physician Advisor, Trinity Medical Center

Sabina A. Braithwaite, MD, MPH, FACEP, NREMTP
EMS System Medical Director, Wichita-Sedgwick County, KS
Clinical Associate Professor of Emergency Medicine, University of Kansas Medical Center, Kansas City
Clinical Associate Professor of Preventive Medicine and Public Health, University of Kansas Medical Center, Wichita
Vice Chair, Board of Directors, International Trauma Life Support

Jeremy J. Brywczynski, MD
Assistant Professor, Emergency Medicine, Vanderbilt University Medical Center, Nashville, TN
Medical Director, Vanderbilt LifeFlight
Medical Director, Vanderbilt FlightComm
Assistant Medical Director, Nashville (TN) Fire Department

John E. Campbell, MD, FACEP
Medical Director, EMS & Trauma, State of Alabama, Retired

Leon Charpentier, EMT-P
Harker Heights (TX) Fire Chief, Retired

James H. Creel, Jr. MD, FACEP
Clinical Associate Professor and Program Director, Department of Emergency Medicine, University of Tennessee College of Medicine (UTCOM)
Chief of Emergency Medicine, Erlanger Health System, Chattanooga, TN

Ann M. Dietrich, MD, FAAP, FACEP
Professor of Pediatrics, Ohio State University, Director of Risk Management, Section of Emergency Medicine, Columbus (OH) Children's Hospital
Pediatric Medical Advisor, Medflight of Ohio

Ray Fowler, MD, FACEP
Professor of Emergency Medicine, Surgery, Emergency Medical Education, and Health Professions, The University of Texas Southwestern Medical Center

Attending Emergency Medicine Faculty, Parkland Memorial Hospital, Dallas, TX

Pam Gersch, RN, CLNC
Program Director, AirMed Team, Rocky Mountain Helicopters, Redding, CA

Martin Greenberg, MD, FAAOS, FACS
Chief of Hand Surgery, Advocate Illinois Masonic Medical Center
Chief of Orthopedic Surgery, Our Lady of the Resurrection Medical Center, Chicago, IL
Reserve Police Officer, Village of Tinley Park, IL
Tactical Physician, South Suburban Emergency Response Team
ITOA Co-Chair, TEMS Committee

Kyee H. Han, MBBS, FRCS, FCEM
Consultant in Accident and Emergency Medicine
Medical Director, North East Ambulance Service NHS Trust
Honorary Clinical Senior Lecturer, The James Cook University Hospital, Middlesbrough, UK

Donna Hastings, MA, EMT-P, CPCC
Chair, ITLS Editorial Board
CEO, Heart and Stroke Foundation of Alberta, NWT and Nunavut, Calgary, Canada

Leah J. Heimbach, JD, RN, EMT-P
Principal, Healthcare Management Solutions, LLC, White Hall, WV

Eduardo Romero Hicks, MD, EMT
Director, Sistema de Urgencias del Estado de Guanajuato, Guanajuato State Emergency System, México
Associate Professor, University of Guanajuato Nursing School, Guanajuato, México
Medical Director, ITLS Guanajuato México Chapter

Ahamed H. Idris, MD
Professor of Surgery and Medicine and Director, DFW Center for Resuscitation Research, UT Southwestern Medical Center at Dallas, TX

David Maatman, NREMT-P/IC
Education Coordinator, American Medical Response, Grand Rapids, MI

Kirk Magee MD, MSc, FRCPC
Associate Professor, Dalhousie Department of Emergency Medicine, Halifax, Nova Scotia

Patrick J. Maloney, MD
Staff Physician, Denver (CO) Health Medical Center and Denver Emergency, Center for Children
Clinical Instructor, University of Colorado School of Medicine, Denver, CO

Leslie K. Mihalov, MD
Chief, Emergency Medicine, and Medical Director, Emergency Services, Nationwide Children's Hospital
Associate Professor of Pediatrics at The Ohio State University College of Medicine

Richard N. Nelson, MD, FACEP
Professor and Vice Chair, Department of Emergency Medicine, The Ohio State University College of Medicine

Jonathan Newman, MD, MMM, FACEP
Assistant Medical Director, United Hospital Center, Bridgeport, WV

Bob Page, BAS, NREMT-P, CCEMT-P, NCEE
Edutainment Consulting and Seminars, LLC

Wm. Bruce Patterson, Platoon Chief/EMT-P
Strathcona County Emergency Services

Andrew B. Peitzman, MD
Mark M. Ravitch Professor
Executive Vice-Chairman, Department of Surgery, and Chief, Division of General Surgery, University of Pittsburgh

Paul E. Pepe, MD, MPH
Professor of Medicine, Surgery, Pediatrics, Public Health and Chair, Emergency Medicine, University of Texas Southwestern Medical Center and Parkland Emergency-Trauma Center
Director, City of Dallas Medical Emergency Services for Public Safety, Public Health and Homeland Security, Dallas, TX

William F. Pfeifer, MD, FACS
Professor of Surgery, Department of Speciality Medicine, Rocky Vista University College of Osteopathic Medicine
Mile High Surgical Specialists, Littleton, CO
Colonel MC USAR (ret)

Art Proust, MD, FACEP
Associate Medical Director, SFVEMSS, Geneva, IL

Mario Luis Ramirez, MD, MPP
Tactical and Prehospital EMS Fellow and Clinical Instructor in Emergency Medicine, Department of Emergency Medicine, Vanderbilt University Medical Center, Nashville, TN

Jonathan M. Rubin, MD, FAAEM
Associate Professor of Emergency Medicine, Medical College of Wisconsin

S. Robert Seitz, MEd, RN, NREMT-P
Assistant Professor, School of Health and Rehabilitation Sciences, Emergency Medicine Program, University of Pittsburgh
Assistant Program Director, Office of Education and International Emergency Medicine, University of Pittsburgh Center for Emergency Medicine
Continuing Education Editor, Journal of Emergency Medical Services, Editorial Board, International Trauma Life Support

Corey M. Slovis, MD, FACP, FACEP, FAAEM
Professor of Emergency Medicine and Medicine and Chairman, Department of Emergency Medicine, Vanderbilt University Medical Center, Nashville, TN
Medical Director, Metro Nashville Fire Department and International Airport

J. T. Stevens, NREMT-P

Ronald D. Stewart, OC, ONS, ECNS, BA, BSc, MD, FACEP, DSc, LLD
Professor Emeritus, Medical Education, and Professor of Emergency Medicine and Anaesthesia, Dalhousie University, Halifax, Nova Scotia

Arlo Weltge, MD, MPH, FACEP
Clinical Associate Professor of Emergency Medicine, University of Texas, Houston Medical School
Medical Director, Program in EMS, Houston Community College

Howard A. Werman, MD, FACEP
Professor of Clinical Emergency Medicine, The Ohio State University
Medical Director, MedFlight of Ohio

Katherine West, BSN, MSEd, CIC
Infection Control Consultant, Manassas, VA

Melissa White, MD, MPH
Assistant Professor, Assistant Residency Director, and Medical Director, John's Creek Fire Department
Medical Director, Emory Emergency Medical Services
Associate Medical Director, Emory Flight/Air Methods, GA
Department of Emergency Medicine, Emory University School of Medicine, Atlanta, GA

Janet M. Williams, MD
Professor of Emergency Medicine, University of Rochester (NY) Medical Center

E. John Wipfler, III, MD, FACEP
Attending Emergency Physician, OSF Saint Francis Medical Center Residency Program
Medical Director, STATT TacMed Unit, Tactical Medicine
Sheriff's Physician, Peoria County (IL) Sheriff's Office
Clinical Associate Professor of Surgery, University of Illinois College of Medicine, Peoria, IL

Arthur H. Yancey II, MD, MPH, FACEP
Deputy Director of Health for EMS, Fulton County Department of Health and Wellness, Atlanta, GA
Associate Professor, Department of Emergency Medicine, Emory University School of Medicine, Atlanta, GA

What's New in This Edition

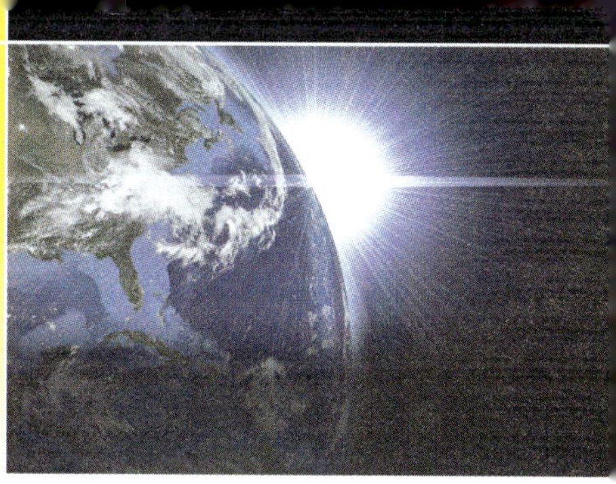

The seventh edition of the ITLS textbook, *International Trauma Life Support for Emergency Care Providers*, has been updated and refined to reflect the latest and most effective approaches to the care of the trauma patient. The text also has been made to conform to the newest AHA guidelines for artificial ventilation and CPR. Other general changes include the addition of key terms, new case presentations for all chapters, updated bibliographies, new photos, and redrawings of many illustrations for a more up-to-date look. There is now also an all new student and instructor resource website. Important chapter-by-chapter changes are as follows:

- In the Introduction it is explained why the concept of the "Golden Period" has replaced the "Golden Hour."
- In Chapter 1, scene safety has been expanded with comments on blast scenes. The discussion of personal watercraft injuries has been updated and expanded. The blast injuries section has been updated to include new terminology.
- In Chapter 2, minor changes have been made in the assessment sequence to make it more practical. Also added is the concept that serious external hemorrhage should be noted in the general impression and control of bleeding must be immediately delegated. The concept of "Fix-It" has been introduced. As the leader performs the assessment, he or she will delegate responses to abnormalities found in the assessment. This is to reinforce the rule that the leader must not interrupt the assessment to deal with problems but must delegate the needed actions to team members. That emphasizes the team concept and keeps on-scene time at a minimum. The order of presentation of the three assessments (ITLS Primary Survey, ITLS Ongoing Exam, and ITLS Secondary Survey) has been changed. The ITLS Ongoing Exam is performed before the ITLS Secondary Survey, a more common situation, and may replace it. The use of finger-stick serum lactate levels and prehospital abdominal ultrasound exams are mentioned as areas of current study to better identify patients that may be in early shock.
- Chapter 3 reflects the changes in Chapter 2.
- In Chapter 4, capnography is stressed as the standard for confirming and monitoring the position of the endotracheal tube. Use of ELM (external larynx manipulation) is introduced as a means of improving the visualization of the vocal chords.
- In Chapter 5, the fact that cyanide poisoning will make a pulse oximeter reading unreliable has been added. Use of ELM is mentioned. Face-to-face intubation is briefly discussed. Fiber optic and video intubation are also mentioned.
- In Chapter 6, a discussion of blast injuries has been added.
- In Chapter 7, recent studies on chest wall thickness and the current controversy over which site to use to decompress a tension pneumothorax are discussed. A procedure for decompression by the lateral approach was added. Also

added is that the decompression needle should be at least 6 cm long and that several needles in this length should be available.

- In Chapter 8, the discussion of hemorrhagic shock has been updated with the experience of the military during the recent conflicts. A description of the use of capnography to monitor shock was also added.
- In Chapter 9, insertion of an IO needle by use of the EZ-IO system was added.
- In Chapter 11, recent studies are discussed that suggest with penetrating injuries to the trunk, taking time to do spinal motion restriction (SMR) doubles the death rate.
- In Chapter 12, the procedure for use of a short backboard was moved to Resource Central, but photo scans of performing SMR for standing patients were added. Photos were updated.
- In Chapter 13, the use of finger-stick serum lactate levels and the use of prehospital abdominal ultrasound exams are mentioned.
- In Chapter 14, the discussion of management of bleeding from extremity injuries has been expanded.
- In Chapter 15, procedures for use of a tourniquet and use of hemostatic agents have been added.
- In Chapter 16, the application of antimicrobial sheets to a burn if there is to be a very long transport is mentioned. The concept of escharotomy not being a prehospital procedure is clarified.
- In Chapter 17, the fact that the laryngeal mask airway and King LT airway are available in pediatric sizes and can be used for rescue airways has been added.
- In Chapter 21, the chapter has been extensively rewritten by new authors.
- In Chapter 22, the chapter has been updated with the latest recommendations for postexposure prophylaxis.

Resource Central

- In "Optional Skills," the use of the PtL airway and use of the FAST1® have been deleted. The procedure for use of the short backboard was added. The term "RSI" was updated to DAI (drug-assisted intubation).
- In "Multicasualty Incidents and Triage," the discussion of various triage schemes has been expanded.
- In "Role of the Medical Helicopter," the data has been updated.
- In "Trauma Scoring in the Prehospital Care Setting," the CDC Trauma Triage Scheme has been added.
- In "Tactical EMS," the bibliography has been updated.

Explore Resource Central

At the beginning of each chapter, we prompt readers to visit Resource Central on www.bradybooks.com for interactive learning exercises on topics discussed. Students will find quizzes, additional web links, games, videos, and more to supplement classroom learning. Through Resource Central, this text also offers instructors a full complement of online supplemental teaching materials such as test banks and PowerPoint lectures to aid in the classroom.

Acknowledgments

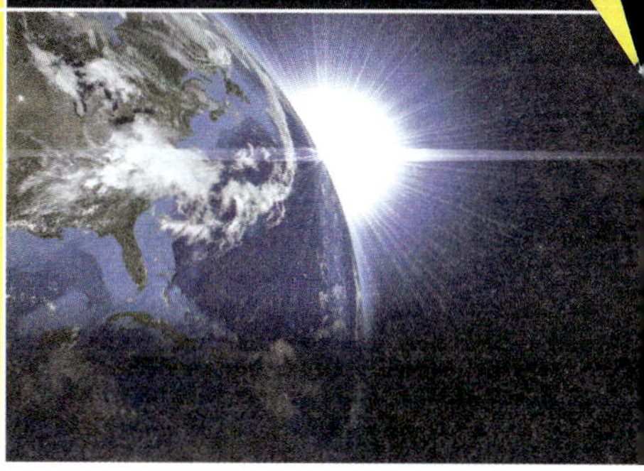

Special thanks to the following friends of ITLS who provided invaluable assistance with ideas, reviews, and corrections of the text. This was such a big job, and there were so many people who contributed, that I am sure I have left someone out. My apologies in advance.

Roy Alson, MD, FACEP
Leon Charpentier, EMT-P
Donna Hastings, EMT-P
Eduardo Romero Hicks, MD
David Maatman, NREMT-P/IC
William Pfeifer, MD, FACS
S. Robert Seitz, MEd, RN, NREMT-P
John T. Stevens, EMT-P

We wish to thank the EMS professionals who reviewed material especially for this seventh edition of International Trauma Life Support for Emergency Care Providers. *Their assistance is appreciated.*

Daniel K. W. Wittrock, EMT-2, NREMT-Basic, Primary Instructor for Danish Emergency Medical Training, ITLS Advanced Instructor, Military Medical Instructor, Slagelse, Denmark
David Borrett, BA, REMT/P, Paramedic Faculty, Century College, MN
Deborah L. Petty, BS, CICP, EMT-P I/C, St. Charles County Ambulance District, St. Peter's, MO
Jeffrey Asher, M.Ed, Chippewa Valley Technical College, Eau Claire, WI
Chris Ebright, B.Ed, NREMT-P, National EMS Academy, Covington, LA
Kevin J. O'Hara, MS EMT-P CIC, Nassau County EMS Academy, East Meadow, NY
Michael Humphrey-Parris, EMT-P, City of Vallejo Fire Department, San Francisco Paramedic Association, Vallejo and San Francisco, CA
Lafe Bush, CCEMTP, AS
K. Lee Darnell, MBA, NREMT-P, CEO, Adrenaline Junkies Education and Consulting, LLC, Pooler, GA
Bil Rosen, NREMT-P, Clinical Coordinator, Capital Health EMS, Trenton, NJ
Carl Voskamp, MBA, Lic-P, Victoria College EMS Program, Victoria, TX
Rudy Garrett, AS, NREMT-P, CCEMT-P, Training Coordinator, Somerset-Pulaski County EMS, Somerset, KY
Valerie D. Simonds MS, RN, NREMT-P, University of Maryland, Maryland Fire and Rescue Institute, College Park, MD

Another special thanks goes to the following photographers who donated their work to help illustrate the text.

Roy Alson, MD, FACEP
Sabina Braithwaite, MD
James Broselow, MD
Brant Burden, EMT-P
Anthony Cellitti, NREMT-P
Leon Charpentier, EMT-P
Stanley Cooper, EMT-P
Delphi Medical

Pamela Drexel, Brain Trauma Foundation
David Effron, MD, FACEP
Ferno Washington, Inc.
Peter Gianas, MD
Peter Goth, MD
KING Airway Systems
Kyee H. Han, MD, FRCS, FFAEM
Michal Heron
Eduardo Romero Hicks, MD
Jeff Hinshaw, MS, PA-C, NREMT-P
Masimo Corporation
Lewis B. Mallory, MBA, REMT-P
Bonnie Meneely, EMT-P
Nonin Medical, Inc.
North American Rescue
Bob Page, NREMT-P
William Pfeifer, MD, FACS
Robert S. Porter
Don Resch
Sam Splints
E. M. Singletary, MD

Introduction to the ITLS Course

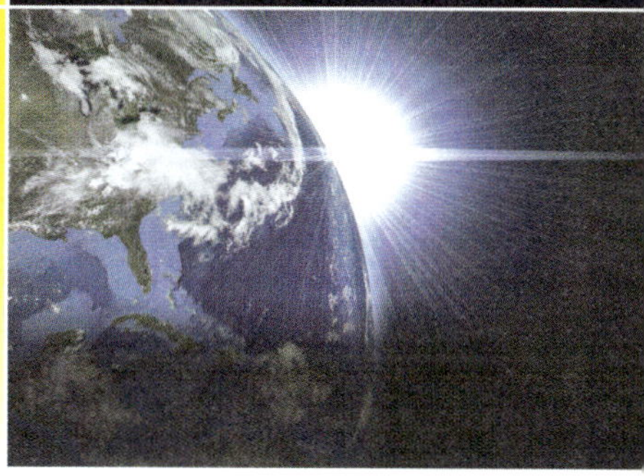

Trauma, the medical term for *injury*, has become the most expensive health problem in the United States and most other countries. In the United States, trauma is the fourth-leading cause of death for all ages and the leading cause of death for children and adults under the age of 45 years. Trauma causes 73% of all deaths in the 15- to 24-year-old age group. For every fatality, there are 10 more patients admitted to hospitals and hundreds more treated in emergency departments. The price of trauma, in both physical and fiscal resources, mandates that all emergency medical services (EMS) personnel learn more about this disease to treat its effects and decrease its incidence.

Because the survival of trauma patients is often determined by how quickly they get definitive care in the operating room, it is crucial that you know how to assess and manage the critical trauma patient in the most efficient way. The purpose of the ITLS course is to teach you the most rapid and practical method to assess and manage critical trauma patients. The course is a combination of written chapters to give you the "why" and the "how" and practical exercises to practice your knowledge and skills on simulated patients so that at the end of the course you feel confident in your ability to provide rapid lifesaving trauma care.

PHILOSOPHY OF ASSESSMENT AND MANAGEMENT OF THE TRAUMA PATIENT

Severe trauma, along with acute coronary syndrome and stroke, is a time-dependent disease. The direct relationship between the timing of definitive (surgical) treatment and the survival of trauma patients was first described by Dr. R Adams Cowley of the famous Shock-Trauma Center in Baltimore, Maryland. He discovered that when patients with serious multiple injuries were able to gain access to the operating room within an hour of the time of injury, the highest survival rate was achieved. He referred to this as the "Golden Hour." Over the years we have found that some patients (such as penetrating trauma to trunk) do not have even a golden "hour" but rather a shorter period of minutes, whereas many patients with blunt trauma may have a golden period longer than an hour. It has been suggested that we now call the prehospital period the "Golden Period" because it may be longer or shorter than an hour.

The Golden Period begins at the moment the patient is injured, not at the time you arrive at the scene. Much of this period has already passed when you begin your assessment, so you must be well organized in what you do. In the prehospital setting it is better to think of the Golden Period for on-scene care as being 10 minutes. In those 10 minutes, you must identify live patients, make treatment decisions, and begin to move patients to the appropriate medical facility. This means that every action must have a lifesaving purpose. Any action that increases scene time but is not potentially lifesaving must be omitted. Not only must you reduce evaluation and resuscitation to the most efficient and critical steps, but you also must develop the habit of assessing and treating every trauma patient in a planned logical and sequential manner so you do not forget critical actions.

When performing patient assessment, it is best to proceed in a "head-to-toe" manner so that nothing is missed. If you jump around during your assessment, you will inevitably forget to evaluate something crucial. Working as a team with your partner is also important because many actions must be done at the same time.

It has been said that medicine is a profession that was created for obsessive-compulsive people. Nowhere is this truer than in the care of the trauma patient. Often the patient's life depends on how well you manage the details. It is very important to remember that many of the details necessary to save the patient occur before you even arrive at the scene of the injury.

You or a member of your team must:

- Know how to maintain your ambulance or rescue vehicle so that it is serviced and ready to respond when needed.
- Know the quickest way to the scene of an injury. Use of global positioning satellite (GPS) navigation has been shown to decrease not only the time to respond but also the time of transport.
- Know how to size up a scene to recognize dangers and identify mechanisms of injury.
- Know which scenes are safe and, if not safe, what to do about them.
- Know when you can handle a situation and when to call for help.
- Know when to approach the patient and when to leave with the patient.
- Know your equipment and maintain it in working order.
- Know the most appropriate hospital and the fastest way to get there. (Organized trauma systems and transfer/bypass guidelines can shorten the time it takes to get a trauma patient to definitive care.)

As if all that were not enough, you also have to:

- Know where to put your hands, which questions to ask, what interventions to perform, when to perform them, and how to perform critical procedures quickly and correctly.

If you think the details are not important, then leave the profession now. Our job is saving lives, a most ancient and honorable profession. If we have a bad day, someone will pay for our mistakes with suffering or even death. Since the early beginnings of emergency medical services (EMS), patients and even rescuers have lost their lives because attention was not paid to the details listed here. Many of us can recall patients that we might have saved if we had been a little smarter, a little faster, or a little better organized. Make no mistake, there is no "high" like saving a life, but we carry the scars of our failures all our lives.

Your mind-set and attitude are very important. You must be concerned but not emotional, alert but not excited, quick but not hasty. Above all, you must continuously strive for what is best for your patient. When your training has not prepared you for a situation, always fall back on the question: *What is best for my patient?* When you no longer care, burnout has set in, and your effectiveness is severely limited. When this happens, seek help. (Yes, all of us need help when the stress overcomes us.) Or seek an alternative profession.

Since 1982, the International Trauma Life Support (ITLS, formerly BTLS) organization has been identifying the best methods to get the most out of those few minutes that prehospital EMS providers have to save the patient's life. Not all patients can be saved, but our goal is never to lose a life that could have been saved. The knowledge in this book can help you make a difference. Learn it well.

John E. Campbell, MD, FACEP
Editor

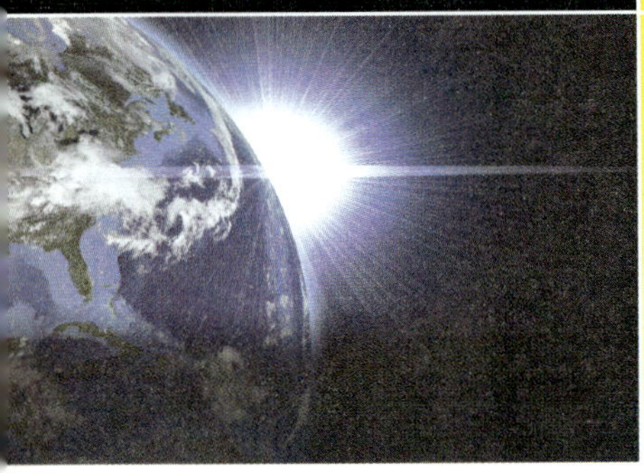

About ITLS

International Trauma Life Support is a global not-for-profit organization dedicated to preventing death and disability from trauma through education and emergency trauma care.

THE SMART CHOICE FOR TRAUMA TRAINING

Train with the best. Train with ITLS. Together, we are improving trauma care worldwide. International Trauma Life Support—a not-for-profit organization dedicated to excellence in trauma education and response—coordinates ITLS education and training worldwide. Founded in 1985 as Basic Trauma Life Support, ITLS adopted a new name in 2005 to better reflect its global role and impact. Today, ITLS has more than 80 chapters and training centers around the world. Through ITLS, hundreds of thousands of trauma care professionals have learned proven techniques endorsed by the American College of Emergency Physicians.

ITLS is the smart choice for your trauma training, because it is:

- *Practical.* ITLS trains you in a realistic, hands-on approach proven to work in the field—from scene to surgery.
- *Dynamic.* ITLS content is current, relevant, and responsive to the latest thinking in trauma management.
- *Flexible.* ITLS courses are taught through a strong network of chapters and training centers that customize content to reflect local needs and priorities.
- *Team centered.* ITLS emphasizes a cohesive team approach that works in the real world and recognizes the importance of your role.
- *Grounded in emergency medicine.* Practicing emergency physicians—medicine's frontline responders—lead ITLS efforts to deliver stimulating content based on solid emergency medicine.
- *Challenging.* ITLS course content raises the bar on performance in the field by integrating classroom knowledge with practical application of skills.

FOCUSED CONTENT THAT DELIVERS

ITLS empowers you with the knowledge and skill to provide optimal care in the prehospital setting. It offers a variety of training options for all levels and backgrounds of emergency personnel around the world. ITLS courses combine classroom learning, hands-on skills stations, and assessment stations that put your learning to work in simulated trauma situations. Not only are courses taught as a continuing education option, but they are also used as essential curricula in many paramedic, EMT, and first responder training programs.

ITLS Programs

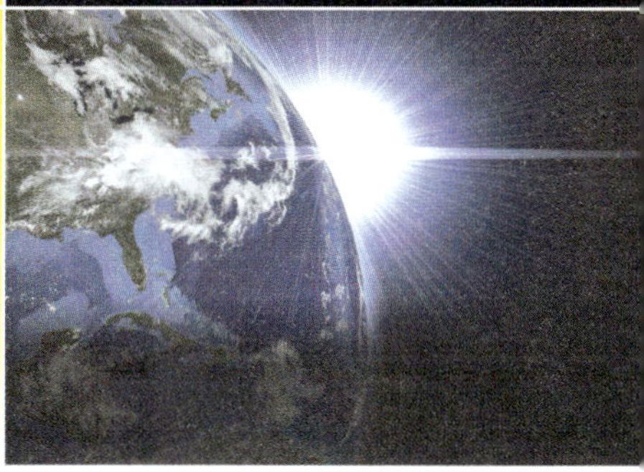

ITLS PROVIDER

ITLS Provider includes 8 hours of classroom instruction, 8 hours of hands-on skills training, and testing for ITLS Basic or Advanced certification. Innovative skills stations let you practice the abilities appropriate for your level of certification:

- Patient assessment and management
- Basic and advanced airway management
- Spinal motion restriction—rapid extrication, short backboard, helmet management, log roll and long backboard/scoop stretcher utilization
- Extremity immobilization and traction splint application
- Needle chest decompression and fluid resuscitation (for Advanced certification)

With its comprehensive approach to core knowledge and skills, ITLS Provider is appropriate for all levels of EMS personnel—from EMT-Bs and first responders to advanced EMTs, paramedics, trauma nurses, and physicians.

ITLS MILITARY

ITLS Military is a custom edition of ITLS Provider, edited by military experts. The military-based scenarios are customized for the challenges faced by military personnel. The text can be used as the course manual for an ITLS Military Provider course or as a stand-alone resource.

ITLS eTRAUMA

ITLS eTrauma presents the 8 hours of ITLS Provider classroom instruction in a self-paced, online format that adapts to your schedule. It reinterprets course lectures with 13 lessons featuring video clips, quiz questions, click-and-drag matching exercises, new case studies, and other interactive tools. You can use ITLS eTrauma for continuing education or as the first step in achieving your ITLS Basic or Advanced Provider certification. Either way, you will maximize your learning and retention with online education that's innovative, flexible, and affordable.

ITLS COMPLETER

ITLS Completer is the perfect next step if you choose ITLS eTrauma to earn your ITLS Provider certification. The Completer Course is an in-person session that features 8 hours of hands-on skill demonstration, practice, and testing, plus the written exam required for Provider certification. You will earn your ITLS Provider certification and card at the completion of this course. Together, ITLS eTrauma and ITLS Completer are your flexible solution for ITLS Provider certification.

ITLS PEDIATRIC

ITLS Pediatric focuses on the special needs of young trauma patients. In 8 hours, you will learn the principles of proper assessment, management, critical interventions, patient packaging, and rapid transport. You also will practice proven techniques for communicating with young patients and their parents. The practical skills you gain will enable you to feel confident and competent when you care for a critically injured child. Hands-on skill stations include:

- Patient assessment and management
- Airway management and thoracic trauma
- Fluid resuscitation
- Spinal motion restriction and extrication, with an emphasis on pediatric immobilization devices

ITLS ACCESS

ITLS Access teaches skills that are critical for EMS crews and first responders at the scene of a motor vehicle collision. In hands-on modules, you will learn how to reach, stabilize, and extricate trapped victims, with a special focus on patient care during extrication. The 8-hour course trains you in how to use hand tools and items found on the scene or carried on an ambulance or first responder unit, instead of hydraulics. In addition to techniques for traditional vehicles, we have expanded the scope to include hybrid vehicles, trucks, buses, and small aircraft.

ITLS INSTRUCTOR

ITLS Instructor courses prepare EMS professionals to teach ITLS courses. To participate as a potential instructor, you need to successfully complete the course you want to teach, demonstrate instructor potential, and meet local ITLS chapter requirements.

ITLS REFRESHER

ITLS Refresher courses keep experienced ITLS providers and instructors up to date with the ITLS curriculum and skills.

CONTINUING EDUCATION CREDIT FOR ITLS COURSES

The Continuing Education Coordinating Board for Emergency Medical Services has accredited ITLS courses to provide continuing education hours to EMS professionals. CECBEMS credit is accepted by numerous national, state, and local organizations, including the National Registry of Emergency Medical Technicians, as the standard in EMS CE.

ENROLLING IN AN ITLS COURSE

ITLS provides its courses through chapters and training centers. The ITLS Course Management System makes it easy to find a course in your area. Log on to cms.itrauma.org to search for courses and contact the course administrator to register.

If you need information about your local chapter or training center, check our list at itrauma.org or call ITLS headquarters at 888-495-ITLS or 630-495-6442 (for international callers). We will put you in touch with your local organization—or help you start the program in your area.

International Trauma Life Support

3000 Woodcreek Drive, Suite 200

Downers Grove, Illinois 60515

Phone: 888-495-ITLS

630-495-6442 (International)

Fax: 630-495-6404

Web: www.itrauma.org

E-mail: info@itrauma.org

ITLS LEADERSHIP

Board of Directors

ITLS LEADERSHIP

Editorial Board

Executive Director

Scene Size-up

James H. Creel, Jr., MD, FACEP

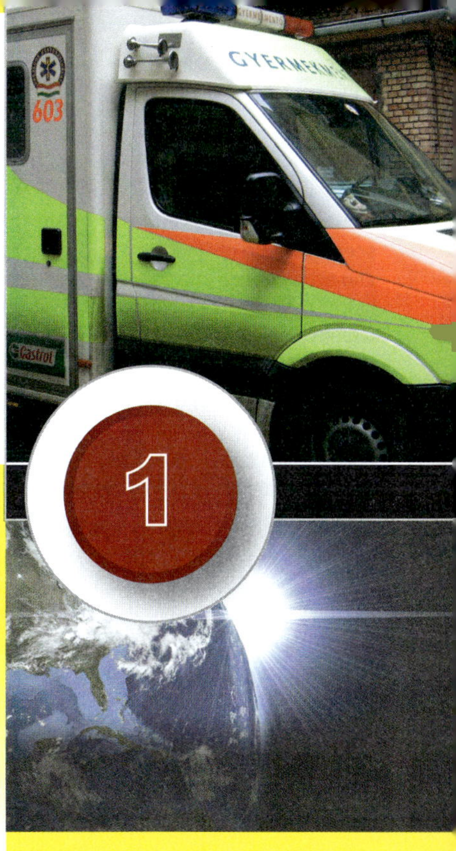

(Photo courtesy of International Trauma Life Support)

Scene Size-up

Valutazione della Scena

Valoración de la Escena

Taille-haut de scène

Ocena miejsca zdarzenia

Beurteilung der Einsatzstelle

Procjena mjesta događaja

مسح الموقع

mesto nesreće

Ocena prizorišča

Helyszínfelmérés

OBJECTIVES

Upon successful completion of this chapter, you should be able to:

1. Discuss the steps of the scene size-up.
2. List the two basic mechanisms of motion injury.
3. Identify the three collisions associated with a motor-vehicle crash (MVC), and relate potential patient injuries to deformity of the vehicle, interior structures, and body structures.
4. Name the five common forms of MVCs.
5. Describe potential injuries associated with proper and improper use of seat restraints, headrests, and air bags in a head-on collision.
6. Describe potential injuries from rear-end collisions.
7. Describe the three assessment criteria for falls, and relate them to anticipated injuries.
8. Identify the two most common forms of penetration injuries, and discuss associated mechanisms and extent of injury.
9. Relate five injury mechanisms involved in blast injuries and how they relate to scene size-up and patient assessment.

KEY TERMS

blast injuries, *p. 23*
essential equipment, *p. 5*
focused exam, *p. 6*
high-energy event, *p. 6*
ITLS Primary Survey, *p. 2*
mechanism of injury, *p. 5*
occupant restraint systems, *p. 15*
OPIM, *p. 3*
personal protective equipment, *p. 3*
rapid trauma survey, *p. 6*
scene size-up, *p. 2*
standard precautions, *p. 2*

scene size-up observations made and actions taken at a trauma scene before actually approaching the patient. It is the initial step in the ITLS Primary Survey.

ITLS Primary Survey a brief exam to find immediately life-threatening conditions. It is made up of the scene size-up, initial assessment, and either the rapid trauma survey or the focused exam.

standard precautions procedures used to prevent contamination by a patient's body fluids. This always entails wearing gloves, frequently requires a face shield, and occasionally requires a protective gown or suit.

Chapter Overview

Scene size-up is the first step in the **ITLS Primary Survey** (Table 1-1). It is a critical part of trauma assessment and begins before you approach the patient. If you fail to perform the preliminary steps of scene size-up, you may jeopardize your life as well as the life of your patient. Scene size-up includes taking **standard precautions** to prevent exposure to blood and other potentially infective material, evaluating the scene for dangers, determining the total number of patients, determining essential equipment needed for this particular scene, and identifying the mechanisms of injuries (Table 1-2). Each of these steps will be covered in detail in this chapter, and there will be special emphasis on how to use your knowledge of the mechanisms of injury to predict occult injuries to the patient. Motion (mechanical) injuries are by and large responsible for the majority of the mortality from trauma in most countries. This chapter reviews the most common mechanisms of motion injuries and stresses the injuries that may be associated with these mechanisms.

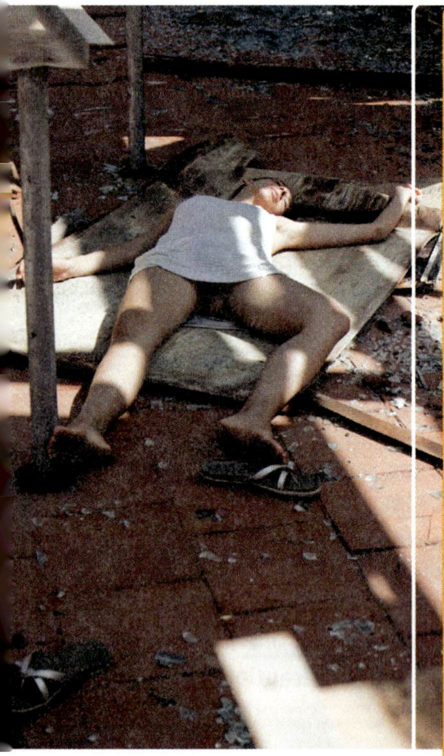

(Photo courtesy of Edw, Shutterstock)

CASE PRESENTATION

An advanced life support (ALS) ambulance has been dispatched by request of the fire service, who is on the scene of an explosion at an abortion clinic. They report multiple victims. The clinic has been the target of numerous organized protests, picketing, death threats, and harassment of the staff. Bomb threat hoaxes have occurred in the past. The team leader immediately calls for more ambulance backup because of the report of multiple patients. On arrival the ambulance is met by the fire service scene commander. The crew can see that the doors and windows have been blown out of the clinic, and debris, dust, and glass are in the street in front of the facility. Two persons are down in the street, and one is sitting up and being helped by firefighters. Firefighters are spraying water on a small fire inside the structure.

- What has happened? Is this a criminal act?
- Are the responders in danger?
- What protective clothing is required?
- What are the potential hazards?
- Should the ambulance team proceed into the scene?
- Is a chemical agent or other toxic material involved?
- What resources are needed?

Keep these questions in mind as you read the chapter. Then, at the end of the chapter, find out how the rescuers completed this call. ■

Table 1-1 ITLS Patient Assessment

ITLS Primary Survey	Perform a scene size-up Perform initial assessment Perform a rapid trauma survey or focused exam Make critical interventions and transport decision Contact medical direction
ITLS Secondary Survey	Repeat initial assessment Repeat vital signs and consider monitors Perform a neurological exam Perform a detailed (head-to-toe) exam
ITLS Ongoing Exam	Repeat initial assessment Repeat vital signs and check monitors Reassess the abdomen Check injuries and interventions

Scene Size-up

Scene size-up begins at dispatch, when you anticipate what you will find at the scene. At that time, you should think about what equipment you may need and whether other resources (more units, special extrication equipment, multicasualty incident [MCI] protocols) may be needed. Although information from dispatch is useful to begin to think about a plan, do not overrely on this information. Information given to the dispatcher is often exaggerated or even completely wrong. Be prepared to change your plan depending on your own survey of the scene.

Standard Precautions

Trauma scenes are among the most likely to subject the rescuer to contamination by blood or other potentially infectious material (**OPIM**). This subject will be covered in more detail in Chapter 22. Not only are trauma patients often bloody, but they also frequently require airway management under adverse conditions. **Personal protective equipment (PPE)** is always needed at trauma scenes. Protective gloves are always needed, and many situations will require eye protection. It is wise for the rescuer in charge of airway management to have a face shield or eye protection and mask. In highly contaminated situations, impervious gowns with mask or face shield also may be needed. In a toxic environment, chemical suits and gas masks may be needed. Remember to protect your patient from contamination by body fluids by changing your gloves between patients.

OPIM short for *other potentially infectious material* to which a rescuer may be exposed (other than blood).

personal protective equipment (PPE) equipment that an EMS rescuer dons for protection from various dangers that may be present at a trauma scene. At a minimum that entails wearing protective gloves. At a maximum the rescuer may require a chemical suit and self-contained breathing apparatus.

Table 1-2 Steps of the Scene Size-up

1. Standard precautions (personal protective equipment)
2. Scene safety
3. Initial triage (total number of patients)
4. Need for more help or equipment
5. Mechanism of injury

Scene Safety

Begin sizing up the scene for hazards as you approach in your vehicle. Your first decision is to determine the nearest safe place to park the ambulance or rescue vehicle. You would like the vehicle as close as possible, and yet it must be far enough away from the scene for you to be safe while you are performing the scene size-up. In some situations you should not enter the scene until it has been cleared by a bomb technician and/or HazMat technician. Try to park facing away from the scene, so if dangers arise, you can load the patient and leave quickly. Next, determine if it is safe to approach the patient. Perform a "windshield survey" before leaving your response vehicle. Consider the following:

- *Crash/rescue scenes.* Is there danger from fire or toxic substances? Is there danger of electrocution? Are unstable surfaces or structures present such as ice, water, slope, or buildings in danger of collapse? Areas with potential for low oxygen levels or toxic chemical levels (sewers, ship holds, silos, and so on) should never be entered until you have the proper protective equipment and breathing apparatus. You should never enter a dangerous area without a partner and a safety line attached.
- *Crime scenes.* Danger may exist even after a crime has been committed. Be alert for persons fleeing the scene, for persons attempting to conceal themselves, and for persons who are armed or who are making threatening statements or gestures. Do not approach a known crime scene if law enforcement personnel are not present. Wait for law enforcement, not only for your own safety and the safety of victims, but also to help preserve evidence. Do not approach the scene if you see that law enforcement personnel are in defensive positions or have their weapons drawn.
- *Blast scenes.* Explosions usually are associated with industrial accidents, but in some countries the proliferation of illegal methamphetamine labs have been associated with an increased incidence of chemical explosions. Also, because the threat of terrorist activity is both common and worldwide, it is a more common concern when approaching the scene of an explosion. If possible, law enforcement personnel, along with a bomb technician and a HazMat technician, should first evaluate the blast scene to make sure the scene is safe to enter and no chemical, biological, or radiological hazards exist. If possible, park your vehicle outside the blast zone (area where glass is broken). If you are not sure of scene safety, call for ambulatory victims to leave the scene and follow a designated emergency responder to a safe area for triage and decontamination.

  If it is necessary to enter the blast zone to save lives, try to do so in protective clothing using respiratory protection (chemical suit and gas mask). Identify those who are still alive prior to entry if possible. Rapidly rescue patients who are too injured to walk using "load-and-go" tactics with expedient spinal motion-restriction techniques. If the scene might be dangerous, the best policy is to do no treatment on scene but rather to immediately remove all living patients. Take the patients directly to the ambulance and begin patient assessment and treatment in the ambulance. If resources are available, those patients should be taken directly from the scene to the appropriate hospital. Leave the dead in place.

  The proper management of blast scenes is beyond the scope of this course, which is focused mainly on assessment and management of the injured patient. Other courses (see bibliography) are available for more in-depth knowledge of this subject.

- *Bystanders.* You and the victims may be in danger from bystanders. Are bystanders talking in loud, angry voices? Are people fighting? Are weapons present? Is there evidence of the use of alcohol or illegal drugs? Is this a domestic-violence scene? You may not be recognized as a rescuer, but as a symbol of authority and thus attacked. Are dangerous animals present? Request law enforcement personnel at any sign of danger from violence.

Consider whether or not the scene poses a continued threat to the patient. If there is danger of fire, water, structure collapse, toxic exposure, and so on, the patient may have to be moved immediately. This does not mean that you should expose yourself or your partners to unnecessary danger. You may need to call for special equipment and proper backup from the police, fire services, or power company. If the scene is unsafe, you should make it safe or try to remove the patients from the scene without putting yourself in danger. Sometimes there is no clearly good way to do this. Use good judgment. You are there to save lives, not give up your own.

Total Number of Patients

Determine the total number of patients now. If there are more patients than your team can effectively handle, call for backup. Remember that you usually need one ambulance for each seriously injured patient. If there are many patients, establish medical command and initiate multicasualty incident (MCI) protocols. Are all patients accounted for? If the patient is unconscious, and there are no witnesses to the incident, look for clues (schoolbooks or diaper bag, passenger list in a commercial vehicle) that other patients might be present. Carefully evaluate the scene for other patients. This is especially important at night or if there is poor visibility.

PEARLS

It is wise to invest in a high-intensity tactical flashlight. It is small enough to carry in your shirt pocket but it is many times brighter than regular flashlights.

Essential Equipment and Additional Resources

If possible, carry all **essential equipment** to the scene. This prevents loss of time returning to the vehicle. Remember to change gloves between patients. The following equipment is always needed for trauma patients.

- Personal protection equipment
- Long backboard with effective strapping and head motion-restriction device
- Appropriately sized rigid cervical extrication collar
- Oxygen and airway equipment, which should include suction equipment and a bag-mask
- Trauma box (bandage material, hemostatic agent, tourniquet, blood pressure cuff, stethoscope)

essential equipment equipment that is worn or carried when the team approaches the trauma patient. It includes personal protective equipment, long backboard and strapping, rigid cervical extrication collar, oxygen and airway equipment, and trauma box.

If special extrication equipment, more ambulances, or additional personnel are needed, call now. You are less likely to call for help when involved in patient care. Be sure to tell additional responders exactly where to respond and of any dangers present.

Mechanism of Injury

Once you determine that it is safe to approach the patient, begin to assess for the **mechanism of injury**. This may be apparent from the scene itself, but it may require questioning the patient or bystanders. Injuries are caused by the transfer of energy. Kinetic energy is equal to the mass (M) of the object in motion multiplied by the square of the velocity (V) divided by two.

mechanism of injury the means by which the patient was injured, such as fall, motor-vehicle collision, or explosion.

$$\text{Kinetic Energy} = \tfrac{1}{2}(M \times V^2)$$

Table 1-3 Mechanisms of Injury and Potential Injury Patterns

Mechanisms of Injury	Potential Injury Patterns
Frontal impact Deformed steering wheel Dashboard knee imprints Spiderweb deformity of windscreen	• Cervical-spine fracture • Flail chest • Myocardial contusion • Pneumothorax • Aortic disruption • Spleen or liver laceration • Posterior hip dislocation • Knee dislocation
Lateral impact (T-bone)	• Contralateral neck sprain • Cervical-spine fracture • Lateral flail chest • Pneumothorax • Aortic disruption • Diaphragmatic rupture • Laceration of spleen, liver, kidney • Pelvic fracture
Rear impact	• Cervical-spine injury
Ejection	• Exposure to all mechanisms and mortality increased
Pedestrian vs. car	• Head injury • Aortic disruption • Abdominal visceral injuries • Fracture lower extremities and pelvis

high-energy event a mechanism of injury in which it is likely that there was a large release of uncontrolled kinetic energy transmitted to the patient, thus increasing the chances for serious injury.

You are not expected to have to calculate how much energy was transferred in a traumatic event but rather to estimate whether the collision was a low-energy event (auto backed into another in a parking lot) or **high-energy event** (auto hit a tree at a speed of 40 miles [64 kilometers] per hour). The formula is shown only to stress that speed (velocity) has a much larger effect on energy than does mass. A small increase in speed causes a large increase in energy transferred. Energy transmission follows the laws of physics; therefore, injuries present in predictable patterns (Table 1-3). Knowledge and appreciation of the mechanism of injury is very helpful in your evaluation of the patient for occult injuries and, along with your assessment of the patient, can predict 90% of injuries. Missed or overlooked injuries may be catastrophic, especially when they become known only after the compensatory mechanisms are exhausted.

Remember that patients who are involved in a high-energy event are at risk for severe injury. Despite normal vital signs and no apparent anatomic injury on the initial assessment, 5% to 15% of those patients will later exhibit severe injuries that are discovered on repeat examinations. Therefore, a high-energy event signifies a large release of uncontrolled energy. Consider the patient injured until you have proven otherwise.

rapid trauma survey a brief exam from head to toe performed to identify life-threatening injuries.

focused exam an exam used when there is a focused (localized) mechanism of injury or an isolated injury. The exam is limited to the area of injury.

It is important to be aware of whether the mechanism is *generalized* (MVC, fall from a height, and so on) or *focused* (stab wound of abdomen, an amputation of a foot). Focused injuries are localized to a discrete area. Generalized mechanisms require a **rapid trauma survey**, whereas focused mechanisms may only require a more limited exam of the affected areas or systems called a **focused exam**. Factors to be considered are direction and speed of impact, patient kinetics and physical

Table 1-4 Basic Mechanisms of Motion Injury

Blunt Injuries	Penetrating Injuries
• Rapid forward deceleration (collisions)	• Projectiles
• Rapid vertical deceleration (falls)	• Knives
• Energy transfer from blunt instruments (baseball bat, blackjack)	• Falls on fixed objects

size, and the signs of energy release (e.g., major vehicle damage). A strong correlation exists between injury severity and automobile velocity changes, as measured by the amount of vehicle damage. It is important that you consider these two questions: What happened? How was the patient injured?

Mechanism of injury is also an important triage tool and is information that you should report to the emergency physician or trauma surgeon. Severity of vehicle damage also has been suggested as a nonphysiologic triage tool. Taking a few brief photos with a digital camera can be helpful for the personnel in the emergency department to recognize the severity of forces involved. It is essential to develop an awareness of mechanisms of injury and thus have a high index of suspicion for occult injuries. Always consider the potential injury to be present until it is ruled out in a hospital setting.

Motion injuries are by and large responsible for the majority of the mortality from trauma in the world. The most common mechanisms of motion injuries and those injuries commonly associated with these mechanisms are discussed in the section that follows. The two basic mechanisms of motion injury are *blunt* and *penetrating* (Table 1-4). Patients may have injuries from both at the same time.

Motor-Vehicle Collisions

Injury patterns from collisions with automobiles, motorcycles, all-terrain vehicles (ATVs), personal watercraft, and tractors are varied. The important concept to appreciate is that energy is neither created nor destroyed but is only changed in form (law of conservation of energy). Thus the kinetic energy of motion must be absorbed, and this absorption of energy is the basic component in producing injury. Motion injury may be blunt or penetrating. Generally, blunt trauma is more common in the rural setting, and penetrating trauma is more common in the urban setting. Rapid forward deceleration is usually blunt but may be penetrating. The most common example of rapid forward deceleration is the motor-vehicle collision (MVC). You should consider all MVCs to occur as three separate events (Figure 1-1). They are

- Machine collision
- Body collision
- Organ collision resulting in rupture, shearing, or bruising

Consider approaching an MVC in which an automobile has hit a tree head-on at 40 miles (64 kilometers) per hour. The tree brings the auto to an immediate stop by transferring the energy into damage to the tree and the automobile. The person inside the auto is still traveling at 40 miles (64 kilometers) per hour until he strikes something that stops him (such as seat belts, steering wheel, windshield, or dashboard). At that point, energy transfers into damage to the person and to the surface struck. The organs inside the person are also traveling

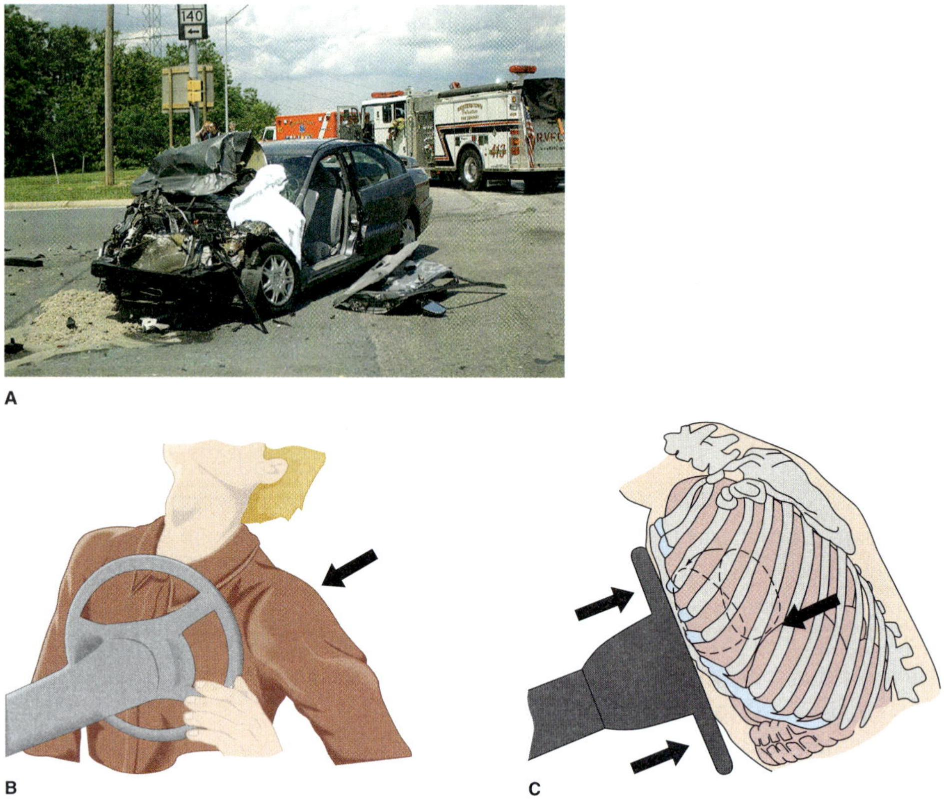

FIGURE 1-1 The three collisions of a motor-vehicle crash. A. Vehicle collision. B. Body Collision. C. Organ collision. *(Photo copyright Mark C. Ide)*

at 40 miles (64 kilometers) per hour until they are stopped by striking a stationary object (such as inside of skull, sternum, steering wheel, dashboard) or by their ligamentous attachments (such as the aorta by ligamentum arteriosum). In this auto-versus-tree example, appreciation of the rapid forward decelerating mechanism (high-energy event) coupled with a high index of suspicion should make you concerned that the victim may have possible head injury, cervical-spine injury, myocardial contusion, any of the "deadly dozen" chest injuries, intra-abdominal injuries, and musculoskeletal injuries (especially fracture or dislocation of the hip).

To explain the forces involved, consider Sir Isaac Newton's first law of motion: "A body in motion remains in motion in a straight line unless acted on by an outside force." Motion is created by force (energy exchange), and therefore force will stop motion. If this energy exchange occurs within the body, tissue damage occurs. This law is well exemplified in the automobile crash. The kinetic energy of the vehicle's forward motion is absorbed as each part of the vehicle is brought to a sudden halt by the impact. Remember that the body of the occupant is also traveling at 40 miles (64 kilometers) per hour until impacted by some structure within the car. With awareness of this mechanism, one can see the multitude of injuries that could occur. Be aware of the following clues:

- Deformity of the vehicle (indication of forces involved—energy exchange)
- Deformity of interior structures (indication of where the patient impacted—energy exchange)
- Deformity or injury patterns of the patient (indication of what parts of the body may have been impacted)

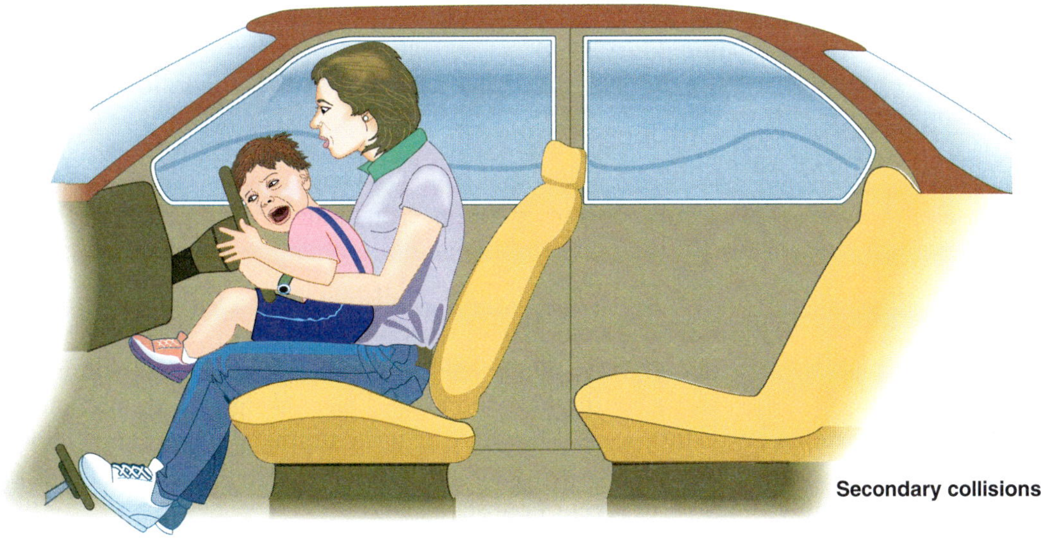

FIGURE 1-2 Secondary collisions in a deceleration motor-vehicle collision. In this case, a secondary collision is the unrestrained body of the mother crushing the child against the steering wheel.

Additional collisions may occur other than the three already mentioned. Objects inside the automobile (books, bags, luggage, and other persons) will become missiles traveling at the original speed of the auto and may strike persons in front of them. They are called *secondary collisions.* A good example of this occurs when an unrestrained parent is holding a child in her lap and crushes the child between her and the dashboard in a deceleration collision (Figure 1-2).

In rear-impact auto collisions, multiple impacts may occur if the auto strikes another auto from the rear and is then in turn struck from behind by another auto following. Also, vehicles frequently deflect from hitting one object and then collide with a second or even third vehicle or stationary object. They are much like a rollover collision in that the persons inside the vehicle are subjected to energy transfer from multiple directions. It is often more difficult to predict injuries in these cases. You must quickly but carefully look for clues inside the vehicle. Remember that in multiple-impact collisions, the airbag only works for the first one.

MVCs occur in several forms, and each form is associated with certain patterns of injury. The five common forms of MVCs are the following:

- Frontal-impact or head-on collision
- Lateral-impact or T-bone collision
- Rear-impact collision
- Rollover collision
- Rotational collision

Frontal-Impact Collision (Head-on)

In an MVC involving a frontal-impact collision, an unrestrained body is brought to a sudden halt. The energy transfer is capable of producing multiple injuries.

Windshield injuries occur in the rapid forward-decelerating type of event, in which the unrestrained occupant impacts the windshield forcefully (Figure 1-3). The possibility for injuries is

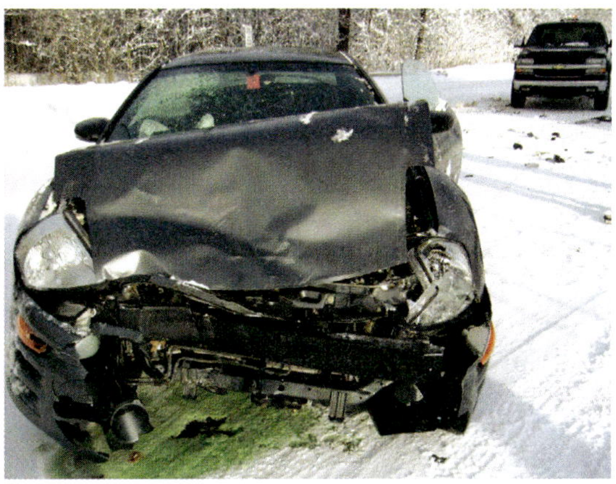

FIGURE 1-3 In a head-on collision, most injuries are inflicted by the windshield, steering wheel, and dashboard. *(Courtesy of Maria Dryfhout, Shutterstock)*

great under those conditions. Of utmost concern is the potential for serious airway and cervical-spine injury.

Remembering the three separate collision events, note the following:

- *Machine collision*—deformed front end
- *Body collision*—spiderweb pattern of windshield
- *Organ collision*—coup/contracoup brain, soft-tissue injury (scalp, face, neck), hyperextension/flexion of cervical spine

From the spiderweb appearance of the windshield and an appreciation of the mechanism of injury, you should maintain a high index of suspicion for possible occult injuries of the cervical spine. The head usually strikes the windshield, resulting in direct trauma to the face and head. External signs of trauma include cuts, abrasions, and contusions. They may be quite dramatic in appearance; however, the key concern is airway maintenance with motion restriction of the cervical spine and evaluation of level of consciousness.

Steering wheel injuries most often occur to an unrestrained driver of a vehicle in a head-on collision. The driver may subsequently also impact with the windshield. The steering wheel is the vehicle's most lethal weapon for the unrestrained driver, and any degree of steering wheel deformity (check under collapsed airbags) must be treated with a high index of suspicion for face, neck, thoracic, or abdominal injury. The two components of this weapon are the ring and column (Figure 1-4). The ring is a semirigid, plastic-covered metal ring attached to a fixed inflexible post—a battering ram.

Utilizing the three-collision concept, check for the presence of the following:

- *Machine collision*—front-end deformity
- *Body collision*—ring fracture/deformity, column normal/displaced
- *Organ collision*—traumatic tattooing of skin

The head-on collision is entirely dependent on the area of the body that impacts with the steering wheel. Signs may be readily visible, with direct trauma such as lacerations of mouth and chin, contusion/bruises of the anterior neck, traumatic tattoos of the chest wall, and bruising of the abdomen. These external signs may be subtle or dramatic in appearance, but more important, they may represent the tip of the iceberg. Deeper structures and organs may harbor occult injuries due to *shearing forces*, *compression forces*, and *displacement of kinetic energy*. Organs that are susceptible to shearing injuries due to their ligamentous attachments are the aortic arch, liver, spleen, kidneys, and bowel. With the exception of small-bowel tears, those injuries are sources for occult bleeds and hemorrhagic shock. Compression injuries are common with the lung, heart, diaphragm, and urinary bladder. An important sign is respiratory distress, which may be due to pulmonary contusions, pneumothorax, diaphragmatic hernia (bowel sounds in chest), or flail chest. Consider a bruised chest wall as a myocardial contusion that requires monitoring of cardiac rhythm and, if available, a 12-lead ECG.

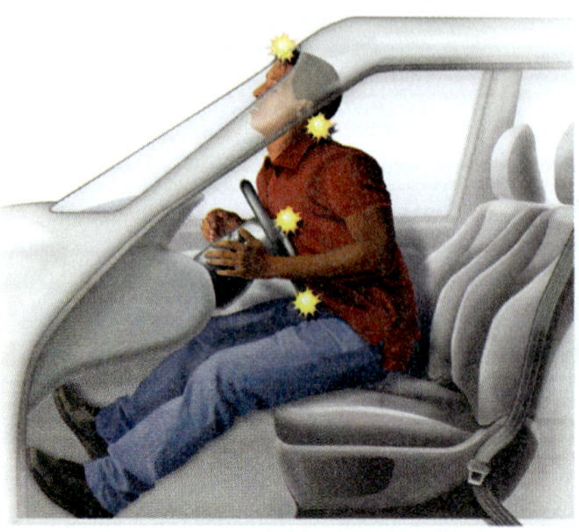

FIGURE 1-4 Steering wheel injuries.

In short, the steering wheel is a lethal weapon capable of producing devastating injuries, many of which are occult. Steering wheel deformity is a cause for alarm and must heighten your index of suspicion. You also must relay this information to the receiving physician.

Dashboard injuries occur most often to an unrestrained passenger. The dashboard has the capability of producing a variety of injuries, depending on the area of the body that strikes the dashboard. Most frequently, injuries involve the face and knees; however, many types of injuries have been described (Figure 1-5).

Applying the three-event concept of collision, you will note

- *Machine collision*—deformity of the car
- *Body collision*—fracture/deformity of the dash
- *Organ collision*—facial trauma, coup/contracoup brain, hyperextension/flexion of the cervical spine, pelvis, hip, and knee trauma

Facial, brain, and cervical-spine injuries have already been mentioned. Like chest contusion, knee trauma may represent only the tip of the iceberg. Knees commonly impact with the dashboard. This may range from the simple contusion noted about the patella to the severe compound fracture of the patella. Frank dislocation of the knees can occur. In addition, kinetic energy may be transmitted proximally and may result in fracture of the femur or fractured/dislocated hip. On occasion, the pelvis can impact with the dash, resulting in acetabulum and pelvic fractures. These injuries are associated

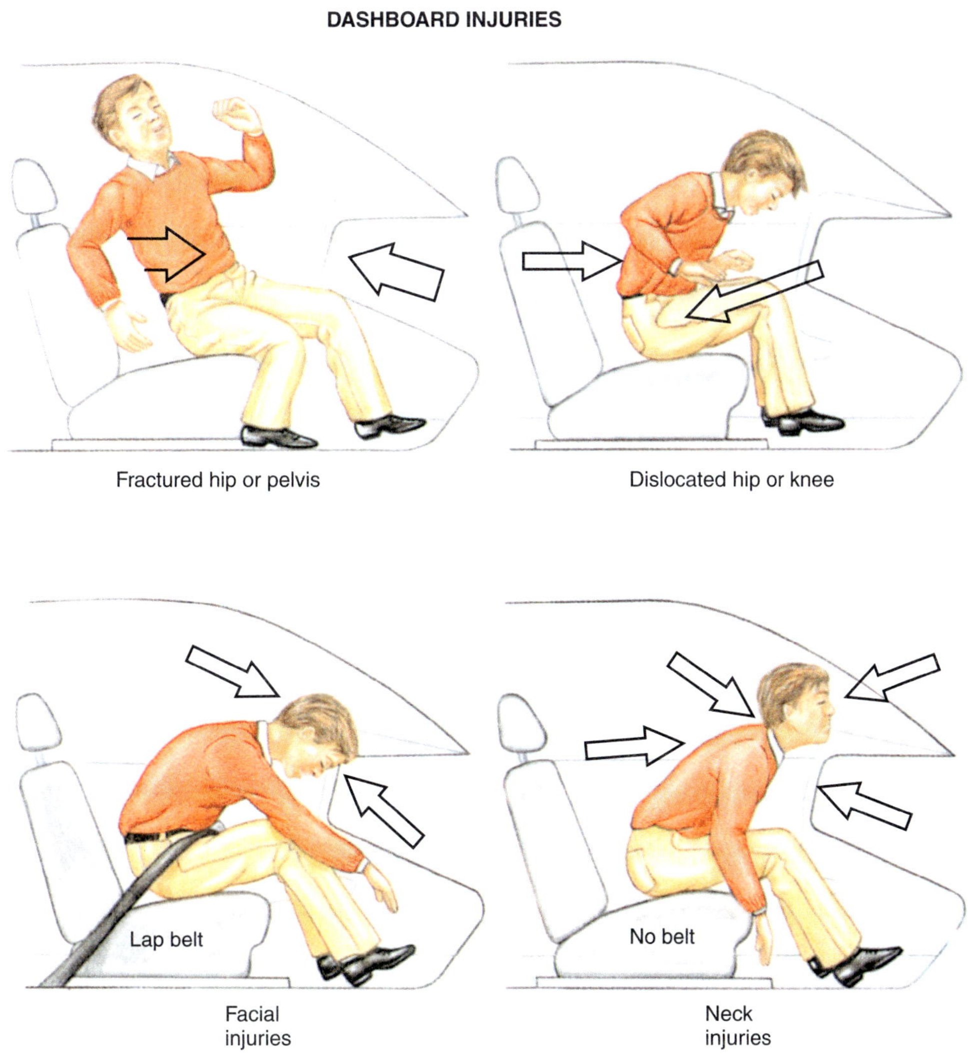

FIGURE 1-5 Dashboard injuries.

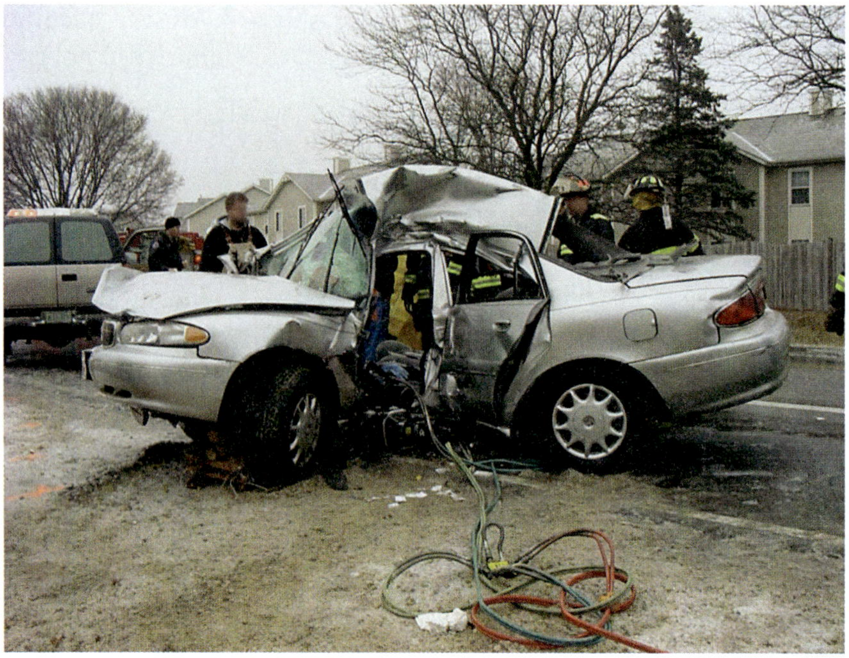

a.

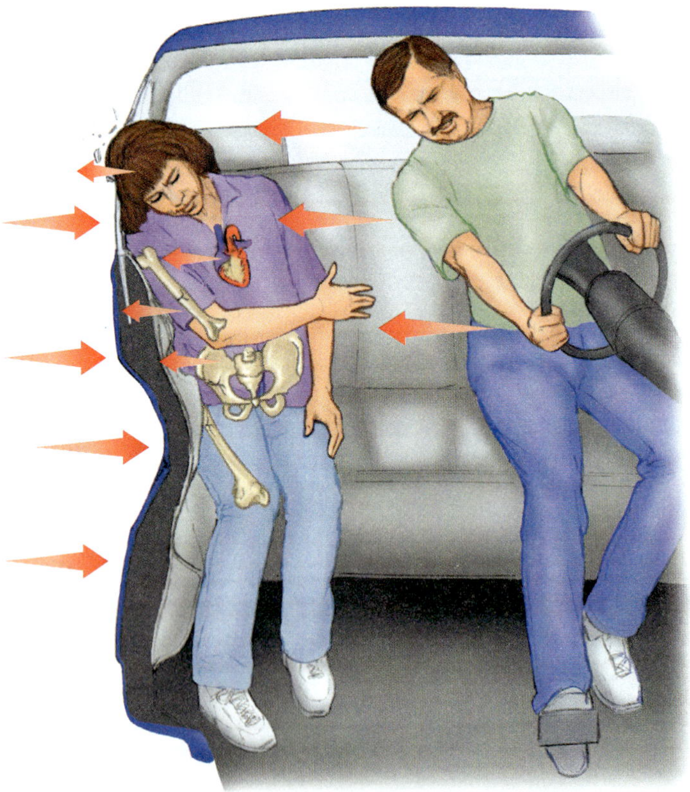

b.

FIGURE 1-6 In a lateral-impact collision, most injuries are inflicted by intrusion of the door, armrest, side window, or door post. *(Photo courtesy of Anthony Cellitti, NREMT-P)* with hemorrhage that may lead to shock. Maintain a high index of suspicion, and always palpate the femurs as well as gently squeeze the pelvis and palpate the symphysis pubis.

Deceleration collisions are the most common to have secondary collisions from people or objects in the back of the vehicle. Secondary missiles can cause deadly injuries.

Lateral-Impact or T-Bone Collision

The mechanism of the lateral-impact collision is similar to that of the frontal-impact collision, with the addition of lateral energy displacement (Figure 1-6). Applying the three-collision concept, look for the presence of the following:

- *Machine collision*—primary deformity of the car—check the impact side (driver/passenger)
- *Body collision*—degree of door deformity (e.g., armrest bent, outward or inward bowing of door)
- *Organ collision*—cannot be predicted by external exam alone; consider organs underneath areas of external injury

Look for the following common injuries.

- *Head.* Coup/contracoup is due to lateral displacement.
- *Neck.* Lateral displacement injuries range from cervical-muscle strain to fracture or subluxation with neurological deficit.
- *Upper arm and shoulder.* Injuries appear on the side of the impact.
- *Thorax/abdomen.* Injury is due to direct force either from inward bowing of door on the side of the impact or from unrestrained passenger being propelled across seat.
- *Pelvis/legs.* Occupants on the side of the impact are likely to have pelvic, hip, or femur fractures.

Injuries of the thorax vary from soft-tissue injuries to flail chest, lung contusion, pneumothorax, or hemothorax. Abdominal injuries include those of solid or hollow organs. Pelvic injuries may include fracture/dislocation, bladder rupture, and urethral injuries. Shoulder girdle or lower extremity injuries are common, depending on the level of the impacting force.

Rear-Impact Collision

In the most common form of rear-impact collision, a stationary car is struck from the rear by a moving vehicle (Figure 1-7). Or a slower-moving car may be impacted from the rear by a faster-moving car. The sudden increase in acceleration produces posterior displacement of the occupants and possible hyperextension of the cervical spine if the headrest is not properly adjusted. If the seat back breaks and falls backward into the rear seat, there is greater chance of lumbar-spine injury. Rapid forward deceleration may also occur if the car suddenly strikes something in the front or if the driver applies the brakes suddenly. Note deformity of the auto anterior and posterior as well as interior deformity and headrest position. The potential for cervical-spine injuries is great (Figure 1-8). Be alert for associated deceleration injuries as well.

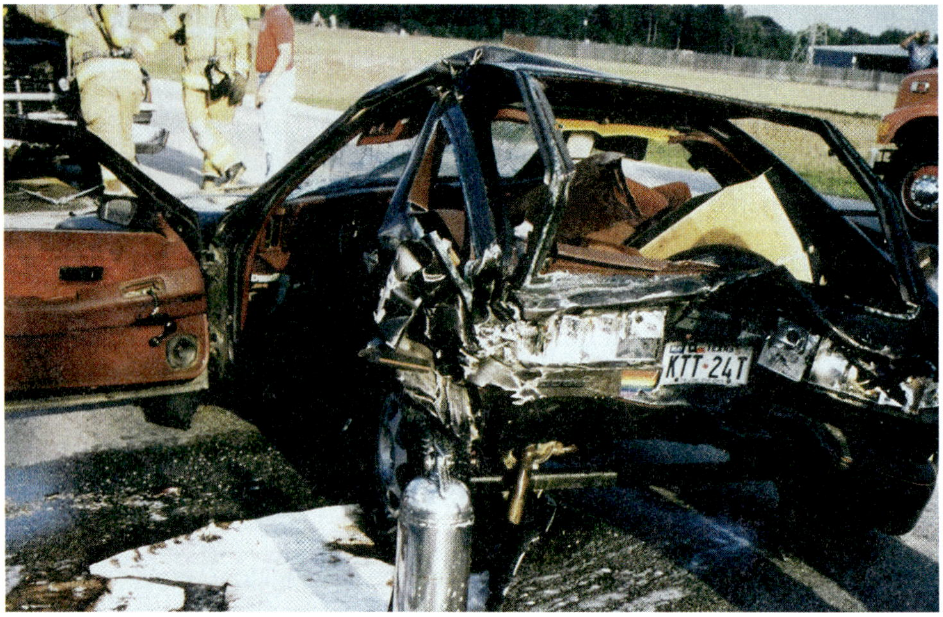

FIGURE 1-7 In a rear-impact collision, the potential exists for neck and back injury. *(Courtesy of Bonnie Meneely, EMT-P)*

Rollover Collision

During a vehicle rollover, the body may be impacted from any direction; thus, the potential for injuries is great (Figure 1-9). The chance for axial-loading injuries of the spine is increased in this form of MVC. Rescuers must be alert for clues that suggest the car turned over (such as roof dents, scratches, debris, and deformity of roof posts). Lethal injuries often occur in this form of collision because of the greater likelihood of occupants being ejected. Occupants ejected from the car are three times as likely to be killed or have serious injuries.

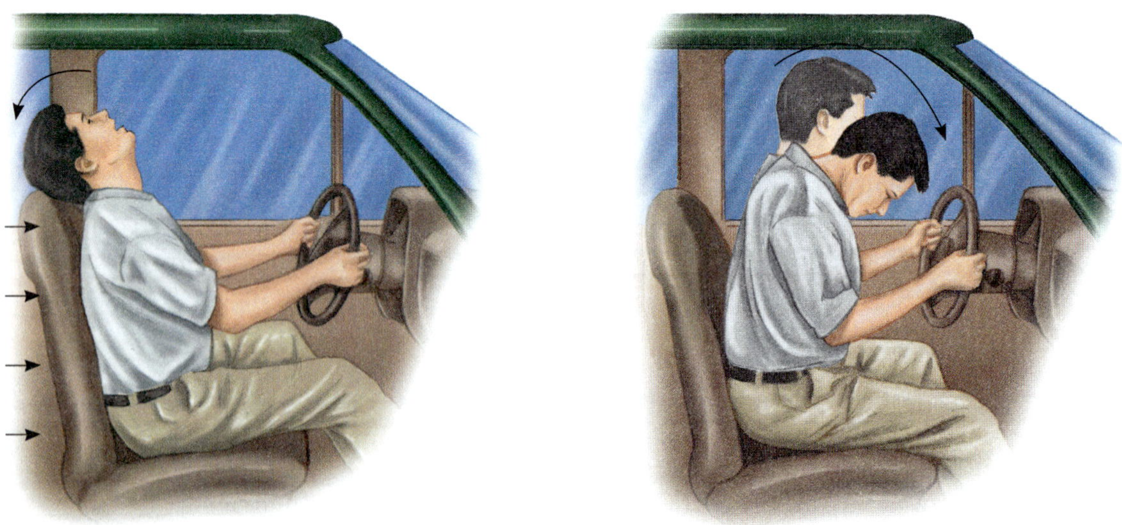

a. Victim moves ahead while head remains stationary. Head rotates backward. Neck extends.

b. Head snaps forward. Head rotates forward. Neck flexes.

FIGURE 1-8 Mechanism of cervical-spine injury in a rear-impact collision.

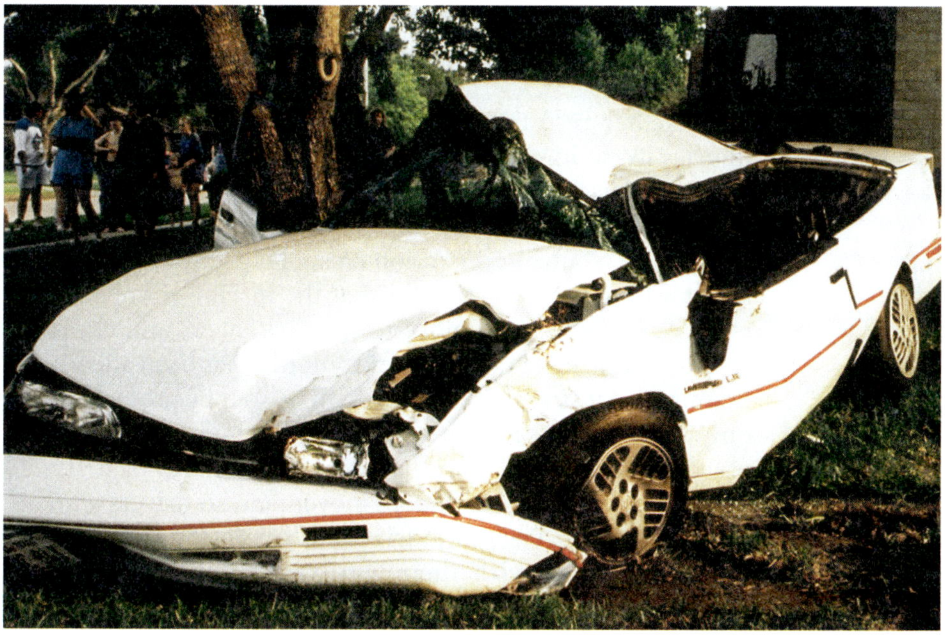

FIGURE 1-9 A rollover collision has a high potential for injury. Many mechanisms are involved, and unrestrained victims are frequently ejected. *(Courtesy of Bonnie Meneely, EMT-P)*

Rotational Collision

A rotational mechanism is best described as what occurs when one part of the vehicle stops and the rest of the vehicle remains in motion. A rotational collision usually occurs when a vehicle is struck in the front or rear lateral area. This converts forward motion to a spinning motion. The results are a combination of the frontal-impact and the lateral-impact mechanisms with the same possibilities of injuries of both mechanisms.

Occupant Restraint Systems

occupant restraint systems systems built into a vehicle to prevent the driver and passengers from being thrown about the interior of the vehicle or from being ejected from the vehicle in the event of a collision.

Restrained occupants are more likely to survive a collision, because they are protected by **occupant restraint systems** from much of the impact inside the auto and are unlikely to be ejected from the auto. Those occupants are, however, still susceptible to certain injuries.

A lap belt is intended to go across the pelvis (iliac crests), not the abdomen. If the belt is in place and the victim is subjected to a frontal deceleration crash, his body tends to fold together like a clasp knife (Figure 1-10). The head may be thrown forward into the steering wheel or dashboard. Facial, head, or neck injuries are common. Abdominal injuries also occur if the lap belt is positioned improperly. The compression forces that are produced when a body is suddenly folded at the waist may injure the abdomen or the lumbar spine.

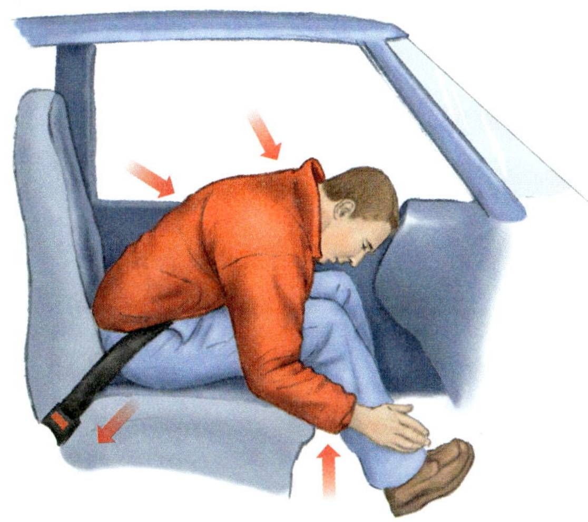

FIGURE 1-10 Clasp-knife effect.

The three-point restraint or cross-chest lap belt (Figure 1-11) secures the body much better than a lap belt alone. The chest and pelvis are restrained, so life-threatening injuries are much less common. The head is not restrained, and therefore the neck is still subjected to stresses that may cause fractures, dislocations, or spinal cord injuries. Clavicular fractures (at the

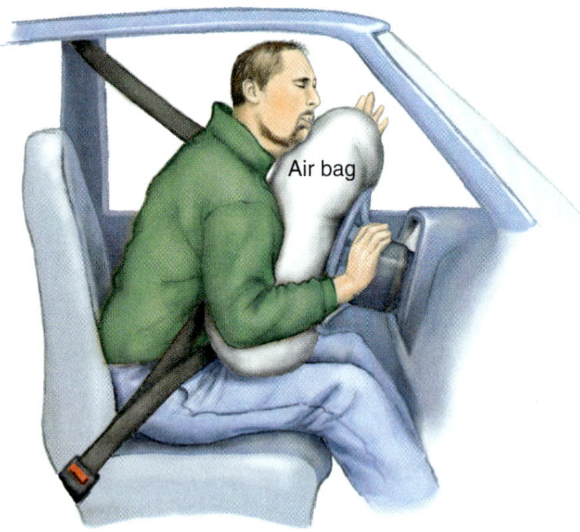
Air bag
Air bag and three-point restraint
prevents collisions 2 and 3.

FIGURE 1-11 Air bag and three-point restraint.

point where the chest strap crosses) are common. Internal organ damage may still occur due to organ movement inside the body.

Like belt restraints, air bags (passive restraints) will reduce injuries in victims of MVCs in most but not all situations. Air bags are designed to inflate from the center of the steering wheel and the dashboard to protect the front-seat occupants in case of a frontal deceleration crash. If functioning properly, they cushion the head and chest at the instant of impact, thus effectively decreasing injury to the face, neck, and chest. Be sure to stabilize the neck, however, until it has been adequately examined. Air bags deflate immediately, so they protect against only one impact. The driver whose car hits more than one object is unprotected after the initial collision. Air bags also do not prevent "down and under" movement, so drivers who are extended (tall drivers and drivers of small, low-slung autos) may still impact with their legs and suffer leg, pelvis, or abdominal injuries.

It is important for occupants to wear chest and lap belts even when the car is equipped with air bags. Researchers have recently shown that some drivers who appear uninjured after deceleration crashes have been later found to have serious internal injuries. A clue to which driver may have internal injuries is the condition of the steering wheel. A deformed steering wheel is just as important a clue in an auto equipped with an air bag as in those that are not. This clue may be missed because the deflated air bag covers the steering wheel. Thus, a quick "lift and look" under the air bag should be part of the routine examination of the steering wheel (Figure 1-12).

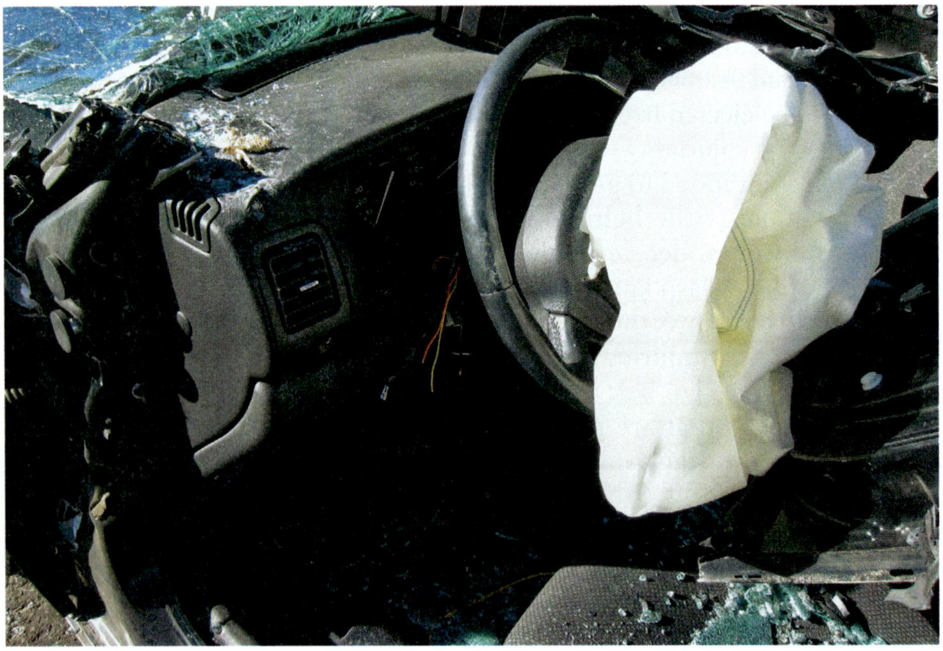

FIGURE 1-12 Lift the collapsed air bag to note whether or not there is a deformity of the steering wheel. *(Courtesy of Olivier Le Queinec, Shutterstock.com)*

Many autos are now equipped with side air bags in the doors. Some have air bags that come down from the roof to protect the head, and at least one make of auto has air bags under the dash to protect the legs. They obviously give much-needed extra protection.

Certain dangers are associated with air bags. Small drivers who bring the seat up close to the steering wheel may sustain serious injuries as the bag inflates. Infants in car seats placed in the front seat may be seriously injured by the air bag.

In summary, when at the scene of an MVC, note the type of collision and the clues (such as deformities of the vehicle) that imply high kinetic energy has been spent. Maintain a high index of suspicion for occult injuries and thus keep scene time to a minimum. In addition, knowledge of anatomy and physiology is essential. Focus on what injuries can be predicted, and appreciate that age and environment may suggest the probability of other injuries. Last, comorbidities (for example, diabetes, cardiovascular disease, chronic obstructive pulmonary disease) and medications (for example, anticoagulants) can make the case more complex and demanding. Those observations and clues are essential to quality patient care and must be relayed to medical direction and the receiving physician.

Tractor Accidents

Another large motorized vehicle with which you must be familiar is the farm tractor. Worldwide about 50% of all farm accident fatalities are from tractor overturns. Each year about 800 people in the United States and over a million worldwide die from tractor accidents. The two basic types of tractors are the two-wheel drive and the four-wheel drive. In both, the center of gravity is high, and thus the tractors are easily turned over (Figure 1-13). The majority of fatal accidents are due to the tractor turning over and crushing the driver. Most overturns (85%) are to the side; these are less likely to pin the driver because he has a chance to jump or be thrown clear. Rear overturns, although less frequent, are more likely to entrap and crush the driver because there is almost no opportunity to jump free. The primary mechanism is the crush injury, and the severity

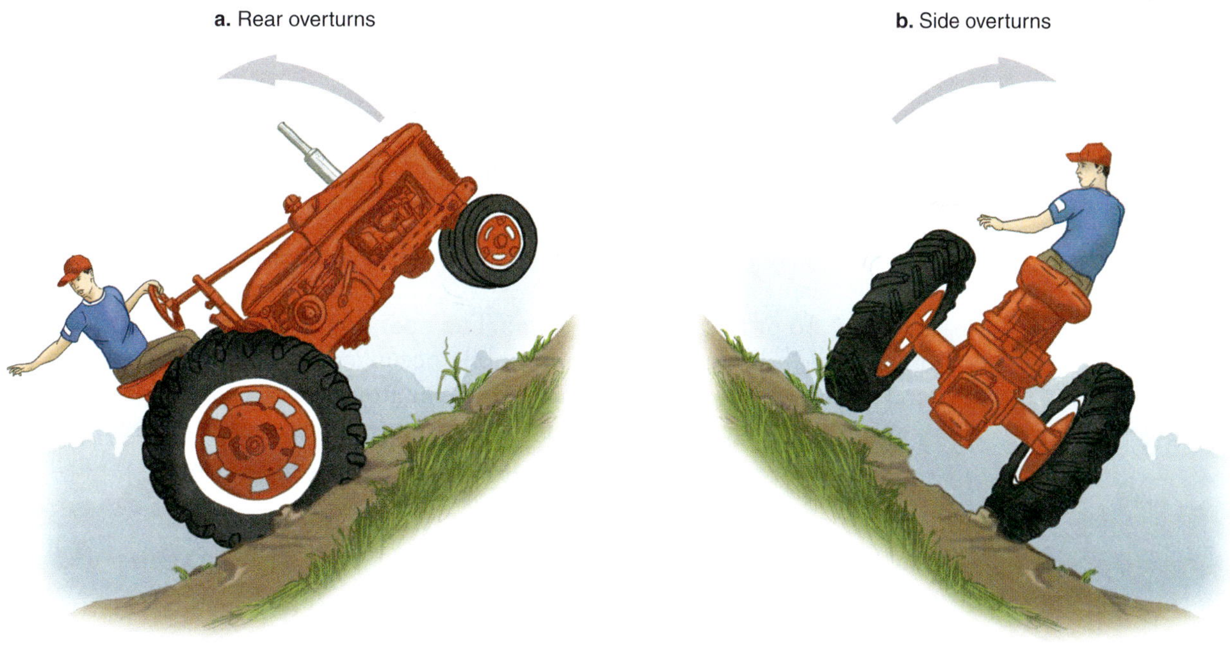

FIGURE 1-13 Tractor accidents.

depends on the part of the anatomy involved. Additional mechanisms are chemical burns from gasoline, diesel fuel, hydraulic fluid, or even battery acid. Thermal burns from hot engine parts or ignited fuel are also common.

Management consists of scene stabilization followed quickly by the primary survey and resuscitation. The following questions are used as a checklist in scene stabilization.

- Is the engine off?
- Are the rear wheels locked?
- Have the fuel situation and fire hazard been addressed?

While you are assessing the patient, other rescuers must stabilize the tractor. The center of gravity must be identified before any attempt is made to lift the tractor. The center of gravity of the two-wheel-drive tractor is located approximately 10 inches (25 cm) above and 24 inches (61 cm) in front of the rear axle. The center of gravity of a four-wheel-drive tractor is closer to the midline of the machine. Because tractors usually overturn on soft ground and their centers of gravity are tricky to determine, great care must be taken during lifting to avoid a second crush injury. Because of the tractor weight and length of time (usually prolonged) the driver is pinned, anticipate serious injuries. Often, the patient will go into profound shock as the compressing weight of the tractor is removed and blood rushes to the formerly compressed tissue.

Rapid, safe management of tractor accidents requires special exercises in lifting heavy machinery as well as good trauma management.

Small-Vehicle Crashes

Other small vehicles that fall into the motion-injury category include the motorcycle, all-terrain vehicle (ATV), personal watercraft (PWC), and snowmobile. The operators of those machines are not encased within them and, of course, wear no restraining devices. When the operator is subjected to the classic head-on, lateral-impact, rear-end, or rollover collision, the only forms of protection are the following:

- Evasive maneuvering
- Helmet usage
- Protective clothing (such as leather clothes, helmet, boots)
- Use of the vehicle to absorb kinetic energy (such as bike slide)

Motorcycles

It is extremely important for motorcycle riders to wear helmets. Helmets help prevent head injury (which causes 75% of motorcycle deaths). Regardless, helmets give no protection to the spine. The operator of a motorcycle involved in a crash is much like an ejected automobile occupant, and severe injuries are common. Injuries depend on the part of the anatomy subjected to kinetic energy. The lack of protective encasement leads to a higher frequency of head, neck, and extremity injuries. Important clues include deformity of the motorcycle, distance of skid, and deformity of stationary objects or cars.

All-Terrain Vehicles

The ATV was designed as a vehicle to traverse rough terrain. The ATV was used initially by ranchers, hunters, and farmers. Unfortunately, some people view it as a fast toy. Careless misuse has resulted in an ever-increasing morbidity and mortality from ATV accidents—sadly and frequently among the very young. The two basic designs are three-wheeled (no longer made and, so, rare) and four-wheeled. The four-wheel design affords reasonable stability and handling, but the three-wheeled ATV has a high center of gravity and is prone to roll over when turned sharply. Listed here are the four most common mechanisms:

- Vehicle rollover
- Fall-off of rider or passenger
- Forward deceleration of rider from vehicle impact with stationary object
- Impact of rider or passenger's head or extremities when passing too close to stationary objects (trees)

The injuries produced depend on the mechanism and the part of the anatomy that is impacted. The most frequent injuries are fractures, about half of which are above and half below the diaphragm. The major bony injuries involve the clavicles, sternum, and ribs. Be very suspicious for head or spinal injury.

Personal Watercraft

The use of PWC, such as the Jet Ski, Sea-Doo, or WaveRunner, has become popular in water recreational activities. Over a million PWCs are in operation in the United States. The U.S. Coast Guard reported in 2006 that 24% of all boating accidents involved one or more PWCs. In the United States, California reports that PWCs represent 16% of all registered vessels but account for 55% of all injuries. The rate of emergency department–treated injuries related to PWCs is about 8.5 times higher than the rate of that of motorboats. The death rate is about three times higher.

The PWC is designed to be operated by a driver who is in a sitting, standing, or kneeling position, with one or more passengers located behind the driver in tandem. PWCs are able to obtain high speeds quickly, but have no braking mechanism. Like motorcycles, PWCs offer no protection to the driver or passengers. Most injuries are caused by PWC collisions, either with other watercraft or with fixed objects such as docks or tree stumps. Most are due to driver inexperience and error.

PWCs are unique in that they are steered by the flow of water through the motor so that when the motor is shut off, the craft cannot be steered. The usual response when approaching an obstruction (tree stump, dock) is to slow down and turn to avoid it. However, with a PWC, when you slow the engine, you lose the ability to steer and often hit the object. (There is no braking mechanism.)

PWC collisions produce injury patterns similar to those encountered with motorcycle–auto collisions. Rectal and vaginal trauma may occur when rear-seat passengers or the driver fall off backward, impacting the water (buttocks first) at high speeds. The likelihood of drowning (even with the use of personal flotation devices) is always a danger. Remember, water is not soft when a body impacts with it at high speeds; therefore, you must assess and practice the same index of suspicion as with any high-energy event.

Snowmobiles

Snowmobiles are used both as recreational and utility vehicles. The snowmobile has a low clearance and a low center of gravity. The injuries common to this vehicle are similar to those that occur with ATVs. Turnovers are somewhat more common, and because the vehicle is usually heavier than an ATV, crush injuries are seen more frequently. Again, the injury pattern depends on the part of the anatomy that is directly involved. Be alert for possible coexisting hypothermia. A common injury with the snowmobile is the "hangman" or "clothesline" injury that results from running under wire fences. Be alert for occult cervical-spine injuries and potential airway compromise.

Pedestrian Injuries

A pedestrian struck by a car almost always suffers severe internal injuries as well as fractures. This is true even if the vehicle is traveling at low speed. The mass of the auto is so large that high speed is not necessary to impart high-energy transfer. When high speed is involved, the results are disastrous.

There are two mechanisms of injury. The first is when the bumper of the auto strikes the body, and the second is when the body, accelerated by the transfer of forces, strikes the ground or some other object. An adult usually has bilateral lower leg or knee fractures plus whatever secondary injuries occur when the body strikes the hood of the car and then later the ground. Children are shorter, so the bumper is more likely to hit them in the pelvis or torso. They usually land on their heads in the secondary impact. When answering a call to an auto–pedestrian accident, be prepared for broken bones, internal injuries, and head injuries.

Falls

The mechanism for falls is vertical deceleration. The types of injuries sustained depend on the following three factors, which you must identify and relay to medical direction:

- Distance of fall
- Anatomic area impacted
- Surface struck

The primary groups involved in vertical falls are adults and children under the age of 5 years old. In children, the falls most commonly involve boys and occur mostly in the summer months in urban high-rise, multiple-occupant dwellings. Predisposing factors include poor supervision, defective railings, and the curiosity associated with that age group. Head injuries are common in falls by children because the head is the heaviest part of the body and thus impacts first.

Adult falls are generally occupational or due to the influence of alcohol or drugs. It is not uncommon for falls to occur during attempts to escape from fire or criminal activity. Generally, adults attempt to land on their feet; thus their falls are more controlled. In this landing form, the victim usually impacts initially on the feet and then falls backward, landing on the buttocks and outstretched hands. Classically, this "lover's leap" fall may result in the following injuries (Figure 1-14):

- Fractures of the feet or legs
- Hip and/or pelvic injuries
- Axial loading to the lumbar and cervical spine
- Vertical deceleration forces to the organs
- Colles fractures of the wrists

The greater the height, the greater is the potential for injury. However, serious injury can occur in a short-distance fall. Surface

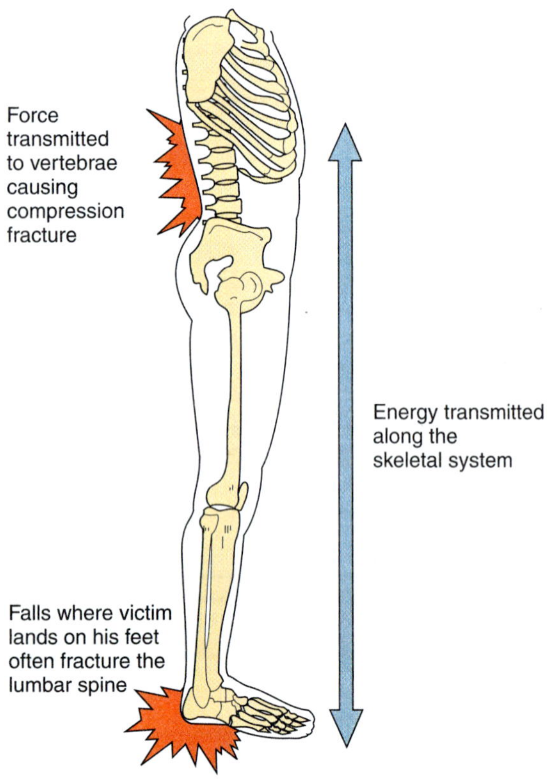

FIGURE 1-14 Axial loading.

density (concrete versus sawdust) and irregularity (gym floor versus staircase) also influence the severity of injury. Relay information about distance fallen and surface struck to medical direction with other pertinent information.

Penetrating Injuries

Numerous objects are capable of producing penetrating injuries. They range from the industrial saw blade that breaks off at an extremely high rate of speed to the foreign body hurled by a lawn mower. Most high-velocity objects are capable of penetrating the thorax or abdomen. Common forms of penetrating wounds come from the knife and gun.

The severity of a knife wound depends on the anatomic area penetrated, length of the blade, and angle of penetration (Figure 1-15). Remember, an upper abdominal stab wound may cause intrathoracic organ injury, and stab wounds below the fourth intercostal space may have penetrated the abdomen. The golden rule with any impaled object is to stabilize it in place. It will be removed at the hospital. Impaled objects in the cheek of the face and those blocking the airway are exceptions to this rule.

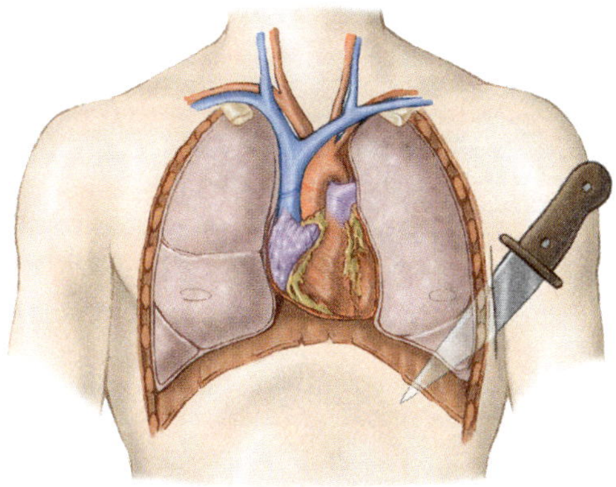

Stab wounds at nipple level or below frequently penetrate the abdomen.

FIGURE 1-15 Stab wounds.

Most penetrating wounds inflicted by firearms are due to handguns, rifles, and shotguns. Important factors to obtain, if possible, are the type of weapon, its caliber, and the distance from which the weapon was fired. However, remember that you must treat the patient and the wound, not the weapon.

Wound Ballistics

Because the kinetic energy produced by a projectile is mostly dependent on velocity, weapons are classified as either high or low velocity. Weapons with velocities less than 2,000 feet (610 meters) per second are considered low velocity and include essentially all handguns and some rifles. Injuries from these weapons are much less destructive than those sustained from high-velocity weapons, such as a military rifle. Low-velocity weapons are certainly capable of lethal injuries, depending on the body area struck. More civilians are killed by low-velocity bullets because they are more often shot by low-velocity weapons. All wounds inflicted by high-velocity weapons carry the additional factor of hydrostatic pressure. This factor alone can increase the injury.

Factors that contribute to tissue damage include the following:

- *Missile size.* The larger the bullet, the more resistance and the larger the permanent tract.
- *Missile deformity.* Hollow point and soft nose flatten out on impact, resulting in the involvement of a larger surface.
- *Semijacket.* The jacket expands and adds to surface area.
- *Tumbling.* Tumbling of the missile causes a wider path of destruction.
- *Yaw.* The missile can oscillate vertically and horizontally (wobble) about its axis, resulting in a larger surface area presenting to the tissue.

The wounds consist of the following three parts:

- *Entry wound.* Usually smaller than the exit wound, it may have darkened, burned edges if the bullet is fired from very close range (Figure 1-16).

PEARLS: Basic Ballistics

Know the information offered here, but remember: Treat the patient, not the weapon.

- *Caliber*—the internal diameter of the barrel; this corresponds to the ammunition used for the particular weapon.
- *Rifling*—a series of spiral grooves in the interior surface of the barrel of some weapons.
- *Ammunition*—case, primer, powder, and bullet.
- *Bullet construction*—usually solid lead alloy; may have a full or partial copper or steel jacket. The shape of the nose of the bullet may be rounded, flat, conical, or pointed. The bullet nose may also be soft or hollow (for expansion or fragmentation).

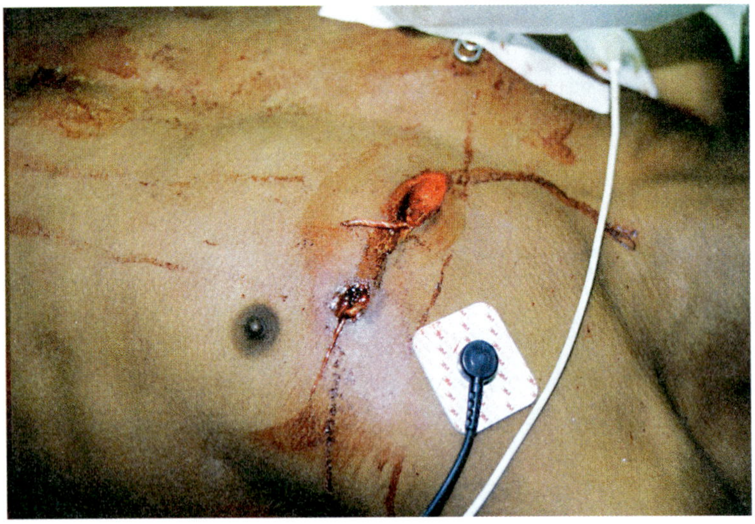

FIGURE 1-16 Comparison of an entrance wound and an exit wound. The entrance wound is lateral, just above the left nipple, and the exit wound is medial at the left of the sternum. *(©Edward T. Dickinson, MD)*

- *Exit wound.* Not all entry wounds will have exit wounds, and on occasion there may be multiple exits due to fragmentation of bone and missile. Generally, the exit wound is larger and has ragged edges.
- *Internal wound.* Low-velocity projectiles inflict damage primarily by damaging tissue that the missile contacts. High-velocity projectiles inflict damage by tissue contact and transfer of kinetic energy to surrounding tissues (Figure 1-17). Damage is related to the following:
  - Shock waves
  - Temporary cavity, which is 30 to 40 times the bullet's diameter and creates immense tissue pressures
  - Pulsation of the temporary cavity, which creates pressure changes in the adjacent tissue

Generally, damage done is proportional to tissue density. Highly dense organs such as bone, muscle, and the liver sustain more damage than less dense organs such as the lungs. A key factor to remember is that once a bullet enters a body, its trajectory will not always be in a straight line. Any patient with a missile penetration of the head, thorax, or abdomen should be transported immediately. Patients who have wounds that are not near the spine do not usually need spinal motion-restriction (SMR), and taking the time to perform SMR actually can increase the death rate because of the prolonged scene time. Personnel who have been shot while wearing a flak vest should be managed with caution; be alert for possible cardiac and other organ contusions.

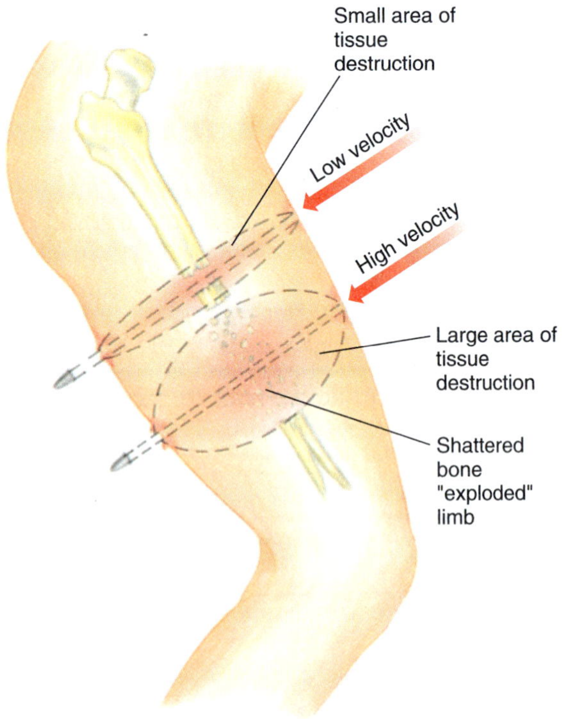

FIGURE 1-17a High-velocity versus low-velocity injury.

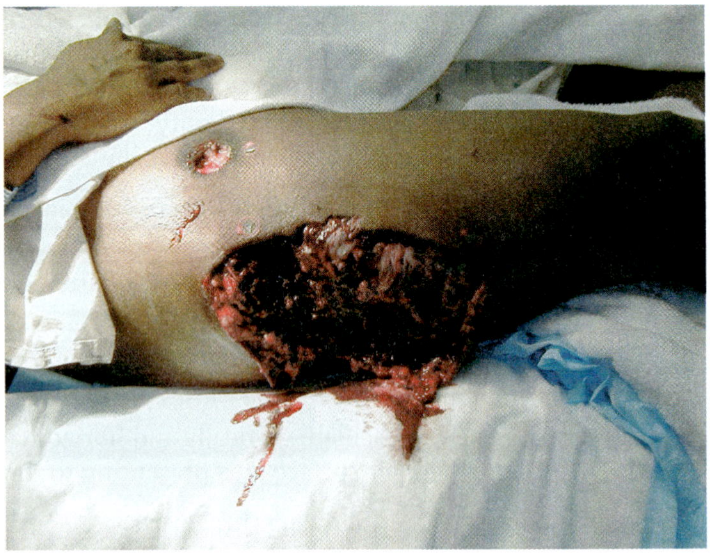

FIGURE 1-17b Example of a high-velocity wound of leg. *(Courtesy of Roy Alson, MD)*

In shotgun wounds, injury is determined by kinetic energy at impact, which is influenced by:

- Powder charge
- Size of pellets
- Choke of muzzle
- Distance to target

Velocity and kinetic energy dissipate rapidly as distance is traveled. At 40 yards, the velocity is one-half the initial muzzle velocity. Remember that at close range shotgun wounds are high energy because the pellets are still tightly grouped and act like a massive single bullet.

Blast Injuries

Blast injuries in this country occur primarily in industrial settings such as grain elevator and gas fume explosions but may be from criminal or terrorist activity.

blast injuries injuries commonly produced by the different mechanism associated with an explosion (air blast, shrapnel, burns, etc.).

The mechanism of injury by blast/explosion is due to three to five factors (Figure 1-18):

- *Primary*—initial air blast. A primary blast injury is caused solely by the direct effect of blast overpressure on tissue. Air is easily compressible, unlike

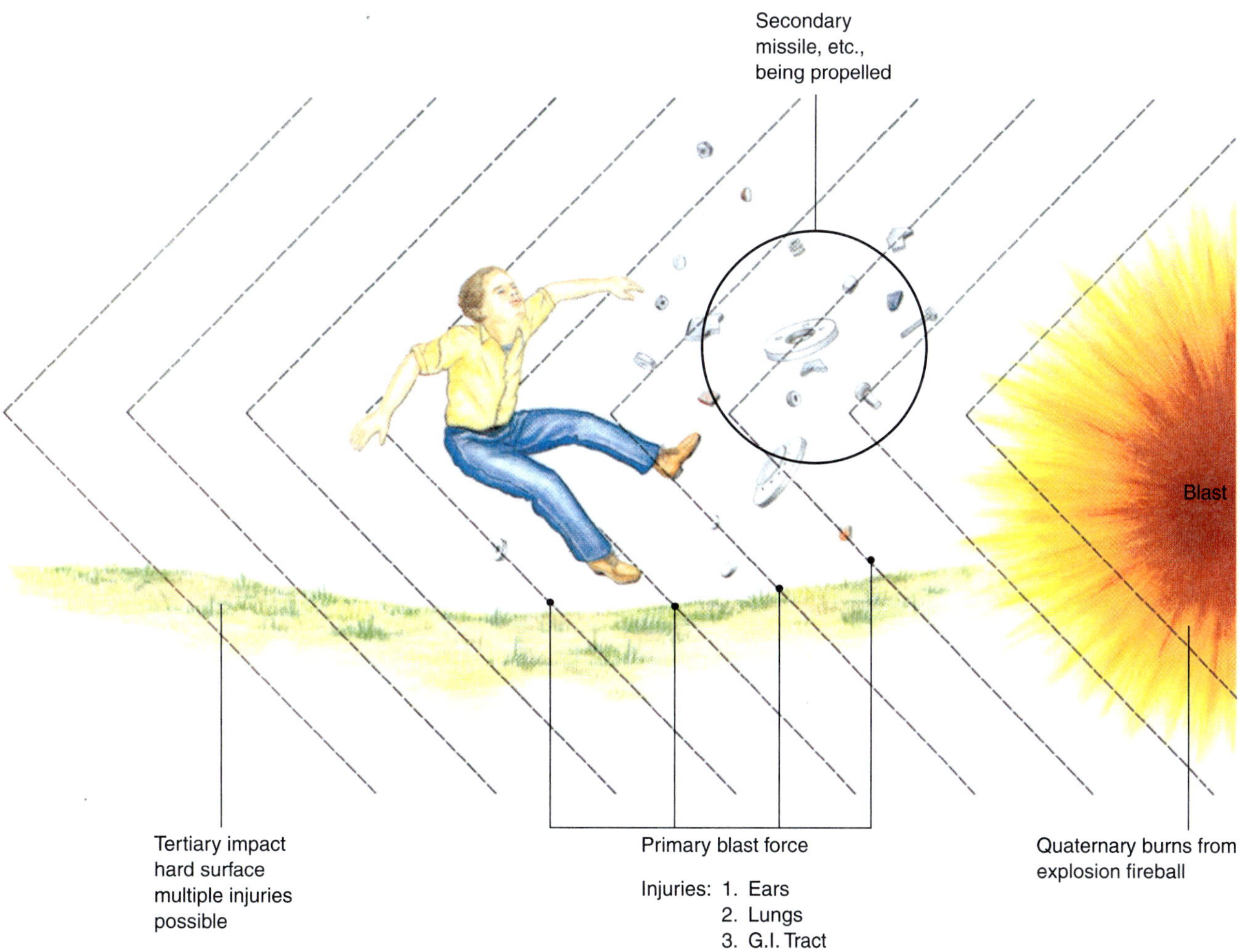

FIGURE 1-18 Explosions can cause injury with the initial blast, when the victim is struck by debris, or by the victim being thrown against the ground or other fixed objects by the blast.

water. As a result, a primary blast injury almost always affects air-filled structures such as the lungs, ears, and gastrointestinal tract.

- *Secondary*—patient being struck by material (shrapnel) propelled by the blast force.
- *Tertiary*—body being thrown and impacting on ground or other object.
- *Quaternary*—thermal burns from the explosion fireball or respiratory injuries from inhalation of toxic dust or fumes.
- *Quinary*—contamination by chemical, biological, or radiological material that was dispersed by the explosion (dirty bomb).

Injuries due to the primary air blast are almost exclusive to the air-containing organs. The auditory system usually involves ruptured tympanic membranes. Lung injuries may include pneumothorax, parenchymal hemorrhage, and especially alveolar rupture. Alveolar rupture may cause air embolus that may be manifested by bizarre central nervous system symptoms. Gastrointestinal tract injuries may vary from mild intestinal and stomach contusions to frank rupture. Always suspect lung injuries in a blast victim.

Injuries caused by the secondary factors may be penetrating or blunt. Fragments of shrapnel from an explosion may attain velocities of 14,000 feet (4,270 meters) per second. This is over four times the velocity of the most powerful high-velocity rifle bullets. A piece of shrapnel traveling at this velocity would impart more than 16 times the energy of a similarly sized high-velocity rifle bullet. Any shrapnel wound should be considered serious.

Tertiary injuries are much the same as when a person is ejected from an automobile or has fallen from a height. The blast wave may propel the person at a high velocity for a varying distance. The injuries will depend on what the person impacts (solid object versus water or soft ground, for example).

Quaternary injuries are seen when there is a large fireball associated with the explosion or when toxic fumes or dust are produced by the explosion. They are more common when the victim is in an enclosed space or has previous lung disease such as asthma or emphysema.

Quinary injuries are relatively new and reflect a terrorist's attempts to make bombs more deadly by using the explosion to disperse toxic chemicals, biological agents, or radiological agents. Such bombs are called "dirty bombs" for that reason.

CASE PRESENTATION (continued)

The EMS team remains in their ambulance until the fire service scene commander confirms the scene is safe and the HazMat tech reports that there are no chemical, biological, or radiological contaminations identified. The bomb went off in the waiting room as the staff was closing the office. Only the three staff members were in the office. The team dons Level D PPE (gloves and eye protection) and quickly evaluates the patients down in the street.

Patient 1 is dead and is left where she was. Patient 2 is responsive only to pain. There is some bleeding from her nose, ears, and mouth, and there are multiple penetrating injuries from shrapnel. This patient also has decreased breath sounds over one side of the chest and is breathing rapidly, is hypotensive, and has distended neck veins. The team leader suspects a tension pneumothorax from blast overpressure. The leader also suspects that this patient may have additional internal injuries such as shock lung and gastrointestinal injury from blast overpressure. The patient improves when the tension pneumothorax is decompressed. She is quickly packaged and transported to the local Level I trauma center by a second ambulance. The sitting third patient is conscious and complaining that she cannot hear. She says she was in the bathroom when the explosion occurred in the waiting room and thus was shielded somewhat. You find no obvious external injuries and suspect blast overpressure has ruptured her eardrums. Her chest is clear, and she has no difficulty breathing at this time. The fire service scene commander confirms that there are no other victims, so the ambulance team transports patient 3 to the trauma center for evaluation.

The emergency physician confirms that patient 2 has a tension pneumothorax and shock lung. He replaces your decompressing needle with a chest tube. She requires extensive surgery for multiple shrapnel injuries plus a ruptured liver. Patient 3 survives with substantial permanent hearing loss in both ears. ■

Summary

Trauma is the most serious disease affecting young people. Being a rescuer is among the most important professions but requires great dedication and continuous training. Saving patients who have sustained severe trauma requires attention to detail and careful management of time. Teamwork is essential because many actions must occur at the same time.

At the scene of an injury, there are certain important steps to perform before you begin care of the patient. Failure to perform a scene size-up will subject you and your patient to danger and may cause you to fail to anticipate serious injuries that your patient may have sustained. Take standard precautions and assess the scene for dangers first. Then determine the total number of patients and the need for additional rescuers or special equipment. If there are more patients than your team can manage, report to dispatch and initiate MCI protocols.

Resource Central

See Multi-Casualty Incidents and Triage for procedures to follow.

Identify the mechanism of injury and consider it as part of the overall management of the trauma patient. Ask yourself: What happened? What type of energy was applied? How much energy was transmitted? What part of the body was affected? If there is an MVC, consider the form of the crash and survey the vehicle's interior and exterior for damage.

Note that tractor accidents require careful stabilization of the machine to prevent a second injury to the patient. Falls require identification of distance fallen, surface struck, and position of the patient on impact. Stab wounds require knowledge of the length of the instrument as well as the angle at which it entered the body. When evaluating a shooting victim, you need to know the weapon, caliber, and distance from which it was fired.

Information about the high-energy event (e.g., falls, vehicle collision) is also important to the emergency physician. Be sure not only to record your findings but also to give a verbal report to the emergency department physician or trauma surgeon when you arrive. With this knowledge and a high index of suspicion, you can give your patient the greatest chance of survival.

Bibliography

1. Almogy, G., Y. Mintz, et al. 2006. Suicide bombing attacks: Can external signs predict internal injuries? *Annals of Surgery* 243(4): 541–46.
2. American College of Surgeons, Committee on Trauma. 2008. Appendix B: Biomechanics of injury. In *Advanced Trauma Life Support for Doctors Student Course Manual*. 8th ed. Chicago: American College of Surgeons.
3. Campbell, J., J. Smith. 2008. Chapter 6: Incendiaries and explosives. In *Homeland Security and Emergency Medical Response*. New York: McGraw-Hill, Inc. 117–139.
4. Committee on Injury and Poison Prevention. 2000. American Academy of Pediatrics: Personal watercraft use by children and adolescents. *Pediatrics* 105(2): 452–53.
5. DeHaven, H. 2000. Mechanical analysis of survival in falls from heights of fifty to one hundred and fifty feet. *Injury Prevention* 6: 62–68.
6. McSwain, N. E. Jr. 2011. Chapter 4: Kinematics of trauma. In *Prehospital Trauma Life Support*. 7th ed. St. Louis: Mosby, Inc. 43–85.
7. Newgard, C., K. Martens, E. Lyons. 2002. Crash scene photography in motor vehicle crashes without air bag deployment. *Academic Emergency Medicine* 9(9): 924–29.
8. Wightman, J., S. Gladish. 2001. Explosions and blast injuries. *Annals of Emergency Medicine* 37(6): 664–78.

Explore Resource Central

For additional review and practice tests, visit **www.bradybooks.com** and click on Resource Central to access book-specific resources for this text. To access Resource Central, follow directions on the Student Access Card provided with this text. If there is no card, go to www.bradybooks.com and follow the Resource Central link to Buy Access from there.

Trauma Assessment and Management

John E. Campbell, MD, FACEP
John T. Stevens, NREMT-P
Leon Charpentier, EMT-P

2

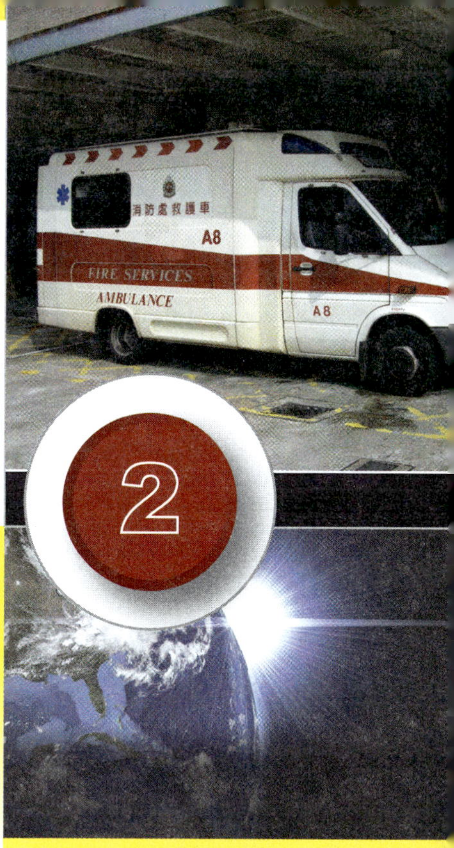

(Photo courtesy of International Trauma Life Support)

Primary Survey

Valutazione Primaria
Reconocimiento Primario
Enquête Primaire
Badanie wstępne
Schnelle Traumauntersuchung
Primarni pregled
التقييم الأولي
primarni pregled
Primarni Pregled
Első áttekintés

OBJECTIVES

Upon successful completion of this chapter, you should be able to:

1. Outline the steps in trauma assessment and management.
2. Describe the ITLS Primary Survey.
3. Explain the initial assessment and how it relates to the rapid trauma survey and the focused exam.
4. Describe when the initial assessment can be interrupted.
5. Describe when critical interventions should be made and where to make them.
6. Identify which patients have critical conditions and how they should be managed.
7. Describe the ITLS Ongoing Exam.
8. Describe the ITLS Secondary Survey.

KEY TERMS

AVPU, *p. 34*
DCAP-BLS, *p. 42*
focused exam, *p. 28*
initial assessment, *p. 28*
ITLS Ongoing Exam, *p. 28*
ITLS Primary Survey, *p. 28*
ITLS Secondary Survey, *p. 28*
patient assessment, *p. 28*
rapid trauma survey, *p. 28*
SAMPLE history, *p. 38*
TIC, *p. 42*

Chapter Overview

ITLS **patient assessment** is made up of the **ITLS Primary Survey**, the ITLS Secondary Survey, and the ITLS Ongoing Exam. The ITLS Primary Survey is made up of the scene size-up, **initial assessment**, and a **rapid trauma survey** or **focused exam**. The purpose of the Primary Survey is to determine if *immediately* life-threatening conditions exist and to identify those patients who should have immediate transport to the hospital. The **ITLS Ongoing Exam** is meant to identify changes in the patient's condition, and the **ITLS Secondary Survey** is an evaluation for all injuries, not just life-threatening ones.

The scene size-up will set the stage for how you will perform the rest of the Primary Survey. If there is a dangerous generalized mechanism of injury (auto crash, fall from a height, etc.) or if the patient is unconscious and the mechanism of injury is unknown, you should extend the Primary Survey to include a rapid examination of the head, neck, chest, abdomen, pelvis, extremities, and back. You would then perform critical interventions and transport. Ongoing Exams and possibly a Secondary Survey would be performed en route.

If there is a dangerous localized mechanism of injury suggesting an isolated injury (bullet wound of thigh, amputation of the hand, etc.), you would perform the initial assessment but the focused exam would be limited to the area affected by the injury. The full rapid trauma survey is not required. You would then perform critical interventions and transport. Ongoing Exams and possibly a Secondary Survey would be performed en route.

If there is no significant life threat in the mechanism of injury (e.g., shot off big toe) you would do the initial assessment and, if normal, go directly to a focused exam based on the patient's chief complaint. The Secondary Survey would not be necessary.

To make the most efficient use of time, ITLS prehospital assessment and management of the trauma patient is divided into three assessments (Primary Survey, Ongoing Exam, and Secondary Survey), and each assessment is made up of certain steps (Figure 2-1). Those assessments are the foundation on which prehospital trauma care is built.

patient assessment the process by which the EMS responder evaluates a trauma patient to determine injuries sustained and the patient's physiologic status; made up of the ITLS Primary Survey, ITLS Ongoing Exam, and ITLS Secondary Survey.

ITLS Primary Survey a brief exam to find immediately life-threatening conditions; made up of the scene size-up, initial assessment, and either the rapid trauma survey or the focused exam.

initial assessment a rapid assessment of airway, breathing, and circulation to prioritize the patient and identify immediately life-threatening conditions; part of the ITLS Primary Survey.

rapid trauma survey a brief exam from head to toe performed to identify life-threatening injuries.

focused exam an exam used when there is a focused mechanism of injury or an isolated injury; an exam that is limited to the area of injury.

ITLS Ongoing Exam an abbreviated exam to determine changes in the patient's condition.

ITLS Secondary Survey a comprehensive heat-to-toe exam to find additional injuries that may have been missed in the ITLS Primary Survey.

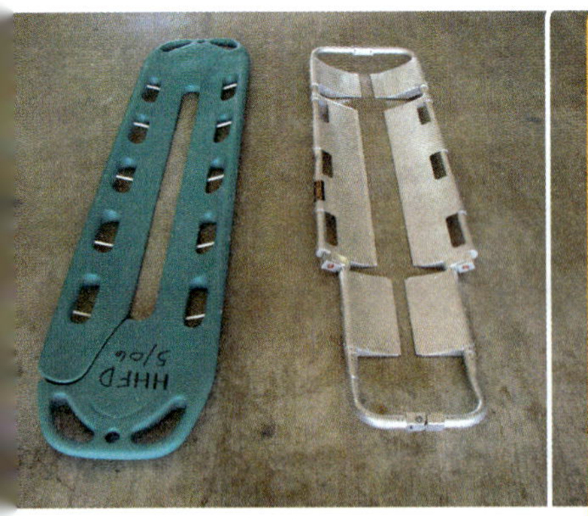

(Courtesy of Leon Charpentier, EMT-P)

CASE PRESENTATION

An ALS ambulance has been dispatched to the scene of a domestic dispute. En route, the team is told that a man has been stabbed with a kitchen knife. *What is their first concern when they arrive?* On arrival, the police, who have the uninjured wife in custody, meet them. The scene commander shows the team a 10-inch kitchen knife with blood on the blade. She says the patient may be found at the foot of the seven-step flight of stairs leading out from the kitchen. *When approaching the patient, what should they be looking for? What is/are the mechanism(s) of injury? What is the first priority? What type of assessment should be performed? Is this a load-and-go situation?* Keep these questions in mind as you read the chapter. Then, at the end of the chapter, find out how the rescuers completed this call. ■

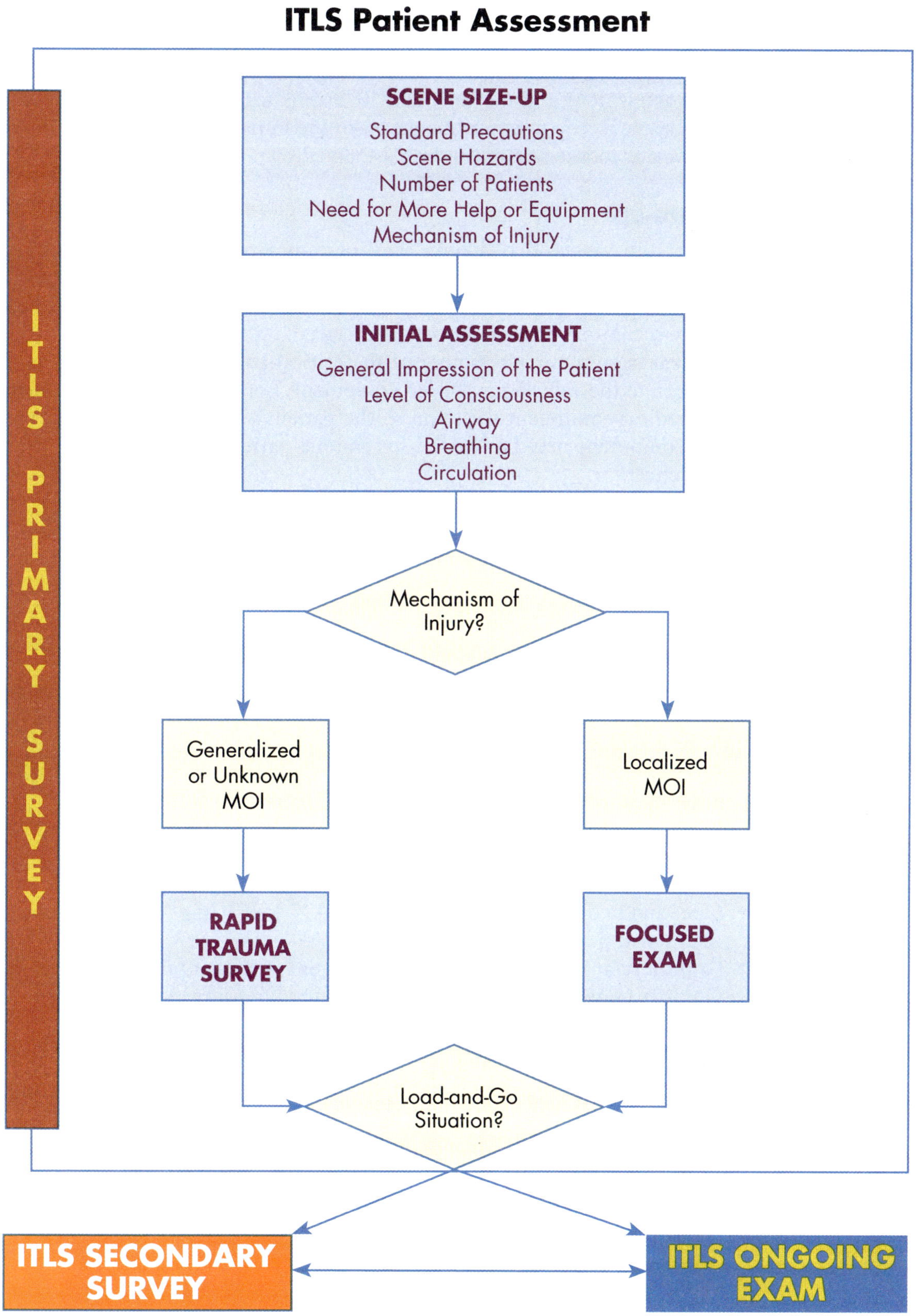

FIGURE 2-1 Steps in the assessment of the trauma patient.

PEARLS: A Systematic Approach

Use the same systematic ITLS approach for each trauma patient.

PEARLS: Safety

Do not approach the patient before doing a scene size-up. Foolish haste may subtract a rescuer and add a patient.

ITLS Primary Survey

The ITLS Primary Survey includes an evaluation of the scene and preparation for patient assessment and management. It begins with the scene size-up and then, if the scene is safe to enter, moves on to the initial assessment and a rapid trauma survey or focused exam (Figures 2-2 and 2-3).

Scene Size-up

On-scene trauma assessment begins with certain actions that are performed before you approach the patient. It cannot be stressed too much that failure to perform preliminary actions can jeopardize your life as well as the patient's life. Perform the scene size-up as described in Chapter 1.

Once you begin your assessment of the critical patient, you may not have time to return to the vehicle for needed equipment. For this reason, always carry essential medical equipment with you to the patient's side. Anticipate that the following equipment may be needed for trauma patients, depending on your level of practice:

- Personal
    - Portable radio
    - Small, high-intensity light
    - Personal protective equipment (gloves, goggles)
    - Spring-loaded punch
    - EMS scissors
    - Stethoscope
    - Pen and pad; felt-tip pen (initial triage marker)
- Trauma Kit (carried by team leader)
    - Airway: hand-powered suction, blind insertion airway device (BIAD), cricothyroidotomy-set endotracheal (ET) intubation kit (including surgical mask/goggles)
    - Bag-mask device (#4/5)
    - Oxygen (D-tank), nonrebreather mask
    - One- and two-inch tape, 10-pack sterile 4 × 4, 4" Kling®, 4" Ace™, one each sterile 5"–9"/8"–10" dressings
    - Commercial tourniquet, hemostatic agent such as Quikclot Combat Gause™ or Quikclot Emergency Dressing™ (both kaolin based)
    - Seal for sucking chest wound, such as Asherman™ Chest Seal, Bolin™ Chest Seal, Halo™ vent, or Vaseline™ Gauze)
    - Device for chest decompression, such as Cook Emergency Pneumothorax Set, Turkel™ Safety Needle, or 14-gauge 3.25 inch (8 cm) angiocath.
    - Rescue or warming blanket (may be contained with stretcher)
- Spinal motion restriction (SMR) package (carried by second rescuer)
    - Long backboard
    - Three to four straps
    - Cervical immobilization device (CID) or sheet rolls + 2" tape
    - Adjustable cervical collar
- Special equipment (brought by EMT or third rescuer based on dispatch information)
    - Stretcher or Stokes basket or "scoop" stretcher
    - Burn sheets/irrigation fluids

ITLS PRIMARY SURVEY

SCENE SIZE-UP

Standard Precautions Hazards, Number of Patients, Need for additional resources, **Mechanism of Injury**

INITIAL ASSESSMENT

GENERAL IMPRESSION
Age, Sex, Weight, General Appearance, Position, Purposeful Movement, Obvious Injuries, Skin Color
Life-threatening Bleeding

LOC
A-V-P-U
Chief Complaint/Symptoms

AIRWAY (WITH C-SPINE CONTROL)
Snoring, Gurgling, Stridor; Silence

BREATHING
Present? Rate, Depth, Effort

CIRCULATION
Radial/Carotid Present? Rate, Rhythm, Quality
Skin Color, Temperature, Moisture; Capillary Refill
Has bleeding been controlled?

RAPID TRAUMA SURVEY

HEAD and NECK
Wounds?
Neck Vein distention? Tracheal Deviation?

CHEST
Asymmetry (Paradoxical Motion?), Contusions, Penetrations, Tenderness, Instability, Crepitation
Breath Sounds
Present? Equal? (If unequal: percussion)
Heart Tones

ABDOMEN
Contusions, Penetration/Evisceration; Tenderness, Rigidity, Distention

PELVIS
Tenderness, Instability, Crepitation

LOWER/UPPER EXTREMITIES
Obvious Swelling, Deformity
Motor and Sensory

POSTERIOR
Obvious wounds, Tenderness, Deformity

If radial pulse present:
VITAL SIGNS
Measured Pulse, Breathing, Blood Pressure

If altered mental status: Brief Neurological exam
PUPILS
Size? Reactive? **Equal?**

GLASGOW COMA SCALE
Eyes, Voice, Motor

FIGURE 2-2 The ITLS Primary Survey including the rapid trauma survey.

ITLS PRIMARY SURVEY

SCENE SIZE-UP
Standard Precautions
Hazards, Number of Patients, Need for additional resources,
Mechanism of Injury

↓

INITIAL ASSESSMENT
GENERAL IMPRESSION
Age, Sex, Weight, General Appearance, Position,
Purposeful Movement, Obvious Injuries, Skin Color
Life-threatening Bleeding

LOC
A-V-P-U
Chief Complaint/Symptoms

AIRWAY
(WITH C-SPINE CONTROL)
Snoring, Gurgling, Stridor; Silence

BREATHING
Present? Rate, Depth, Effort

CIRCULATION
Radial/Carotid Present? Rate, Rhythm, Quality
Skin Color, Temperature, Moisture; Capillary Refill
Has bleeding been controlled?

↓

FOCUSED EXAM
Focused exam of the identified injury
Also evaluate the spine if distracting injury and any possibility of spinal injury

If radial pulse present:
VITAL SIGNS
Measured Pulse, Breathing, Blood Pressure

If altered mental status: Brief Neurological exam
PUPILS
Size? Reactive? **Equal?**

GLASGOW COMA SCALE
Eyes, Voice, Motor

FIGURE 2-3 The ITLS Primary Survey including the focused exam.

- Spinal extrication device
- Monitor/defibrillator
- Additional heavy dressings

PEARLS: Interruptions

The team leader should delegate any intervention required during the ITLS Primary Survey and should not interrupt the completion of the survey except for airway obstruction, cardiac arrest, or scene danger.

Once the scene is safe to enter, as team leader, you must focus your attention on the rapid assessment of your patient. All decisions on treatment require that you have identified life-threatening conditions. Remember, once you begin patient assessment in the ITLS Primary Survey, only three things should cause you to interrupt completion of the assessment. You may interrupt the assessment sequence only if (1) the scene becomes unsafe, (2) you must treat an airway obstruction, or (3) you must treat cardiac arrest. (Respiratory arrest, dyspnea, or bleeding may be delegated to other team members while you continue assessment of the patient.)

For critical patients, the goal should be to complete the Primary Survey in less than two minutes and to have on-scene times of five minutes or less. Internal bleeding can usually be stopped only in the operating room, so all scene interventions should be lifesaving or should be delayed until the patient is in the ambulance on the way to the hospital.

The "Fix It" Process

Experience has shown that most mistakes occur because the team leader stops to perform an intervention and forgets to perform part of the assessment. To prevent this, when immediate interventions are needed, delegate them to your team members while you continue the assessment. This is an important concept that immediately addresses problems encountered and yet does not interrupt the assessment sequence and does not increase scene time. It is what teamwork is all about. Think of it as the "Fix It" process.

As you perform your assessment, you will have interventions that need to be performed immediately by your partners. For example, when you check the airway, the "Fix It" may be a nonrebreather mask at 15 LPM, or it may be endotracheal intubation. When you check the neck, the "Fix It" may be to apply a cervical collar. As you read the patient assessment sequence, look for the "Fix Its" that can be done on scene.

Initial Assessment

The purpose of the initial assessment is to prioritize the patient and to determine the existence of immediately life-threatening conditions. The information gathered is used to make decisions about critical interventions and time of transport. Once you determine that the patient may be safely approached, assessment should proceed quickly and smoothly. The next steps in the Primary Survey (initial assessment and rapid trauma survey) should take less than two minutes. As you begin, you will place the trauma bag beside the patient and direct Rescuer 2 to stabilize the patient's neck (if needed) and to assume responsibility for the airway. Rescuer 3 will place the backboard beside the patient and address any bleeding while you are proceeding with your exam. This team approach makes the most efficient use of time and allows you to rapidly perform the initial assessment without performing interventions yourself, which can interrupt your thought process.

The initial assessment is made up of your general impression on approaching the patient, an evaluation of the patient's level of consciousness (LOC), manual stabilization of the cervical spine (if needed), and an assessment of the patient's airway, breathing, and circulation (ABCs).

Form a General Impression of the Patient on Approach

You have already sized up the scene, determined the total number of patients, and initiated multicasualty incident (MCI) protocols if there are more patients than your team can effectively handle (see Chapter 1). As you approach (try to approach the patient from the front so he does not turn his head to see you), note the patient's approximate age, sex, weight, and general appearance. The old and the very young are at increased risk. Female patients may be pregnant. Observe the position of the patient, both body position and position in relation to surroundings. Note the patient's activity. (Is the patient aware of surroundings, moving purposefully, anxious, obviously in distress, etc.?) Does the patient have any obvious major injuries or major bleeding?

Resource Central

See Multi-Casualty Incidents and Triage for more procedures related to such incidents.

(This changes priority to C-A-B-C.) The first *C* stands for *control bleeding*. (Do not confuse this with the American Heart Association's CAB for cardiac arrest, where the *C* stands for *compressions*.) If your patient has major external bleeding, you must immediately direct another team member to control it ("Fix It").

Your observation of the patient in relation to the scene and the mechanism of injury will help you prioritize the patient. If there are multiple patients, rapidly triage them. Triage will be different for a small group than for a mass-casualty event in which the number of patients exceeds the care available. When there are only a few patients, the main decision is which patient will be treated and transported first, whereas in a mass-casualty situation the decision must be made as to who will receive care and who will not.

Evaluate Initial Level of Consciousness While Obtaining Cervical-Spine Stabilization

Assessment begins immediately, even if the patient is being extricated. If there is a mechanism of injury that suggests spinal injury, Rescuer 2 immediately and gently but firmly stabilizes the head and neck ("Fix It") in a neutral position. Holding the head (with hands or knees) rather than holding the neck keeps the hands from being in the way when another team member applies a cervical collar later. As team leader, you may need to initially stabilize the neck if there is not a second rescuer immediately available. If you elect to do this, you should immediately turn this responsibility over to the first rescuer arriving to help you. (You cannot stabilize the neck and perform an adequate assessment at the same time.) If the head or neck is held in an angulated position and the patient complains of pain on any attempt to straighten it, you should stabilize it in the position found. The same is true of the unconscious patient whose neck is held to one side and does not move when you gently attempt to straighten it. *The rescuer stabilizing the neck must not release it until he or she is relieved or a suitable motion-restriction device is applied.*

The team leader should say to the patient, "My name is _____. We are here to help you. Can you tell me what happened?" The patient's reply gives immediate information about both the airway and the level of consciousness. If the patient responds appropriately to questioning, you can assume that the airway is open and the LOC is normal. If the response is not appropriate (the patient is unconscious or awake but confused), make a mental note of the LOC using the **AVPU** scale (Table 2-1). Anything below "A" (alert) should trigger a systematic search for the causes during the rapid trauma survey. Loss or decrease in LOC can be caused by many things, including obstructed airway, respiratory failure, shock, increased intracranial pressure, as well as drugs or metabolic disorders. The rapid trauma survey leads you in a systematic, organized way.

AVPU an abbreviated description of the patient's level of consciousness. AVPU stands for alert, responds to verbal stimuli, responds to pain, and unresponsive.

Table 2-1 Levels of Mental Status (AVPU)

A—Alert (awake, oriented, and obeys commands)
V—Responds to Verbal stimuli (awake but confused, or unconscious but responds in some way to verbal stimuli)
P—Responds to Pain (unconscious but responds in some way to touch or painful stimuli)
U—Unresponsive (no gag or cough reflex)

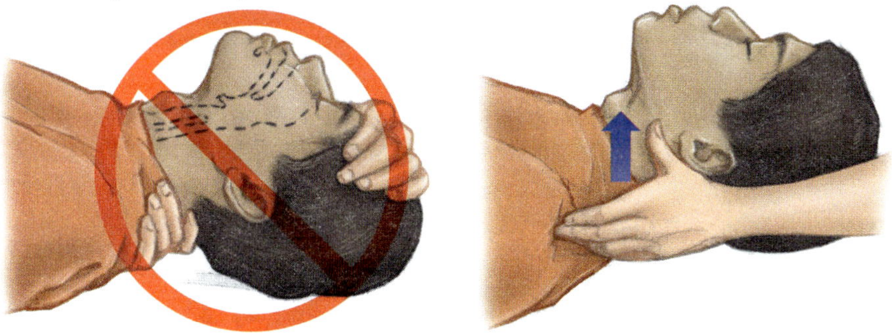

FIGURE 2-4 Opening the airway using the modified jaw thrust. Maintain in-line stabilization while pushing up on the angles of the jaw with your thumbs.

Assess the Airway

If the patient cannot speak or is unconscious, further evaluation of the airway should follow. Look, listen, and feel for movement of air. Rescuer 2 should position the airway as needed. Because of the ever-present danger of spinal injury, avoid extending the neck to open the airway of a trauma patient. If the airway is obstructed (apnea, snoring, gurgling, stridor), use an appropriate method (reposition, sweep, suction) to open it immediately ("Fix It") (Figure 2-4). Failure to quickly provide an open airway is one of the three reasons to interrupt the patient assessment part of the ITLS Primary Survey. If simple positioning and suctioning fail to provide an adequate airway, or if the patient has stridor, advanced airway techniques may be necessary immediately ("Fix It").

Assess Breathing

Look, listen, and feel for movement of air. If the patient is unconscious, place your ear over the patient's mouth so you can judge both the depth (tidal volume; see Chapter 4) and rate of ventilations. Look at the movement of the chest (or abdomen), listen to the sound of air movement, and feel both the movement of air on your cheek and the movement of the chest wall with your hand. *If the chest is moving but you do not feel air at the mouth or nose, the patient is NOT breathing adequately.* Notice if the patient uses accessory muscles to breathe. If ventilation is inadequate (Table 2-2), Rescuer 2 should begin to assist ventilation immediately ("Fix It"), using his knees to restrict movement of the patient's neck and free his hands to apply oxygen or a bag-mask to assist ventilation (Figure 2-5). When assisting or providing ventilation, be sure that the patient gets an adequate ventilatory rate (one breath every six to eight seconds) and an adequate volume (about 500 cc). Rescuers tend to ventilate too fast. If you monitor ventilation with capnography (recommended), you should maintain the end tidal CO_2 ($ETCO_2$) at about 35–45. All patients who are breathing too fast should receive supplemental

Table 2-2 Normal and Abnormal Respiratory Rates

	Normal	Abnormal
Adult	10–20	<8 and >24
Small child	15–30	<15 and >35
Infant	25–50	<25 and >60

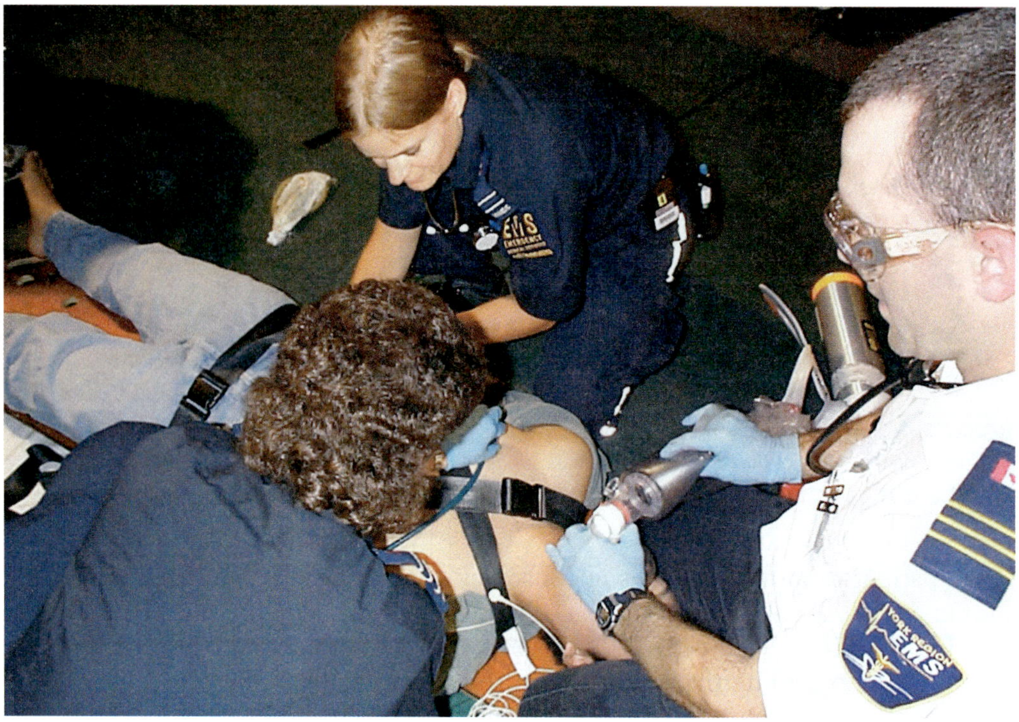

FIGURE 2-5 Using your knees to maintain stabilization of the neck will free your hands to assist ventilation. *(Courtesy of ITLS Ontario, Steve McNenly, Jennifer Lundren, and Sheryl Jackson)*

high-flow oxygen. As a general rule, all patients with multisystem trauma should receive supplemental high-flow oxygen ("Fix It"). Recently, there has been some evidence that too much oxygen may be harmful, so it would be prudent to try to keep the pulse oximeter reading around 95% rather than 100%.

Assess Circulation

Has the external bleeding been controlled? Most bleeding can be stopped by direct pressure or pressure dressings. Tourniquets have been discouraged in the past, but recent military experience has found that, for bleeding not adequately controlled with pressure, an appropriate tourniquet should be used immediately. If a dressing becomes blood soaked, remove the dressing and redress once to be sure direct pressure is being placed on the bleeding area. Hemostatic agents such as QuikClot Combat Gauze (kaolin based) should be used in this situation ("Fix It"). Use of elevation and pressure points is now discouraged due to lack of evidence that they are effective. It is important to report excessive bleeding to the receiving physician. Do not use clamps to stop bleeders; this may cause injuries to other structures. (Nerves are present alongside arteries.)

Now note the rate and quality of the pulses at the wrist (brachial in the infant). Quickly note whether the rate is too slow (< 60 in an adult) or too fast (> 120). Also note its quality (thready, bounding, weak, irregular). While at the wrist, note skin color, temperature, and condition (and capillary refill in an infant or small child). Pale, cool, clammy skin, thready radial pulse, and decreased LOC are the best early assessments of decreased perfusion (shock). If the pulse is not palpable at the wrist, check for the presence of a carotid pulse. If pulses are absent at the neck, immediately start CPR ("Fix It") unless there is massive blunt trauma. Immediately transport the patient. This is also one of the three reasons to interrupt assessment during the ITLS Primary Survey.

Rapid Trauma Survey or Focused Exam

The choice between the rapid trauma survey and the focused exam depends on (1) the mechanism of injury and (2) the results of the initial assessment. If there is a dangerous generalized mechanism of injury (such as an auto crash or fall from a height), you should do a rapid trauma survey (Figure 2-2). You also should do a rapid trauma survey if the patient is unconscious and you do not know the mechanism of injury. If there is a dangerous *focused* mechanism of injury suggesting an isolated injury (bullet wound of thigh or amputation of the hand, for example), you may perform the focused exam (Figure 2-3), which is limited to the area affected by the injury. As a practical matter, remember that where there appears to be only one isolated injury (stab or bullet wound), there may be others of which the patient is not aware. You should have a low threshold for doing a rapid trauma survey rather than a focused exam. Finally, if there is no significant mechanism of injury (e.g., dropped a rock on a toe) and the initial assessment is normal (alert with no loss of consciousness, normal breathing, radial pulse less than 120, and no complaint of dyspnea, chest, abdominal, or pelvic pain), you may move directly to the focused exam based on the patient's chief complaint.

If you identify a priority (high-risk) patient, you need to find the cause of the abnormal findings and identify if this is a load-and-go patient.

You have identified a priority patient if you find any of the following:

- Dangerous mechanism of injury
- High-risk group (very young, very old, chronically ill)
- History that reveals
  - Loss of consciousness
  - Difficulty breathing
  - Severe pain of head, neck, or torso
- Initial assessment reveals
  - Altered mental status
  - Abnormal breathing
  - Abnormal circulation (shock or uncontrolled bleeding)

Rapid Trauma Survey

The rapid trauma survey is a brief exam done to find all life threats (Figure 2-2). A more thorough assessment—the ITLS Secondary Survey—will follow later if time permits. Having completed the initial assessment, begin obtaining a brief, targeted history (What happened? Where do you hurt?). Quickly assess (look and feel) head and neck for obvious wounds.

Evaluate neck veins, which if engorged, indicate positive pressure in the chest (possible tension pneumothorax or cardiac tamponade). If they are distended, look and palpate at the sternal notch for tracheal deviation. A rigid cervical extrication collar may be applied at this time ("Fix It").

Expose and examine the chest. Look to see if it is moving symmetrically. If not, is there paradoxical motion? Are there contusions or abrasions? Are there penetrations or sucking wounds? Briefly palpate for tenderness, instability, or crepitation. Then listen to see if breath sounds are present and equal bilaterally. Listen with the stethoscope over the lateral chest about the fourth intercostal space in the midaxillary line on both sides. If breath sounds are not equal (decreased or absent on one side), percuss the chest to determine whether the patient is just splinting from pain or if a pneumothorax (hyperresonant) or a hemothorax (dull) is present. If abnormalities are found during the chest exam (open chest wound, flail chest, tension pneumothorax, hemothorax), treat them as you discover them. Delegate the appropriate intervention (seal open wound, hand stabilize flail) to another team member ("Fix It"). If a tension pneumothorax is identified, and the patient (1) has altered mental status, (2) is cyanotic, and (3) has absent radial pulses, prepare to decompress immediately ("Fix It"). Before moving to the abdominal exam, very briefly notice the heart sounds so you will have a baseline for changes such as development of muffled heart sounds.

Briefly examine the abdomen, looking for bruises, penetrating wounds, or impaled objects. Palpate briefly for tenderness, rigidity, or distention. Be aware that an unconscious patient or one with a cervical-spine injury may have a false-negative exam.

Briefly palpate the pelvic girdle for tenderness, instability, or crepitation by gently pressing down on the symphysis and gently squeezing in on the anterior iliac crests. Note that tenderness is not the same thing as being unstable. The pelvis may be tender and yet stable. If the pelvis is unstable, you can feel the pelvic ring collapse as you apply pressure ("Fix It"). If the pelvis is unstable, direct another team member to get the scoop stretcher and possibly the pelvic compression belt. If the pelvis is unstable, do not check again!

Very quickly, examine the lower and upper extremities for gross deformity or swelling. An unstable pelvis and bilateral femur fractures indicate an unstable patient at risk for shock. Before moving the patient, check to make sure he can feel and move his feet and hands

At this point, transfer the patient to a long backboard, checking the posterior of the patient as you do this. If the patient has an unstable pelvis or bilateral femur fractures, to prevent further injuries, use a scoop stretcher (Figure 2-6) to transfer the patient to a long backboard. A scientific study has shown that at least one brand of scoop stretcher (Ferno) provides stabilization equal or superior to a rigid backboard, and you may simply use it instead of a backboard (Krell, 2006). Remember that if you use a scoop stretcher, you are still responsible to do your best to evaluate the posterior side of the patient. Transfer your patient to the ambulance as soon as you have her secured to the backboard.

SAMPLE history the minimum amount of information needed for a trauma patient; the letters in SAMPLE stand for symptoms, allergies, medications, past medical history, last oral intake medical history, last oral intake, and events preceding the incident.

You now obtain baseline vital signs (blood pressure, pulse, and respiratory rate) and the rest of the **SAMPLE history** (see the following section). If a critical situation is present, transport *now* and obtain the vital signs during transport.

If the patient has an altered mental status, do a brief neurological exam to identify possible increased intracranial pressure (ICP). It is critical to identify this condition (see Chapter 10) because it will have important implications with respect to

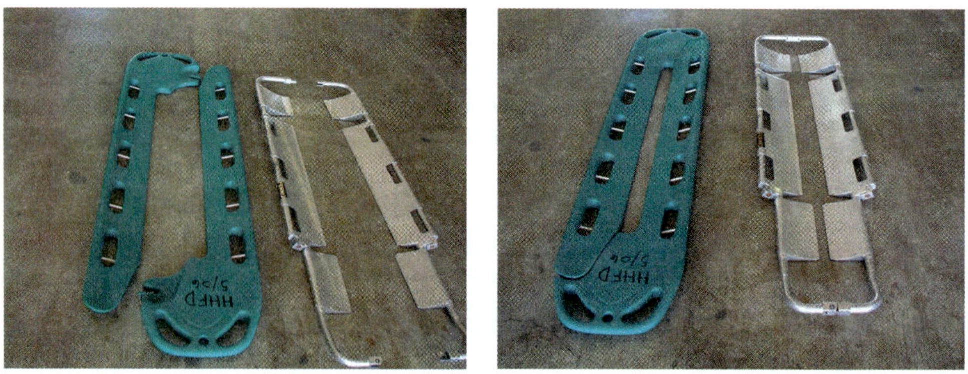

a. b.

FIGURE 2-6 Scoop stretchers may be used to transfer backboard patients who should not be logrolled. The newer, more rigid scoop stretchers (as shown) can replace standard backboards. *(Photos courtesy of Leon Charpentier, EMT-P)*

Table 2-3 SAMPLE History

S	—Symptoms
A	—Allergies
M	—Medications
P	—Past medical history (Other illnesses?)
L	—Last oral intake (When was the last time there was any solid or liquid intake?)
E	—Events preceding the incident (Why did it happen?)

the rate at which you provide ventilation, your aggressiveness in treating shock, and very possibly the destination of the patient. This exam should include the pupils, Glasgow Coma Scale (GCS) score, and signs of cerebral herniation (see Chapter 10). Also look for medical identification devices. Head injury, shock, and hypoxia are not the only things that cause altered mental status; also think about nontraumatic causes such as hypoglycemia and drug or alcohol overdose. All patients with altered mental status should have a finger-stick glucose performed as soon as they are placed in the ambulance.

SAMPLE History

At the same time as you are performing the patient assessment part of the ITLS Primary Survey (initial assessment and rapid trauma survey or focused exam), you or one of the other rescuers should obtain a SAMPLE history (Table 2-3). This is especially important if you must gather information from bystanders because they will not be going with you when you transport the patient.

Remember, prehospital providers are the only ones who get to see the scene and also may be the only ones who get to take a history because many patients who are initially alert lose consciousness before arriving at the hospital. You are not only making interventions to deliver a living patient to the hospital, but you also must be the detective who figures out what happened and why. Pay special attention to the patient's complaints (symptoms) and events prior to the incident (the *S* and *E* of the SAMPLE history). A more detailed history may be taken later during the ITLS Secondary Survey. The patient's symptoms can suggest other injuries, and this will affect further examination. It is important to know as much about the mechanism as possible. (Was she restrained? How far did she fall? What caused her to fall?) Look for clues to serious injury such as history of loss of consciousness, shortness of breath, or pain in the neck, back, chest, abdomen, or pelvis.

Critical Interventions and Transport Decision

When you have completed the initial assessment and rapid trauma survey or focused exam, enough information is available to decide if a critical situation is present. Patients with critical trauma situations are transported immediately. Most treatment interventions will be done during transport.

If your patient has any of the following critical injuries or conditions, transport immediately.

- *Initial assessment reveals*
  - Altered mental status
  - Abnormal breathing
  - Abnormal circulation (shock or uncontrolled bleeding)

PEARLS: On Scene Time

Survival of many trauma patients is time-dependent. Critical trauma patients often need definitive care in the operating room. Delegate interventions that *must* be done on scene. If possible, do interventions during transport.

- *Signs discovered during the rapid trauma survey of conditions that can rapidly lead to shock*
  - Penetrating wounds of the torso
  - Abnormal chest exam (flail chest, open wound, tension pneumothorax, hemothorax)
  - Tender, distended abdomen
  - Pelvic instability
  - Bilateral femur fractures
- *Significant mechanism of injury and/or poor general health of patient.* Even though the patient appears to be stable, if there is a dangerous mechanism or other dangers (such as age, poor general health, death of another passenger in the same auto), consider early transport. "Stable" patients can become unstable quite rapidly.

If the patient has one of the critical conditions listed, after the rapid trauma survey or focused exam, immediately load her into an ambulance, and transport rapidly to the nearest appropriate emergency facility. When in doubt, transport early.

The following procedures are done at the scene, and most of them can be delegated to team members to perform while you continue the ITLS Primary Survey.

Procedures that are not lifesaving, such as splinting, bandaging, insertion of IV lines, or even elective endotracheal intubation, must not hold up transport of the critical patient. At this point, the ITLS Primary Survey is over, and the team leader may help the other rescuers with patient care.

Contacting Medical Direction

Resource Central

See Communications with the Receiving Hospital.

When you have a critical patient, it is extremely important to contact medical direction as early as possible. It takes time to get the appropriate surgeon and the operating room team in place, and the critical patient may have no time to wait. Always notify the receiving facility of your estimated time of arrival (ETA), the condition of the patient, and any special needs on arrival.

ITLS Ongoing Exam

Ongoing assessment and management includes the critical procedures performed on scene and during transport and communication with medical direction. The ITLS Ongoing Exam is an abbreviated exam to assess for changes in the patient's condition. In contrast to the ITLS Secondary Survey, which is performed only once, the Ongoing Exam may be performed multiple times during a long transport. In critical cases with short transport times, there may not be time to perform a Secondary Survey; the Ongoing Exam may take its place. It should be performed and recorded no less than every five minutes for critical patients and every 15 minutes for stable patients. The Ongoing Exam also should be performed as follows:

- Each time the patient is moved
- Each time an intervention is performed
- Any time the patient's condition worsens

This exam is meant to find any changes in the patient's condition, so concentrate on reassessing only those things that may change. For example, if you have applied a traction splint, reassess the limb for decreased pain and for the presence of distal pulses, motor function, and sensation (PMS). On the other hand, if you decompress a chest, you must reassess almost everything in the initial assessment and rapid trauma survey down through the abdominal exam.

Having moved the patient to the ambulance and completed the ITLS Primary Survey and vital signs (including a brief neurological exam if the patient is not alert), transport the patient and begin the ITLS Ongoing Exam, completing exposure of the patient if he is unstable. In the critical, multitrauma patient, the first Ongoing Exam may essentially be a repeat of the Primary Survey, including the initial assessment and rapid trauma survey.

PROCEDURE

Performing an Ongoing Exam

The ITLS Ongoing Exam should be performed in the following order:

1. Ask the patient if there have been any changes in how he feels. Complete the SAMPLE history if not already done.
2. Reassess mental status (LOC and pupils). If the patient has an altered mental status, check a finger-stick glucose and recheck the GCS.
3. Reassess the ABCs.
   a. Reassess the airway.
      (1) Recheck patency.
      (2) If this is a burn patient, assess for signs of inhalation injury.
   b. Reassess breathing and circulation.
      (1) Recheck vital signs.
      (2) Note skin color, condition, and temperature.
      (3) Check the neck for jugular venous distention (JVD) and tracheal deviation. (If a cervical collar has been applied, remove the front to examine the neck.)
      (4) Recheck the chest. Notice the quality of breath sounds. If breath sounds are unequal, evaluate for splinting, pneumothorax, and hemothorax. Listen to the heart to see if the sounds have become muffled.
4. Reassess the abdomen, if mechanism suggests possible injury. Note the development of tenderness, rigidity, or distention.
5. Check each of the identified injuries (lacerations for bleeding, PMS distal to all injured extremities, flails, pneumothorax, open chest wounds, and so on).
6. Check interventions.
   a. Check ET tube for patency and position.
   b. Check oxygen for flow rate.
   c. Check IVs for patency and rate of fluid.
   d. Check seals on sucking chest wounds.
   e. Check patency of tension pneumothorax decompression needle.
   f. Check splints and dressings.
   g. Check impaled objects to be sure they are well stabilized.
   h. Check body position of pregnant patients.
   i. Check cardiac monitor, capnograph, and pulse oximeter.

Accurately record what you see and what you do. Record changes in the patient's condition during transport. Record the time that you perform each intervention. Extenuating circumstances or significant details should be recorded in the comments or remarks section of the written report.

Resource Central

Review the information in Documentation: The Patient Care Record.

Resource Central

See Trauma Scoring in the Prehospital Care Setting for more information on the use of the Glasgow Coma Scale.

DCAP-BLS short for deformities, contusions, abrasions, penetrations, burns, lacerations, and swelling.

TIC short for tenderness, instability, and crepitus.

ITLS Secondary Survey

The ITLS Secondary Survey is a more comprehensive exam meant to pick up additional injuries that might have been missed in the brief ITLS Primary Survey. This assessment also establishes the baseline from which treatment decisions will eventually be made. It is important to record the information discovered in this assessment. Whether or not to perform a Secondary Survey as well as when to perform one depends on the situation:

- Critical patients should have this assessment done during transport rather than on scene.
- If there is a short transport and you must perform interventions, you may not have time to do the Secondary Survey.
- If the ITLS Primary Survey does not reveal a critical condition, the ITLS Secondary Survey may be performed on scene. Stable patients with no dangerous mechanism of injury (e.g., dropped rock on toe) do not require a Secondary Survey.

When you perform the Secondary Survey, you should always begin by quickly repeating the initial assessment. You can do this as your team member is checking the vital signs.

You should have obtained the SAMPLE history during the ITLS Primary Survey and Ongoing Exam, but now you can obtain further information if needed. Perform your Secondary Survey while you are obtaining the rest of the history (if the patient is conscious).

PROCEDURE

Performing a Secondary Survey

The exam should contain the following elements (Figure 2-7).

1. Repeat the initial assessment.
2. Consider using monitors (cardiac, pulse oximeter, CO_2). These are usually applied during transport.
3. Record vital signs again. Record pulse rate, respiratory rate, and blood pressure. Remember, the pulse pressure is as important as the systolic pressure. Many people now consider the pulse oximetry and capnography readings as part of the vital signs. These are useful tools, but you must know their limitations. (See Chapters 4 and 5.)
4. Do a brief neurological exam. It gives important baseline information that is used in later treatment decisions. This exam should include the following:
   a. *Level of consciousness:* If the patient is conscious, describe her orientation, emotional status, and whether she follows commands. If she has an altered mental status, record her level of coma (for Glasgow Coma Scale score, see Table 2-4). If there is altered mental status, check finger-stick blood glucose (if not already done) and check the oxygen saturation level. If there is any chance of narcotic overdose, give 2 mg of Naloxone IV. For elderly or other special-needs patients, try to determine from a caretaker if the patient is at the usual baseline level of alertness and responsiveness.
   b. *Pupils:* Note the size of the pupils and whether they are equal or unequal. Do they respond to light?
   c. *Motor:* Can the patient move fingers and toes?

ITLS ONGOING EXAM

PATIENT HISTORY
Complete S.A.M.P.L.E. History if not already done

LOC
A-V/P-U
Pupils

If altered mental status:
Finger-stick Glucose
GLASCOW COMA SCALE
Eyes, Voice, Movement

VITAL SIGNS
Measured Pulse, Respiratory Rate, Blood Pressure
Pulse Oximeter, Cardiac Monitor, CO_2 Monitor, Temperature

AIRWAY
Patency? If burn patient assess for signs of inhalation injury

BREATHING
Present? Rate, Depth, Effort

CIRCULATION
Skin Color, Temperature, Moisture; Capillary Refill

BLEEDING STILL CONTROLLED?

Examine Neck
Obvious Wounds, Tenderness, Swelling
Neck Vein Distention? Tracheal Deviation?

Examine CHEST
Asymmetry (Paradoxical Motion?), Contusions, Penetrations, Tenderness, Instability, Crepitation

BREATH SOUNDS
Present? Equal? (If unequal: **Percussion)**
Heart Tones

Examine ABDOMEN
Contusions, Penetration/evisceration; Tenderness, Rigidity, Distention

Recheck Identified INJURIES

Check INTERVENTIONS
ET tube, Oxygen, IVs, seals on chest wounds, decompression needle, splints & dressings, impaled objects, position of pregnant patients

Recheck MONITORS
Cardiac, Capnograph, Pulse Oximeter

FIGURE 2-7 ITLS Ongoing Exam.

d. *Sensation:* Can she feel you when you touch her fingers and toes? Does the unconscious patient respond when you pinch her fingers and toes?

5. Perform a detailed (head-to-toe) exam. Pay particular attention to the patient's complaints and also recheck the injuries that you found previously. The exam should consist of inspection, auscultation, palpation, and sometimes percussion.
   a. Begin at the head examining for deformities, contusions, abrasions, penetrations, burns, lacerations, and swelling (**DCAP-BLS**), and palpating for tenderness, instability, and crepitus (**TIC**). Also

Table 2-4 Glasgow Coma Scale

Eye Opening	Points	Verbal Response	Points	Motor Response	Points
Spontaneous	4	Oriented	5	Obeys commands	6
To voice	3	Confused	4	Localizes pain	5
To pain	2	Inappropriate words	3	Withdraws	4
None	1	Incomprehensible sounds	2	Abnormal flexion	3*
		Silent	1	Abnormal extension	2**
				No movement	1

* Decorticate posturing to pain
** Decerebrate posturing to pain

check for raccoon eyes, Battle's sign, and drainage of blood or fluid from the ears or nose. Assess the mouth. Assess the airway again.

b. Check the neck for DCAP-BLS, TIC, distended neck veins, and deviated trachea.
c. Check the chest for DCAP-BLS, TIC. Also check for paradoxical movement of the chest wall. Be sure that breath sounds are present and equal on each side (check all four fields). Note rales, wheezing, or "noisy" breath sounds. Notice if heart sounds are as loud as before. (A noticeable decrease in heart sounds may be an early sign of cardiac tamponade.) Recheck seals over open wounds. Be sure flails are well stabilized. If you detect decreased breath sounds, percuss to determine whether the patient has a pneumothorax or hemothorax.
d. Perform an abdominal exam. Look for signs of blunt or penetrating trauma. Feel all four quadrants for tenderness or rigidity. Do not waste time listening for bowel sounds; it gives you no useful information. If the abdomen is painful to gentle pressure during examination, you can expect the patient to be bleeding internally. If the abdomen is both distended and painful, you can expect hemorrhagic shock to occur very quickly.
e. Assess pelvis and extremities (unstable pelvis noted in Rapid Trauma Survey is not rechecked). Examine for DCAP-BLS and feel for TIC. Be sure to check and record pulse, motor function, and sensation (PMS) on all fractures. Do this before and after straightening any fracture. Angulated fractures of the upper extremities are usually best splinted as found. Most fractures of the lower extremities are gently straightened and then stabilized using traction splints or air splints. Critical patients have all splints applied during transport.

Transport immediately if the ITLS Secondary Survey reveals the development of any of the critical trauma situations. After you finish the Secondary Survey, you should finish bandaging and splinting.

Adjuncts for Trauma Patient Assessment

One of the decisions to be made when assessing a trauma patient is determining the level of trauma center to which to take the patient. Patients with unstable vital signs and those with serious anatomical injuries are usually taken to trauma centers, but the decision can be more difficult for patients with normal vital signs and normal a level of consciousness who also have a significant mechanism of injury.

Ideally you should take the most severely injured patients to the appropriate trauma centers as quickly as possible because it has been shown to have the best patient outcomes. However, avoid taking every injured patient to a trauma center, overloading this resource with patients who do not have critical injuries.

ITLS SECONDARY SURVEY

INITIAL ASSESSMENT

GENERAL IMPRESSION
Does the patient appear better, worse, or unchanged?

LOC
A-V/P-U

AIRWAY
(WITH C-SPINE CONTROL)
Snoring, Gurgling, Stridor, etc; Silence

BREATHING
Present? Rate, Depth, Effort

RADIAL PULSE – CAROTID if no radial
Present? Rate, Rhythm, Quality
Skin Color, Temperature, Moisture; Capillary Refill

BLEEDING STILL CONTROLLED?

DETAILED EXAM

PATIENT HISTORY
Complete S.A.M.P.L.E. History if not already done

VITAL SIGNS
Measured Pulse, Respiratory Rate, Blood Pressure
Consider Pulse Oximeter, Cardiac Monitor, CO_2 Monitor, Blood Sugar, Temperature, prn

GLASCOW COMA SCALE
(Eyes, Voice, Movement); Emotional State

Examine Head
DCAP-BLS, TIC
(Pupils, Battles Sign, Raccoon Eyes, Drainage from ears or nose

Examine Neck
DCAP-BLS, TIC Neck Vein Distention? Tracheal Deviation?

Examine CHEST
Asymmetry, Paradoxical motion, DCAP-BLS, TIC

BREATH SOUNDS
Present? Equal? (If unequal: **Percussion**) Abnormal Breath Sounds?
Heart Tones

Examine ABDOMEN
Contusions, Penetration/evisceration; Tenderness, Rigidity, Distention

Examine PELVIS
DCAP-BLS, TIC

Examine LOWER/UPPER EXTREMITIES
DCAP-BLS, TIC, Distal PMS

POSTERIOR
Examine only if not done in Primary Survey
DCAP-BLS, TIC

FIGURE 2-8 ITLS Secondary Survey.

Better tools are needed to distinguish between patients who have injuries that are either not severe or not time critical and will remain stable, and those who appear stable initially and then decompensate later, requiring emergent transfer to a trauma center. There are at least two adjuncts for trauma triage that may prove to be helpful in that situation by distinguishing between the two patient groups: serum lactate and ultrasound.

Serum lactate is a marker for tissue hypoxia and has been used in the hospital setting to monitor critical patients. In the field it appears to be useful to predict which patients with normal vital signs are having occult internal bleeding and will soon develop hemorrhagic shock. Multiple services have been using prehospital finger-stick serum lactate levels to predict who will develop shock. If further studies confirm its predictive value, it will be very useful.

Portable ultrasound can be used to assess for intraabdominal hemorrhage and cardiac tamponade among other things. Abdominal trauma sonography is very commonly used in the initial assessment of trauma patients in the emergency department and is called the *FAST exam* (focused assessment with sonography in trauma). It is noninvasive and only takes from one to three minutes to perform. In many emergency departments FAST has replaced the diagnostic peritoneal lavage in the initial assessment for blood in the abdomen after blunt trauma. Because it is portable and not difficult to learn to use for simple exams like the FAST exam, it is being used in the field by some ground and air services (especially in Europe), and the information obtained is being used to determine which patients are transported directly to a trauma center and which are transported to a community hospital instead. Initial studies are reporting that it has a very high (90% and higher) predictive value for intra-abdominal bleeding. Studies of its use in moving ambulances and helicopters have been mixed, and as with most procedures, success depends on the skill and training of the operator.

Hopefully, those and other assessment adjuncts will prove to give emergency responders more options to improve patient care and health-care resource utilization.

CASE PRESENTATION (continued)

An ALS ambulance has been dispatched to the scene of a domestic dispute. En route, the team is told that a man has been stabbed with a kitchen knife. Upon arrival they see that the scene is safe and the police have the uninjured wife in custody. The scene commander shows the team a 10-inch kitchen knife with blood on the blade. She says the patient may be found at the foot of the seven-step flight of stairs leading out from the kitchen.

The team grabs their essential equipment and heads for the patient. As they approach, they see an adult male who appears to be about 30 years old, lying at the foot of the steps. He is wearing only a pair of briefs and is lying on his left side in a pool of blood. He is awake, ashen, and sweaty. The team leader instructs team member 3 to attend to the bleeding from a large laceration just under the patient's right buttock. The leader introduces himself and tells the patient he is going to have team member 2 control movement of his head and neck to prevent possible injury. He notes that the patient is alert and his airway is open and clear.

They gently logroll the patient onto the backboard. The leader assesses the patient's breathing, finding it rapid, unlabored, with adequate tidal volume, but notes that he has a rapid carotid but no radial pulses. Maintaining neck stability with her knees, team member 2 begins to administer oxygen via nonrebreather mask. The leader quickly checks the bleeding and sees that team member 3 has controlled the bleeding with direct pressure and is now applying a pressure dressing.

Asked what happened, the patient states that his wife found a note in his pants when he was taking a shower. She accused him of having an affair with another woman and came after him with the knife. She caught him and cut the back of his upper leg as he was trying to run out the door. He then stumbled out the door and fell down the stairs. He denies loss of consciousness and states he does not think he was hurt by the fall down the stairs.

The team leader, having determined the patient to be a "load-and-go," quickly begins a rapid trauma survey. (If the patient has not fallen down the stairs, the team would have had to do only a focused exam.) The leader checks for neck tenderness and venous distention, then examines and palpates the chest, finding no asymmetrical movement, bruises, or penetrations. He auscultates breath sounds, finding them present and bilaterally equal. He notes no marks on the abdomen and after palpating, finds no tenderness, rigidity, or distention. He then briefly palpates the pelvic girdle, finding no tenderness, instability, or crepitation, and notes that the pressure dressing is controlling the bleeding. He briefly palpates the extremities for deformity or swelling. While team members 2 and 3 secure the patient to the spine board, the leader asks about allergies (none), medications (none), and when was last oral intake (four hours previously). Spinal motion restriction would not have been indicated if the patient had not had the fall and distracting injury.

The team quickly transfers the patient to the ambulance. The leader instructs team member 3 to transport the patient to the trauma center. While the leader begins the ITLS Ongoing Exam, team member 2 obtains a set of vital signs (pulse, 132; respiration 30; blood pressure 76/48) and a finger-stick blood sugar (168). Explaining to the still alert patient what they are doing, they establish two large-bore IVs running wide open in an attempt to improve signs of decreased peripheral circulation and bring the systolic blood pressure up to 80–90 mm Hg. While team member 2 attaches a cardiac monitor and a pulse oximeter, the leader checks the wound again to confirm that bleeding is still controlled, and then calls the emergency department at the trauma center to advise them of their ETA and the status of the patient.

If there is time during transport, the leader will conduct a thorough ITLS Secondary Survey in search on any additional injuries. ■

Summary

Patient assessment is key to trauma care. The interventions required are not difficult, but their timing often is critical. If you know what questions to ask and how to perform the exam, you will know when to perform the lifesaving interventions without unnecessarily prolonging time on scene. This chapter has described a rapid, orderly, and thorough examination of the trauma patient with examination and treatment priorities always in mind. The continuous practice of approaching the patient in the way described will allow you to concentrate on the patient, rather than on what to do next. Optimum speed is achieved by teamwork. Teamwork is achieved by practice. You should plan regular exercises in patient evaluation to perfect each team member's role. Current research may provide future assessment adjuncts to help us make better decisions about the level of care our patients may need.

Bibliography

1. Alam, H. B., et al. 2005. Hemorrhage control in the battlefield: Role of new hemostatic agents. *Military Medicine* 170: 63–69.
2. Brooke, M., et al. 2010. Paramedic application of ultrasound in the management of patients in the prehospital setting: a review of the literature. *Emergency Medicine Journal* 27(9): 702–707.
3. Jansen, T. C., J. van Bommel, et al. 2008. The prognostic value of blood lactate levels relative to that of vital signs in the pre-hospital setting: a pilot study. *Critical Care* 12(6):160–166.
4. Korner, M., M. Krotz, et al. 2008 Current role of emergency ultrasound in patients with major trauma. *Radiographics* 28(1): 225–242
5. Krell, J. M., et al. 2006. Comparison of the Ferno scoop stretcher with the long backboard for spinal immobilization. *Prehospital Emergency Care* 10: 46–51.
6. MacKenzie, E. J., F. Rivara, et al. 2006. A national evaluation of the effect of trauma center care on mortality. *New England Journal of Medicine* 354(4): 366–378.
7. van Beest, P. A., J. Mulder, et al. 2009. Measurement of lactate in a prehospital setting is related to outcome. *European Journal of Emergency Medicine* 16(6): 318–322.

Explore Resource Central

For additional review and practice tests, visit www.bradybooks.com and click on Resource Central to access book-specific resources for this text. To access Resource Central, follow directions on the Student Access Card provided with this text. If there is no card, go to www.bradybooks.com and follow the Resource Central link to Buy Access from there.

Assessment Skills

Donna Hastings, EMT-P
Eduardo Romero Hicks, MD

Patient Assessment

Valutazione del paziente

Evaluación del Paciente

D'évaluation des Patients

Ocena stanu chorego

Patientenbeurteilung

Pregled ozljeđenika

تقييم حالة المصاب

procena pacijenta

Ocena stanja pacienta

Sérültvizsgálat

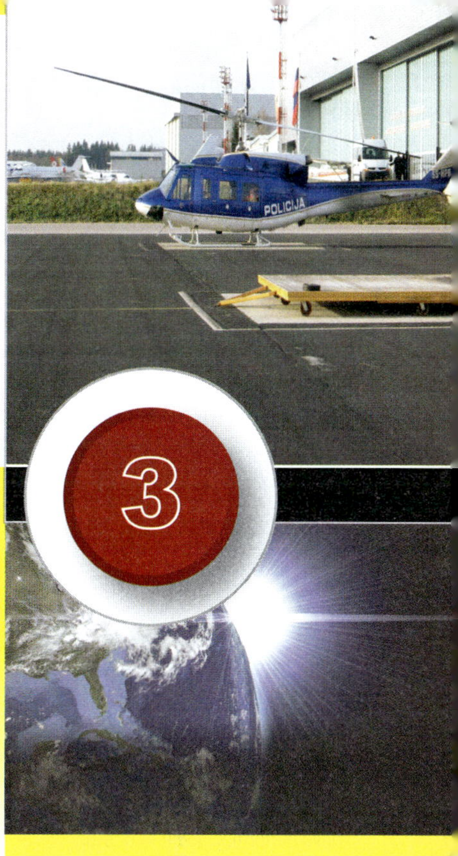

(Photo courtesy of International Trauma Life Support)

OBJECTIVES

Upon successful completion of this chapter, you should be able to:

ITLS Primary Survey

1. Correctly perform the ITLS Primary Survey.
2. Identify within two minutes which patients require load and go.
3. Describe when to perform critical interventions.

ITLS Ongoing Exam and ITLS Secondary Survey

4. Correctly perform the ITLS Ongoing (reassessment) Exam.
5. Correctly perform the ITLS Secondary Survey.
6. Describe when to perform critical interventions.
7. Demonstrate proper communications with medical direction.

Assessment and Management of the Trauma Patient

8. Demonstrate the proper sequence of rapid assessment and the management of the multiple-trauma patient.

PROCEDURE

ITLS Primary Survey

Short written scenarios will be used along with a model (to act as the patient). You will divide into teams to practice performing the initial assessment, critical interventions, and transport decision. Each member of the team must practice being team leader at least once. The critical information represents the answers you should be seeking at each step of the survey. The Treatment Decision Tree at the end of the chapter represents the actions that should be taken (personally or delegated) in response to your assessment.

PEARLS: ITLS Primary Survey

- Do not approach the patient until you have performed a scene size-up.
- Do not interrupt the ITLS Primary Survey except for airway obstruction, cardiac arrest, or if the scene becomes too dangerous. Team members may perform other critical interventions while you complete the survey.
- Give any ventilation instructions as soon as you assess airway and breathing.
- Prophylactic hyperventilation is not recommended for patients with decreased LOC. Use it only for head-injury patients who show signs of the cerebral herniation syndrome.
- Assist ventilations in anyone who is hypoventilating (less than eight breaths per minute or $ETCO_2$ of greater than 45).
- Give oxygen to all multiple-trauma patients. If in doubt, give oxygen.
- Endotracheal tubes are the best method to protect the airway and ventilate the adult patient.
- Transfer the patient to the backboard as soon as the ITLS Primary Survey is completed.
- When the ITLS Primary Survey is completed, decide if the patient is critical or stable.
- Call medical direction early if you have a critical patient. (Other physicians may have to be called from home to treat the patient.)
- If the patient has a critical trauma situation, load him into the ambulance and transport. (Transport pregnant patients with the backboard tilted slightly to the left. Do not let them roll over onto the floor.)

(continued on page 52)

ITLS Primary Survey—Critical Information

If you ask the right questions, you will get the information you need to make the critical decisions necessary in the management of your patient. The following questions are presented in the order in which you should ask yourself as you perform the Primary Survey. *This is the* minimum *information that you will need as you perform each step of the ITLS Primary Survey* (Figure 3-1).

Scene Size-up

- Have I taken standard precautions?
- Do I see, hear, smell, or sense anything dangerous?
- Are there any other patients?
- Are additional personnel or resources needed?
- Do we need special equipment?
- What is the mechanism of injury here?
- Is it generalized or focused?
- Is it potentially life threatening?

Initial Assessment

General Impression

- What is my general impression of the patient as I approach?
- Is there life-threatening bleeding that must be addressed now?

Level of Consciousness (AVPU)

- Introduce yourself and say: "We are here to help you. Can you tell us what happened?"
- From the patient's response, what is the AVPU (alert, voice, pain, unresponsive) rating?

Airway

- Is the airway open and clear?
- Is the sound of breathing abnormal (snoring, gurgling, stridor)?

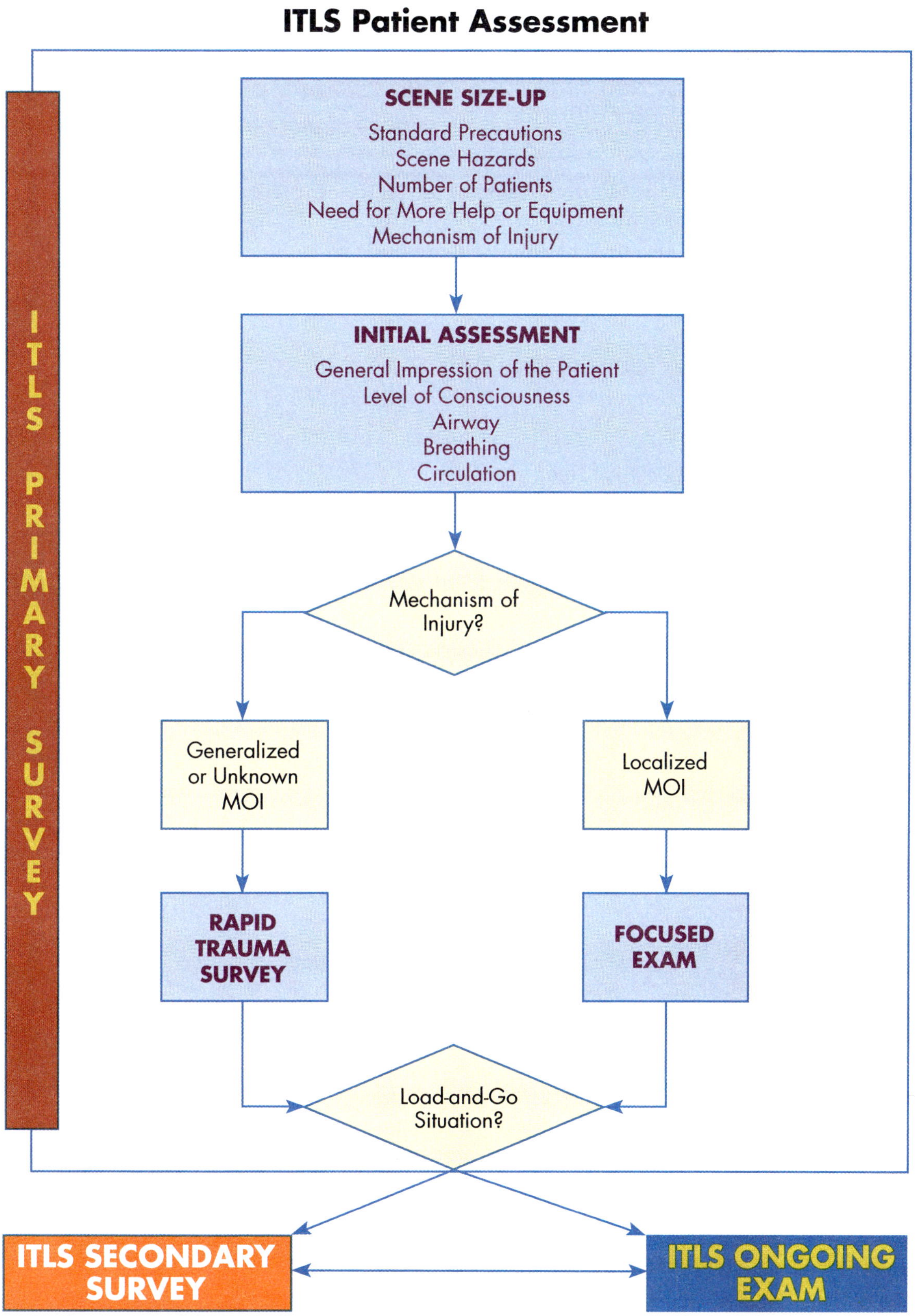

FIGURE 3-1 Steps in the assessment of the trauma patient.

PEARLS: ITLS Primary Survey (*Continued*)

- If absolutely necessary, certain critical interventions may have to be done before transport. Remember that you are trading minutes of the patient's Golden Period for those procedures. Use good judgment.
- The indications to decompress a tension pneumothorax include signs of a tension pneumothorax and more than one of the following: respiratory distress and cyanosis, loss of radial pulse (obvious shock), loss of consciousness or an obviously decreasing level of consciousness.
- Start IVs in the ambulance en route unless the patient is entrapped or the ambulance has not arrived on scene.

Breathing

- Is the patient breathing?
- What is the rate and depth of respiration?
- Is breathing labored?

Circulation

- What is the rate and quality of the pulse at the wrist (and at the neck, if not palpable at the wrist)?
- Is major external bleeding still present?
- What are the skin color, condition, and temperature?

Decision

- Is this a critical situation (Table 3-1)?
- Are there interventions that I must delegate now?

Table 3-1 Trauma Assessment–Treatment Decision Tree

Assessment	Action
SCENE SIZE-UP	
Safety	Put on gloves, protective clothing. Remove hazards or patient from hazards.
Number of patients	Call for help if needed.
Extrication needed	Call for special equipment if needed.
Mechanisms of injury	Suspect appropriate injuries (e.g., cervical spine).
GENERAL IMPRESSION	Begin to establish priorities.
Age, sex, weight	
Position (in surroundings, body position/posture)	
Activity	
Obvious major injuries	
Major bleeding	Direct pressure, tourniquet, hemostatic agent, as needed
LEVEL OF CONSCIOUSNESS	
Alert/responsive to voice	Maintain cervical-spine motion restriction.
Unresponsive to voice	Modified jaw thrust prn.
AIRWAY	
Snoring	Modified jaw thrust.
Gurgling	Suction.
Stridor	Intubate, confirm tube placement with waveform capnography if available.
Silence	Attempt to ventilate. If unsuccessful:
	– Reposition; rapid extrication if still in a vehicle.
	– Visualize.
	– Suction.
	– Consider Heimlich maneuver.
	– Intubate confirm tube placement with waveform capnography if available.
	– Consider translaryngeal jet ventilation or needle crycothyroidotomy.

(*Continued*)

Table 3-1 *(Continued)*

Assessment	Action
BREATHING	
Absent	Ventilate twice (check pulse before continuing ventilation at 8–10 + oxygen).
< 8	Assist ventilation at 8–10 + oxygen.
Low tidal volume	Assist ventilation.
Labored	Oxygen by nonrebreather at 15 liters/minute
Normal or rapid	Consider oxygen.
CIRCULATION	
RADIAL PULSE	
Absent	Check carotid pulse (see below). Note late shock.
Present	Note rate and quality.
Bradycardia	Consider spinal shock, head injury.
Tachycardia	Consider hypovolemic shock. Consider need for pain management. Consider cardiac monitor.
CAROTID PULSE	Done if no radial pulse.
Absent	CPR + bag-mask + oxygen, load and go. Quick look and defibrillate if ventricular fibrillation. If PEA, consider needle decompression bilaterally. If asystole, consider termination of resuscitation.
Present	Note rate and quality.
Bradycardia	Consider spinal shock, head injury.
Tachycardia	Consider late shock.
SKIN	COLOR AND CONDITION
Pale, cool, clammy	Consider hypovolemic shock.
Cyanosis	Reconsider intubation/ventilation; check oxygen.
MAJOR BLEEDING	Consider intubation. Direct pressure, pressure dressing. Consider tourniquet and/or hemostatic agent.
HEAD	
Major facial injuries	Consider intubation.
NECK	
Swelling, bruising, retracting	Consider intubation.
Neck vein distention	Consider tamponade, tension pneumothorax.
Tracheal deviation	Consider tension pneumothorax.
Tenderness, deformity, or generalized mechanism of injury	APPLY CERVICAL COLLAR NOW.
CHEST	Inspect and palpate.
Symmetrical, stable	Continue exam.
Bruises, crepitation	Consider early cardiac monitoring.
Penetrating wounds	Occlusive dressing.
Paradoxical motion	Stabilize flail; consider early intubation.
BREATH SOUNDS	
Present and equal	Continue exam.

(Continued)

Table 3-1 Trauma Assessment–Treatment Decision Tree (*Continued*)

Assessment	Action
Unequal	Percuss chest to determine pneumothorax versus hemothorax.
With decreased LOC, absent radial pulses, cyanosis, JVD, possible tracheal deviation.	Consider needle decompression.
HEART TONES	Note for comparison later.
Muffled with JVD and bilateral breath sounds	Consider pericardial tamponade.
ABDOMEN, PELVIS, UPPER LEGS	
If tender abdomen, unstable pelvis, or bilateral femur fractures	Expect development of shock.
MOVEMENT/SENSATION IN EXTREMITIES	
Present	Record.
Decreased or absent.	Suspect spinal injury.
POSTERIOR	
Injuries identified.	Appropriate management of identified injuries. Transfer to backboard. TRANSPORT IMMEDIATELY IF CRITICAL TRAUMA SITUATION PRESENT.
SAMPLE HISTORY	Record.
VITAL SIGNS	Measure and record pulse, respirations. Auscultate and record blood pressure.
Systolic < 90 with signs of shock	Consider IV fluid therapy en route.
Systolic < 80	IV fluid therapy en route.
Systolic < 60	IV fluid therapy en route.
Pulse pressure > 60 with decreased LOC	Consider increased intracerebral pressure. Maintain systolic blood pressure of 110–120.
PUPILS	
Unequal	Suspect head injury unless patient is alert, then suspect eye injury. Give 100% oxygen.
Unequal or dilated and fixed with GCS ≤ 8	Give 100% oxygen; do not let patient get hypotensive. (Target systolic BP of 110–120.) Intubation and hyperventilation (20 breaths per minute or at rate to maintain $ETCO_2$ of about 30). (Unequal pupils or dilated and fixed pupils and GSC 8 or less are suggestive of cerebral herniation.)
Pinpoint (with respiratory rate < 8)	Consider naloxone.
Dilated/reactive (with GCS ≤ 8)	Give 100% oxygen; consider intubation. Ventilate at 6–8 breaths per minute or to maintain $ETCO_2$ of 35–45.
GLASGOW COMA SCALE score (for decreased LOC)	
≤ 8	Give 100% oxygen. Do not let patient get hypotensive (target systolic BP of 110–120). Intubation en route is indicated. Consider hyperventilation only if patient shows signs of cerebral herniation: – GCS ≤ 8 with extensor posturing – GCS ≤ 8 with pupillary asymmetry or nonreactivity – GCS ≤ 8 with a subsequent drop of more than 2 points
ALL PATIENTS WITH DECREASED LOC	Check for medical identification devices. Do blood-glucose check.

Rapid Trauma Survey

(See Figure 3-2.)

Head and Neck

- Are there obvious wounds of the head or neck?
- Is there deformity or tenderness of the neck?
- Are the neck veins distended?
- Does the trachea look and feel midline or deviated?

Chest

- Is the chest symmetrical? Is there paradoxical movement? Is there any obvious blunt or penetrating trauma?
- Are there any sucking (open) wounds?
- Is there TIC of the ribs?
- Are the breath sounds present and equal?
- If breath sounds are not equal, is the chest hyperresonant (pneumothorax) or dull (hemothorax)?
- Are heart sounds normal or decreased?

Abdomen

- Are there obvious wounds?
- Is the abdomen tender, rigid, or distended?

Pelvis

- Are there obvious wounds or deformity?
- Is there tenderness, instability, or crepitation?

Upper Legs

- Are there obvious wounds, swelling, or deformity?
- Is there tenderness, instability, or crepitation?

Lower Legs and Arms

- Are there obvious wounds, swelling, or deformity?
- Is there tenderness, instability, or crepitation?
- Can the patient feel/move fingers and toes?

Posterior

This exam is performed during transfer to the backboard.

- Are there any wounds, tenderness, or deformity of the patient's posterior side?

Decision

- Is there a critical situation?
- Should I move the patient to the ambulance now?
- Are there interventions that I must delegate or perform now?

History

- What is the SAMPLE history (if not already obtained)

FIGURE 3-2 The ITLS Primary Survey including the rapid trauma survey.

ITLS PRIMARY SURVEY

SCENE SIZE-UP

Standard Precautions Hazards, Number of Patients, Need for additional resources, **Mechanism of Injury**

INITIAL ASSESSMENT

GENERAL IMPRESSION
Age, Sex, Weight, General Appearance, Position, Purposeful Movement, Obvious Injuries, Skin Color
Life-threatening Bleeding

LOC
A-V-P-U
Chief Complaint/Symptoms

AIRWAY
(WITH C-SPINE CONTROL)
Snoring, Gurgling, Stridor; Silence

BREATHING
Present? Rate, Depth, Effort

CIRCULATION
Radial/Carotid Present? Rate, Rhythm, Quality
Skin Color, Temperature, Moisture; Capillary Refill
Has bleeding been controlled?

RAPID TRAUMA SURVEY

HEAD and NECK
Wounds?
Neck Vein distention? Tracheal Deviation?

CHEST
Asymmetry (Paradoxical Motion?), Contusions, Penetrations, Tenderness, Instability, Crepitation
Breath Sounds
Present? Equal? (If unequal: percussion)
Heart Tones

ABDOMEN
Contusions, Penetration/Evisceration; Tenderness, Rigidity, Distention

PELVIS
Tenderness, Instability, Crepitation

LOWER/UPPER EXTREMITIES
Obvious Swelling, Deformity
Motor and Sensory

POSTERIOR
Obvious wounds, Tenderness, Deformity

If radial pulse present:
VITAL SIGNS
Measured Pulse, Breathing, Blood Pressure

If altered mental status: Brief Neurological exam
PUPILS
Size? Reactive? **Equal?**

GLASGOW COMA SCALE
Eyes, Voice, Motor

Baseline Vital Signs

- Are the vital signs abnormal?

Disability

Perform this exam now if there is altered mental status. Otherwise, postpone this exam until you perform the ITLS Secondary Survey.

- Are the pupils equal and reactive?
- What is the Glasgow Coma Scale score?
- Are there signs of cerebral herniation (unconscious, dilated pupil(s), hypertension, bradycardia, posturing)?
- Does the patient have a medical identification device?
- What is the finger-stick glucose?

PROCEDURE

ITLS Ongoing Exam

Short written trauma scenarios will be used along with a model (to act as the patient). You will divide into teams to practice performing the ITLS Ongoing (reassessment) Exam, making critical decisions and interventions. Each member of the team must practice being team leader at least once. The critical information represents the answers you should be seeking at each step of the exam.

ITLS Ongoing Exam—Critical Information

The following questions are presented in the order in which you should ask yourself as you perform the Ongoing Exam. This is the minimum information that you will need as you perform each step of the exam (Figure 3-3).

Subjective Changes

- Are you feeling better or worse now?

Mental Status

- What is the LOC?
- What is pupillary size? Are they equal? Do they react to light?
- If altered mental status, what is the finger-stick glucose (if not already done), and what is the Glasgow Coma Scale score now?

Reassess ABCs

- Record vital signs (pulse, respiratory rate, and blood pressure)
- Airway
    - Is the airway open and clear?
    - Is the sound of breathing abnormal (snoring, gurgling, stridor)?
    - If there are burns of the face, are there signs of inhalation injury?
- Breathing and circulation
    - What is the rate and depth of respiration?
    - What is the rate and quality of the pulse?

PEARLS: ITLS Ongoing Exam

- Repeat the ITLS Ongoing Exam:
    - If the patient's condition changes
    - If you make an intervention
    - If you move the patient (scene to ambulance, ambulance to hospital emergency department)
- Remain calm and think. Your knowledge, training, and concern are the most important tools you carry.

FIGURE 3-3 The ITLS Ongoing Exam.

ITLS ONGOING EXAM

PATIENT HISTORY
Complete S.A.M.P.L.E. History if not already done

LOC
A-V/P-U
Pupils

If altered mental status:
Finger-stick Glucose
GLASCOW COMA SCALE
Eyes, Voice, Movement

VITAL SIGNS
Measured Pulse, Respiratory Rate, Blood Pressure
Pulse Oximeter, Cardiac Monitor, CO_2 Monitor, Temperature

AIRWAY
Patency? If burn patient assess for signs of inhalation injury

BREATHING
Present? Rate, Depth, Effort

CIRCULATION
Skin Color, Temperature, Moisture; Capillary Refill

BLEEDING STILL CONTROLLED?

Examine Neck
Obvious Wounds, Tenderness, Swelling
Neck Vein Distention? Tracheal Deviation?

Examine CHEST
Asymmetry (Paradoxical Motion?), Contusions, Penetrations,
Tenderness, Instability, Crepitation

BREATH SOUNDS
(Present? Equal? (If unequal: **Percussion)**
Heart Tones

Examine ABDOMEN
Contusions, Penetration/evisceration; Tenderness, Rigidity, Distension

Recheck Identified INJURIES

Check INTERVENTIONS
ET tube, Oxygen, IVs, seals on chest wounds, decompression needle,
splints & dressings, impaled objects, position of pregnant patients

Recheck MONITORS
Cardiac, Capnograph, Pulse Oximeter

- What is the blood pressure?
- What are the skin color, condition, and temperature (capillary refill in children)?
- Is any external bleeding controlled?

■ Neck
- Are the neck veins normal, flat, or distended?
- If distended, is the trachea midline or deviated?
- Is there increased swelling of the neck?

- Chest
  - Are the breath sounds present and equal?
  - If breath sounds are unequal, is the chest hyperresonant or dull?
  - Are heart sounds still normal, or have they become muffled?
- Abdomen (if mechanism suggests possible injury)
  - Is there any tenderness?
  - Is the abdomen tender, rigid, or distended?
- Assessment of identified injuries
  - Have there been any changes in the condition of any of the injuries that I have found?
- Check interventions. (Ask the appropriate question for your patient.)
  - Is the endotracheal tube still patent and in the correct position?
  - Is the oxygen rate correct?
  - Is the oxygen tubing connected?
  - Are the IVs running at the correct rate?
  - Does the IV bag contain the correct fluid?
  - Is the open chest wound still sealed?
  - Is the decompression needle still working?
  - Are any of the dressings blood soaked?
  - Are the splints in good position?
  - Is the impaled object still well stabilized?
  - Is the pregnant patient tilted 20 to 30 degrees to the patient's left?
  - Is the cardiac monitor attached and working?
  - Is the pulse oximeter attached and working?
  - If intubated, is the capnograph attached and working?

PROCEDURE

ITLS Secondary Survey

Short written scenarios will be used along with a model (to act as the patient). You will divide into teams to practice performing the ITLS Secondary Survey. Each member of the team must practice being team leader at least once. The critical information represents the answers you should be seeking at each step of the exam.

ITLS Secondary Survey—Critical Information

As a general rule, you should quickly repeat the initial assessment before you begin the ITLS Secondary Survey. You can do this as your teammate checks the vital signs. If you ask the right questions, you will get the information you need to make the critical decisions necessary in the management of your patient. The following questions are presented in the order in which you should ask yourself as you perform the Secondary Survey. This is the minimum information that you will need as you perform each step of the exam (Figure 3-4).

SAMPLE History

Complete the SAMPLE history now if you have not already done so.

- What is the patient's history?

PEARLS: ITLS Secondary Survey

- Critical patients get an ITLS Secondary Survey en route to the hospital if time permits.
- Stable patients may get an ITLS Secondary Survey at the scene (on the backboard).
- Transport immediately if your detailed exam reveals any of the critical trauma situations.
- Critical patients should not have traction splints applied at the scene. They take too long.

ITLS SECONDARY SURVEY

INITIAL ASSESSMENT

GENERAL IMPRESSION
Does the patient appear better, worse, or unchanged?

LOC
A-V/P-U

AIRWAY
(WITH C-SPINE CONTROL)
Snoring, Gurgling, Stridor, etc; Silence

BREATHING
Present? Rate, Depth, Effort

RADIAL PULSE – CAROTID if no radial
Present? Rate, Rhythm, Quality
Skin Color, Temperature, Moisture; Capillary Refill

BLEEDING STILL CONTROLLED?

DETAILED EXAM

PATIENT HISTORY
Complete S.A.M.P.L.E. History if not already done

VITAL SIGNS
Measured Pulse, Respiratory Rate, Blood Pressure
Consider Pulse Oximeter, Cardiac Monitor, CO_2 Monitor, Blood Sugar, Temperature, prn

GLASCOW COMA SCALE
(Eyes, Voice, Movement); Emotional State

Examine Head
DCAP-BLS, TIC
(Pupils, Battles Sign, Raccoon Eyes, Drainage from ears or nose

Examine Neck
DCAP-BLS, TIC Neck Vein Distention? Tracheal Deviation?

Examine CHEST
Asymmetry, Paradoxical motion, DCAP-BLS, TIC

BREATH SOUNDS
Present? Equal? (If unequal: **Percussion**) Abnormal Breath Sounds?
Heart Tones

Examine ABDOMEN
Contusions, Penetration/evisceration; Tenderness, Rigidity, Distension

Examine PELVIS
DCAP-BLS, TIC

Examine LOWER/UPPER EXTREMITIES
DCAP-BLS, TIC, Distal PMS

POSTERIOR
Examine only if not done in Primary Survey
DCAP-BLS, TIC

FIGURE 3-4 The ITLS Secondary Survey.

Vital Signs and Repeat Initial Assessment

- General Impression
  - Does the patient appear better, worse, or unchanged?
- Airway
  - Is the airway open and clear?
  - Is the sound of breathing abnormal (snoring, gurgling, stridor)?
- Breathing
  - What is the rate and depth of respiration?
  - Is the breathing labored?
- Circulation
  - What is the pulse rate and blood pressure?
  - What are the skin color, condition, and temperature (capillary refill in children)?
  - Is all external bleeding still controlled?

Neurological Exam

- What is the LOC?
- If altered mental status, what is the blood glucose (if not already done)?
- Are the pupils equal? Do they respond to light?
- Can the patient move his fingers and toes?
- Can the patient feel me touch his fingers and toes?
- What is the Glasgow Coma Scale score (if altered mental status)?

Detailed Exam

- Head
  - Is there DCAP-BLS or TIC of the face or head?
  - Are Battle's sign or raccoon eyes present?
  - Is there blood or fluid draining from the ears or nose?
  - Is there pallor, cyanosis, or diaphoresis?
- Neck
  - Is there DCAP-BLS or TIC of the neck?
  - Are the neck veins normal, flat, or distended?
  - Is the trachea midline or deviated?
- Chest
  - Is there DCAP-BLS of the chest?
  - Is there any TIC of the ribs?
  - Are there any open wounds or paradoxical movement?
  - Are the breath sounds present and equal?
  - Are there abnormal breath sounds?
  - If breath sounds are not equal, is the chest hyperresonant or dull?
  - Are heart sounds normal or decreased?
  - If patient is intubated, is the endotracheal tube still in good position?
- Abdomen
  - Is there DCAP-BTLS of the abdomen?
  - Is the abdomen tender, rigid, or distended?
- Pelvis

If the pelvis has already been examined during the ITLS Primary Survey, no further exam should be done.

- Lower Extremities
  - Is there DCAP-BLS or TIC of the legs?
  - Is there normal PMS?
  - Is range of motion normal? (optional)
- Upper Extremities
  - Is there DCAP-BTLS of the arms?
  - Is there normal PMS?
  - Is range of motion normal? (optional)

PROCEDURE

Patient Assessment and Management

Short written trauma scenarios will be used along with a model (to act as the patient). You will be divided into teams to practice the management of simulated trauma situations using the principles and techniques taught in the course. You will be evaluated in the same manner on the second day of the course. You will be expected to use all the principles and techniques taught in this course while managing these simulated patients. To familiarize yourself with the evaluation procedure, you will be given a copy of a scenario and a grade sheet. Review Chapter 2 and the previous surveys in this chapter.

Ground Rules for Teaching and Evaluation

1. You will be allowed to stay together in three-member groups (different-sized groups are optional) throughout the practice and evaluation stations.
2. You will have three practice scenarios. This allows each member of the team to be team leader once.
3. You will be evaluated as team leader once.
4. You will assist as a member of the rescue team during two scenarios in which another member of your team is being evaluated as team leader. You may assist, but the team leader must do all assessments. This gives you a total of six scenarios from which to learn: three practices, one evaluation, and two assists while others are evaluated.
5. Wait outside the door until the instructor comes out and gives you your scenario.
6. You will be allowed to look over your equipment before you start your exam.
7. Be sure to ask about scene safety if not provided in the scenario.
8. Be sure to apply your personal protective equipment.
9. If you have a live model for a patient, you must talk to that person just as you would a real patient. It is best to explain what you are doing as you examine the patient. Be confident and reassuring.
10. You must ask your instructor for things you cannot find out from your patient. Examples are blood pressure, pulse, and breath sounds.
11. Wounds and fractures must be dressed or splinted just as if they were real. Procedures must be done correctly (such as blood pressure, logrolling, strapping, and splinting).

12. If you need a piece of equipment that is not available, ask your instructors. They may allow you to simulate the equipment.
13. During practice and evaluation, you may be allowed to go (or may be directed) to any station, but you cannot go to the same station twice.
14. You will be graded on the following:
    a. Assessment of the scene
    b. Assessment of the patient
    c. Management of the patient
    d. Efficient use of time
    e. Leadership
    f. Judgment
    g. Problem-solving ability
    h. Patient interaction
15. When you finish your testing scenario, there is to be no discussion of the case. If you have any questions, they will be answered after the faculty meeting at the end of the course.

Explore Resource Central

For additional review and practice tests, visit www.bradybooks.com and click on Resource Central to access book-specific resources for this text. To access Resource Central, follow directions on the Student Access Card provided with this text. If there is no card, go to www.bradybooks.com and follow the Resource Central link to Buy Access from there.

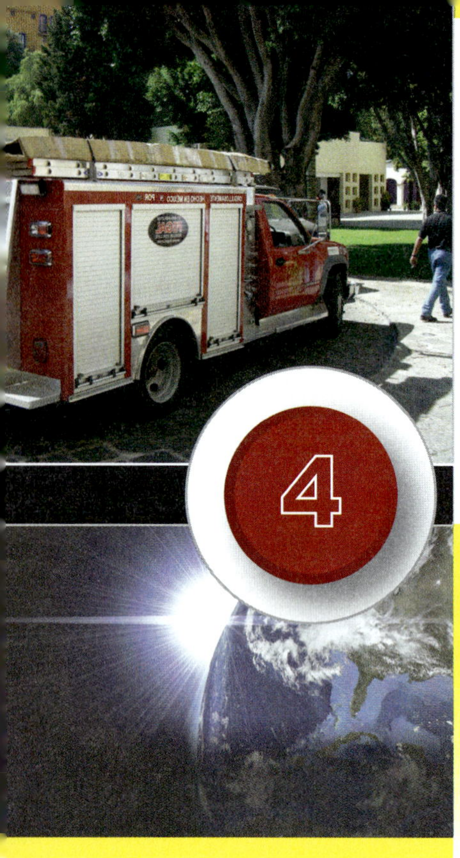

4

(Photo courtesy of International Trauma Life Support)

Airway Management

Kirk Magee, MD, MSc, FRCPC
Ronald D. Stewart, OC, BA, BSc, MD, FRCPC

Airway Vie Aeree Vía Aérea Voie Respiratoire
Drogi oddechowe Atemweg Dišni put مجرى الهواء
disajni put Dihalna pot Légút

KEY TERMS

BIAD, *p. 73*
capnography, *p. 72*
external laryngeal manipulation (ELM), *p. 67*
flow-restricted oxygen-powered ventilation device (FROPVD), *p. 78*
hypoventilation, *p. 78*
lung compliance, *p. 72*
minute volume, *p. 78*
MMAP, *p. 76*
normal ventilation, *p. 78*
patent airway, *p. 71*
pulse oximeter, *p. 78*
rapid sequence intubation (RSI), *p. 75*
Sellick maneuver, *p. 67*
tidal volume, *p. 72*
ventilation, *p. 65*

OBJECTIVES

Upon successful completion of this chapter, you should be able to:

1. Describe the anatomy and physiology of the respiratory system.
2. Explain the importance of observation as it relates to airway control.
3. Describe methods to deliver supplemental oxygen to the trauma patient.
4. Briefly describe the indications, contraindications, advantages, and disadvantages of the following airway adjuncts:
    a. Nasopharyngeal airways
    b. Oropharyngeal airways
    c. Bag-masks
    d. Flow-restricted oxygen-powered ventilation devices
    e. Blind insertion airway devices
    f. Endotracheal intubation
5. Describe the predictors of difficult mask ventilation and endotracheal intubation.
6. Describe the Sellick maneuver.
7. Describe the essential components of an airway kit.

Chapter Overview

Of all the tasks expected of field teams caring for the trauma patient, none is more important than that of airway control. Maintaining an open airway and adequate **ventilation** in the trauma patient can be a challenge in any setting, but it can be almost impossible in the adverse environment of the field with its poor lighting, the chaos that often surrounds the event, the position of the patient, and perhaps hostile onlookers.

Airway control is a task that you must master because it frequently cannot wait until you get to the hospital. Patients who are cyanotic, underventilated, or both, are in need of immediate help—help that only you can give them in the initial stages of their care. It falls to you, then, to be familiar with the basic structure and function of the airway, to be versed in how to achieve and maintain an open airway, and to know how to oxygenate and ventilate a patient.

Because of the unpredictable nature of the field environment, you will be called on to manage patient airways in almost every conceivable situation: in wrecked cars, dangling above rivers, in the middle of a shopping center, or at the side of a busy highway. You therefore need *options* and alternatives from which to choose. What will help one patient may not work for another. One patient may require a simple jaw-thrust maneuver to open an airway, whereas another may require a surgical procedure to prevent impending death.

Airway management is not simply "passing the tube." It is about maintaining and achieving effective oxygenation and ventilation. Whatever the methods required, you must always start with the basics. It is of little value—and in some cases it may be downright dangerous—to apply "advanced" techniques of airway control before beginning basic maneuvers. The discussion of airway control in the trauma patient will be rooted in several fundamental truths: Air should go in and out, oxygen is good, and blue is bad. Everything else follows from this.

This chapter begins with the basics (anatomy and physiology) and progresses through the concepts of the patent airway and basic techniques for artificial ventilation on to advanced airway techniques and monitoring devices. It then reinforces what you have learned by allowing you to practice those techniques in the Airway Management Skill Station (Chapter 5).

ventilation the movement of air or gases in and out of the lungs.

CASE PRESENTATION

An ALS ambulance has been called to a home where there is a "man down." Their scene size-up reveals that the scene is safe, and they are met by a young woman who says her husband was mowing the grass and was stung multiple times by "bees." He is now in the house on the couch, and she thinks he is dying. *How would you approach this patient? What is the mechanism of injury? What type of assessment would you perform? What would you do first? Is this a load-and-go situation?* Keep these questions in mind as you read the chapter. Then, at the end of the chapter, find out how the rescuers completed this call. ■

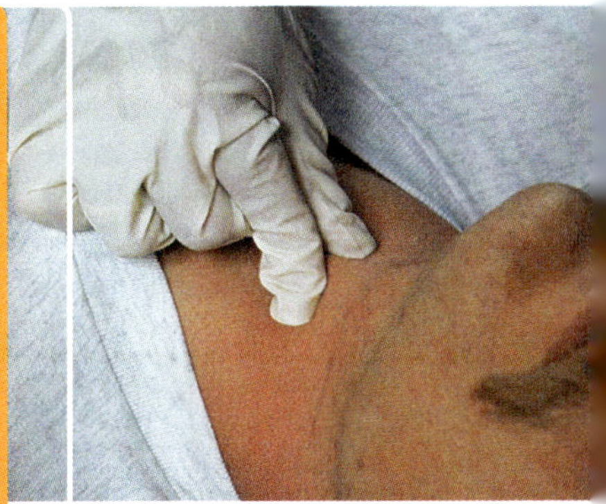

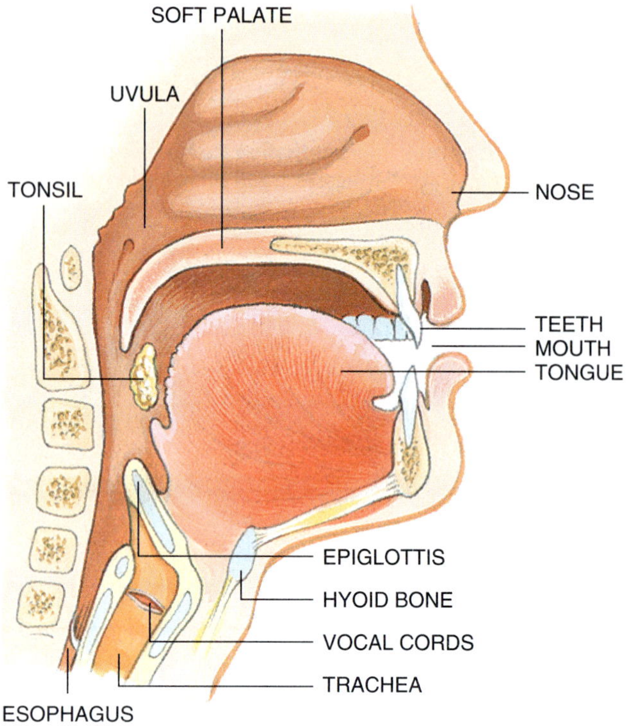

FIGURE 4-1 Anatomy of the upper airway. Note that the tongue, hyoid bone, and epiglottis are attached to the mandible by a series of ligaments. Lifting forward on the jaw will therefore displace all these structures anteriorly.

Anatomy and Physiology

The airway begins at the tip of the nose and the lips and ends at the *alveolocapillary membrane*, through which gas exchange takes place between the air sacs of the lung (the *alveoli*) and the lung's capillary network. The airway consists of chambers and pipes, which conduct air with its 21% oxygen content to the alveoli and carry away the waste *carbon dioxide* that diffuses from the blood into the alveoli.

Nasopharynx

The beginning of the respiratory tract (the nasal cavity and oropharynx) is lined with moist mucous membranes (Figure 4-1). This lining is delicate and highly vascular. It deserves all the respect that you can give it, and that means preventing undue trauma by using liberally lubricated tubes and avoiding unnecessary poking about. The *nasal cavity* is divided by a very vascular midline *septum*, and on the lateral walls of the nose are "shelves" called the *turbinates*. Those projections can get in the way when tubes or other devices need to be inserted into the nostrils. Carefully sliding a well-lubricated tube's bevel along the floor or the septum of the nasal cavity will usually prevent traumatizing the turbinates.

Oropharynx

The teeth are the first obstruction we meet in the oral part of the airway. They may be more obstructive in some patients than in others. In any case, the same general principle always applies: *Patients should have the same number and condition of teeth at the end of an airway procedure as they had at the beginning.*

The tongue is mostly a large chunk of muscle and represents the next potential obstruction. It is attached to the jaw anteriorly and through a series of muscles and ligaments to the *hyoid bone*, a wishbone-like structure just under the chin from which the cartilage skeleton (the larynx) of the upper airway is suspended. The *epiglottis* also is connected to the hyoid, so elevating the hyoid will lift the epiglottis upward and open the airway further.

Hypopharynx

The epiglottis is one of the main anatomic landmarks in the airway. You must be familiar with it and be able to identify it by sight and by touch. It looks like a floppy piece of cartilage covered by mucosa—which is exactly what it is—and it feels like the tragus, the cartilage at the opening of the ear canal. Its function is unclear, but it is nonetheless important when you must assume control of the airway.

The epiglottis is attached to the hyoid and thence to the mandible by a series of ligaments and muscles. In the unconscious patient, the tongue can produce some airway obstruction by falling back against the soft palate and even the posterior pharyngeal wall. However, it is the epiglottis that will produce complete airway obstruction in the supine unconscious patient whose jaw is relaxed and whose head and neck are in the neutral position. In such patients the epiglottis will fall down against the glottic opening and prevent ventilation.

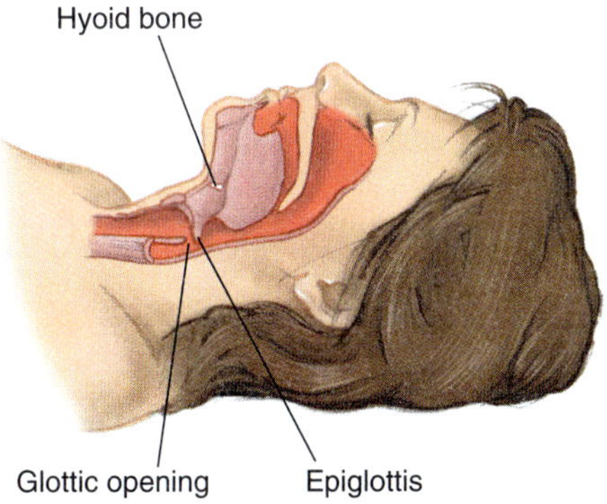

FIGURE 4-2a The epiglottis is attached to the hyoid and then to the mandible. When the mandible is relaxed and falls back, the tongue falls upward and against the soft palate and the posterior pharyngeal wall, whereas the epiglottis falls over the glottic opening.

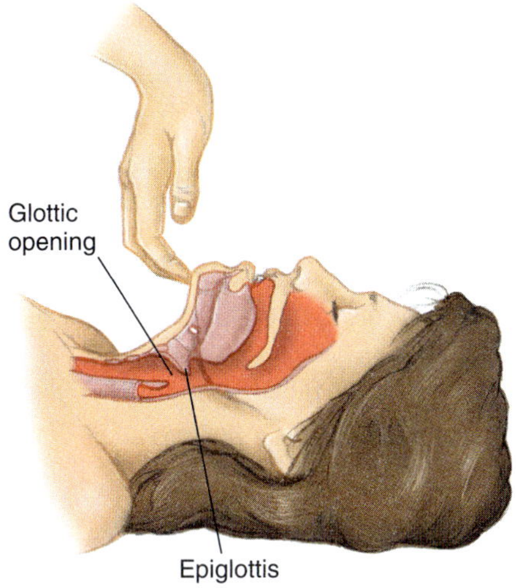

FIGURE 4-2b Extension of the head and lifting the chin will pull the tongue and the epiglottis upward and forward, exposing the glottic opening and ensuring the patent airway. In the trauma patient, only the jaw, or chin and jaw, should be displaced forward, and the head and neck should be kept in alignment.

It is essential to understand this crucial fact in the management of the airway. To ensure an open (patent) airway in an unconscious supine patient, displace the hyoid anteriorly by lifting forward on the jaw (chin lift, jaw thrust) or by pulling on the tongue. This will lift the tongue out of the way. It also will keep the epiglottis elevated and away from the posterior pharyngeal wall and glottic opening (Figure 4-2). Both nasotracheal and orotracheal intubation require elevation of the epiglottis by a laryngoscope or the fingers, by pulling on the tongue or by lifting forward on the jaw.

Larynx

On either side of the epiglottis is a recess called the *pyriform fossa*. An endotracheal tube can "catch up" in either one. Pyriform fossa placement of an endotracheal tube can be identified easily by "tenting" of the skin on either side of the superior aspect of the *laryngeal prominence* (Adam's apple) or by transillumination if a lighted stylet (or "lightwand") is being used to intubate.

The vocal cords are protected by the *thyroid cartilage*, a boxlike structure shaped like a *C*, with the open part of the *C* representing its posterior wall. That wall is covered with muscle. In some patients, the cords can close entirely in *laryngospasm*, producing complete airway obstruction. The thyroid cartilage can easily be seen in most people on the anterior surface of the neck as the laryngeal prominence. Manipulating the thyroid cartilage can help bring the vocal cords into view during endotracheal intubation. This is called **external laryngeal manipulation (ELM)**. The movement is usually pressing the thyroid cartilage backward against the esophagus (much like the **Sellick maneuver** described next) and then upward and slightly to the patient's right side.

external laryngeal manipulation (ELM) a maneuver to improve visualization of the vocal cords during endotracheal intubation.

Sellick maneuver a maneuver (posterior pressure on the cricoid cartilage) to prevent gastric insufflation and vomiting.

Inferior to the thyroid cartilage is another part of the larynx, the *cricoid*. The cricoid is a cartilage shaped like a signet ring with the ring in front and the signet behind. It can be palpated as a small bump on the anterior surface of the neck

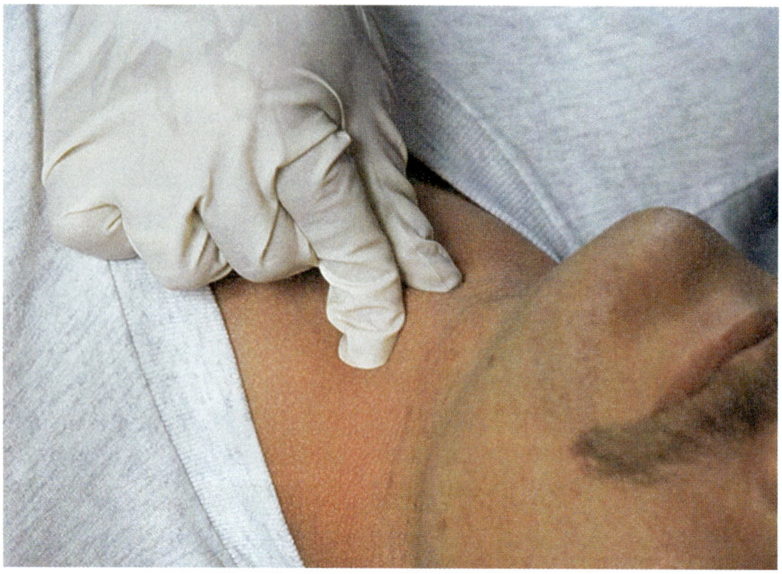

FIGURE 4-3 The Sellick maneuver.

inferior to the laryngeal prominence. The esophagus is just behind the posterior wall of the cricoid cartilage. Pressure on the cricoid at the front of the neck will close off the esophagus to pressures as high as 100 cm H_2O. This is the *Sellick maneuver* (Figure 4-3). It can be used to reduce the risk of gastric regurgitation during the process of intubation and to prevent insufflation of air into the stomach during positive pressure ventilation by mouth-to-mouth, bag-mask, or flow-restricted oxygen-powered ventilation device. If there is any danger of cervical-spine injury, you must carefully support and stabilize the neck while performing ELM or the Sellick maneuver.

Connecting the inferior border of the thyroid cartilage with the superior aspect of the cricoid is the *cricothyroid membrane*. This membrane is a very important landmark through which you can gain direct access to the airway below the cords. You can palpate the cricothyroid membrane on most patients by finding the most prominent part of the thyroid cartilage. Then slide your index finger down until you feel a second "bump," just before your finger palpates the last depression before the *sternal notch*. That second bump is the *cricoid cartilage*. At its upper edge is the *cricothyroid membrane* (Figure 4-4). In some patients, especially those with a thick neck, you may find the cricoid cartilage more easily by going from the sternal

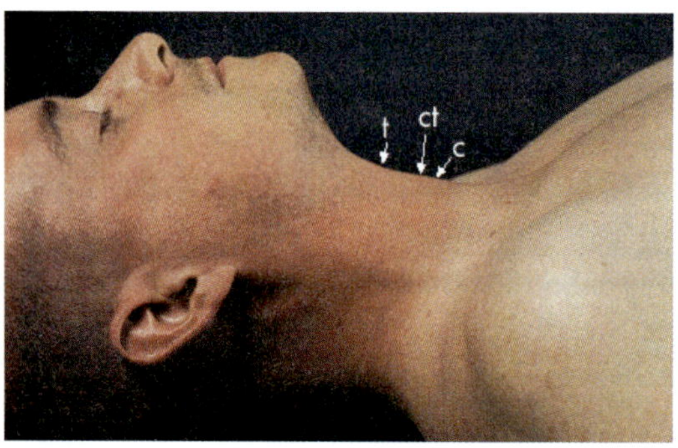

FIGURE 4-4a External view of the anterior neck, showing the surface landmarks for the thyroid cartilage (laryngeal) prominence, the cricothyroid membrane, and the cricoid cartilage.

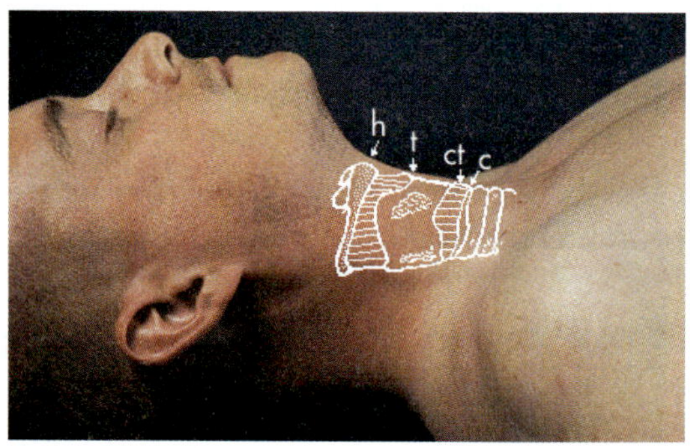

FIGURE 4-4b Cutaway view showing the important landmarks of the larynx and upper airway: hyoid, thyroid cartilage, cricothyroid membrane, and cricoid cartilage.

notch upward until you feel the first prominent cartilage "bump." Just over the "top" of this bump is the cricothyroid membrane. The sternal notch is an important landmark as well. It is the point at which the cuff of a properly placed endotracheal tube should lie (Figure 4-5). The sternal notch is readily palpated at the junction of the clavicles with the upper edge of the sternum.

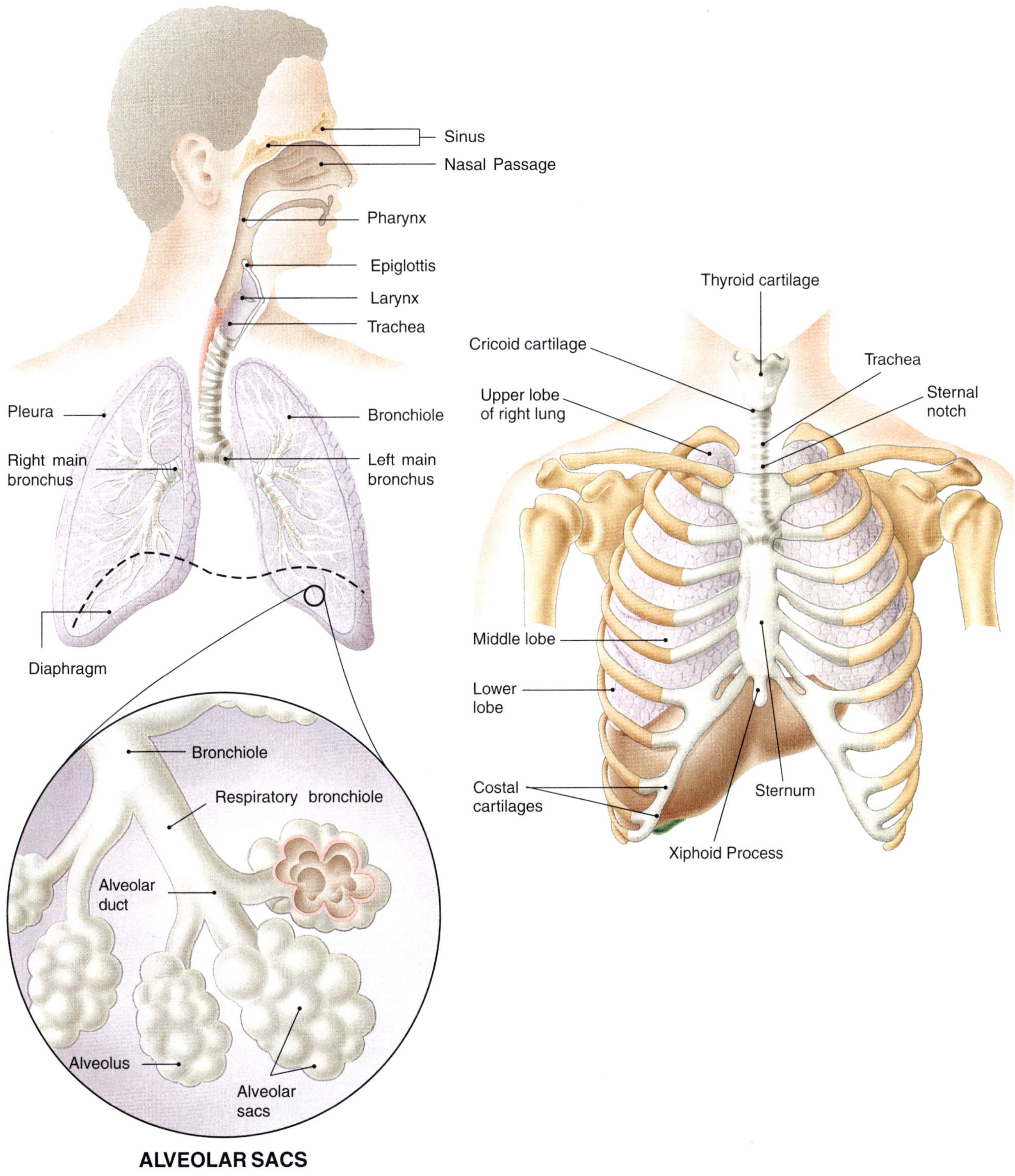

FIGURE 4-5 The respiratory system. Notice the sternal notch, at which point the clavicles join the sternum. It marks the position of the tip of a well-placed endotracheal tube.

Trachea and Bronchi

The *tracheal rings* (C-shaped cartilaginous supports for the trachea) continue beyond the cricoid cartilage. The trachea soon divides into the left and right *mainstem bronchi*. The point at which the trachea divides is called the *carina*. It is important to note that the right mainstem bronchus takes off at an angle that is slightly more in line with the trachea. As a result, tubes or other foreign bodies usually end up in the right mainstem bronchus. One of the goals of a properly performed endotracheal intubation is to avoid a right (or left) mainstem bronchus intubation.

You should know how far some of the major anatomic landmarks are from the teeth. This knowledge will help you place an endotracheal tube at the correct level, and by remembering only three numbers you will be able to detect a tube that is too far into the airway or not in far enough. The three numbers to remember are 15, 20, and 25. The first number, *15*, is the distance (in centimeters) from the teeth to the vocal cords of the average adult. The number *20* (5 cm farther down the airway) is the sternal notch. About 5 cm farther again at *25* is the carina (Figure 4-6). Those are average distances and can vary by several centimeters.

Extension or flexion of the head of an intubated patient will move the endotracheal tube up or down as much as 2 to 2.5 cm. Tubes can easily become dislodged. Detection of misplacement can be difficult unless you are monitoring oxygen saturation and expired CO_2. Taping the head down or guarding against movement will lessen the risk of tube displacement. (This is even more important in children.) It also will reduce trauma to the tracheal mucosa. Less movement of the tube will result in less stimulation to the patient's airway reflexes. It also may result in a more stable cardiovascular system and intracranial pressure in the patient.

To help protect the airway from becoming blocked and to reduce the risk of aspiration, the body has developed brisk reflexes that will attempt to expel any offending foreign material from the oropharynx, the glottic opening, or the trachea. Those areas are well supplied by sensitive nerves that can activate the swallowing, gag, and cough reflex. Activation of swallowing, gagging, or coughing by stimulation of the upper airway can cause significant cardiovascular stimulation as well as elevation in intracranial pressure. You can protect patients from such

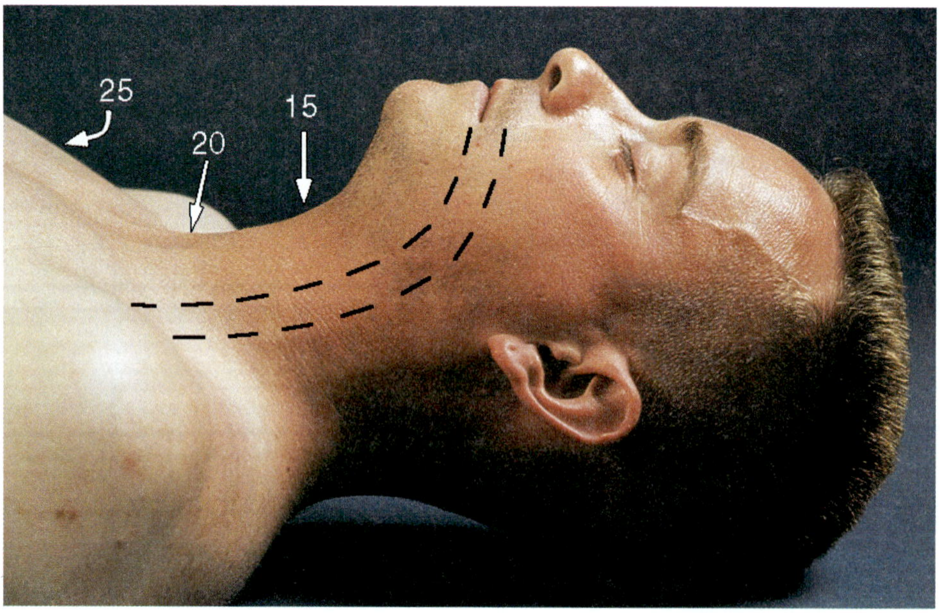

FIGURE 4-6 Major airway landmarks and distances from the teeth: 15 = 15 cm from teeth to cords, 20 = 20 cm from teeth to sternal notch, 25 = 25 cm from teeth to carina.

unwanted effects by suppressing the reflexes through the use of topical lidocaine. (See Chapter 5.)

The Lungs

The *lungs* are the organs through which gas exchange takes place. They are contained within a "cage" formed by the ribs, and usually fill up the *pleural space*, which is the *potential space* between the internal chest wall and the lung surface. The lungs have only one opening to the outside, the *glottic opening*, which is the space between the vocal cords. Expansion of the chest wall (the cage) and movement of the diaphragm downward cause the lungs to expand (because the pleural space is airtight), and air rushes in through the *glottis*. The air travels down the smaller and smaller tubes to the alveoli, where gas exchange (respiration) takes place.

The Patent Airway

One of the first maneuvers essential to caring for a patient is ensuring a *patent* or *open airway*. Without this, all other care is of little use. This must be done quickly because patients cannot tolerate hypoxia for more than a few minutes. The effect of hypoxia and inadequate ventilation in an unconscious injured patient can be devastating. If they are compounded by the absence of adequate perfusion, the patient is in even more difficult straits. Patients suffering from head trauma not only may have hypoxic brain damage from airway compromise but may also build up high levels of carbon dioxide that can increase blood flow to the injured brain, causing swelling and increased intracranial pressure.

patent airway an open airway.

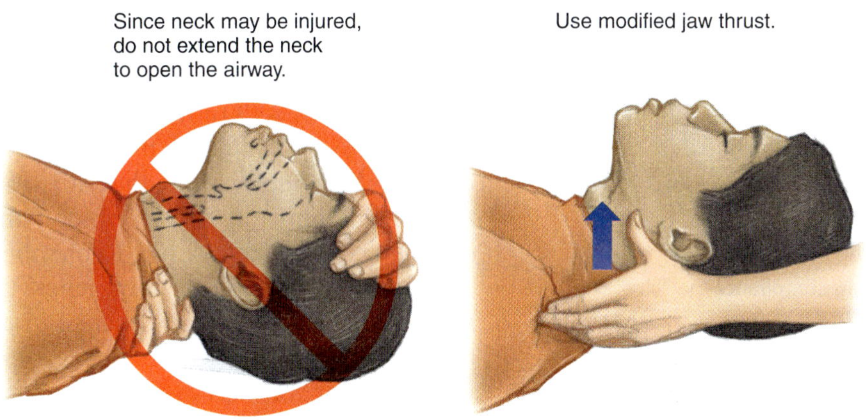

FIGURE 4-7a Opening the airway using a modified jaw-thrust maneuver. Maintain in-line stabilization while pushing up on the angle of the jaw with your thumbs.

Ensuring an open airway in a patient can be a major challenge in the prehospital setting. Not only can trauma disrupt the anatomy of the face and airway, but it also can result in bleeding, which can lead to airflow obstruction and obscure airway landmarks. Add to this the risk of cervical-spine injury, and the challenge is readily apparent. You also must remember that some airway maneuvers, including suction and insertion of nasopharyngeal and oropharyngeal airways, may stimulate a patient's protective reflexes and increase the likelihood of vomiting and aspiration, cardiovascular stimulation, and increased intracranial pressure.

The first step in providing a **patent airway** in the unconscious patient is to ensure that the tongue and epiglottis are lifted forward and maintained in that position. This is done by using the modified jaw-thrust (Figure 4-7a) or the jaw-lift maneuver (Figure 4-7b). Either will prevent the tongue from falling backward against the soft palate or posterior pharyngeal wall. Either will pull forward on the hyoid, lifting the epiglottis up out of the way. They are essential

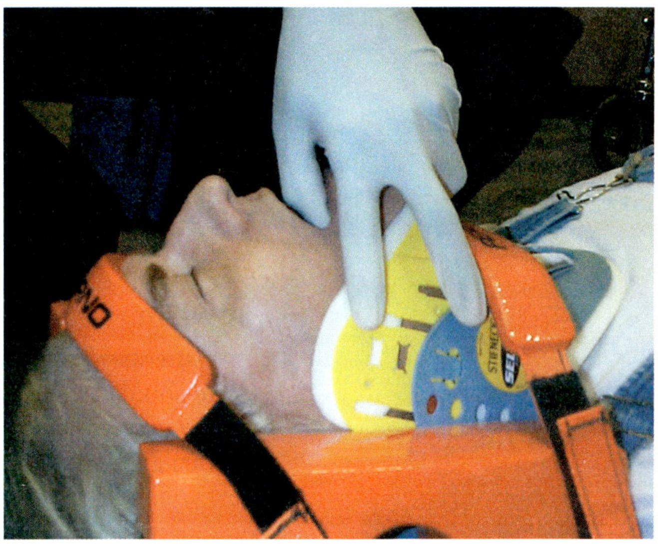

FIGURE 4-7b Jaw lift. *(Courtesy of Buddy Denson, EMT-P)*

maneuvers for both basic and advanced airway procedures. Done properly, they will open the airway without tilting the head backward or moving the neck.

Constant vigilance and care are required to maintain a patent airway in your patient. Following are essentials for this task:

capnography a noninvasive device that detects or measures the amount of carbon dioxide in the expired breath of a patient.

- Continual observation of the patient to anticipate problems, frequently requiring monitoring devices such as pulse oximetry and **capnography**
- An adequate suction device with large-bore tubing and attachment
- Airway adjuncts

Observation

The patient who is injured is at risk of airway compromise even if completely conscious and awake. This is partially due to the fact that many patients have full stomachs, are anxious, and are prone to vomiting. Some patients also will be bleeding into their oropharynx and thus swallowing blood. In view of these facts, you should constantly observe your patient for airway problems following injury. One team member must be responsible for both airway control and adequate ventilation for any patient who might be at risk of airway compromise.

tidal volume the amount of air that is inspired and expired during one respiratory cycle.

The general appearance of a patient, the respiratory rate, and any complaints must be noted and addressed. In a patient who is breathing spontaneously, you must check frequently for adequate **tidal volume** by feeling over the mouth and nose and by observing chest wall movements. Bare the chest—at least below the breasts—is a good rule to follow. Check the supplemental oxygen line periodically to ensure that oxygen is being delivered to the patient at a given flow rate or percentage.

Always immediately clear blood and secretions. You also must be alert for sounds that indicate trouble. Remember: *Noisy breathing is obstructed breathing.*

lung compliance the "give" or elasticity of the lungs

If the patient has an endotracheal tube in place, monitor **lung compliance** and search for the cause of any change in compliance. If possible, monitor endotracheal tube position by pulse oximetry and continuous expiratory CO_2 monitoring. (For more on capnography, see Chapter 5.) Use of waveform capnography is rapidly becoming the gold standard for monitoring ET tube placement during transport of critically ill patients and is strongly recommended in all intubated patients. By use of nasal sensors capnography also can be used to monitor the ventilation status of the nonintubated patient. A trend to elevation of the expired CO_2 is evidence that the patient is hypoventilating and will need ventilatory assistance. The use of pulse oximetry is recommended in all trauma patients. (See Chapter 5.) The development of confusion or combativeness can be a sign that the patient is hypoxic and needs an airway procedure such as ET intubation, or if intubated, the tube may no longer be in the trachea and needs to be reinserted. Consider combative patients to be hypoxic until a systematic and rapid evaluation rules it out.

Suction

All patients who are injured and who have cervical motion-restriction devices in place should be considered at high risk for airway compromise. In addition, one of the greatest threats to the patent airway is that of vomiting and aspiration, particularly in patients who have recently eaten a large meal washed down with large quantities of alcohol. As a result, portable suction devices should be considered basic equipment for field trauma care. A portable suction device should have the following characteristics (Figure 4-8):

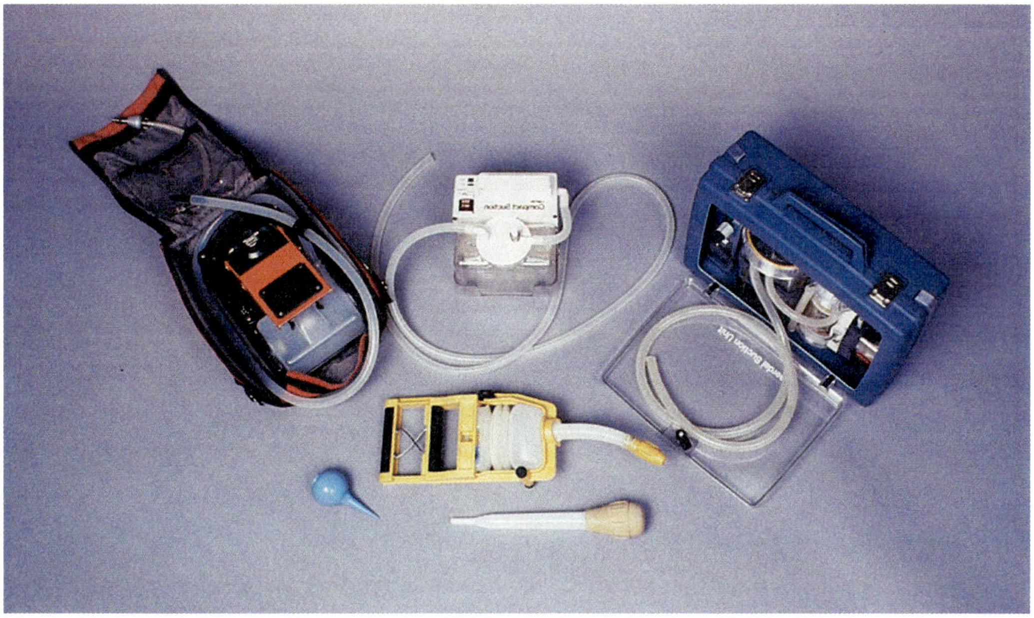

FIGURE 4-8 Examples of suction apparatus.

- It can be carried in an airway kit with an oxygen cylinder and other airway equipment. It should not be separated or stored remote from oxygen; otherwise, it represents an "extra" piece of equipment requiring extra hands.
- It can be hand powered or battery powered rather than oxygen driven. Hand powered is preferred. You should always have a hand-powered suction as a backup if you use a battery-powered suction.
- It can generate sufficient suction and volume displacement to remove pieces of food, blood clots, and thick secretions from the oropharynx.
- It has tubing of sufficient diameter (0.8–1 cm) to handle whatever is suctioned from the patient.

Suction tips should be of large bore, such as the rigid "tonsil-tip" suckers that can handle most clots and bleeding. In some cases the suction tubing itself can be used to withdraw large amounts of blood or gastric contents. A 6-mm endotracheal tube can be used with a connector as a suction tip. The tube's side hole removes the necessity for a proximal control valve to interrupt suction. Usually team member 2 (see Chapter 2) assumes responsibility for the airway. As the VO (vomit officer), team member 2 must be constantly alert to prevent the patient from aspirating.

Airway Adjuncts

Equipment to help ensure a patent airway will include various nasopharyngeal (NPA), oropharyngeal (OPA), blind insertion airway devices (**BIAD**), and endotracheal airways. Insertion of these devices must be reserved for patients whose protective reflexes are sufficiently depressed to tolerate them. Care must be taken to avoid provoking vomiting or gagging, since both occurrences are bad for these patients.

BIAD a blind insertion airway device, such as the King Airway, which can be inserted without having to visualize the larynx. BIADs are also called *supraglottic airways.*

Nasopharyngeal Airways

Nasopharyngeal airways (NPAs) should be soft and of appropriate length. They are designed to prevent the tongue and epiglottis from falling against the posterior

PEARLS: Preventing Deaths

- Become skilled at recognizing when
  - Active airway management is necessary. The need to intubate is not the same as the need to ventilate!
  - The patient needs assistance with ventilation.
- Use capnography to ensure adequate ventilation and prevent inadvertent hyperventilation when:
  - An airway device is placed incorrectly.
  - An airway device that was placed correctly has become displaced. (The pulse oximeter and capnograph are critical for this.)
- Become competent in intubating the trachea. Be prepared to use a rescue airway (e.g., Combitube®, King LT-D™ airway) if you are unable to intubate.
- Prevent aspiration of gastric contents. Suction must be immediately available. Be prepared for equipment failure by having backup equipment available.
- Failure to manage the airway can be a fatal error.

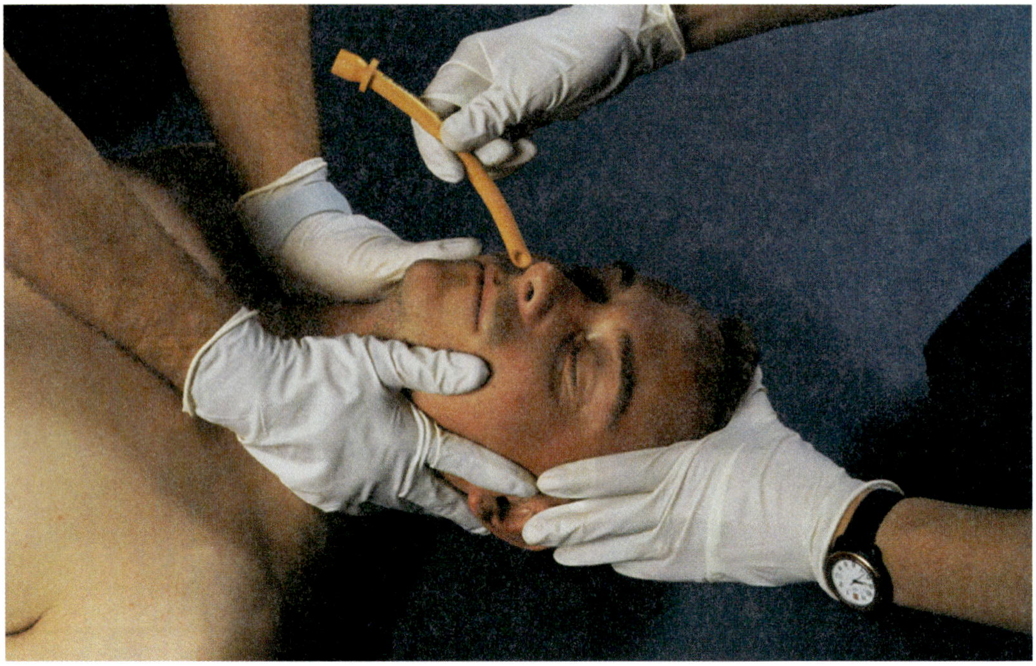

FIGURE 4-9a The nasopharyngeal airway is inserted with the bevel slid along the septum or floor of the nasal cavity.

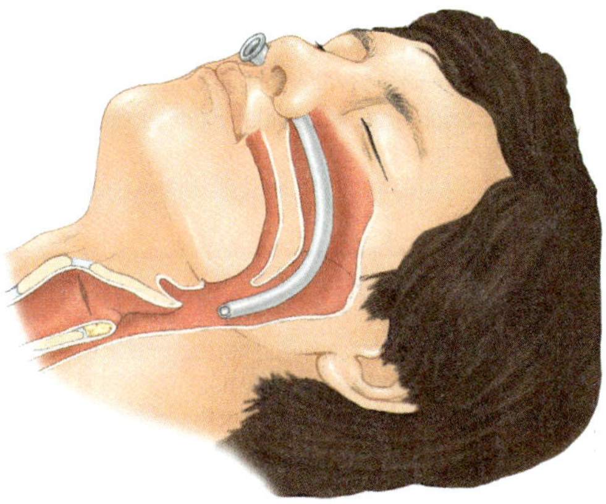

FIGURE 4-9b The nasopharyngeal airway rests between the tongue and the posterior pharyngeal wall.

pharyngeal wall. (See Chapter 5 for insertion technique.) In a pinch, a 6-mm or 6.6-mm endotracheal tube can be cut and serve as an NPA. With light lubrication and gentle insertion, there should be few problems with this airway (Figure 4-9). However, bleeding and trauma to the nasal mucosa are common. Mild hemorrhage from the nose after insertion of the airway is *not* an indication to remove it. In fact, it is probably better to keep an NPA in place so as not to disturb the clot or reactivate the bleeding. The NPA will be better tolerated than the oropharyngeal one and thus can usually be used in patients who still have a gag reflex.

Oropharyngeal Airways

Oropharyngeal airways (OPAs) are designed to keep the tongue off the posterior pharyngeal wall and thereby help maintain a patent airway (Figure 4-10). Successful placement of an OPA should not give you a false sense of security. Patients who are easily able to tolerate an OPA should be considered candidates for endotracheal intubation because their protective reflexes are so depressed that they cannot protect their lower airways from aspiration. One OPA, the S.A.L.T. (supraglottic airway laryngopharyngeal tube) airway system is not only an OPA, but also, when inserted into the pharynx, serves as a guide to insert an endotracheal tube and then serves as the ET tube holder and protector (Figure 4-11).

Resource Central

See Optional Skills for more information on BIADs.

Blind Insertion Airway Devices

Esophageal tracheal combitube (Combitube®), King LT-D™ airway, intubating laryngeal airway (ILA; air-Q™), and the laryngeal mask airway (LMA) are all blind insertion airway devices (BIADs). This means the advanced EMS provider can properly insert the device without having to visualize the larynx.

BIADs are not as effective as endotracheal intubation in preventing aspiration or ensuring ventilation. Thus they are not recommended for advanced EMS providers except as rescue devices in cases in which you are unable to ventilate the patient using a bag-mask or you are unsuccessful in intubating the trachea. Evidence is mounting that single-tube devices such as the King LT-D™ and the ILA may be better suited for the prehospital environment than the more complicated esophageal tracheal combitube.

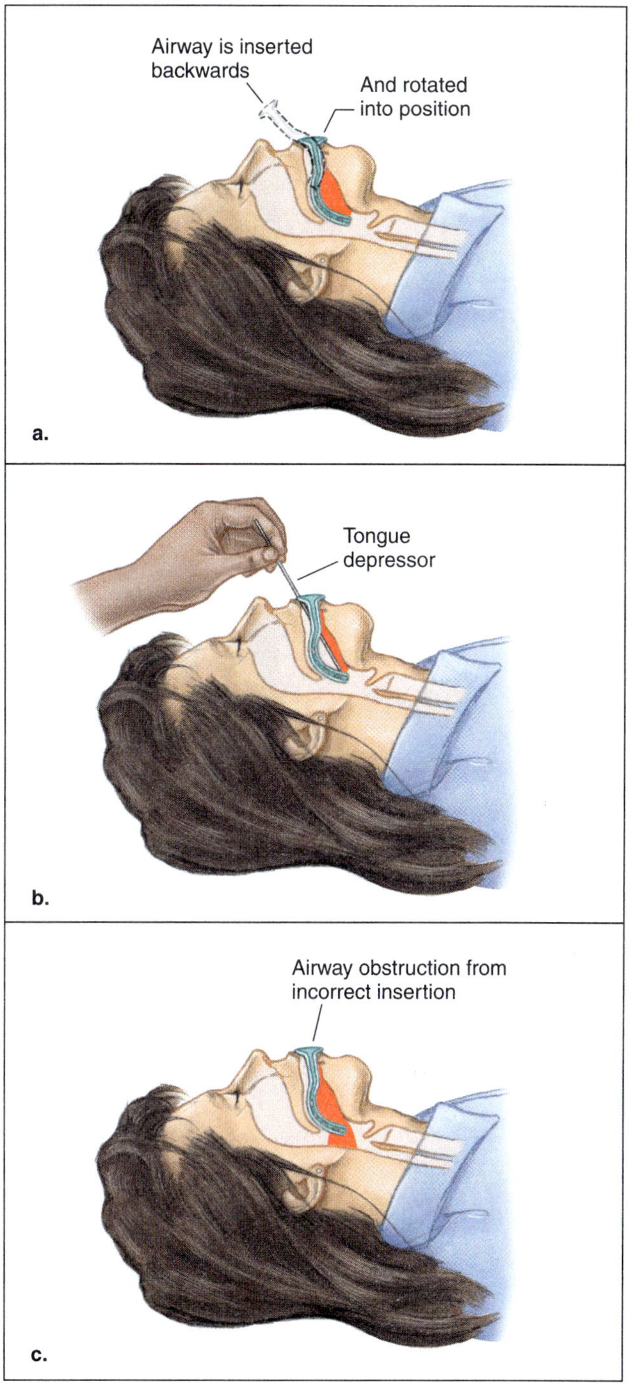

FIGURE 4-10 Insertion of an oropharyngeal airway.

Endotracheal Tubes

Endotracheal intubation is the gold standard of airway care in patients who cannot protect their airways or in those needing assistance with breathing. However, it is not always the most appropriate choice for airway management in the prehospital setting. Several problems will face you when you decide to intubate a trauma patient. Intubation frequently must be done under the most difficult circumstances—on the side of the road, in a crashed vehicle, or under a train. In addition, the patient may still have a gag reflex or the patient's spine may need to be motion restricted with a cervical collar or other equipment. This may so restrict movement and visualization of the airway that you have to consider alternative methods of intubation.

The original method of intubation was tactile or digital. That was changed by the invention of the laryngoscope, which allowed visualization of the upper airway and placement of the tube under direct vision. The ability to see the actual passage of the tube through the glottic opening rendered tactile orotracheal intubation obsolete, and its practice largely died out until interest in it was revived in the last two decades.

There are several choices to facilitate intubation in the trauma patient, ranging from awake intubation using topical anesthetics to deep sedation and **rapid sequence intubation (RSI).** RSI refers to the use of paralytic agents to quickly facilitate tube placement and to minimize the risk of aspiration. However, you must be cognizant of the fact that both deep sedation and RSI inhibit the normal muscle tone of the airway and thus may make it impossible to effectively mask-ventilate the patient. In this situation, it is necessary to immediately place an endotracheal tube to achieve successful ventilation, or failing this, a surgical airway may be required. For that reason, you must be very familiar with the predictors of difficult laryngoscopy and intubation before deciding to intubate a patient who is already breathing on his own. *Remember, patients who have spontaneous yet inadequate respiratory effort are better off than the patient who has been given a paralytic and can neither be mask-ventilated nor intubated.*

rapid sequence intubation (RSI) a technique to improve the likelihood of intubating a difficult patient by administering a sedative and paralytic agent. Also called *rapid sequence induction* and *drug-assisted intubation.*

Although it is not always possible to guess every time which patient will have a difficult airway, certain physical features allow us to predict which patients might potentially have difficult laryngoscopy and intubation. The mnemonic

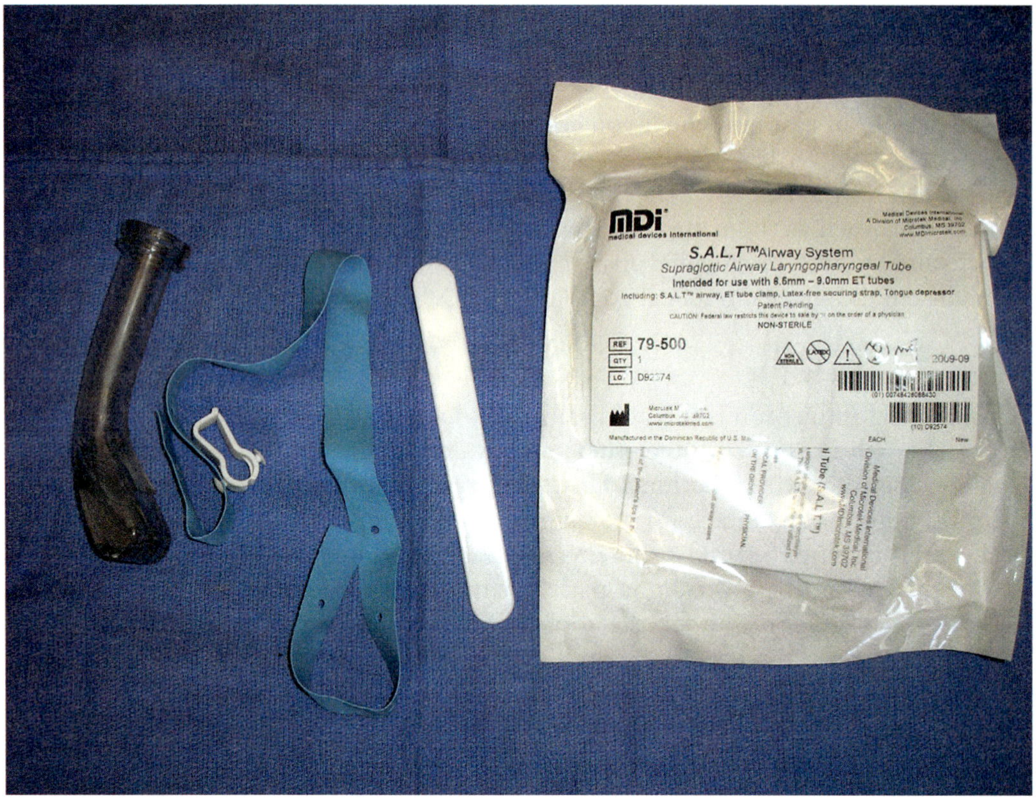

FIGURE 4-11 The S.A.L.T. airway system is not only an oropharyngeal airway, but it also can help guide an endotracheal tube into the trachea.

MMAP a technique for predicting when a patient will be difficult to intubate; MMAP stands for Mallampati, measurement 3-3-1, atlanto-occipital extension, and pathology.

"**MMAP**" has been proposed to identify these features. MMAP stands for Mallampati, measurement 3-3-1, atlanto-occipital extension, and pathology:

M—*Mallampati.* The Mallampati score ranges from I to IV and is dependent on what structures can be viewed when the mouth is opened (Table 4-1). Generally, the higher the grade, the more difficult it will be to perform laryngoscopy.

M—*Measurement 3-3-1.* This measurement also can aid in predicting the difficult airway. Ideally, you should be able to fit three fingers under the patient's chin between the hyoid bone and the mentum of the chin. The patient should be able to open his mouth so that three fingers fit between the upper and lower incisors. Last, the patient should be able to protrude the lower jaw such that the lower teeth are 1 cm beyond the upper teeth.

A—*Atlanto-occipital extension.* In patients in whom cervical-spine injury is *not* suspected, the ability to extend the head at the atlanto-occipital junction to achieve the "sniffing position" will aid in visualizing the vocal cords.

P—*Pathology.* Finally, pathology refers to any clinical evidence of anatomic airway obstruction. Airway obstruction can result from medical or traumatic conditions, such as edema, infection, burns, and penetrating or blunt injuries. This is particularly important because upper airway obstructive pathology, often evidenced by stridor, is a relative contraindication to RSI.

As for all clinicians responsible for emergency airway management, the appropriate decision regarding whom and how to intubate will ultimately be related to several factors. These include the assessment of the patient and the particular clinical presentation, the skill set of the individual health-care professionals present,

Table 4-1 Estimating Difficulty of Intubation

Mallampati Score
View pharynx with mouth open and tongue not protruding.
Scoring: I. Entire tonsil or tonsillar bed is visible. II. Upper half of tonsil or tonsillar bed is visible. III. Soft and hard palate are clearly visible. IV. Only hard palate is visible.
The higher the score, the higher the degree of difficulty.

and the system in which they work. An additional factor unique to the prehospital setting is time. Ventilation with a bag-mask and immediate transport of the patient may be a better option in certain instances than taking the additional time required to perform RSI. Remember, airway management can occur without RSI, but RSI cannot occur without airway management!

Although *direct-vision orotracheal intubation* should be considered the primary method of placing a tube in the trachea, the procedure is not always easy, nor is it indicated in all patients. In the management of trauma patients particularly, options must be available to permit successful intubation in even the most challenging of situations and patients. There is evidence that the technique of *direct-vision orotracheal intubation* results in movement of the head and neck. The question therefore arises of whether the use of this method presents an added risk in possible cervical-spine injuries. Controversy exists as to whether such movement is either substantial or of real clinical significance. In short, the method of intubation should be suited to each patient. Those with a low risk of cervical-spine injury can be intubated in the conventional way, using a laryngoscope. Intubation by the nasotracheal route, the tactile or transillumination methods, or a combination of the two should be reserved for patients with specific indication for alternative techniques. (See Chapter 5.)

Resource Central

See Optional Skills for how to perform alternative techniques.

Translaryngeal jet ventilation (TLJV) can provide a quick, reliable, and relatively safe temporary method of adequate oxygenation and ventilation when the airway cannot be maintained because of obstruction or partial obstruction above the cords, and access below the level of the cords is needed. A special cannula is inserted through the cricothyroid membrane, and the patient is ventilated using a special manual jet ventilator device.

Resource Central

See Optional Skills for more information on the TLJV method.

Supplemental Oxygen

Patients who are injured need supplemental oxygen, especially if they are unconscious. It is well recognized that patients suffering from head injury are frequently hypoxic. Furthermore, supplemental oxygen significantly reduces nausea and vomiting during ambulance transport. Supplemental oxygen can be supplied by a simple face mask run at 10–12 liters per minute. This will provide the patient with about 40% to 50% oxygen. Nonrebreathing masks with a reservoir bag and oxygen flow rates into the bag of 12–15 liters per minute can provide 60% to 90% oxygen to the patient. They are recommended for all trauma patients requiring supplemental oxygen. Nasal oxygen cannulae are well tolerated by most patients, but provide only about 25% to 30% oxygen to the patient. They are recommended only for those patients who refuse to accept an oxygen mask.

Supplemental oxygen must be used to ensure adequate oxygenation when you perform positive pressure ventilation. Oxygenation must be supplemented during mouth-to-mask ventilation by running oxygen at 10–12 liters per minute through the oxygen nipple attached to most masks or by placing the oxygen tubing under the mask and running it at the same rate. Alternatively, you can increase the oxygen percentage delivered during mouth-to-mask breathing by placing a nasal cannula on yourself. This increases the delivered oxygen percentage from 17% to about 30%.

Bag-mask devices or resuscitator bags with a large (2.5 liters) reservoir bag and an oxygen flow rate of 12–15 liters per minute will increase the delivered oxygen from 21% (air) to 90% or 100%. Adding a reservoir bag to a bag-mask will increase the delivered oxygen from 40% to 50% to 90% to 100% and thus always should be used.

flow-restricted oxygen-powered ventilation device (FROPVD) an artificial ventilation device that provides 100% oxygen at a flow rate of 40 L/min at a maximum pressure of 50 + 5 cm water.

A **flow-restricted oxygen-powered ventilation device (FROPVD)** will provide 100% oxygen at a flow rate of 40 liters per minute at a maximum pressure of 50 cm ± 5 cm water.

Ventilation

Normal Ventilation

The movement of air or gases in and out of the lungs is called *ventilation*. This should not be confused with *respiration*, which is the exchange of oxygen at the alveoli. At rest, adults normally take in about 400 to 600 cc air with each breath. This is called the *tidal volume*. Multiplying that value by the number of breaths per minute (the respiratory rate) gives the **minute volume**, the amount of air breathed in (and, of course, out) each minute. This is an important value and is normally 5–12 liters per minute. **Normal ventilation** by healthy lungs will produce an oxygen level of about 100 mm Hg and a carbon dioxide level of 35 to 45 mm Hg. A carbon dioxide level below 35 mm Hg indicates hyperventilation, and values greater than 45 mm Hg indicate **hypoventilation**.

minute volume the volume of air breathed in and out in one minute. This varies from 5 to 12 liters per minute.

normal ventilation the movement of air into and out of the lungs is able to maintain the carbon dioxide level between 35 and 45 mm Hg.

hypoventilation the movement of air in and out of the lungs is unable to maintain the carbon dioxide level below 45 mm Hg.

The clinical terms *hypoventilation* and *hyperventilation* do not refer to oxygenation but to the level of carbon dioxide maintained. It is easier for carbon dioxide to diffuse across the alveolocapillary membrane of the lungs than it is for oxygen to do so. This makes it easier to excrete carbon dioxide than to oxygenate the blood. Thus, if the chest or lungs are injured, the body may be able to maintain normal levels of carbon dioxide in the blood and yet the cells can be hypoxic. A patient with a contused lung might have a respiratory rate of 36, a carbon dioxide level of 30 mm Hg, and an oxygen level of only 80 mm Hg. Although hyperventilating, this person is still hypoxic. He does not need to breathe faster; he needs to have supplemental oxygen. When in doubt, give your patient oxygen.

pulse oximeter a noninvasive device for measuring the oxygen saturation of the blood.

Devices to measure oxygen saturation (**pulse oximeters**) have been available for several years and expired CO_2 monitors (capnographs) are now available for prehospital use. Pulse oximeters measure oxygen saturation and should be used on almost all trauma patients, whereas CO_2 monitors are most useful for continuously monitoring endotracheal tube placement (though they have many other uses. (See Chapters 8 and 10.) These devices will be discussed in Chapter 5.

Positive Pressure (Artificial) Ventilation

Normal breathing takes place because the negative pressure inside the (potential) pleural space "draws" air in through the upper airway from the outside. In any patient who is unable to do this, or whose airway needs protecting, you may need to "pump" air or oxygen in through the glottic opening. This is called *intermittent positive pressure ventilation (IPPV)*. IPPV in trauma patients can take various forms, from mouth-to-mouth to bag-mask-endotracheal tube ventilation. *NOTE: "Pumping" air into the oropharynx is no guarantee that it will go through the glottic opening and into the lungs.*

The oropharynx leads to the esophagus. Pressure in the oropharynx of greater than 25 cm H_2O will open the esophagus and lead to air being pumped into the stomach (gastric insufflation). Bag-masks and FROPVDs can produce pressures greater than this, which is why the Sellick maneuver (posterior pressure on the cricoid cartilage) is so very important as a basic airway maneuver.

When you need to ventilate a patient using IPPV, you should know approximately what the *delivered volume* is. Delivered volume is how much volume you are delivering with each breath you give. You can estimate the minute volume by multiplying delivered volume by the ventilatory rate. A FROPVD that delivers oxygen at the rate of 40 liters per minute will have a delivered volume of about 700 cc each second that the valve is activated. Unless the Sellick maneuver is used, delivering this volume at a pressure of 50 cm H_2O will almost guarantee gastric insufflation and all the complications resulting from it. Bag-mask ventilation is no better because pressures generated by squeezing the bag may equal or exceed 60 cm H_2O.

Delivered volumes are usually less with bag resuscitators than with FROPVDs. There are two reasons for this. The average resuscitator bag holds only 1,800 cc of gas, which is the absolute limit to the volume that could be delivered if you were able to squeeze the bag completely. Using one hand, the best an average adult can squeeze is approximately 1,200 cc. Most people will squeeze only 800 to 1,000 cc with one hand. The other reason for greater delivered volumes with FROPVDs is that they have a trigger that allows the rescuer to hold a mask on the face with both hands, thus decreasing mask leak. Keep in mind that these volumes, delivered from the ventilating port of these devices, equal the volumes delivered to the patient only if an endotracheal tube is in place. In other words, they do not take into account mask leak. When performing IPPV with a mask, keep the following essentials in mind:

- Supplemental oxygen must be provided for the patient during IPPV.
- Suction must be *immediately* available.
- Ventilation must be done carefully to avoid gastric distention and to reduce the risk of regurgitation and possible aspiration. You can help prevent these complications by using the Sellick maneuver and by timing ventilation with the patient's native respiration.
- Pulse oximetry and end-tidal CO_2 monitoring (capnography) are the most reliable methods of monitoring effectiveness of ventilation. The pulse oximeter measures the oxygen saturation of the blood, and the capnograph measures the CO_2 level. Use the end-tidal CO_2 level to judge whether to increase or decrease the rate of ventilation. If you adjust your respiratory rate to keep the expired CO_2 level between 35 and 45, you can be sure you are neither hypo- nor hyperventilating the patient.

In the case of bag-mask breathing, up to 40% mask leak can be expected. Balloon mask designs can reduce this, and a two-person technique, in which one rescuer holds the mask in place with both hands while a second squeezes the bag, may better ensure adequate delivered volumes. During the stress of an emergency situation, you will tend to ventilate patients at an increased rate. Normal rates should be 10 to 12 times per minute, but if the patient is intubated, the rate usually can be 8 to 10 times per minute. Your pulse oximeter and end-tidal CO_2 monitor are most important in getting the correct rate for each patient.

Compliance

When air, or air containing oxygen, is delivered by positive pressure into the lungs of a patient, the "give," or elasticity, of the lungs and chest wall will influence how easy it will be for the patient to breathe. If you are performing mask ventilation, a normal elasticity of the lungs and chest wall will allow air to enter the glottic opening, and little gastric distention should result. However, if the elasticity is poor, ventilation will be harder to achieve and gastric distention more likely. The ability of the lungs and chest wall to expand and therefore ventilate a patient is known as *compliance*. It is simpler to speak of "good compliance" or "bad compliance" rather than "high" or "low" compliance because the latter terms can be somewhat confusing.

Compliance is an important concept because it governs whether or not you can adequately ventilate a patient. Compliance can become bad (i.e., low) in some disease states of the lung or in patients who have an injury to the chest wall. In cardiac arrest, compliance will become bad due to poor circulation to the muscles. This makes ventilating the patient all the more difficult. With an endotracheal tube in place, the patient's compliance becomes an important clinical sign and may reveal airway problems. Keep in mind that with an endotracheal tube in place and with bag-mask ventilation, you have a kind of "pressure-detection" device much like a tire-pressure gauge. That is, you can "feel" with your fingers and hand a *change* in compliance, either worsening or improving. A worsening of compliance may be the first sign of a tension pneumothorax. Poor compliance also will be felt in right (or left) mainstem bronchus intubation—pulling back on the tube will result in an immediate improvement in the ability to ventilate (i.e., better compliance).

Ventilation Techniques

Mouth-to-Mouth

Mouth-to-mouth ventilation is the most reliable and effective method, with the advantage of requiring no equipment and a minimum of experience and training. Delivered volumes are consistently adequate because mouth seal is effectively and easily maintained. In addition, compliance can be "felt" more accurately, and high oropharyngeal pressures are therefore less likely. This method is almost never used because of the fear of disease transmission. However, it is appropriate for many patients, especially those with whom you are familiar (such as family members). Because of its effectiveness and universal availability, you should be familiar with the technique.

Mouth-to-Mask

Though not quite as effective as mouth-to-mouth ventilation, mouth-to-mask ventilation can overcome the slight danger of disease transmission by interposing a face mask between your mouth and that of the patient. Commercially designed pocket face masks, which fold into a small case that can be carried in your pocket, are particularly suited for the initial ventilation of many types of patients. Some have a side port for supplemental oxygen. Pocket ventilating masks have consistently been shown to deliver larger volumes than bag-mask devices and do so with a greater percentage of oxygen than mouth-to-mouth ventilation. Mouth-to-mask ventilation has significant advantages over bag-mask devices and should be more widely used. (See Chapter 5.)

Flow-Restricted Oxygen-Powered Ventilating Device

In the past, the high-pressure, oxygen-powered ventilators (demand valves) were considered too dangerous to use in multiple-trauma patients. Experience with the newer FROPVDs that meet American Heart Association guidelines (oxygen flow rate of 40 liters per minute at a maximum pressure of 50 ± 5 cm H_2O) suggests that these may now be the equal of bag-mask devices for ventilation (Figure 4-12). They have the advantage of delivering 100% oxygen and allowing use of two hands while using face-mask ventilation. FROPVDs are no worse than bag-masks at producing gastric distention. However, because it is more difficult to feel lung compliance when ventilating with the FROPVD, there is still some controversy about its use. FROPVD ventilation, like bag-mask ventilation, can cause or worsen a pneumothorax. Follow your medical director's advice on the use of an FROPVD.

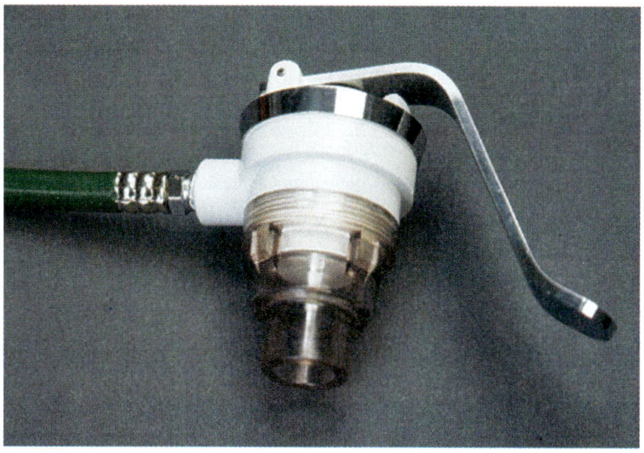

FIGURE 4-12 The flow-restricted oxygen-powered ventilation device. This valve delivers a set flow of 40 liters per minute at maximum pressure of 50 ± 5 cm H_2O. Do not use it unless it meets these standards and your medical director approves.

Bag-Mask Device

The bag-mask, a descendant of the anesthetic bag, is a fixed-volume ventilator with an average delivered volume of about 800 cc of air or oxygen. With a two-handed squeeze, over one liter can be delivered to the patient. It should be used with a reservoir bag or tubing. Plain bag-masks without reservoir bag or tubing can only deliver 40% to 50% oxygen and thus should be replaced with reservoir bags.

The most important problem associated with the bag-mask device is the volume delivered. Mask leak is a serious problem, decreasing the volume delivered to the oropharynx by sometimes 40% or more. In addition, old masks of conventional design have significant dead space beneath them, thus increasing the challenge to provide an adequate volume to the patient. The newer balloon mask has a design that eliminates dead space beneath the mask and provides an improved seal over the nose and mouth. It has been shown in mannequin studies to decrease mask leak and to improve ventilation. It is recommended particularly for trauma patients (Figure 4-13).

A better seal can sometimes be obtained, and larger volumes delivered, in either the balloon or conventional mask, with the use of extension tubing attached to the ventilating port of the bag-mask device. This permits the mask to be better seated on the face without a levering effect from the rigid ventilating port connector that tends to unseat the mask. With the extension in place, the bag can be more easily compressed, even against the knee or thigh, thus increasing the delivered volume and overcoming any mask leak (Figure 4-14). The two-person technique where

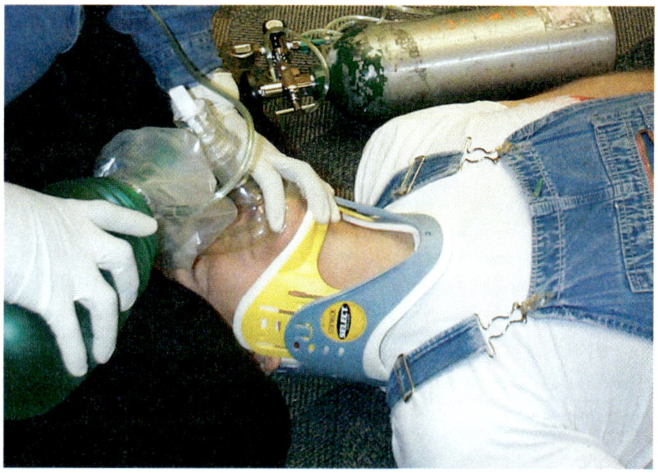

FIGURE 4-13 The inflated balloon mask has been shown to reduce mask leak and provide greater volumes during ventilation with bag-mask devices. *(Courtesy of Buddy Denson, EMT-P)*

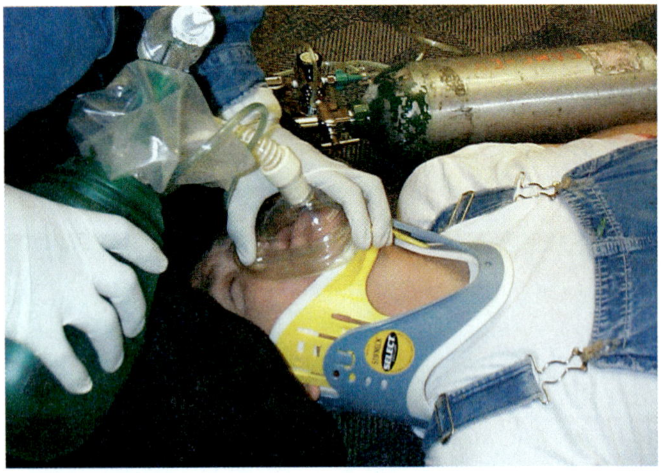

FIGURE 4-14 A ventilating port extension attached to a ventilating bag permits a better mask seal and therefore greater delivered volumes. There is more dead space when using extension tubing, so a higher volume of air must be given. Compressing the bag against the thigh, as shown here, will also increase the delivered volume. *(Courtesy of Buddy Denson, EMT-P)*

one person holds the mask seal and another ventilates is another way to improve ventilations where mask seal is an issue or hand size is small. Capnography should be used to ensure adequate ventilation and prevent inadvertent hyperventilation.

Effective ventilation with a bag-mask requires a high degree of skill and is not without problems. Prehospital personnel must be prepared for situations where mask ventilation is difficult and be able to respond to these challenges. Predictors of difficult mask ventilation can be remembered using the "BOOTS" mnemonic.

B—Beards
O—Obesity
O—Older patients
T—Toothlessness
S —Snores or stridor

All these signs suggest that the patient will not be easy to ventilate. Facial hair and the lack of teeth make mask seal more difficult. Obesity increases both lung and chest compliance. In older patients and in those in whom cervical-spine control is essential, it is more difficult to get proper head and neck positioning. Finally, the presence of snoring or stridor or wheezes should alert the rescuer to the presence of airway obstruction and the need to extend expiratory time for patients with obstructed airway disease.

If unable to ventilate a patient using a bag-mask, the first step should be to reposition the airway by performing an exaggerated head-tilt/chin-lift (if not contraindicated) and an aggressive jaw-thrust. Insert an OPA or NPA. If you are still unsuccessful, the next step is to initiate two-person bag-mask ventilation with extra emphasis on the jaw-thrust maneuver to maximize airway opening. If cricoid pressure is being applied, ease up or release entirely. Consider changing the mask size or type. Continued problems with mask ventilation should prompt the consideration of airway obstruction as a potential cause. Ultimately, the placement of a "rescue" ventilation device (BIAD such as, laryngeal mask airway) or endotracheal tube may be required to definitively ventilate the patient in the worst-case scenario (Figure 4-15).

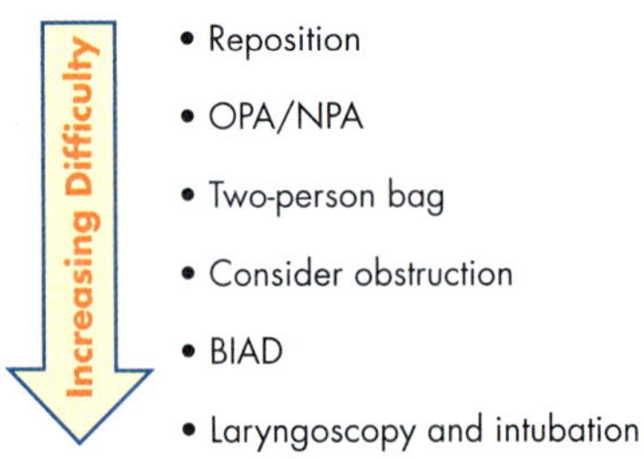

FIGURE 4-15 Response to difficult bag-mask ventilation.

Airway Equipment

The most important rule to follow in regard to airway equipment is that it should be in good working order and immediately available. It will do the patient no good if you have to run back to the ambulance to get the suction apparatus. In other words, be prepared. This is not difficult. Five basic pieces of equipment are necessary for the initial response to all prehospital trauma calls. They are

- Personal protection equipment (See Chapter 1.)
- Long backboard with attached head motion-restriction device
- Appropriately sized rigid cervical extrication collar
- Airway kit (See the following information.)
- Trauma box (See Chapter 1.)

The *airway kit* should be completely self-contained and should contain everything needed to secure an airway in any patient. Equipment now available is lightweight and portable. Oxygen cylinders are aluminum, and newer suction devices are less bulky and lighter. It is no longer acceptable to have suction units that are bulky and stored separately from a source of oxygen. Suction units should be contained in a kit with oxygen and other essential airway tools. A lightweight airway kit should consist of the following (Figure 4-16):

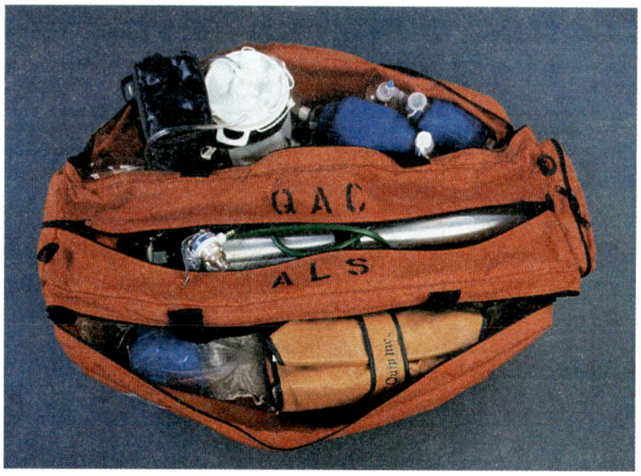

FIGURE 4-16 An airway kit containing the essentials for airway management. Note that portable suction is included in this design. The total weight (with aluminum "D" oxygen cylinder) is approximately 10 kg (22 lb), about the same as a steel "E" cylinder.

- Oxygen D cylinder, preferably aluminum
- Portable battery-powered and hand-powered suction units
- Oxygen cannulae and masks
- Oropharyngeal and nasopharyngeal airways
- Endotracheal intubation kit
- Rescue airway device such as the esophageal tracheal combitube (Combitube®), King LT-D™ airway, intubating laryngeal airway (ILA/air-Q™), or laryngeal mask airway (LMA)
- Bag-mask ventilating device (with reservoir bag)
- Pocket mask with supplemental oxygen intake
- Pulse oximeter
- CO_2 monitor (preferably a waveform capnograph, which allows you to analyze airway problems)
- Translaryngeal oxygen cannula and manual ventilator

The contents of the airway kit are critical. Check all equipment each shift, and have a card attached to be initialed by the person checking it.

CASE PRESENTATION (continued)

An ALS ambulance has been called to a home where there is a "man down." Their scene size-up reveals that the scene is safe, and they are met by a young woman who says her husband was mowing the grass and was stung multiple times by "bees." He is now in the house on the couch, and she says she thinks he is dying.

As the team enters the house, they see a man who appears to be in his 20s. He is lying on the couch and is pale and diaphoretic with audible wheezing. He has swelling of the lips and eyelids.

The team leader begins his initial assessment by introducing the team, while team member 2 prepares to apply a nonrebreather oxygen mask. When questioned about what happened, the man, who is obviously struggling to breathe, is unable to talk. He is beginning to develop some stridor. The wife states he has never had any allergies to medicine or stings and has been stung by wasps before without any serious effects. The team leader, who is unable to feel a peripheral pulse, recognizes that the patient is in anaphylactic shock and is about to lose his airway.

Realizing that is one of the reasons to interrupt the Primary Survey, he has team member 2 immediately give 0.3 mg of 1:1000 epinephrine IM and then start a large-bore IV. The leader immediately opens the airway kit and prepares to perform endotracheal intubation. The patient loses consciousness just as the leader begins the intubation. The leader selects a #7 endotracheal tube because he knows there will be swelling of the larynx. Team member 3 performs the Sellick maneuver, and the leader is able to slide the ET tube through the rapidly closing glottis. By now the IV is running, and he has team member 2 give 50 mg of diphenhydramine and then give a 500-cc bolus of normal saline. The patient is immediately moved to the ambulance, and transport is begun. The patient is given a nebulizer treatment with albuterol en route. The patient improves by the time they arrive at the emergency department and makes a full recovery.

This is an example of an airway problem caused by anaphylactic reaction to a hymenoptera sting (probably from disturbing a yellow jacket nest) that, if not promptly recognized and managed, may require surgical intervention to save the patient's life. ■

Summary

Trauma patients provide the greatest challenge in airway management. To be successful you must have a clear understanding of the anatomy of the airway and be proficient in techniques to open and maintain your patient's airway. You must have the correct equipment organized in a kit that is immediately available when you begin assessment of the trauma patient. To provide adequate ventilation for your patient, you must understand the concepts of tidal volume, minute volume, and lung compliance. Finally, you must become familiar with the various options for monitoring and control of the airway and develop and maintain expertise in performing using them.

Bibliography

1. American College of Emergency Physicians Policy Statement. Verification of endotracheal tube placement. http://www.acep.org/webportal/PracticeResources/PolicyStatements/pracmgt/VerificationofEndotrachealTubePlacement.htm
2. Biebuyck, J. F. 1991. Management of the difficult adult airway. *Anesthesiology* 75: 1087–1110.
3. Donald M. J., B. Paterson. End tidal carbon dioxide monitoring in prehospital and retrieval medicine: a review. 2006. *Emergency Medicine Journal* 23: 728–730.
4. Hüter L., K. Schwarzkopf , J. Rödiger , N. P. Preussler , T. Schreiber. 2009. Students insert the laryngeal tube quicker and more often successful than the esophageal-tracheal combitube in a manikin. *Resuscitation* 80(8): 930–934.

5. International Liaison Committee on Resuscitation. 2005. International Consensus on Cardiopulmonary Resuscitation and Emergency Cardiovascular Care Science with Treatment Recommendations. *Circulation* 112: III-1-III-136.
6. Kober, A., R. Fleischackl, T. Scheck, F. Lieba, H. Strasser, A. Friedmann, D. I. Sessler. 2002. A randomized controlled trial of oxygen for reducing nausea and vomiting during emergency transport of patients older than 60 years with minor trauma. *Mayo Clinical Proceedings* 77: 35–38.
7. Kovacs, G., A. Law. *Airway management in emergency medicine.* New York: McGraw-Hill. In Press. 2007.
8. Langeron, O., E. Masso, C. Huraux, M. Guggiari, A. Bianchi, B. Coriat, et al. 2000. Prediction of difficult mask ventilation. *Anesthesiology* 92(5): 1229–1236.
9. Lecky F., D. Bryden, R. Little, N. Tong and C. Moulton. 2008. Emergency intubation for acutely ill and injured patients. *Cochrane Database of Systematic Reviews* Apr 16(2): CD001429.
10. Mosesso, V. N., K. Kukitsch, et al. 1994. Comparison of delivered volumes and airway pressures when ventilating through an endotracheal tube with bag-valve versus demand-valve. *Prehospital and Disaster Medicine* 9(1): 24–28.
11. O'Connor, R. E., R. A. Swor. 1999. Verification of endotracheal tube placement following intubation. National Association of EMS Physicians Standards and Clinical Practice Committee. *Prehospital Emergency Care* 3: 248–50. [III]
12. Ravussin, P., J. Freeman. 1985. A new transtracheal catheter for ventilation and resuscitation. *Canadian Anaesthesiology Society Journal* 32: 60–64.
13. Robinson, N., M. Clancy. 2001. In patients with head injury undergoing rapid sequence intubation, does pretreatment with intravenous lignocaine/lidocaine lead to an improved neurological outcome? A review of the literature. *Emergency Medicine Journal* 18(6): 453–457.
14. Salem, M. R., A. Y. Wong, M. Mani, et al. 1974. Efficacy of cricoid pressure in preventing gastric inflation during bag-mask ventilation in pediatric patients. *Anesthesiology* 40: 96–98.
15. Sivestri, S., G. Ralls, B. Krauss, et al. 2005. The effectiveness of out-of-hospital use of continuous end-tidal carbon dioxide monitoring on the rate of unrecognized misplaced intubation within a regional emergency medical services system. *Annals of Emergency Medicine* 45(5): 497–503.
16. Stewart, R. D., R. M. Kaplan, B. Pennock, et al. 1985. Influence of mask design on bag-mask ventilation. *Annals of Emergency Medicine* 14: 403–406.
17. Stockinger, Z. T., N. E. McSwain. 2004. Prehospital endotracheal intubation for trauma does not improve survival over bag-valve-mask ventilation. *Journal of Trauma* 56(3): 531–536.
18. Tumpach E. A., M. Lutes, D. Ford, E. B. Lerner. 2009. The King LT versus the Combitube: flight crew performance and preference. *Prehospital Emergency Care* 13(3): 324–328.
19. Ufbert J., J. Bushra, D. Karras, et al. 2005. Aspiration of gastric contents: Association with prehospital intubation. *The American Journal of Emergency Medicine* 23: 379–382.
20. Wang, H., T. Sweeney, R. O'Conner, et al. 2001. Failed prehospital intubations: An analysis of emergency department courses and outcomes. *Prehospital Emergency Care* 5(2): 131–141.

21. White, S. J., R. M. Kaplan, R. D. Stewart. 1987. Manual detection of decreased lung compliance as a sign of tension pneumothorax (abstr). *Annals of Emergency Medicine* 16: 518.

22. Zsolt, T., N. E. McSwain. 2004. Prehospital endotracheal intubation for trauma does not improve survival over bag-valve mask ventilation. *Journal of Trauma* 56: 531–536.

Explore Resource Central

For additional review and practice tests, visit **www.bradybooks.com** and click on Resource Central to access book-specific resources for this text. To access Resource Central, follow directions on the Student Access Card provided with this text. If there is no card, go to www.bradybooks.com and follow the Resource Central link to Buy Access from there.

Airway Skills

Roy L. Alson, PhD, MD
Donna Hastings, MA, EMT-P, CPCC
Bob Page, CCEMT-P, NCEE

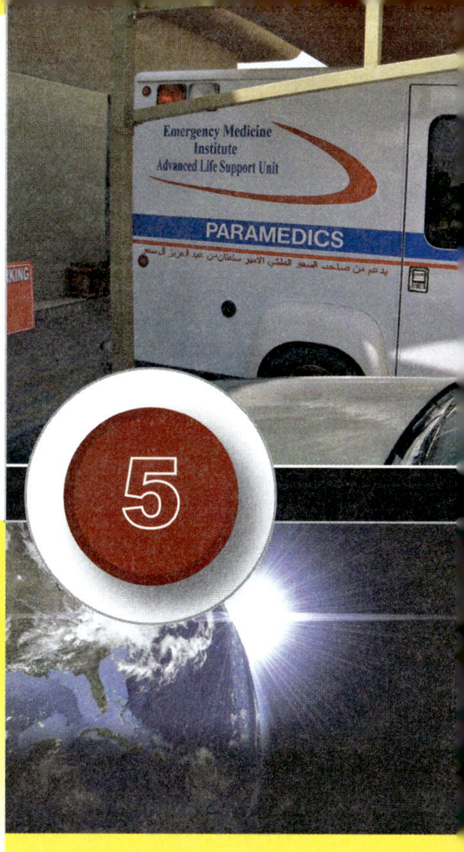

5

Airway Vie Aeree Vía Aérea Voie Respiratoire
Drogi oddechowe Atemweg Dišni put مجرى الهواء
disajni put Dihalna pot Légút

(Photo courtesy of International Trauma Life Support)

OBJECTIVES

Upon successful completion of this chapter, you should be able to:

1. Suction the airway.
2. Insert a nasopharyngeal and oropharyngeal airway.
3. Use the pocket mask.
4. Use the bag-mask.
5. Use the pulse oximeter.
6. Prepare for endotracheal intubation.
7. Perform laryngoscopic orotracheal intubation.
8. Perform nasotracheal intubation.
9. Confirm placement of the endotracheal tube.
10. Use capnography to confirm placement of the endotracheal tube.
11. Anchor the endotracheal tube.

Chapter Overview

Loss of airway is the leading cause of preventable trauma death. It is imperative that emergency personnel know how to assess and manage the airway in the trauma patient. This chapter reviews the necessary skills to open and stabilize the airway of the trauma patient. It is essential that during airway management all team members communicate clearly with each other to ensure a smooth process and successful outcome. One should never be in a "rush" to secure an airway; finesse is often more important than force during airway procedures.

Basic Airway Management

PROCEDURES

Suctioning the Airway

1. Attach the suction connecting tubing to the portable suction machine.
2. Turn the device on and test it.
3. Insert the suction tip through the nose (soft or whistle tip catheter) or mouth (soft or rigid) without activating the suction.
4. Activate the suction and withdraw the suction tube.
5. Repeat the procedure as necessary.

NOTE: Although the intent is to suction foreign matter, air and oxygen also are being suctioned out of the patient. Never suction for greater than 15 seconds. After suctioning, reoxygenate the patient as soon as possible.

Inserting the Nasopharyngeal Airway (NPA)

The nasopharyngeal airway (NPA) is made to go into the right nostril. Avoid use of the NPA if the patient has facial fractures or raccoon eyes. To insert the NPA into the patient's right nostril:

1. Choose the appropriate size. It should be as large as possible but still fit easily through the patient's external nares. The size of the patient's little finger can be used as a rough guide (Figure 5-1).
2. Lubricate the tube with a water-based lubricant.
3. Insert the tube straight back through the right nostril, along the floor of the nose, with the beveled edge of the airway toward the septum.
4. Gently pass it into the posterior pharynx with a slight rotating motion until the flange rests against the nares.

NOTE: If resistance to passage of the NPA is felt, DO NOT FORCE the NPA in, as injury may occur. Remove NPA and attempt insertion in the other nostril. To insert the NPA into the left nostril:

1. Turn the airway upside down so that the bevel is toward the septum.
2. Insert straight back through the nostril until you reach the posterior pharynx.
3. Turn the airway over 180 degrees and insert it down the pharynx.

NOTE: If the tongue is occluding the airway, a jaw thrust or chin lift must be performed to allow the nasopharyngeal airway to go under the tongue.

Inserting the Oropharyngeal Airway (OPA)

1. Choose the appropriate-size OPA. The distance from the corner of the mouth to the lower part of the external ear or to angle of the jaw is a good estimate. The presence of a gag reflex is a contraindication to use of an OPA (Figure 5-2).
2. Open the mouth.
   a. Scissor maneuver
   b. Jaw-lift
   c. Tongue blade
3. Insert the airway gently without pushing the tongue back into the pharynx.
   a. Insert the airway under direct vision using a tongue blade. This is the preferred method and is safe for adults and children.
   b. Insert the airway upside down or sideways and rotate into place after tip of airway passes the tongue. This method should not be used for children.
4. If the OPA causes gagging, remove it and replace it with an NPA.

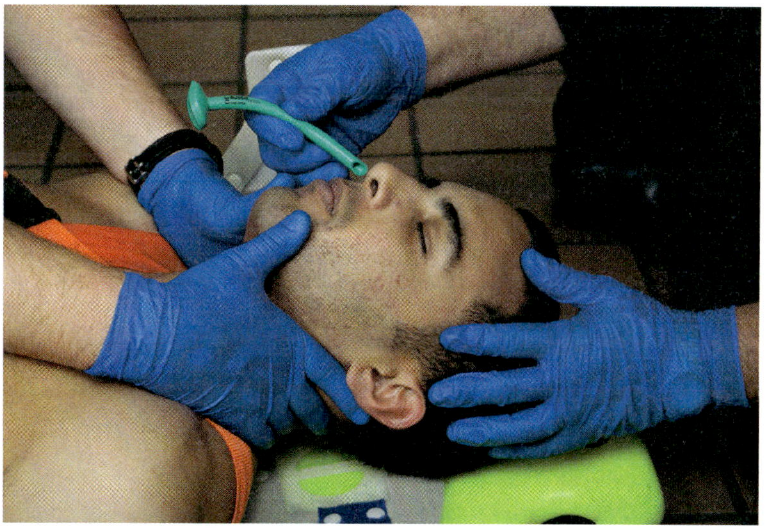

a.

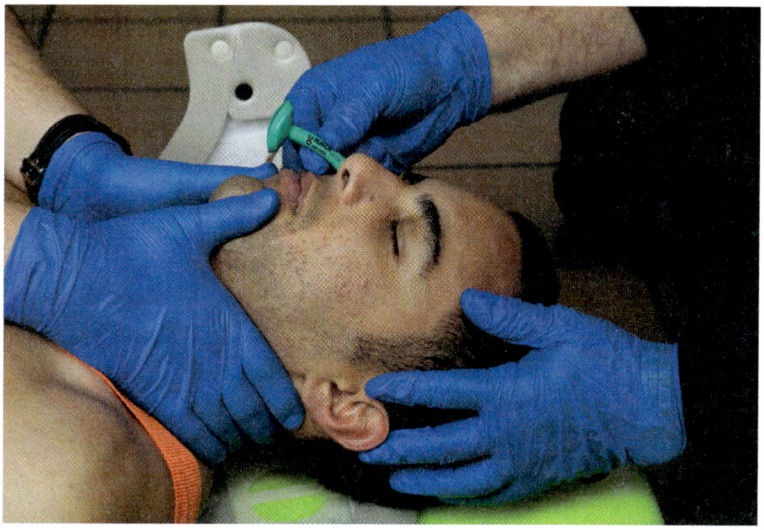

b.

FIGURE 5-1 The nasopharyngeal airway should be the largest size that will easily fit through the external nares. *(Photos courtesy of Lewis B. Mallory, MBA, REMT-P)*

Using a Pocket Mask with Supplemental Oxygen

1. Stabilize the patient's head in a neutral position.
2. Connect the oxygen tubing to the oxygen cylinder and the mask.
3. Open the oxygen cylinder and set the flow rate at 15 liters per minute.
4. Open the mouth.
5. Insert an OPA or NPA, if available. Otherwise use the chin-lift or jaw-thrust maneuver.
6. Place the mask on the face and establish a good seal. Make sure the mask is the proper size for your patient. The mask should cover the nose and mouth and make a good seal (Figure 5-3). Facial hair, lack of teeth, obesity, or advanced age may make it difficult to get a good mask seal.
7. Ventilate mouth-to-mask with enough volume (8–12 cc/kg) to cause adequate chest rise. Ventilate at a rate of 8 to 10 breaths per minute. The inspiratory phase should last 1.5 to 2 seconds. Let the patient exhale for 1.5 to 4 seconds.

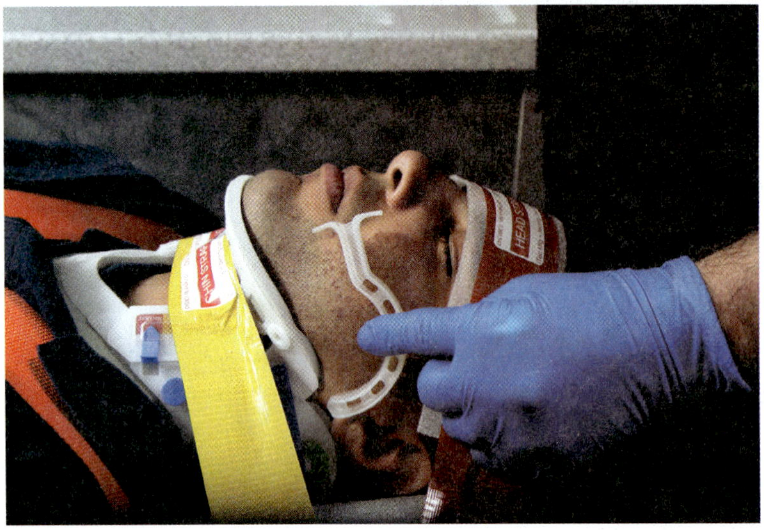

FIGURE 5-2 The distance from the corner of the mouth to the lower part of the external ear or to angle of the jaw is a good estimate for the correct size oropharyngeal airway. *(Courtesy of Lewis B. Mallory, MBA, REMT-P)*

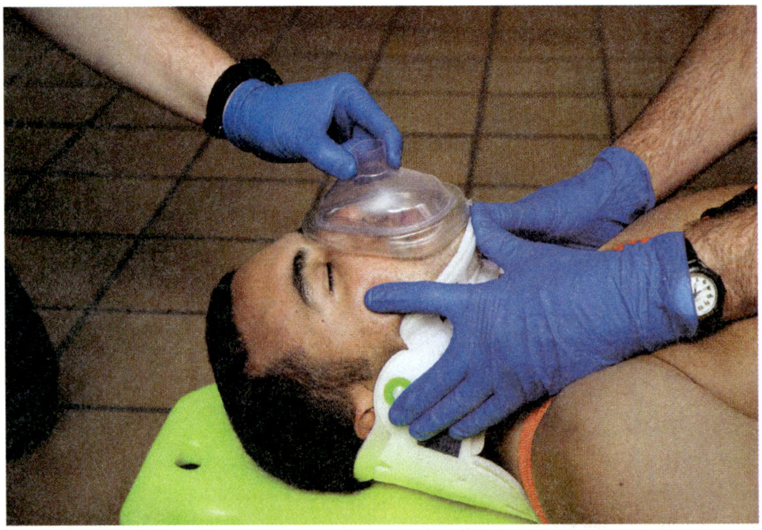

FIGURE 5-3 The mask should cover the nose and mouth and make a good seal. *(Courtesy of Lewis B. Mallory, MBA, REMT-P)*

Using the Bag-Mask

1. Stabilize the patient's head in a neutral position.
2. Connect the oxygen, connecting tubing to the bag-mask system and oxygen cylinder.
3. Attach the oxygen reservoir to the bag-mask.
4. Open the oxygen cylinder and set the flow rate at 12 liters per minute.
5. Select the proper size mask and attach it to the bag-mask device.
6. Open the mouth.
7. Insert an OPA (or an NPA, if the patient has a gag reflex).
8. If available, apply capnography cannula or attach an airway adapter between the bag and the mask.
9. Place the mask on the patient's face and have your partner establish and maintain a good seal. Facial hair, lack of teeth, obesity, or advanced age might make it difficult to get a good mask seal.
10. Using both hands, ventilate with about 10 cc/kg (about 750 cc for an adult) of 100% oxygen at a rate of 8 to 10 breaths per minute. If you are getting good bilateral chest rise, you are giving adequate tidal volume. Use capnography to ensure adequate breathing and prevent inadvertent hyperventilation. As a general rule, keep the end-tidal CO_2 ($ETCO_2$) between 35 and 45 mm Hg.
11. If you are forced to ventilate without a partner, use one hand to maintain a face seal and the other hand to squeeze the bag. This decreases the volume of ventilation because less volume is produced by only one hand squeezing the bag.

The Pulse Oximeter

A pulse oximeter is a noninvasive photoelectric device that measures the arterial oxygen saturation and pulse rate in the peripheral circulation. It consists of a portable monitor and a sensing probe that clips onto the patient's finger, toe, or earlobe (Figure 5-4). The device displays the pulse rate and the arterial oxygen saturation in a percentage value (% SaO_2). This useful device should be used on

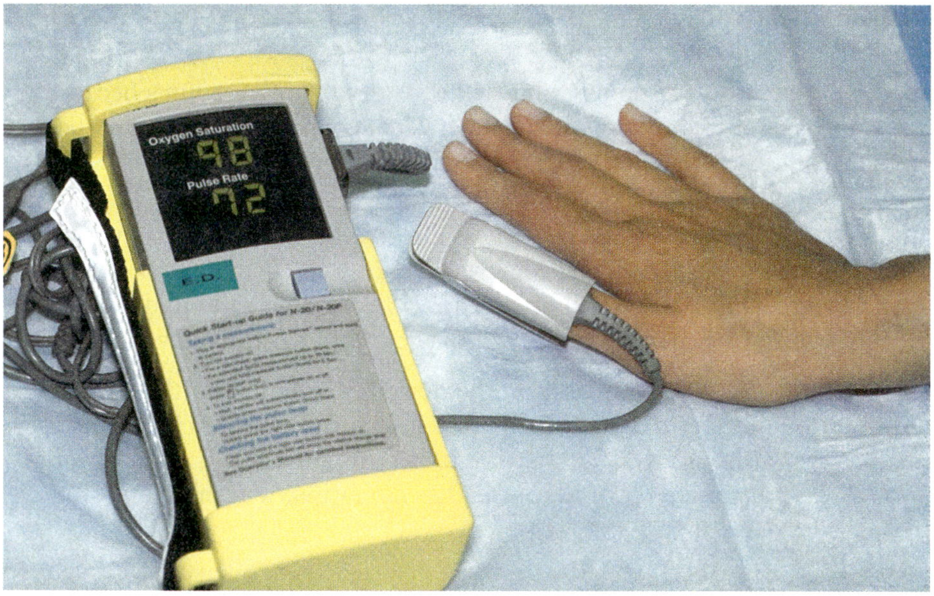

FIGURE 5-4 Portable pulse oximeter. *(Courtesy of David Effron, MD)*

all patients with any type of respiratory compromise. The pulse oximeter is useful to assess the patient's respiratory status, the effectiveness of oxygen therapy, and the effectiveness of bag-mask or flow-restricted oxygen-powered ventilation device (FROPVD) ventilation.

Remember that the device measures percent of SaO_2, not the arterial partial pressure of oxygen (PaO_2). The hemoglobin molecule is so efficient at carrying oxygen that it is 90% saturated (90% SaO_2) when the partial pressure of oxygen is only 60 mm Hg (100 is normal). If you are used to thinking about PaO_2 (where 90–100 mm Hg is normal), then you may be fooled into thinking that an SaO_2 reading (pulse oximeter) of 90% is normal when it is actually critically low. As a general rule, any pulse oximeter reading below 92% is cause for concern and requires some sort of intervention (such as opening the airway, suction, oxygen, assisted ventilation, intubation, decompression of tension pneumothorax). A pulse oximeter reading below 90% is critical and requires immediate intervention to maintain adequate tissue oxygenation. Try to maintain a pulse oximeter reading of 95% or higher. However, do not withhold oxygen from a patient with a pulse oximeter reading above 95% who also shows signs and symptoms of hypoxia or difficulty breathing.

The following are conditions that make the pulse oximeter reading unreliable:

- Poor peripheral perfusion (shock, vasoconstriction, hypotension). Do not attach the sensing probe onto an injured extremity. Try not to use the sensing probe on the same arm that you are using to monitor the blood pressure. Be aware that the pulse oximeter reading will go down while the blood pressure cuff is inflated.
- Severe anemia or exsanguinating hemorrhage
- Hypothermia
- Excessive patient movement
- High ambient light (bright sunlight, high-intensity light on area of the sensing probe)

- Nail polish or a dirty fingernail, if you are using a finger probe. Use acetone to clean the nail before attaching the probe.
- Carbon monoxide poisoning. This will give falsely high readings because the sensing probe cannot distinguish between oxyhemoglobin and carboxyhemoglobin. If carbon monoxide poisoning is suspected, one must use a specific monitor and sensor to measure levels.
- Cyanide poisoning. Cyanide poisons at the cellular level by preventing the cells from using oxygen to make energy. Because the body is using no oxygen, the circulating blood will usually be 95% to 100% saturated. The patient will still be dying from lack of oxygen (at the cellular level).

To use the pulse oximeter, turn on the device, clean the area that you are to monitor (earlobe, fingernail, or toenail), and attach the sensing clip to the area. Remember that although very useful, the pulse oximeter is just another tool to help you assess the patient. Like all tools, it has limitations and should not replace careful physical assessment.

Advanced Airway Management

Preparation for Intubation

Whatever the method of intubation used, both patients and rescuers should be prepared for the procedure. The following equipment is considered basic to all intubation procedures (Figure 5-5):

- *Gloves.* Latex or nitrile examining (not necessarily sterile) gloves should be worn for all intubation procedures.
- *Eye protection.* Providers must wear goggles or face shield.
- *Oxygenation.* All patients should be ventilated by way of a bag-mask or should breathe high-flow oxygen (12 liters per minute) for several minutes

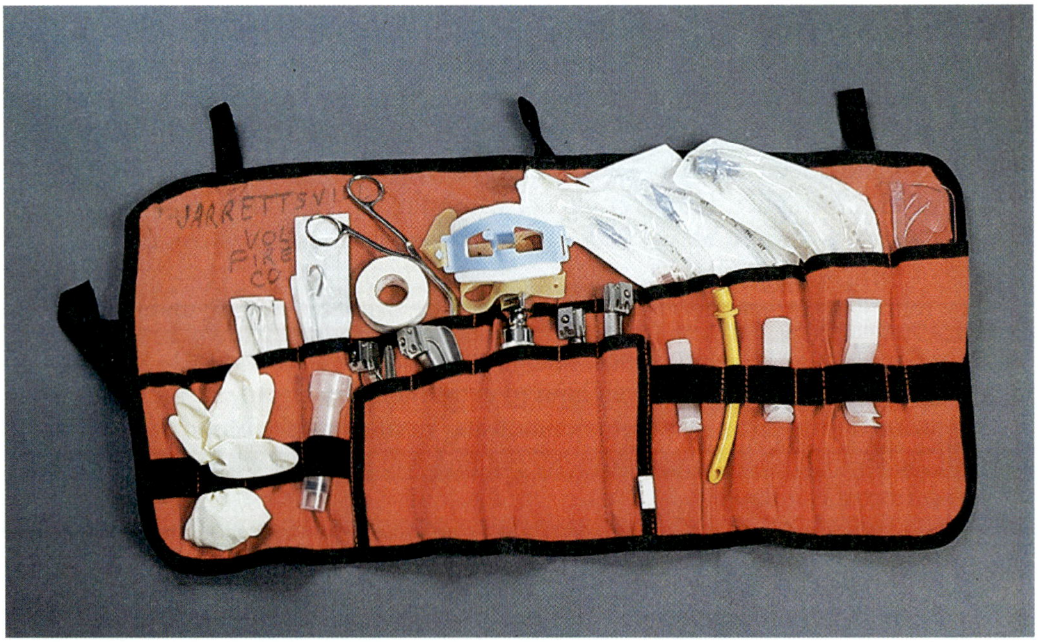

FIGURE 5-5 An intubation wrap contains the essentials for carrying out endotracheal intubation. The kit folds on itself and is compact and portable. When opened, it provides a clean working surface.

prior to the attempt. This will "wash out" residual nitrogen in the lungs and decreases risk of hypoxia during the intubation process

- *Equipment*. Check all equipment, and keep at hand in an organized kit. For laryngoscopic intubation, the endotracheal tube should be held in a "field hockey stick" or open "J" shape by a malleable stylet that is first lubricated and inserted until the distal end is just proximal to the side hole of the endotracheal tube. Check the cuff of the endotracheal tube by inflating it with 10 cc of air. Completely remove the air and leave the syringe filled with air attached to the pilot tube. Lubricate the cuff and distal end of the tube.
- *Capnography*. Have the unit turned on and the waveform visible on the monitor. Record the baseline waveform and CO_2 levels while oxygenating the lungs prior to intubation.
- *Suction*. Suction must be immediately at hand.
- *Assistant*. An assistant should be available to help in the procedure and may apply the Sellick maneuver to reduce gastric insufflation and risk of aspiration, during ventilation and the subsequent intubation attempt. The assistant also may help hold the head and neck in a neutral position or perform external laryngeal manipulation to help make the cords visible to the intubator. Some intubators prefer the assistant to count aloud to 30 during the intubation procedure. You may prefer to simply hold your breath (when you need to breathe, the patient really needs a breath) while performing intubation.
- *Lidocaine*. Topical lidocaine sprayed into the posterior pharynx before intubation attempts can decrease the adverse cardiovascular and intracranial pressure effects of the intubation procedure.

Laryngoscopic Orotracheal Intubation

For laryngoscopic orotracheal intubation, the upper airway and the glottic opening are visualized, and the tube is slipped gently through the cords. The advantages of this method include the ability to see obstructions and to visualize the accurate placement of the tube. It has the disadvantage of requiring a relatively relaxed patient without anatomic distortion and with minimal bleeding or secretions.

The equipment needed for a laryngoscopic orotracheal intubation includes the following:

- Straight (Miller) or curved (Macintosh) blade and laryngoscope handle, all in good working order (checked daily)
- Transparent endotracheal tube, 28 to 33 cm in length and 7, 7.5, or 8 mm in internal diameter for the adult patient
- Stylet to help mold the tube into a field hockey stick shape
- Water-soluble lubricant—no need for it to contain a local anesthetic
- 10 or 12 cc syringe
- Magill forceps
- Tape and tincture of benzoin or endotracheal tube holder
- Suction equipment in good working order
- Pulse oximeter and capnography unit
- If available, a bougie (tracheal tube introducer) for difficult intubations

PROCEDURE

Laryngoscopic Orotracheal Intubation

Intubation in the trauma patient differs from usual endotracheal intubation in that the patient's neck must be stabilized in the neutral position during the procedure. This does make it more difficult to visualize the vocal cords during laryngoscopy. After ventilation and initial preparations, the following steps should be carried out (Figure 5-6; Scan 5-1):

1. An assistant stabilizes the head and neck, performs the Sellick maneuver, and counts slowly aloud to 30 (at your request).
2. In the supine patient, lift the chin and slide the blade into the right side of the patient's mouth. Push the tongue to the left and "inch" the blade down along the tongue in an attempt to see the epiglottis. A key maneuver must be performed here: The blade must pull forward (up) on the tongue to lift up the epiglottis and bring it into view.
3. Use the laryngoscope blade to lift the tongue and epiglottis up and forward in a straight line. "Levering" the blade is a common error novices make and can result in broken teeth and other trauma. The laryngoscope is essentially a "hook" to lift the tongue and epiglottis up and out of the way so that the glottic opening can be identified. Remember that the Miller (straight) blade is used to lift the epiglottis directly, whereas the Macintosh (curved) blade is inserted into the vallecula and lifts the epiglottis indirectly.

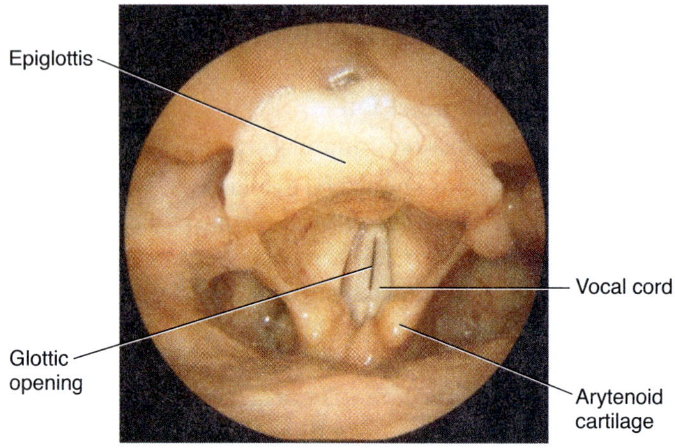

FIGURE 5-6 Landmarks during intubation.

4. Advance the tube along the right side of the oropharynx once the epiglottis is seen. When the glottic opening (or even just the arytenoid cartilages) is identified, pass the tube through to a depth of about 5 cm beyond the cords.
5. While the tube is still held firmly, remove the stylet, inflate the cuff, attach a bag-mask, and check the tube for placement using the immediate confirmation protocol given in the paragraphs that follow.
6. Begin ventilation using adequate oxygen concentration and tidal volume. Maintain an $ETCO_2$ level between 35 and 45 mm Hg. In the rare case where the patient has a closed head injury with elevated intracranial pressure (ICP) and meets criteria for hyperventilation (see Chapter 10), then $ETCO_2$ levels should be titrated between 30 and 35 mm Hg

For difficult intubations where you cannot see the cords or where the angle is such that it is difficult to get the tube through the cords, a bougie or tracheal tube introducer can be very helpful (Scan 5-2). Insert the bougie through the cords and then slip the tube over the bougie and slide it down through the cords. This technique works best when the intubator keeps the blade inserted and the assistant threads the ET tube on to the bougie and holds the end of the bougie. The intubator then threads the ET tube down the bougie through the cords. By maintaining direct visualization, the chance of the ET tube becoming caught on the tongue or epiglottis is reduced. Then remove the bougie and perform steps 5 and 6 listed earlier.

If still having difficulty visualizing the vocal cords, the intubator must take his right hand and, using gentle pressure, manipulate the thyroid (laryngeal) cartilage to bring the vocal cords into view. This process is known as *external laryngeal manipulation (ELM)*. The assistant is then instructed to maintain the positioning of the cartilage, and the intubator passes the tube.

SCAN 5-1 Orotracheal Intubation

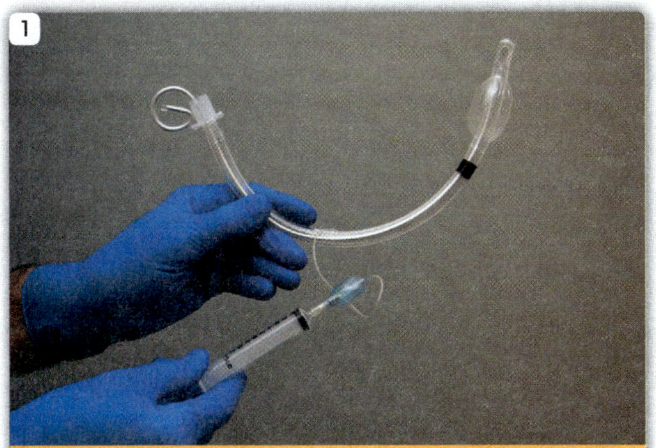

1 Assemble, prepare, and test all equipment. *(Courtesy of Lewis B. Mallory, MBA, REMT-P)*

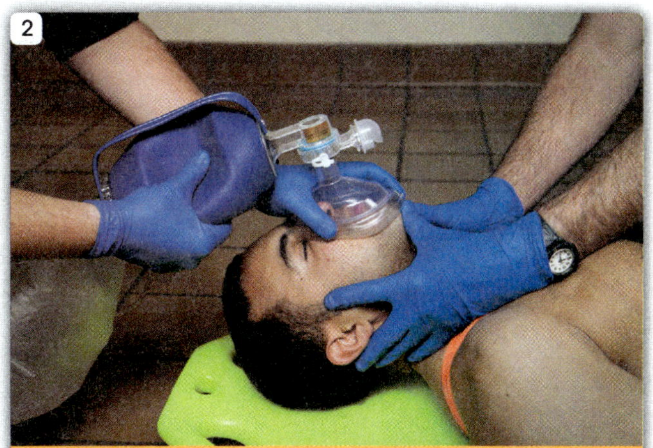

2 Position the patient's head and ventilate him with 100% oxygen. Do not hyperventilate. *(Courtesy of Lewis B. Mallory, MBA, REMT-P)*

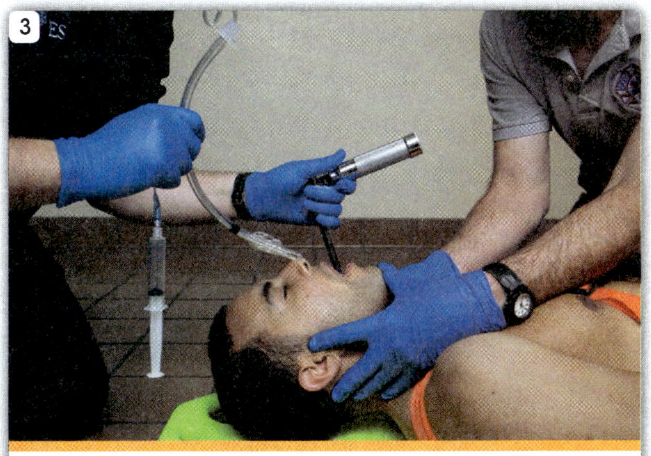

3 Insert the laryngoscope blade. *(Courtesy of Lewis B. Mallory, MBA, REMT-P)*

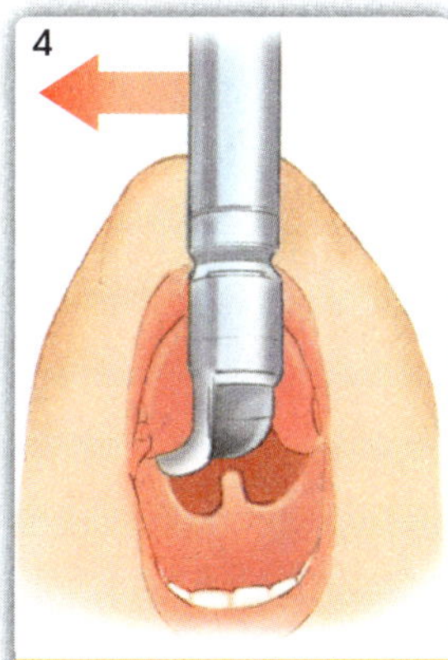

4 Lift the tongue and epiglottis to bring the glottic opening into view.

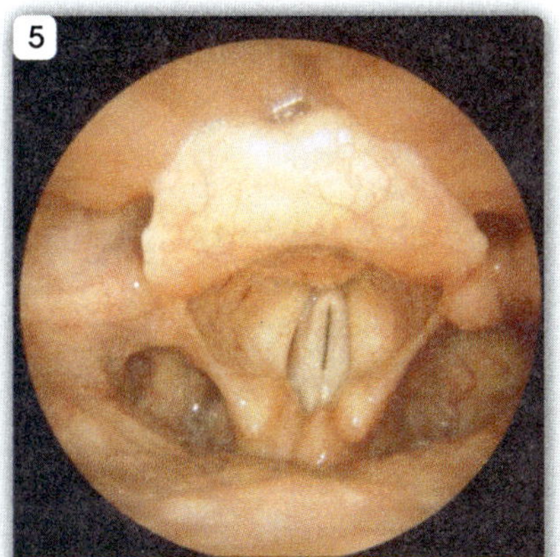

5 Visualize the cords and glottic opening, and insert the ET tube with stylet through the cords.

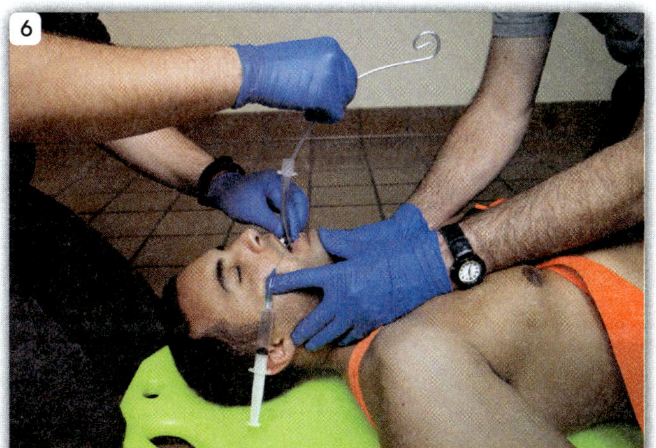

6 When the tube is in place and firmly held, remove the stylet. *(Courtesy of Lewis B. Mallory, MBA, REMT-P)*

(*Continued on next page*)

SCAN 5-1 Continued

7

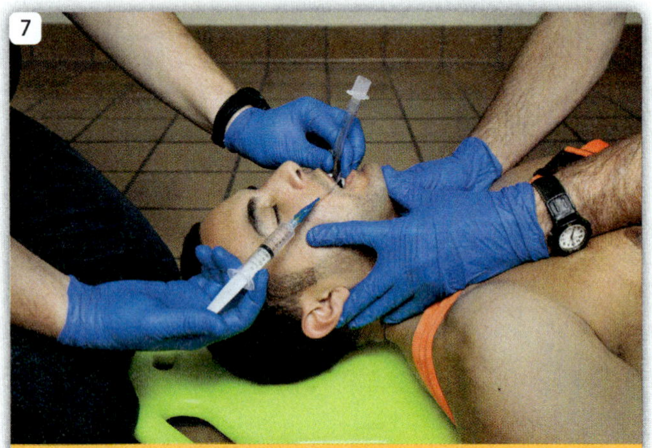

Continuing to hold tube firmly, inflate the cuff with 5 to 10 cc of air. *(Courtesy of Lewis B. Mallory, MBA, REMT-P)*

8a

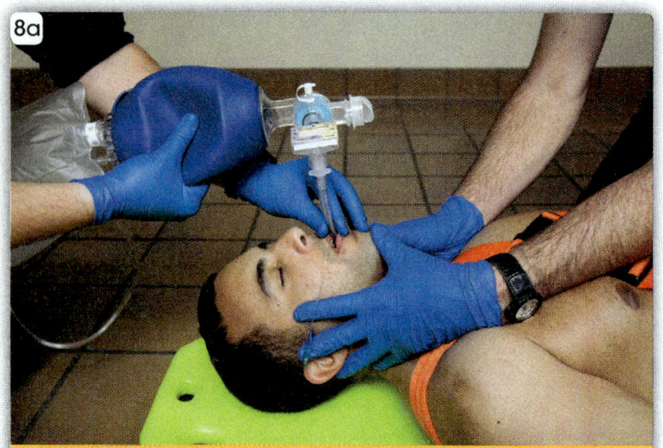

If capnography is not available, begin ventilation with colorimetric CO_2 detector. *(Courtesy of Lewis B. Mallory, MBA, REMT-P)*

8b

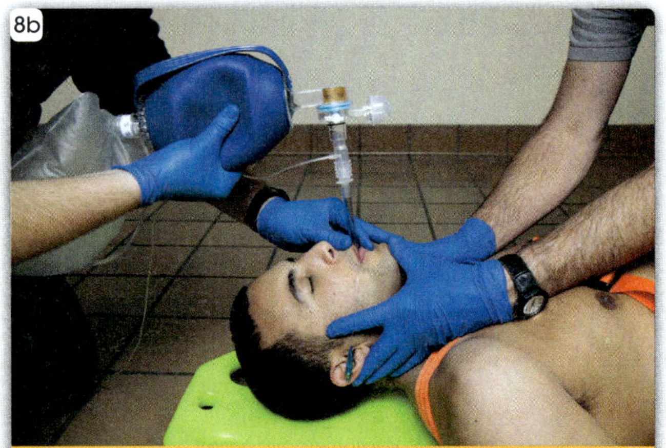

If capnography is available, begin ventilation with capnography monitor. *(Courtesy of Lewis B. Mallory, MBA, REMT-P)*

9

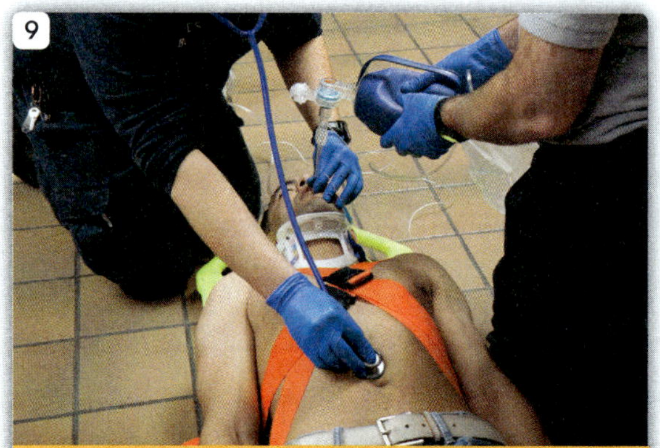

Perform manual confirmation of tube position using a stethoscope. *(Courtesy of Lewis B. Mallory, MBA, REMT-P)*

10a

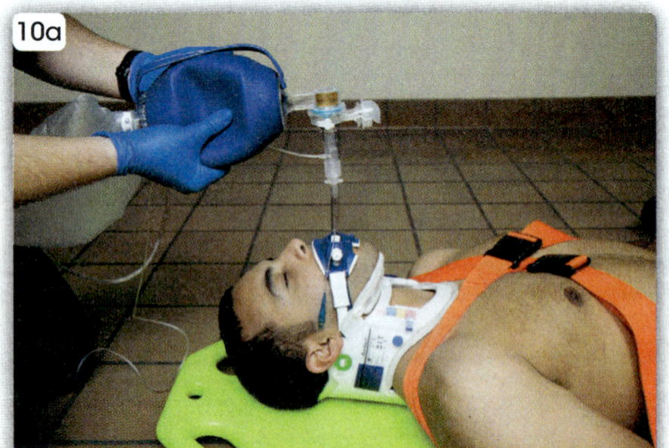

Secure the tube in place and continue ventilating. *(Courtesy of Lewis B. Mallory, MBA, REMT-P)*

10b

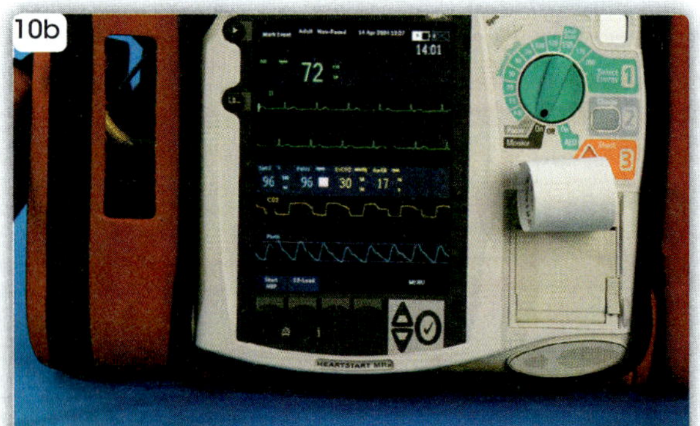

Monitor with capnography, if it is available. *(Courtesy of Lewis B. Mallory, MBA, REMT-P)*

SCAN 5-2 Orotracheal Intubation Using Bougie

1

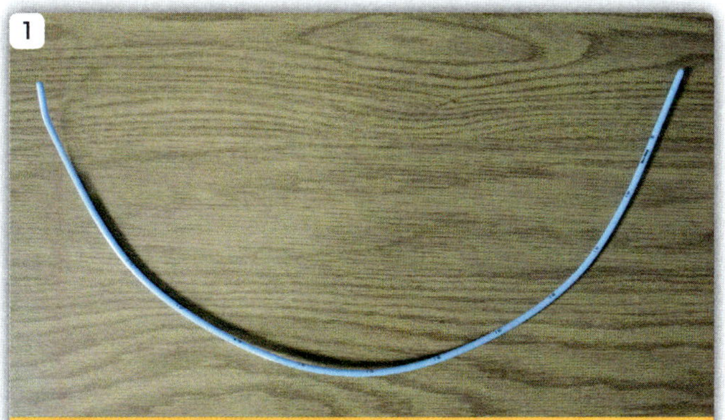

Bougie. *(Courtesy of Stanley Cooper, EMT-P)*

2

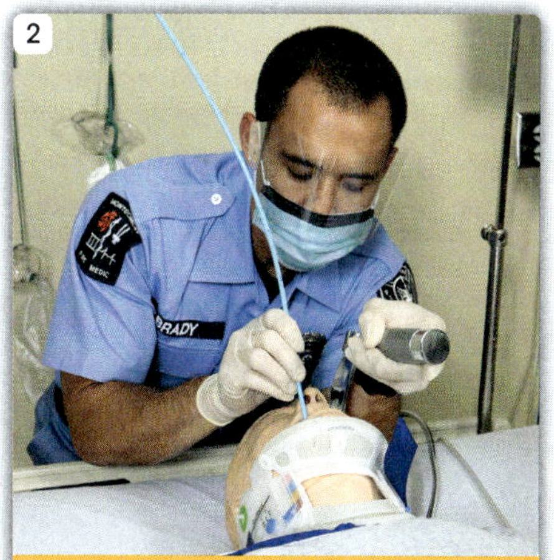

Inserting the bougie into the trachea. *(Courtesy of Stanley Cooper, EMT-P)*

3

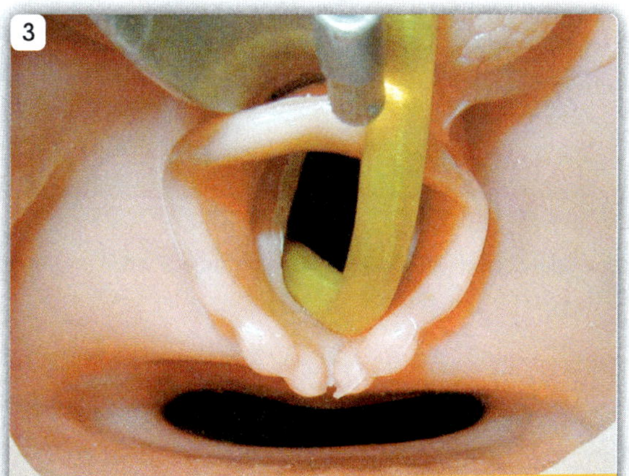

The bougie going between the cords and through the glottic opening. *(Courtesy of Roy Alson, MD)*

4

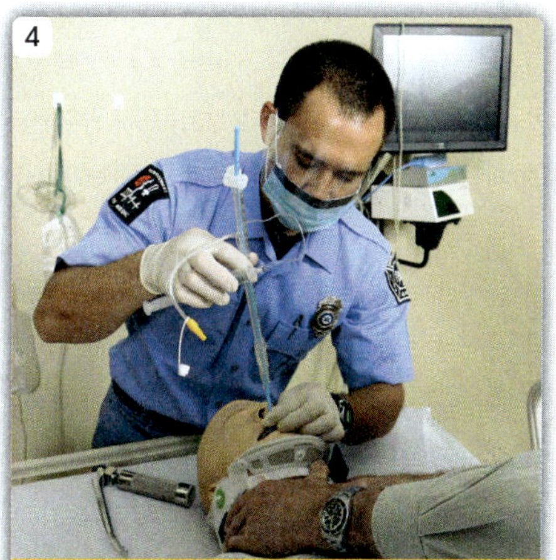

While holding bougie firmly, slide the ET tube over the bougie and into the trachea. *(Courtesy of Stanley Cooper, EMT-P)*

5

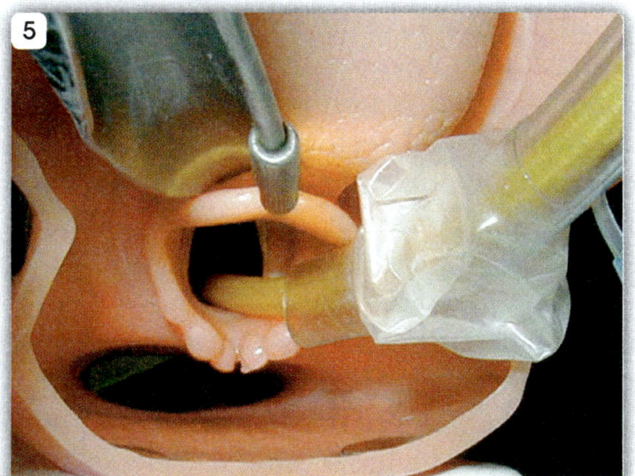

Sliding the ET tube down the bougie and through the cords. *(Courtesy of Roy Alson, MD)*

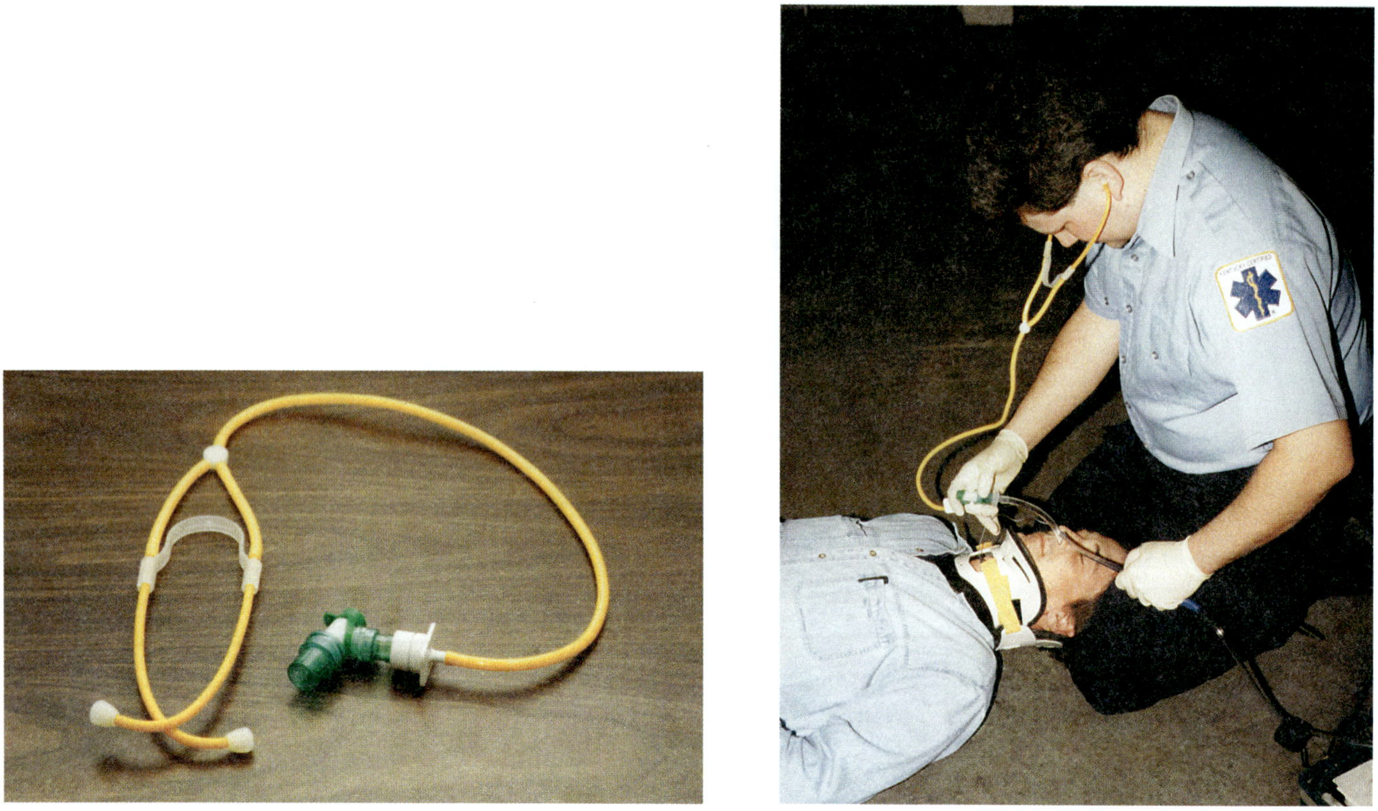

a. b.

FIGURE 5-7 (a) Example of a commercial nasotracheal tube auscultation device (Burden nasoscope) used to (b) better hear breath sounds while inserting the nasotracheal tube. *(Photos courtesy of Brant Burden, EMT-P)*

Nasotracheal Intubation

The nasotracheal route of endotracheal intubation in a prehospital setting may be justified when you cannot open the adult patient's mouth because of clenched jaws and when you cannot ventilate the patient by other means. The disadvantages of this method are its relative difficulty, depending as it does on the appreciation of the intensity of the breath sounds of spontaneously breathing patients, the longer duration to achieve intubation, and the need for the patient to be breathing on his own. It is a blind procedure and as such requires extra skill and care to successfully perform proper intratracheal placement. With the advent of pharmacologically assisted intubation, this technique is being used less frequently. Facial fractures, head injury, and a patient who is taking anticoagulants are all relative contraindications to using nasotracheal intubation.

Guidance of the tube through the glottic opening is a question of you perceiving the intensity of the sound of the patient breathing out. You can, with some difficulty, guide the tube toward the point of maximum intensity and slip it through the cords. You can hear and feel the breath sounds better with your ear placed against the proximal opening of the tube. Commercial adaptors are now available to do this without contaminating yourself or your equipment (Figure 5-7).

The success of this method also will depend on an anterior curve to the tube that will prevent its passing into the esophagus. Prepare two tubes prior

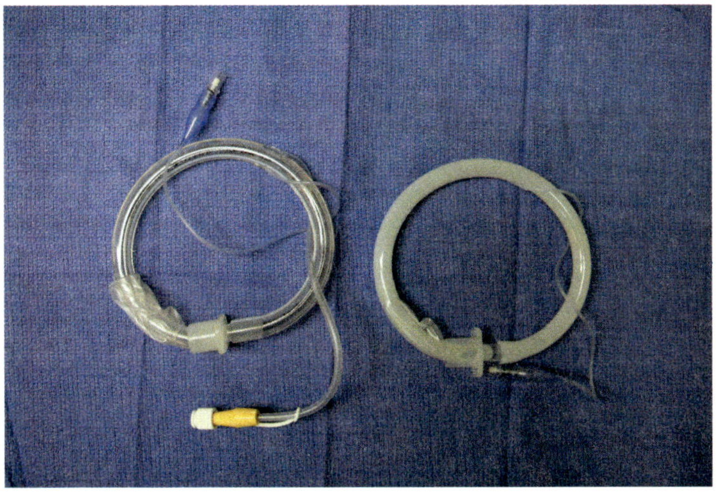

FIGURE 5-8 Prepare a tube for nasotracheal intubation by inserting the distal end of a 7-mm tube into its proximal opening, thus molding it into a formed circle. *(Courtesy of Stanley Cooper, EMT-P)*

to carrying out the intubation attempt. Insert the distal end of the 7-mm tube into its proximal opening, thus molding it into a formed circle (Figure 5-8). Preparing two tubes allows the immediate use of the second, more rigid tube should the first plastic tube become warm with body temperature, thus losing its anterior curve. Some commercial endotracheal tubes can be made to assume this curved shape by pulling on an embedded nylon cord (Figure 5-9). Displacing the tongue and jaw forward also can help in achieving placement because this maneuver lifts the epiglottis anteriorly out of the way of the advancing tube.

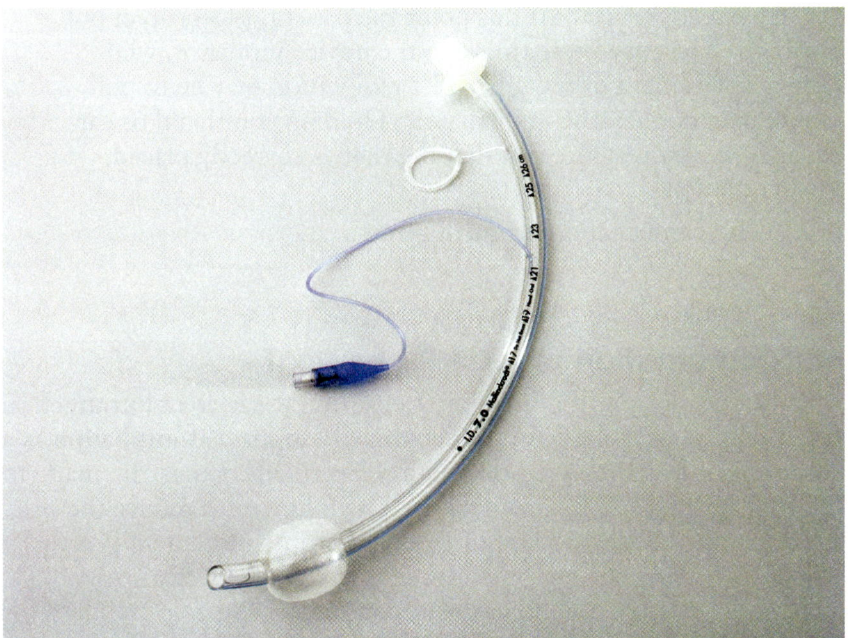

FIGURE 5-9 Commercial ET tube made for performing nasotracheal intubation. *(Image used with permission from Nellcor Puritan Bennett LLC, Boulder, Colorado, doing business as Covidien)*

PROCEDURES

Face-to-Face Intubation

On occasion the location of the victim may prevent access to his head to allow for intubation from the conventional position. A "face-to-face" approach (also called the "tomahawk method") has been described and used successfully. Using this method, the intubator faces the patient and usually utilizes the Macintosh (curved) laryngoscope blade. An assistant maintains neutral position of the cervical spine, if possible. The intubator holds the laryngoscope in his hand with the blade end of the handle emerging from the thumb side of the fist, so that the blade can "hook" the tongue.

Preparation of equipment is as previously mentioned, including having suction immediately available. Entering from the right side of the mouth, the tongue is swept to the left of the mouth, and the jaw and tongue are pulled toward the intubator, allowing for visualization of the larynx and insertion of the ET tube. This technique is very effective with patients in a seated position, such as one trapped in a motor vehicle. It also can be used with morbidly obese patients on whom the intubator is not able to generate sufficient leverage to move the jaw forward.

Nasotracheal Intubation

1. Perform routine preparation procedures.
2. Lubricate the cuff and distal end of a 7-mm or 7.5-mm endotracheal tube. With the bevel against the floor or septum of the nasal cavity, slip the tube distally through the largest naris. Insert along the floor of the nasal cavity at a 90-degree angle to the face.
3. When the tube tip reaches the posterior pharyngeal wall, take great care on "rounding the bend," and then direct the tube toward the glottic opening.
4. By watching the neck at the laryngeal prominence, you can judge the approximate placement of the tube. Tenting of the skin on either side of the prominence indicates that the tube is caught up in the pyriform fossa, a problem solved by slight withdrawal and rotation of the tube to the midline. Bulging and anterior displacement of the laryngeal prominence usually indicate that the tube has entered the glottic opening and has been correctly placed. At this point the patient, especially if not deeply comatose, will cough, strain, or both. This may be alarming to the novice intubator, who might interpret this as laryngospasm or misplacement of the tube. The temptation may be to pull the tube and ventilate because the patient may not breathe immediately. Holding your hand or ear over the opening of the tube to detect airflow may reassure you that the tube is correctly placed, and you may inflate the cuff and begin ventilation.
5. Confirm tube placement using the immediate confirmation protocol given next.

Immediate Confirmation of Tube Placement

One of the greatest challenges of intubation is ensuring the correct intratracheal placement of endotracheal tubes. An unrecognized esophageal intubation is a lethal complication of this lifesaving procedure. Every effort must be made to avoid this catastrophe, and a strict protocol must be followed to reduce the risk.

Although the most reliable method of ensuring proper placement is actually visualizing the tube passing through the glottic opening, even this is not 100% sure. In fact it is only reliable for the moment you see it. The gold standard for confirming and monitoring endotracheal tube placement is waveform capnography. (See later discussion.) If you do not have capnography available, the following protocol can be used but is not reliable. When you use this protocol, you should recognize the unreliable nature of auscultation as the sole method of confirming intratracheal placement. Correct intratracheal placement should be suspected from the following initial signs:

- An anterior displacement of the laryngeal prominence is visible as the tube is passed distally.
- There is coughing, bucking, or straining on the part of the patient. Note: Phonation—any noise made with the vocal cords—is absolute evidence that the tube is in the esophagus, and the tube should be removed immediately.
- There is normal compliance with bag ventilation. (The bag does not suddenly "collapse," but rather there is some resilience to it and resistance to lung inflation.)
- No cuff leak is seen after inflation. (Persistent leak indicates esophageal intubation until proven otherwise.)
- Adequate chest rise occurs with each ventilation.
- There is breath condensation on the tube with each ventilation—not a very reliable method.

The following procedure should then be carried out immediately to prove correct placement.

PROCEDURES

Immediate Confirmation of Tube Placement

1. Auscultate three sites as shown in Figure 5-10.
   a. Epigastrium—the most important—should be silent, with no sounds heard.
   b. Right and left midaxillary lines
2. Inspect for full movement of the chest with ventilation.
3. Check position using suction bulb or syringe AKA esophageal detector device (EDD) or one of the CO_2 detecting devices.
4. Watch for any change in the patient's skin color or in the pulse oximeter reading. Also observe the ECG monitor for changes.

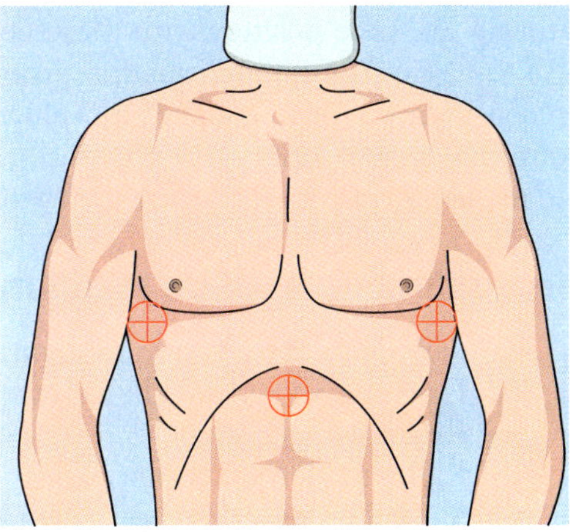

FIGURE 5-10 Sites to auscultate when performing immediate confirmation of ET tube placement.

Commercial suction bulbs or EDDs have been used for confirmation of tube placement (Figure 5-11). Recent research suggests that they are less reliable than capnography, which has become the gold standard for confirming initial tube placement. (Capnography is the best method for confirming ET placement and allows for constant monitoring of tube position.) To use a bulb detector, squeeze the bulb and insert the end into the 15-mm adapter on the endotracheal tube. Do this before you inflate the cuff on the ETT. Release the bulb. If the tube is in the trachea, the bulb will expand immediately. If the tube is in the esophagus, the bulb will remain collapsed. If you are using the EDD, you will be able to withdraw the EDD syringe plunger easily if the tube is in the trachea, but you will not be able to withdraw the plunger if the tube is in the esophagus. Note: Literature about those devices warn that patients with obstructed airway diseases, congestive heart failure, obesity, or right mainstem intubation may have a false reading due to decreased air available for aspiration.

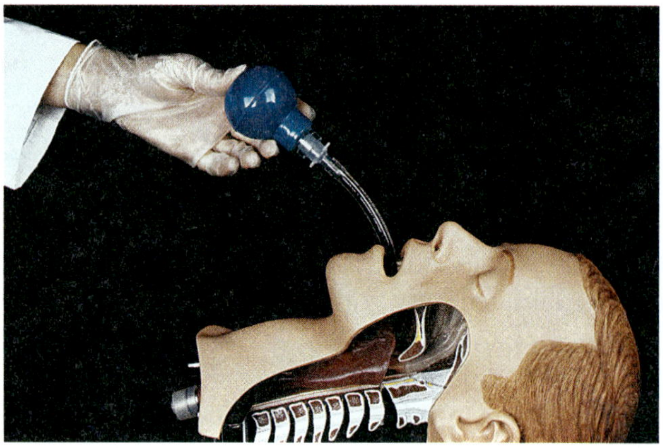

a.

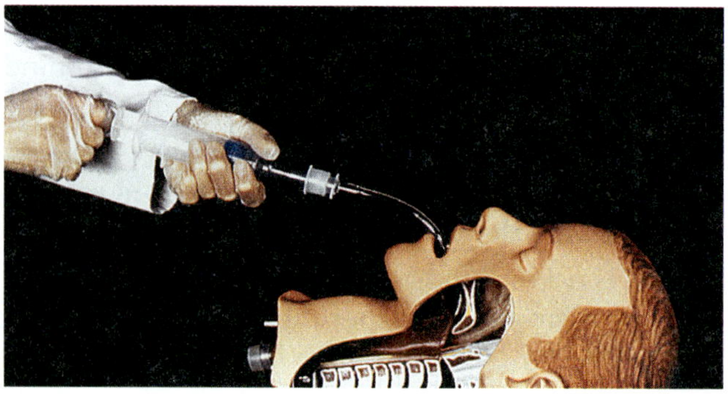

b.

FIGURE 5-11 (a) Esophageal intubation detector device, bulb style. (b) Esophageal intubation detector device, syringe style.

Commercial CO_2 detectors also are available to attach in-line between the endotracheal tube and the bag-mask or FROPVD. Three different kinds are available:

- Qualitative (colorimetric) CO_2 detectors
- Quantitative CO_2 monitors
- Quantitative waveform CO_2 monitors

(See the detailed discussion of the monitors in the following section, "Using Capnometry and Capnography to Confirm and Monitor ET Tube Position.")

Apply the protocol for confirmation of tube placement immediately following intubation. If you are using a quantitative CO_2 monitor or quantitative waveform CO_2 monitor, then you may continue monitoring ET tube position with those devices. If you are not using one of those devices, then repeat the ET tube position reconfirmation protocol after several minutes of ventilation. Thereafter, repeat the reconfirmation protocol after movement of the patient from the ground to the stretcher, after loading onto the ambulance, when you perform the ITLS Secondary Survey and ITLS Ongoing Exam, and immediately prior to arrival at the hospital.

Reconfirming ET Tube Position

1. Auscultate the sites shown in Figure 5-12.
   a. Epigastrium—should be silent with no sounds heard.
   b. Right and left apex
   c. Right and left midaxillary lines
   d. Sternal notch—"tracheal" sounds should be readily heard here.
2. Inspect the chest for full movement of the chest with ventilation.
3. Gently palpate the tube cuff in the sternal notch while compressing the pilot balloon between the index finger and thumb. A pressure wave should be felt in the sternal notch.
4. Use adjuncts such as CO_2 detectors (or a suction bulb, if part of local protocol) to help confirm placement.

Any time placement is still in doubt despite the preceding protocol, visualize directly or remove the tube. Never assume that the tube is in the right place—always be sure and record that the protocol has been carefully followed.

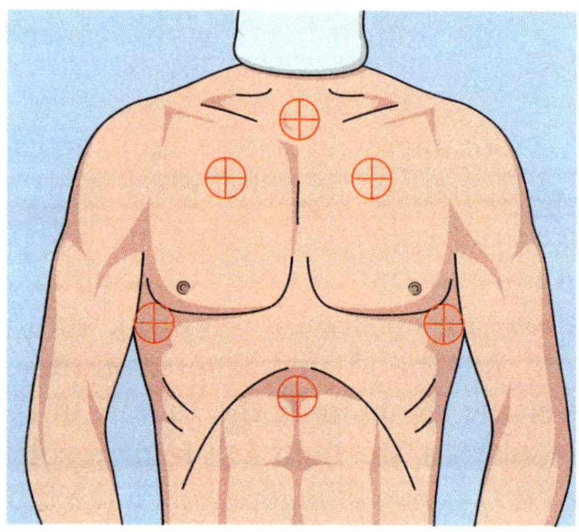

FIGURE 5-12 Sites to auscultate when performing reconfirmation of ET tube placement.

Using Capnometry and Capnography to Confirm and Monitor ET Tube Position

Capnometry represents a major clinical upgrade in the assessment and monitoring of the ventilatory status of the patients. It is important for you to understand the differences between simple detection of $ETCO_2$ called *colorimetric* or *qualitative capnometry*, *quantitative capnometry* (a value without a waveform), and the most useful and diagnostic form known as *quantitative waveform capnography*.

Colorimetric CO_2 detectors (qualitative capnometry) are simple devices designed to detect $ETCO_2$ (Figure 5-13). They do not accurately measure the amount of CO_2. Typically, the devices use a special piece of "litmus paper" that changes color from purple to yellow as it detects CO_2. If a device of this type is used as a confirming device, you must be aware of the following:

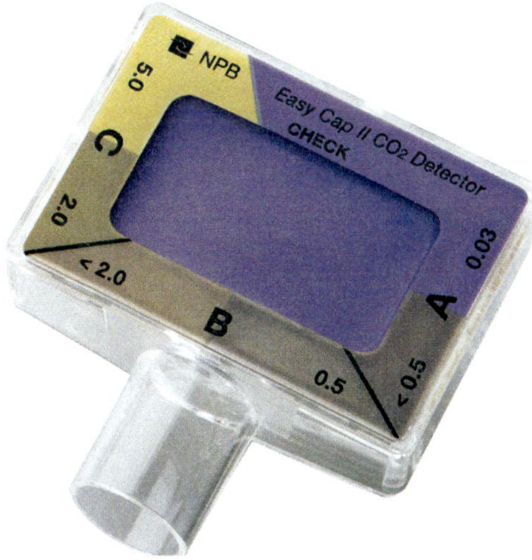

FIGURE 5-13 Colorimetric CO_2 detector. *(Image used by permission from Nellcor Puritan Bennett LLC, Boulder, Colorado, doing business as Covidien)*

- It may not be accurate in poor perfusion states, such as shock or cardiac arrest, due to very small amounts of CO_2 returning to the lungs. In those cases, another confirming device is necessary. In cases of cardiac arrest, best results will be obtained if good compressions are being done at the time the device is used.
- You must bag six breaths through it before using it to confirm the CO_2 as being from the trachea. It is a fact that CO_2 can be detected from the esophagus, and it would take about six breaths to purge it.
- If the device gets wet, it will not be useful.
- Once intubated, the device can be used for spot checks only because it will stay yellow after a few minutes of continuous use, not changing colors with each breath.
- Because the device only detects $ETCO_2$, but does not measure it, it cannot be used as a monitor of ventilation.

Quantitative capnometry actually measures the amount of CO_2 in expired air ($ETCO_2$). More than just detection, the device can be used to monitor the adequacy of ventilations and help the provider to accurately "titrate" the $ETCO_2$ levels in patients where CO_2 levels are critical, such as those with closed head injuries. They are often combined with a pulse oximeter. Quantitative capnometry refers to $ETCO_2$ measurement without a waveform. If the devices are used to confirm tube placement, you must be aware of the following limitations:

- In poor perfusion states or arrest, the numbers will be very low and may take up to 30 seconds to display a number. If this is the case, it may not be useful to initially confirm tube position. Rather, it could be used to monitor the tube after that.
- As in colorimetric devices, they also can detect esophageal CO_2, so six breaths are necessary to actually confirm tracheal CO_2.
- In cases of cardiac arrest, best results are obtained if good compressions are being performed while the device is being used.

Quantitative waveform capnography is the ultimate confirmation device and is a standard of care in surgical suites and many EMS systems. The devices not only detect and measure the $ETCO_2$, but they also provide you with a diagnostic waveform that can confirm (by the shape of the waveform)

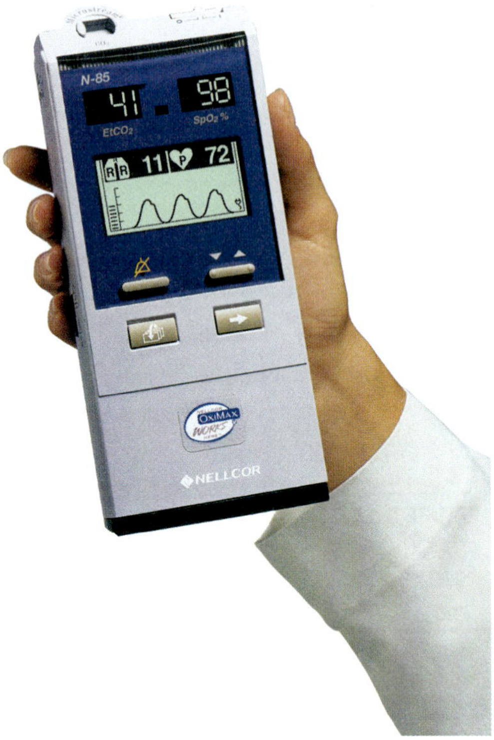

FIGURE 5-14 Quantitative waveform CO_2 monitor incorporated into cardiac monitor. *(Image used by permission from Nellcor Puritan Bennett LLC, Boulder, Colorado, doing business as Covidien)*

endotracheal placement even in low perfusion states. The waveforms will appear within two seconds of the actual breath. Furthermore, the devices can be built into existing cardiac monitors, which will allow you to continuously monitor the waveform and value (Figure 5-14). They also will allow you to print out a real-time waveform that is time and date stamped for absolute documentation of correct tube placement. Capnography has many other uses in nonintubated patients, including perfusion monitor, airway monitor, and ventilation monitor.

In using capnography to confirm endotracheal tube placement, you must be aware of the following limitations:

- Like all CO_2 detection devices, low perfusion states will result in low CO_2 readings and subsequently small waveforms (Figure 5-15). In arrest situations, good compressions should be done as the waveforms are being evaluated. This will increase the size of the waveform.
- To use the devices in conjunction with your cardiac monitors, you must enable the waveform display on the monitor screen before intubation. A delay of 10 to 30 seconds for warm-up (depending on the monitor) will ensue if you wait to activate it after placing the tube. For best results, have the capnography waveform default when the monitor is turned on.

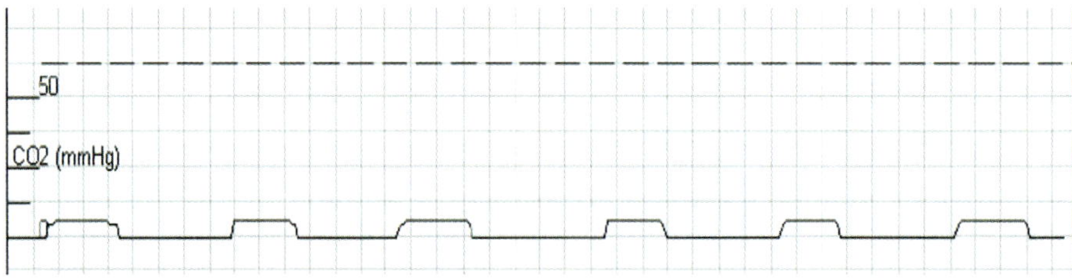

FIGURE 5-15 Small capnography waveform means poor perfusion or severe acidosis.

PROCEDURE

Confirming and Monitoring ET Tube Placement with Capnography

1. Prepare all equipment for intubation. Turn on monitor and attach capnography filter line or wires to the monitor. (This will vary depending on the brand of capnograph.) It is advisable to apply and record baseline capnography during preoxygenation prior to intubation attempt.
2. Place the endotracheal tube and inflate the cuff. In cases of arrest, compressions should not be interrupted to perform this procedure.
3. Attach the capnography airway adapter on the endotracheal tube, and then attach the bag-mask to the airway adapter.
4. Ventilate the patient and observe the waveform. The presence of a "square" pattern confirms tracheal placement (Figure 5-16). Print out the waveform, if possible (for documentation). If the

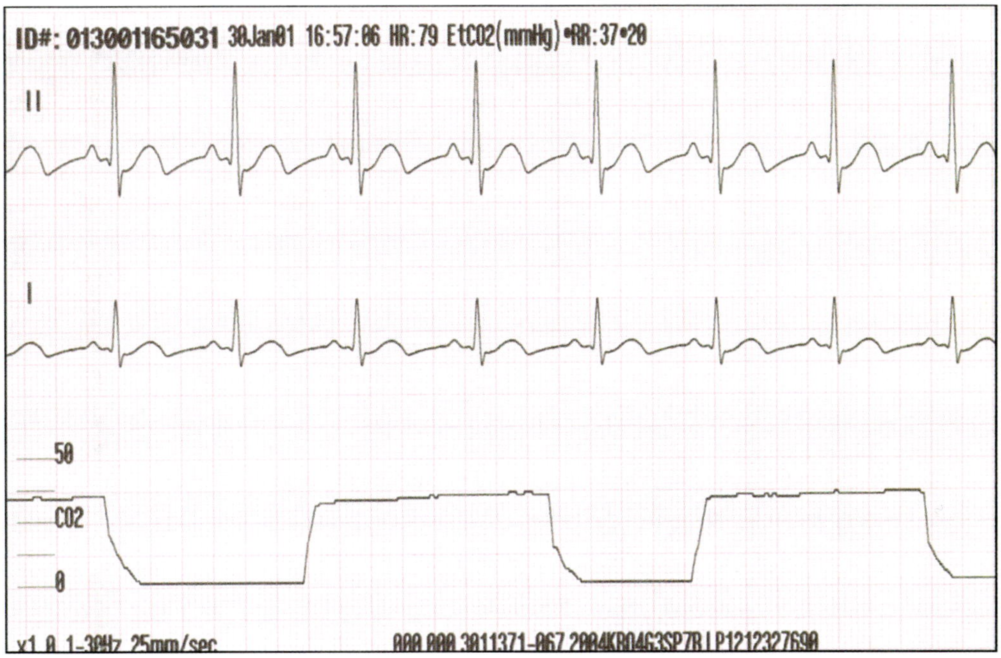

FIGURE 5-16 "Square" waveform is normal.

waveform is nonexistent or appears in gross and irregular waveform patterns, the tube is possibly in the esophagus or hypopharynx. In pediatrics, small tube size may limit CO_2 readings because some air may go around the tube and, thus, is not detectable by the capnogram. Use a cuffed tube in those cases and the waveform and CO_2 readings should improve.

5. Listen for breath sounds midaxillary on each side to rule out right mainstem intubation.
6. Secure the tube and continually monitor the waveforms during transport.
7. On arrival at the receiving facility, print out another waveform (if available) to prove correct placement at the time of patient transfer.
8. On your run report, document the visualization of the vocal cords, attach the waveform printout(s) or document the presence, and document equal breath sounds.

Troubleshooting while monitoring:

- *Loss of waveform completely.* Apnea, or tube is dislodged or obstructed, or air may be leaking around the cuff.
- *Waveforms and values getting smaller.* Hyperventilation (check the depth and rate of ventilation) or hypoperfusion (shock, or loss of pulses). Remember, it is very easy to hyperventilate an intubated patient because the ventilating bag is not squeezed as fast or deep as it is with bag-mask-only techniques. Also, airway pressure increases in the lungs following intubation. It is expected that hypoperfusion will have hypocapnia. However, rarely will you have hypoperfusion with normal or high $ETCO_2$.

Anchoring the Endotracheal Tube

Anchoring an endotracheal tube can be a frustrating exercise. Not only does it require some fine movements of the hands when you appear to be all thumbs, but it is difficult to perform when ventilation, movement, or extrication is being carried out. Keep one thing in mind: There is no substitute for the human anchor. That is, rescuer 2 should be held responsible for ensuring that the tube is held fast and that it does not migrate in or out of the airway. To lose a tube can be a catastrophe, especially if the patient is rather inaccessible or the intubation was a difficult one to begin with.

Fixing the endotracheal tube in place is important for several reasons. First, movement of the tube in the trachea will produce more mucosal damage and may increase the risk of postintubation complications. In addition, movement of the tube will stimulate the patient to cough, strain, or both, leading to cardiovascular and intracranial pressure changes that could be detrimental. Most important, there is a greater risk in the prehospital setting of dislodging a tube and losing control of the airway if it is not anchored solidly in place.

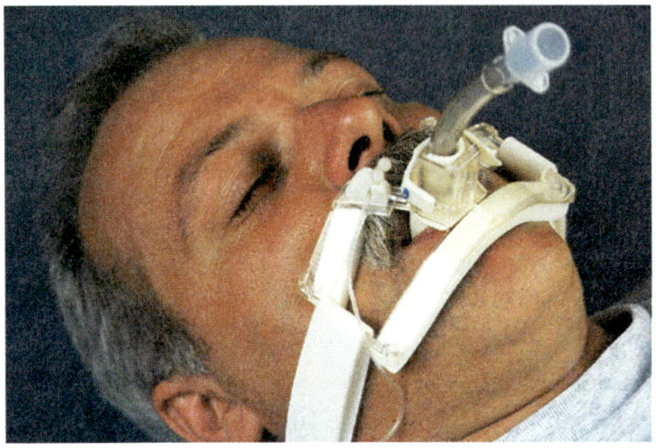

FIGURE 5-17 A commercial endotracheal tube holder.

The endotracheal tube can be secured in place by either tape or a commercially available holder. Although taping a tube in place is convenient and relatively easily done, it is not always effective. There is often a problem with the tape sticking to skin wet with rain, blood, airway secretions, or vomitus. If you are using tape, several principles should be followed:

- Insert an oropharyngeal airway to prevent the patient from biting down on the tube.
- Dry the patient's face and apply tincture of benzoin to better ensure proper adhesion of the tape.
- Carry the tape right around the patient's neck when anchoring the tube. Do not move the neck. Do not tie it so tight that it occludes the external jugular veins.
- Anchor the tube at the corner of the mouth, not in the midline.

Because of the difficulty of fixing the tube in place with tape, it may be better to use a commercial endotracheal tube holder that uses a strap to fix the tube in a plastic holder, which also acts as a bite block (Figure 5-17). Because flexion or extension of the patient's head can move the tube in or out of the airway by 2 or 3 cm, it is good practice to restrict head and neck movement of any patient who has an endotracheal tube in place. (This is even more important in children.) If the patient is spinal motion-restricted because of the risk of cervical-spine injury, flexion and extension should be less of a concern.

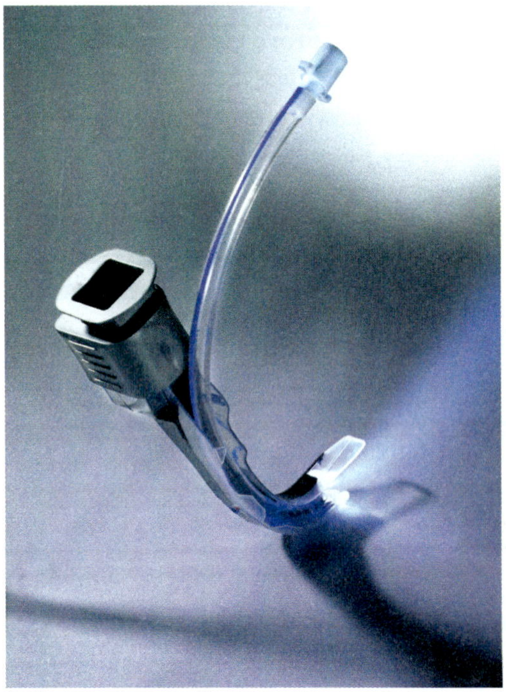

FIGURE 5-18 Example of fiberoptic intubation device (Airtraq Optical Laryngoscope). *(Airtraq® is a registered trademark of Prodol Meditec S.A. Las Arenas Vizcaya Spain)*

Fiberoptic and Video Intubation

Over the last few years there has been an exponential growth in the number and type of devices designed to improve visualization of the larynx and cords during intubation. For example, fiberoptic endoscopic intubation has been used for many years in the operating room. However, the size and complexity of the equipment limited its applicability in the field setting. Some of today's new systems use a variant of the optical scopes, which allows direct visualization of the cords and passage of the ET tube off the scope into the cords (Figure 5-18). Other systems make use of newly developed miniature video cameras that have the image projected on the screen that is either attached to the scope or adjacent to it (Figure 5-19).

Studies have shown an excellent success rate with many of the devices, and they have been proven to be very helpful in intubation of

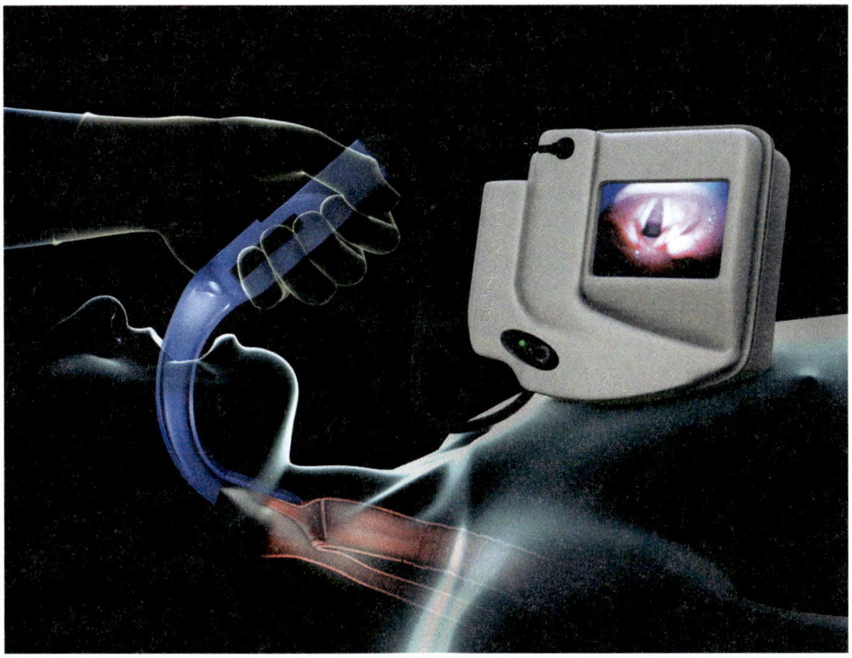

FIGURE 5-19 Example of video intubation device (Glidescope Ranger). *(Courtesy of Verathon©)*

patients with "difficult airways." The major drawback with many of the systems has been the cost of the equipment. As more manufacturers enter the market, the cost per unit should continue to decrease, and with that, more of those types of devices will be in field use.

At this time, the use of the devices should not be considered a "standard" of care in the field setting nor do the authors of this text favor any particular system. For emergency response organizations that have adopted intubating devices, use of those devices should be incorporated into airway management protocols. If available during training courses, personnel should be trained in the use of the devices, so long as such training does not detract from the instruction in the conventional devices used for airway management and stabilization.

Explore Resource Central

For additional review and practice tests, visit www.bradybooks.com and click on Resource Central to access book-specific resources for this text. To access Resource Central, follow directions on the Student Access Card provided with this text. If there is no card, go to www.bradybooks.com and follow the Resource Central link to Buy Access from there.

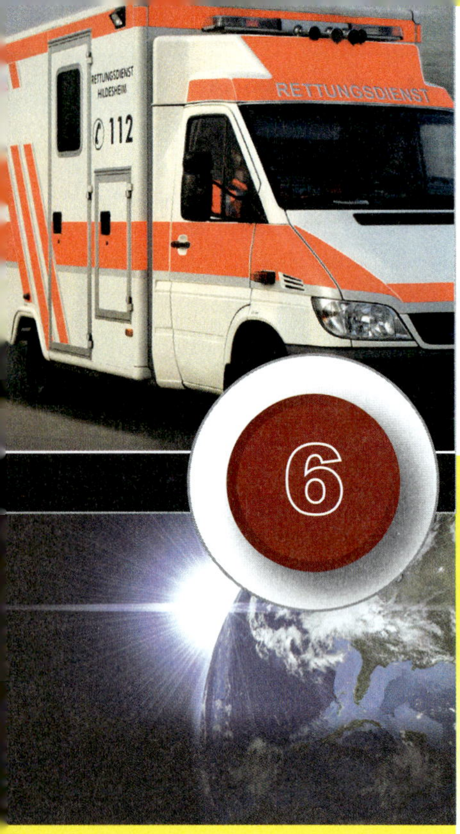

(© Maria P., Fotolia, LLC)

Thoracic Trauma

Graciela M. Bauzá, MD
Andrew B. Peitzman, MD, FACS

Thoracic Trauma

Trauma Toracico

Traumatismo Torácico

Traumatisme Thoracique

Urazy klatki piersiowej

Thorax Trauma

Ozljeda prsnog koša

إصابات القفص الصدري

torakalna trauma

Poškodbe prsnega koša

Mellkasi sérülés (as Injury Pattern)

KEY TERMS

Beck's triad, *p. 121*
flail chest, *p. 113*
massive hemothorax, *p. 117*
mediastinum, *p. 109*
open pneumothorax, *p. 115*
paradoxical pulse, *p. 121*
pericardial tamponade, *p. 120*
pleural space, *p. 109*
tension pneumothorax, *p. 119*

OBJECTIVES

Upon successful completion of this chapter, you should be able to:

1. Identify the major symptoms of thoracic trauma.
2. Describe the signs of thoracic trauma.
3. List the immediate life-threatening thoracic injuries.
4. Define flail chest in relation to associated physical findings and management.
5. Explain the pathophysiology and management of an open pneumothorax.
6. Explain the hypovolemic and respiratory compromise pathophysiology and management in massive hemothorax.
7. Describe the clinical signs of a tension pneumothorax in conjunction with appropriate management. Contrast those with the clinical signs of massive hemothorax.
8. List three indications to perform emergency chest decompression.
9. Identify the physical findings (including Beck's triad) of cardiac tamponade.
10. Explain the cardiac involvement and management associated with blunt injury to the chest.

Chapter Overview

The thoracic cage protects multiple vital organs. They include not only the lungs, heart, great vessels, and spinal cord, but also the liver, stomach, spleen, pancreas, kidneys, and transverse colon. Injury to those organs may result in early deaths. However, when thoracic injuries are recognized and treated appropriately, many of the patients will survive. Injuries to the chest may be caused by motor-vehicle collisions (MVCs), motorcycle collisions (MCCs), falls, firearms, knives, crush, and other blunt and penetrating mechanisms. Thoracic trauma is common in the multiple-trauma patient and is responsible for 20% to 25% of all trauma-related deaths. You must quickly assess for life-threatening injuries (causing hypoxia or hemorrhage), perform lifesaving maneuvers, and transport the patient to the appropriate trauma center without delaying care. This chapter will discuss the critical injuries to the chest and associated organs and the interventions by which you may give your patient the best chance for survival.

CASE PRESENTATION

An ALS ambulance has been dispatched to a bar where a patron has been stabbed. The scene size-up reveals that the police are on scene, have cleared the bar, and are questioning bystanders outside. There is a single male victim who is sitting in a chair and holding his chest. Because the scene is safe and the mechanism of injury (stab wound) is readily apparent, the team dons personal protective equipment. As they approach the patient, each carries essential trauma care equipment. How would you approach this patient? What type of assessment would you perform? What would you do first? Is this a load-and-go situation? *Keep these questions in mind as you read the chapter. Then, at the end of the chapter, find out how the rescuers completed this call.*

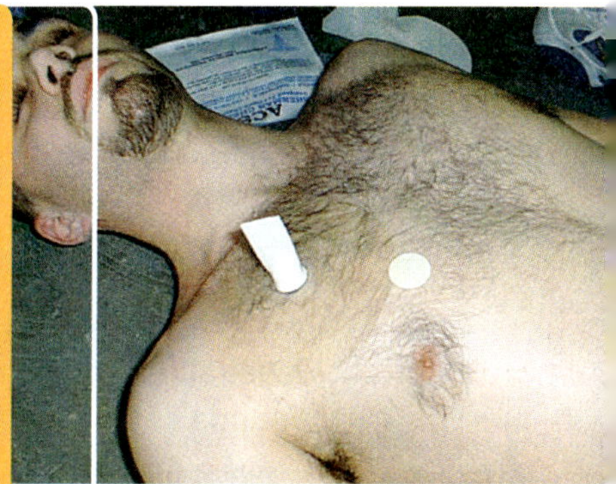

Anatomy of the Thorax

The thoracic organs are protected by 12 pairs of ribs that encircle them from spine to sternum (Figure 6-1). The chest wall is comprised of skin, subcutaneous tissue, muscle, ribs, and the neurovascular bundle (Figure 6-2). Note that the neurovascular bundle runs around the lower border of the rib. This is an important anatomical feature if you have to perform needle decompression of the chest. The structures within the chest but above the diaphragm include the lungs, the lower trachea and main stem bronchi, the heart and great vessels, and the esophagus. The adult thoracic cavity can contain up to three liters of blood on each side.

The lungs are a pair of spongy and elastic organs lined by the pleura, a thin slippery membrane. The visceral pleura lines the lungs directly, whereas the parietal pleura makes up the inner lining of the chest wall. Together they form a potential space (**pleural space**) in which air (pneumothorax), fluid, or blood (hemothorax) may accumulate.

Within the midline of the thoracic cavity is the **mediastinum**, which includes the heart, the aorta and pulmonary artery, superior and inferior vena cava, trachea,

pleural space the potential space between the visceral and parietal pleura within the thorax. In disease or injury states this space can accumulate air, fluid, or blood.

mediastinum the anatomic region within the thorax, located between the lungs, that contains the heart and great vessels, trachea, major bronchi, and the esophagus.

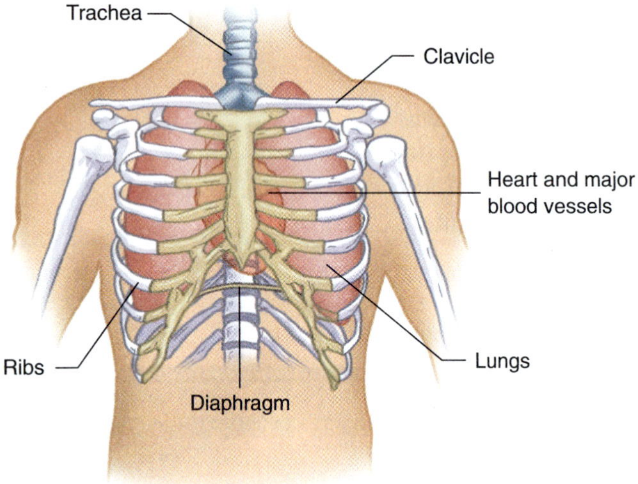

FIGURE 6-1 Thorax.

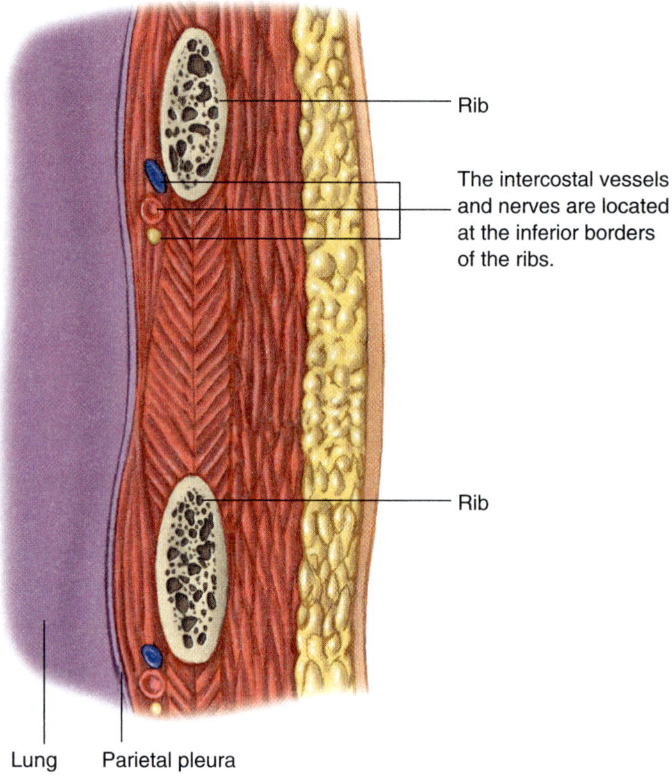

FIGURE 6-2 Rib with intercostal vessels and nerves.

> **PEARLS:** Penetrating Chest Wounds
>
> Patients who have penetrating chest trauma and shock are at the top of the list of load-and-go patients. Nothing should delay transport.

major bronchi, and the esophagus. Penetrating injuries that traverse the mediastinum are particularly dangerous because the heart, great vessels, and tracheobronchial structures are close together in this area, and there is a higher likelihood of fatal injuries. Deceleration injuries such as in head-on collisions or falls from a height are also of concern because they can result in fatal thoracic aortic injuries. Prompt management and transport of these patients can be lifesaving.

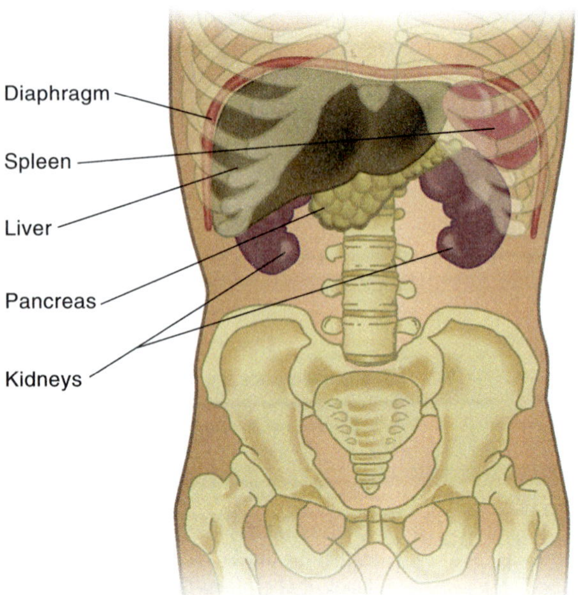

FIGURE 6-3 Intrathoracic abdomen.

The lower aspect of the chest protects the upper abdominal organs (stomach, spleen, liver, kidneys, and pancreas), which are divided from the thoracic cavity by the diaphragm (Figure 6-3). The diaphragm (a thin sheet of muscle) has its origin on the lower six ribs and the xyphoid process of the sternum. Its main function is respiration, and it is innervated by the phrenic nerve, which begins at cervical levels C3 to C5. This is very important because a cervical spinal-cord injury below the fifth cervical vertebrae will cause paralysis from the neck down, yet allow the victim to continue to breathe using his diaphragm, whereas a cord injury above the third cervical nerve will render the patient unable to breathe at all. Clinically speaking, any blunt or penetrating injury below the level of the nipples (T4, or fourth intercostal space) may cause both intrathoracic and intra-abdominal injuries.

Pathophysiology

In the trimodal distribution of trauma deaths (immediate, hours, weeks), injuries to the chest are responsible for most deaths at the scene (immediate deaths) and those within a few hours (early deaths). Immediate scene deaths usually involve disruption of the heart or great vessels. The second peak of deaths is usually due to airway obstruction, tension pneumothorax, hemorrhage, or cardiac tamponade. Only 10% to 15% of patients with chest trauma will require operative intervention. This means that timely prehospital care can save lives.

Chest injury may result from different mechanisms. Blunt trauma is the result of rapid deceleration, shearing forces, and crush injuries. Typically, the aorta, lungs, ribs, and less commonly the heart and esophagus can be injured in predictable fashion from blunt trauma. Conversely, penetrating trauma is unpredictable. A bullet may take an erratic path and can cause damage beyond its path, depending on firing distance, velocity, tumble, and yaw. The depth and direction of knife wounds are difficult to assess on external examination alone. However, obvious trajectory of a penetrating injury can at least suggest the organs most likely to be at risk of injury.

When evaluating the trauma patient always follow the ITLS Primary Survey as discussed in Chapter 2. The Primary Survey is designed to identify life-threatening injuries, and thoracic injuries make up the majority of those. Injuries to the organs within the thoracic cavity may result in decreased oxygenation and massive hemorrhage, both of which can lead to tissue hypoxia (shock) and death. Tissue hypoxia can result from the following:

- Inadequate oxygen delivery to the tissues secondary to airway obstruction
- Hypovolemia from blood loss
- Ventilation/perfusion mismatch from lung parenchymal injury
- Compromise of ventilation and/or circulation from a tension pneumothorax
- Pump failure from severe myocardial injury or pericardial tamponade

Emergency Care of Chest Injuries

The major symptoms of chest injury are shortness of breath and chest pain. The signs indicative of chest injury found on inspection include chest wall contusion, open wounds, subcutaneous emphysema, hemoptysis, distended neck veins, tracheal deviation, asymmetrical chest movement, including paradoxical motion, cyanosis, and shock. In addition, palpation may reveal tenderness, instability, and crepitation (TIC). Listen to the lung fields for the presence and equality of breath sounds. Using the ITLS Primary Survey, including the rapid trauma survey, will guide you in an organized fashion to discovery of those injuries (Figure 6-4).

Life-threatening thoracic injuries should be identified immediately during the ITLS Primary Survey. Major thoracic injuries to identify are listed next and may be remembered as the "deadly dozen":

ITLS Primary Survey

- Airway obstruction
- Flail chest
- Open pneumothorax
- Massive hemothorax
- Tension pneumothorax
- Cardiac tamponade

ITLS Secondary Survey or during hospital evaluation

- Myocardial contusion
- Traumatic aortic rupture

FIGURE 6-4 ITLS Primary Survey.

ITLS PRIMARY SURVEY

SCENE SIZE-UP

Standard Precautions Hazards, Number of Patients, Need for additional resources, **Mechanism of Injury**

↓

INITIAL ASSESSMENT

GENERAL IMPRESSION

Age, Sex, Weight, General Appearance, Position,
Purposeful Movement, Obvious Injuries, Skin Color

Life-threatening Bleeding

|

LOC

A-V-P-U

Chief Complaint/Symptoms

|

AIRWAY

(WITH C-SPINE CONTROL)

Snoring, Gurgling, Stridor; Silence

|

BREATHING

Present? Rate, Depth, Effort

|

CIRCULATION

Radial/Carotid Present? Rate, Rhythm, Quality

Skin Color, Temperature, Moisture; Capillary Refill

Has bleeding been controlled?

↓

RAPID TRAUMA SURVEY

HEAD and NECK

Wounds?

Neck Vein distention? Tracheal Deviation?

|

CHEST

Asymmetry (Paradoxical Motion?), Contusions, Penetrations, Tenderness, Instability, Crepitation

Breath Sounds

Present? Equal? (If unequal: percussion)

Heart Tones

|

ABDOMEN

Contusions, Penetration/Evisceration; Tenderness, Rigidity, Distension

|

PELVIS

Tenderness, Instability, Crepitation

|

LOWER/UPPER EXTREMITIES

Obvious Swelling, Deformity

Motor and Sensory

|

POSTERIOR

Obvious wounds, Tenderness, Deformity

|

If radial pulse present:

VITAL SIGNS

Measured Pulse, Breathing, Blood Pressure

|

If altered mental status: Brief Neurological exam

PUPILS

Size? Reactive? **Equal?**

|

GLASGOW COMA SCALE

Eyes, Voice, Motor

- Tracheal or bronchial tree injury
- Diaphragmatic tears
- Pulmonary contusion
- Blast injuries

Airway Obstruction

Airway management remains a major challenge in the care of any multiple-trauma patient. Hypoxia secondary to airway obstruction (foreign body, tongue, aspiration of vomitus, or blood) is a common cause of preventable trauma death. Management of the airway has been discussed in Chapter 4, so nothing further is added here other than to stress its importance.

PEARLS: Rib Fractures

Multiple rib fractures with or without flail chest can cause hypoxia from mechanical ventilatory problems as well as pulmonary contusion. The patient, especially the older patient, must be closely monitored for hypoxia and respiratory failure. Monitoring with pulse oximetry and capnography is very helpful.

Flail Chest

Flail chest occurs with the fracture of two or more adjacent ribs in two or more places (Figure 6-5), causing instability of the chest wall and paradoxical movement of the "flail segment" in a spontaneously breathing patient. The unstable section of ribs will suck in when the patient breathes in and will push out when the patient breathes out (Figure 6-6). Positive pressure ventilation reverses the movement of the flail segment. Flail segments are not usually seen in the posterior chest because the heavy back muscles usually prevent movement of a flail segment. The patient is at risk for development of a hemothorax or pneumothorax and will always have a pulmonary contusion (Figures 6-7 and 6-8).

Large flails decrease the ability of the patient to create a negative intrathoracic pressure, and thus he may not be able to ventilate and may be in marked respiratory distress. Movement of the broken ribs is very painful and will contribute to the difficulty with ventilation. Large flails are best treated with endotracheal intubation and assisted ventilation with positive end-expiratory pressure (PEEP). For smaller flails, oxygen and continuous positive airway pressure (CPAP) ventilation may be sufficient.

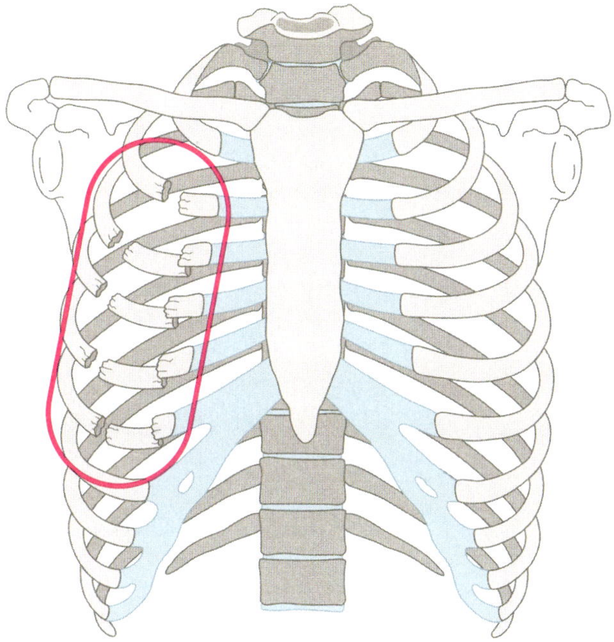

FIGURE 6-5 Flail chest occurs when two or more adjacent ribs fracture in two or more places.

flail chest the fracture of two or more adjacent ribs in two or more places, causing instability of the chest wall and paradoxical movement of the "flail segment" in a spontaneously breathing patient.

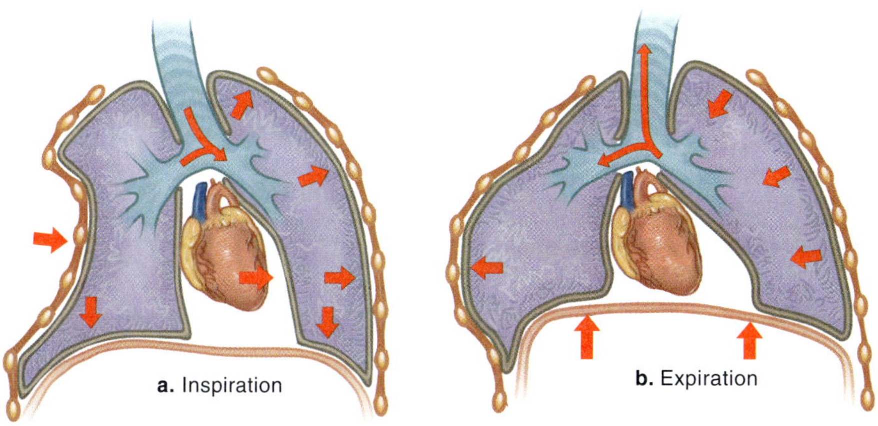

FIGURE 6-6 Pathophysiology of flail chest showing paradoxical motion

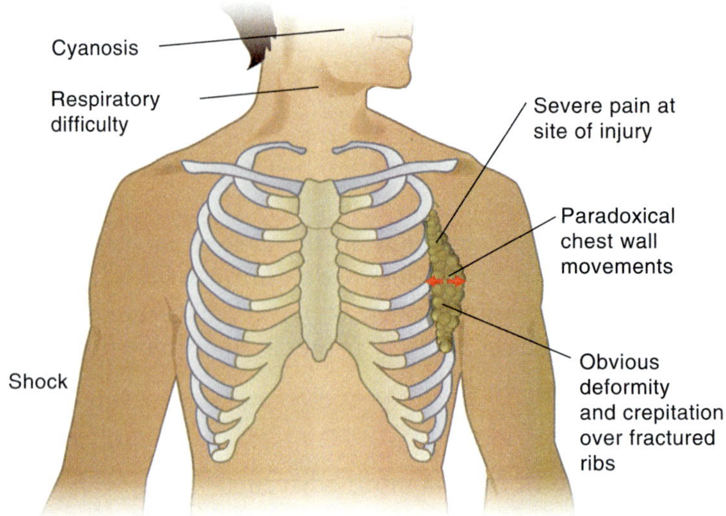

FIGURE 6-7 Physical findings of flail chest.

FIGURE 6-8 Flail chest may be identified during the ITLS Primary Survey.

FLAIL CHEST

SCENE SIZE-UP
T-bone collision? Intrusion of door?

INITIAL ASSESSMENT
LOC
Often unconscious
Airway
Possibly snoring or gurgling
Breathing
Apneic, or shallow and guarded; often NO tidal volume
Pulses
Rapid/thready
Skin cool/clammy; cyanotic

RAPID TRAUMA SURVEY
Neck Veins
Flat
Trachea
Midline
Chest
Asymmetrical with paradoxical motion on affected side
Breath Sounds
Usually decreased on affected side (may be heard on both sides)
Abdomen
Pain of broken ribs may mask abdominal tenderness
Check carefully

PROCEDURE

Management of Flail Chest

1. Ensure an open airway.
2. Assist ventilation.
3. Administer high-flow oxygen.

4. Initially, stabilize the flail segment with manual pressure. Then stabilize it with bulky dressings taped to the chest wall (Figure 6-9). However, this is usually not necessary until the patient is placed on a backboard. Remember that trying to maintain manual pressure on a flail segment while performing a logroll can compromise a stable spine.
5. Load and go.
6. Transport rapidly to the appropriate hospital.
7. Notify medical direction early.
8. Consider intubation early to provide PEEP. CPAP could be used here if available.
9. Administer adequate pain relief, avoiding respiratory depression.
10. If shock is present, use care to prevent fluid overload, which could worsen hypoxemia.

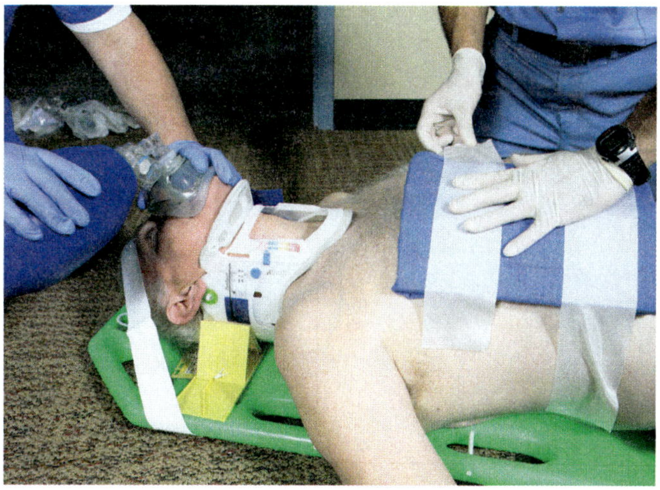

FIGURE 6-9 Stabilizing flail chest. *(Courtesy of Stanley Cooper, EMT-P)*

Remember that intubation and positive pressure ventilation are the best way to stabilize a flail chest, but this may be very difficult in the field if the patient still has a gag reflex. Drug-assisted intubation (DAI) is useful here if available. Also keep in mind that a pneumothorax is commonly associated with a flail chest. Be alert for development of tension pneumothorax.

Open Pneumothorax

An **open pneumothorax** results in the accumulation of air in the potential space between the visceral and parietal pleura secondary to penetrating injury presenting as an open or *sucking chest wound* (>3 cm in diameter). The persistent open wound equalizes intrathoracic pressure and atmospheric pressures resulting in partial or complete lung collapse. The size of the pneumothorax and resultant symptoms are usually proportional to the size of the chest wall defect (Figures 6-10 and 6-11). Normal ventilation involves the creation of

Resource Central

See Optional Skills for further discussion on this topic.

open pneumothorax accumulation of air in the pleural space secondary to penetrating injury presenting as an open or sucking chest wound (>3 cm in diameter).

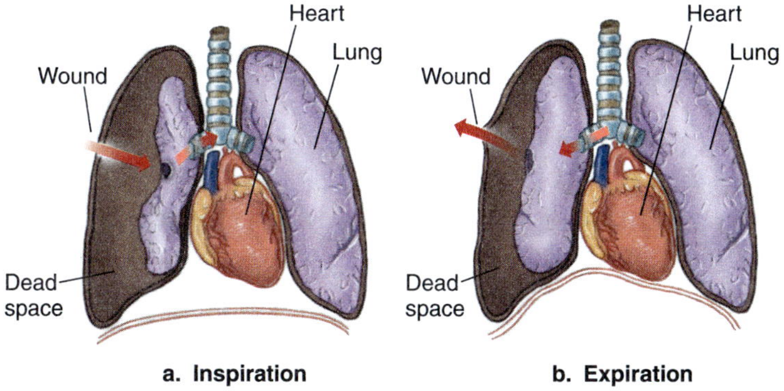

FIGURE 6-10 Open pneumothorax. If the wound is larger than the opening to the trachea, air will preferentially go into dead space rather than the lung.

OPEN PNEUMOTHORAX

SCENE SIZE-UP
Is the scene SAFE?

↓

INITIAL ASSESSMENT
LOC
Possibly decreased
Airway
Possibly gurgling
Breathing
Rapid and shallow, possibly labored, but often poor or NO tidal volume
Pulses
Rapid/thready
Skin cool/clammy; cyanotic

↓

RAPID TRAUMA SURVEY
Neck Veins
Flat
Trachea
Midline
Chest
Asymmetrical with penetration(s)
Breath Sounds
Decreased on affected side
Heart Tones
Note for comparison later
Abdomen
Where did the penetrating object go?
Back
Where did the penetrating object go?

FIGURE 6-11 Open pneumothorax may be identified during the ITLS Primary Survey.

negative intrathoracic pressure by diaphragmatic contraction to draw air into the airways and lungs. If the open wound is greater than two-thirds the diameter of the trachea, air will follow the path of least resistance through the chest wall defect into the intrathoracic dead space resulting in severe hypoxia and hypoventilation

PROCEDURE

Management of Open Pneumothorax

1. Ensure an open airway.
2. Administer high-flow oxygen. Assist ventilation as necessary.
3. Initially, seal the wound with your gloved hand. Then place a commercial chest seal (one with an exit valve is needed, such as Asherman Chest Seal, Bolin Chest Seal, or Halo vent) (Figure 6-12) over the defect, or you may make a seal from a sterile occlusive dressing taped on three sides to act as flutter-type valve (Figure 6-13). Do not tape on all four sides because this could convert an open pneumothorax into a tension pneumothorax.

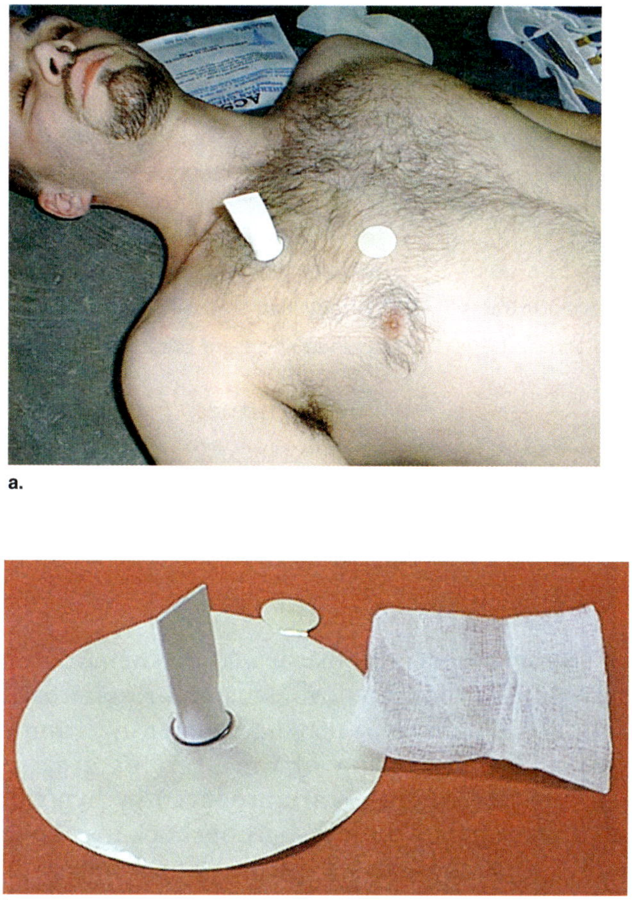

FIGURE 6-12 (a) Sealing a sucking chest wound with (b) the Asherman Chest Seal. *(Photo b courtesy of Teleflex Incorporated, all rights reserved. No other use shall made of the image without the prior written consent of Teleflex Incorporated.)*

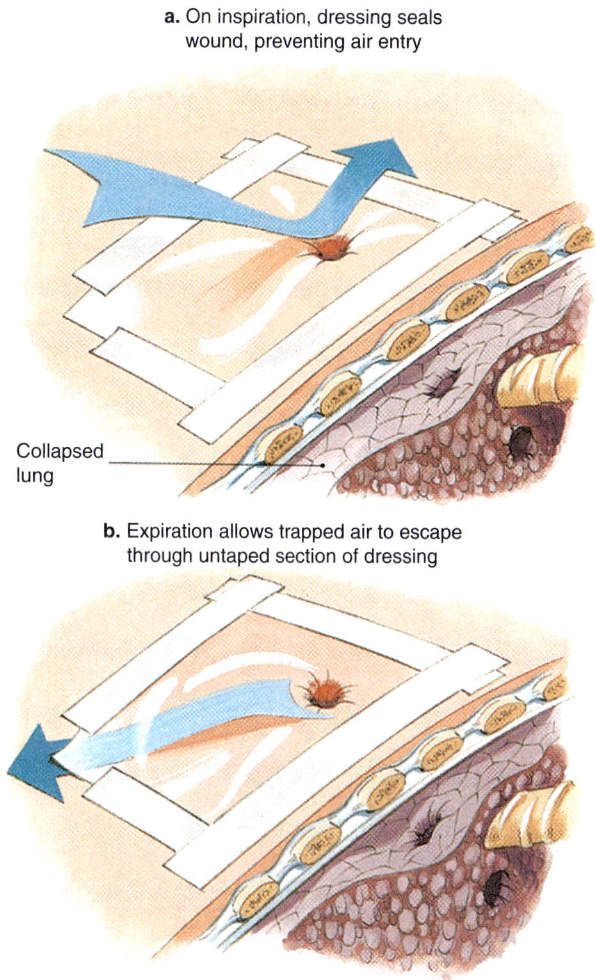

FIGURE 6-13 Treatment of sucking chest wound with impervious dressing taped on three sides to allow air to escape but not enter.

4. Load and go.
5. Insert a large-bore IV.
6. Monitor the heart and note heart tones for comparison later.
7. Monitor oxygen saturation with a pulse oximeter and expiratory CO_2 with capnography (if available).
8. Transport rapidly to the appropriate hospital.
9. Notify medical direction early.

Massive Hemothorax

Blood in the pleural space is a hemothorax (Figure 6-14). A **massive hemothorax** occurs as a result of at least a 1,500 cc blood loss into the pleural space within the thoracic cavity. Each thoracic cavity may contain up to 3,000 cc of blood. Massive hemothorax is more often due to penetrating trauma than to

massive hemothorax the presence of at least 1,500 cc of blood loss into the pleural space of the thoracic cavity.

Table 6-1 Primary Survey of Tension Pneumothorax Contrasted to Massive Hemothorax

	Tension Pneumothorax	Massive Hemothorax
Scene Size-up (LOC)	Seat belt? Steering wheel?	Scene safe? Penetrating vs. blunt trauma
Level of consciousness	Decreased	Decreased
Breathing	Rapid/shallow; labored	Rapid/shallow; labored
Pulses	Weak/thready; absent radials	Weak/thready; absent radials
Skin	Cool/clammy/diaphoretic; cyanotic	Cool/clammy/diaphoretic; pale/ashen
Neck	Neck vein distension; possible tracheal deviation (rare)	Neck veins flat; trachea midline
Breath sounds	Decreased or absent breath sounds on affected side	Decreased or absent breath sounds on affected side
Percussion note	Hyperresonant on affected side	Dull on affected side

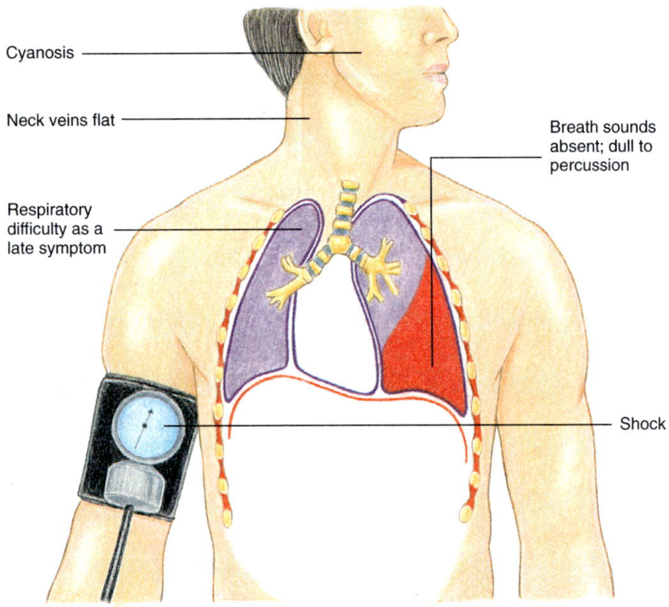

FIGURE 6-14 Physical findings of massive hemothorax.

blunt trauma, but either injury may disrupt a major pulmonary or systemic vessel. As blood accumulates within the pleural space, the lung on the affected side is compressed.

Signs and symptoms of massive hemothorax are produced by both hypovolemia and respiratory compromise. The patient may be hypotensive from blood loss and compression of the heart or great veins. Anxiety and confusion are produced by hypovolemia and hypoxemia. Clinical signs of shock may be apparent. The neck veins are usually flat secondary to profound hypovolemia, but may very rarely be distended due to mediastinal compression. Other signs of hemothorax include decreased breath sounds and dullness to percussion on the affected side. The massive hemothorax may be identified during the ITLS Primary Survey. (See Table 6-1 for comparison of tension pneumothorax and massive hemothorax.)

PROCEDURE

Management of Massive Hemothorax

1. Secure an open airway.
2. Apply high-flow oxygen.
3. Load and go.
4. Notify medical direction early.
5. Treat for shock. Replace volume carefully after IV insertion en route. Try to keep the blood pressure just high enough to maintain a peripheral pulse (80–90 mm Hg systolic). Although the major problem in massive hemothorax is usually hemorrhagic shock, elevating the blood pressure will increase the bleeding into the chest.
6. Observe closely for the possible development of a tension hemopneumothorax, which would require acute chest decompression.

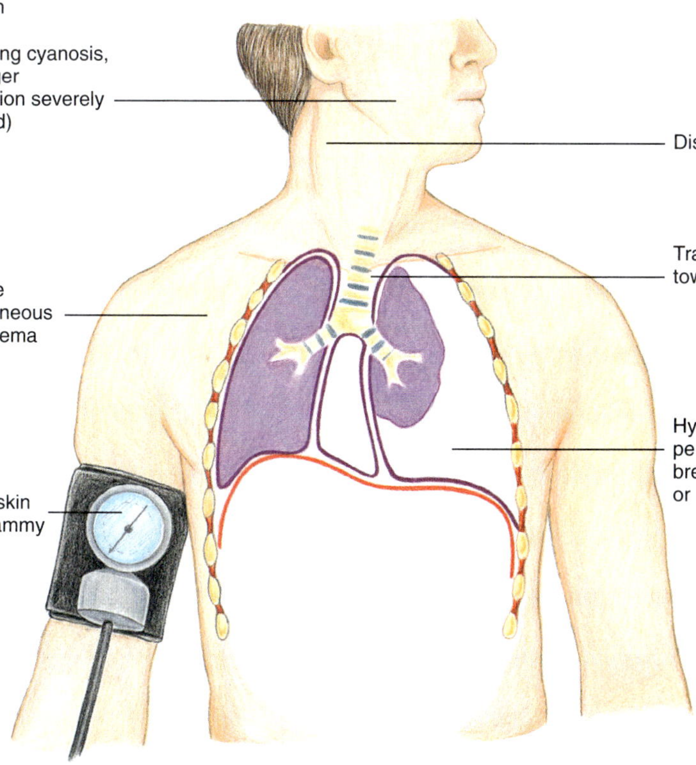

FIGURE 6-15 Physical findings of tension pneumothorax.

> **PEARLS: Simple Pneumothorax**
>
> Reassess patients with chest injuries frequently to prevent progression of a simple pneumothorax or open pneumothorax to a tension pneumothorax. The pulse oximeter and waveform capnography can be helpful.

tension pneumothorax a condition in which air continuously leaks out of the lung into the pleural space. The air continues to accumulate without means of exit, resulting in increasing intrathoracic pressure on the affected side and eventual collapse of the superior and inferior vena cava as well as the lung.

Tension Pneumothorax

A pneumothorax is accumulation of air in the potential space between the visceral and parietal pleura, resulting in complete lung collapse. In a **tension pneumothorax**, air continues to accumulate without means of exit, resulting in increasing intrathoracic pressure on the affected side, displacing the heart and trachea to the opposite side, and collapsing the superior and inferior vena cava, thus occluding venous return to the heart (Figure 6-15).

Clinical signs of a tension pneumothorax include dyspnea, anxiety, tachypnea, distended neck veins, and possibly tracheal deviation away from the affected side. Auscultation will reveal diminished breath sounds on the affected side and will be accompanied by hyperresonance when percussed (Figure 6-16). Shock with hypotension will follow. In a review of 108 field patients diagnosed with tension pneumothorax and requiring needle decompression, none were recorded as having a deviated trachea.

The development of decreased lung compliance (difficulty in squeezing the bag-mask device) in the intubated patient should always alert you to the possibility of a tension pneumothorax. Intubated patients with a history of chronic obstructive pulmonary disease (COPD) or asthma are at increased risk for development of tension pneumothorax from positive pressure ventilation.

TENSION PNEUMOTHORAX

SCENE SIZE-UP
Seat belt? Steering wheel?

↓

INITIAL ASSESSMENT
LOC
Decreased
Airway
Open? Movement of air?
Breathing
Rapid/shallow; labored
Pulses
Weak/thready → Absent radials
Skin cool/clammy, cyanotic

↓

RAPID TRAUMA SURVEY
Head/Neck
Neck vein distention; possible tracheal deviation
Chest
Absent or decreased breath sounds on affected side
Hyperresonant on affected side

FIGURE 6-16 The tension pneumothorax may be identified during the ITLS Primary Survey.

PROCEDURE

Management of Tension Pneumothorax

1. Establish an open airway.
2. Administer high-flow oxygen.
3. Decompress the affected side of the chest, if indicated. The indication for performing emergency decompression is the presence of a tension pneumothorax with decompensation as evidenced by more than one of the following:
   a. Respiratory distress and cyanosis
   b. Loss of the radial pulse (late shock)
   c. Decreasing level of consciousness
4. Load and go.
5. Rapidly transport to the appropriate hospital.
6. Notify medical direction early.

If you are not authorized to decompress the chest, the patient must be transported rapidly to the hospital so decompression can be performed. A chest tube will be necessary on arrival to the hospital. Needle decompression is a temporary, but lifesaving, measure. (See Chapter 7.)

pericardial tamponade the rapid collection of blood between the heart and pericardium from a cardiac injury. The accumulating blood compresses the ventricles of the heart preventing the ventricles from filling between contractions and causing cardiac output to fall.

Cardiac Tamponade

The pericardial sac is an inelastic membrane that surrounds the heart. If blood collects rapidly between the heart and pericardium from a cardiac injury, the ventricles of the heart will be compressed, making the heart less able to refill, and cardiac output falls. A small amount of pericardial blood (as little as 75–100 cc) may compromise cardiac filling and cause signs of **pericardial tamponade** (Figure 6-17).

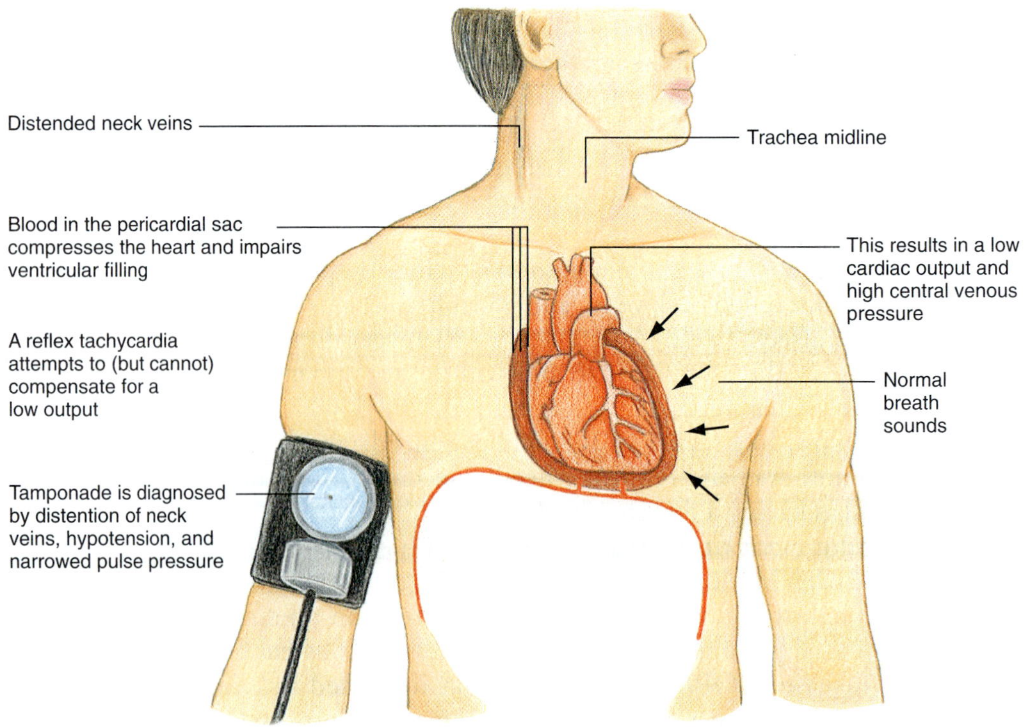

FIGURE 6-17 Pathophysiology and physical findings of cardiac tamponade.

CARDIAC TAMPONADE

SCENE SIZE-UP
Trauma (blunt or penetrating) to anterior chest?

↓

INITIAL ASSESSMENT
LOC
Decreased
Breathing
Rapid/shallow
Pulses
Weak/thready → Absent radials
Possible paradoxical pulse
Skin
Cool/clammy/diaphoretic

↓

RAPID TRAUMA SURVEY
Head/Neck
Neck vein distention; trachea midline
Chest
Sternal contusion or fracture?
Penetrating wound of chest?
Breath sounds usually present and equal
May be unequal if associated pneumothorax or hemothorax
Heart Sounds
Muffled (may develop over time)

FIGURE 6-18 Cardiac tamponade may be identified during the ITLS Primary Survey.

Diagnosis of cardiac tamponade classically relies on the presence of hypotension with narrow pulse pressure, and **Beck's triad**, a combination of distended neck veins, muffled heart sounds, and *pulsus paradoxus*. (If the patient loses the peripheral pulse during inspiration, this is suggestive of a **paradoxical pulse** and the presence of cardiac tamponade.) Muffled heart sounds may be very difficult to appreciate in the prehospital setting, but if you briefly listen to the heart when performing the ITLS Primary Survey, you may notice a change later.

The major differential diagnosis in the field is tension pneumothorax. With cardiac tamponade, the patient will be in shock with equal breath sounds and a midline trachea (Figure 6-18), unless there is an associated pneumothorax or hemothorax.

Other life-threatening thoracic injuries exist that may not be apparent during the ITLS Primary Survey, or at all in the prehospital environment. However, you should remain alert for clues, which may point to the following conditions.

Beck's triad the three clinical signs of cardiac tamponade (distended neck veins, muffled heart sounds, and *pulsus paradoxus*).

paradoxical pulse a clinical sign of cardiac tamponade. It is an exaggeration of the normal variation of the strength of the pulse during the inspiratory phase of respiration, in which the blood pressure decreases as one inhales and increases as one exhales. The paradox is that, in the case of a pericardial tamponade with decreased cardiac output, the palpated radial pulse disappears during inspiration. Also called *pulsus paradoxus.*

PROCEDURE

Management of Cardiac Tamponade

1. Ensure an open airway.
2. Administer high-flow oxygen.
3. Load and go.
4. Transport rapidly to the appropriate hospital.
5. Notify medical direction early.

6. Monitor the heart early, especially with chest pain or an irregular pulse.
7. If available, perform a 12-lead ECG (including V_{4R}).
8. Treat for shock. An IV infusion of electrolyte solution (en route) may increase the filling of the heart and increase cardiac output. However, because there may be associated intrathoracic bleeding, give only enough fluid to maintain a pulse (80–90 mm Hg systolic).
9. Treat dysrhythmias as they present.
10. Watch for other complications, including hemothorax and pneumothorax.

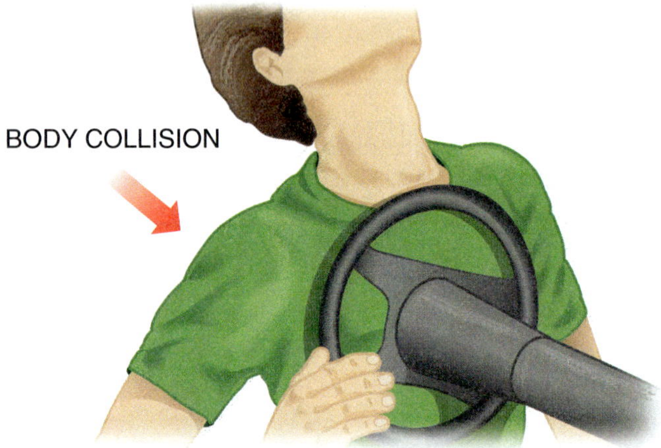

FIGURE 6-19 Pathophysiology of blunt cardiac injury, a collision of the heart against the sternum.

Myocardial Contusion

Blunt cardiac injury (BCI) includes a number of diagnoses, including myocardial contusion, dysrhythmias, acute heart failure, valvular injury, or cardiac rupture. The mechanism is blunt trauma to the anterior chest as in a deceleration MVC or a fall from a height. Among them, myocardial contusion is something that you may suspect and possibly identify as a result of your ITLS Secondary Survey.

Myocardial contusion is a potentially lethal lesion resulting from blunt chest injury. Blunt injury to the anterior chest is transmitted via the sternum to the heart, which lies immediately posterior to it (Figure 6-19). Cardiac injuries from this mechanism may include valvular rupture, pericardial tamponade, or cardiac rupture, but contusion of the right atrium and right ventricle occurs most commonly (Figure 6-20). This bruising of the heart

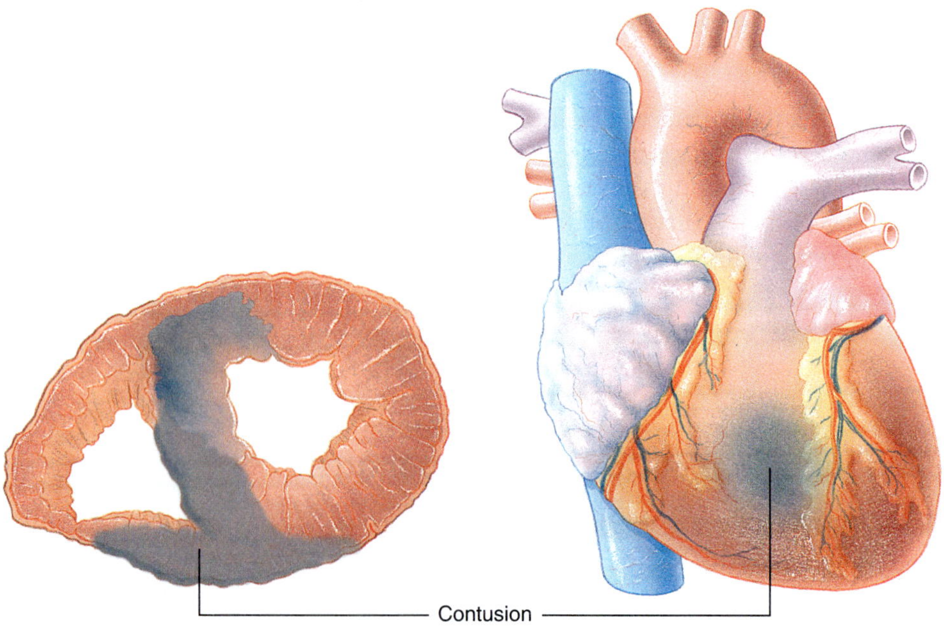

FIGURE 6-20 Myocardial contusion most frequently affects the right atrium and ventricle as they collide with the sternum in the "third collision." This can cause cardiac dysrhythmia.

is basically the same injury as an acute myocardial infarction and likewise presents with chest pain, dysrhythmias, or cardiogenic shock (rare).

If the patient complains of chest pain, is found to have an otherwise unexplained irregular pulse, exhibits neck vein elevation, especially in the presence of blunt force trauma to the anterior chest (bruised or flail sternum), cardiac contusion should be suspected. Those signs are similar to pericardial tamponade and cannot be differentiated in the field so are treated the same. If available, a 12-lead ECG should be performed, which may indicate an injury pattern to the right ventricle (STEMI in leads II, III, aVr, V_1, and V_{4R})

PROCEDURE

Management of Cardiac Contusion

1. Ensure an open airway.
2. Administer high-flow oxygen.
3. Load and go.
4. Transport rapidly to the appropriate hospital.
5. Notify medical direction early.
6. Monitor the heart early, especially with chest pain or an irregular pulse.
7. If available, perform a 12-lead ECG (including V_{4R}).
8. Treat for shock. An IV infusion of electrolyte solution (en route) may increase the filling of the heart and increase cardiac output. However, because there may be associated intrathoracic bleeding, give only enough fluid to maintain a pulse (80–90 mm Hg systolic).
9. Treat dysrhythmias as they present.
10. Watch for other complications, including hemothorax and pneumothorax.

Traumatic Aortic Rupture

Traumatic aortic rupture is a tear in the wall of the aorta. Eighty-five percent of tears occur at the ligamentum arteriosum or the take off of the left subclavian artery; 80% die at the scene. These are usually free ruptures. For the 10% to 20% who do not exsanguinate immediately, the aortic tear will be contained temporarily by surrounding tissue and adventitia. However, usually this will rupture within hours unless recognized and surgically repaired. The diagnosis of a contained thoracic aortic laceration is impossible in the field, so you should have a high index of suspicion for it if the patient has a mechanism of rapid deceleration.

This injury should be suspected in patients with blunt mechanism associated with rapid deceleration such as falls from a height and high-speed MVCs (front and lateral impacts, ejected occupants). There may be no symptoms, or the patient may complain of chest pain or scapular pain. Be suspicious if the patient has asymmetric blood pressure measurements in upper extremities, or upper extremity hypertension, widened pulse pressure, and diminished lower extremity pulses.

PROCEDURE

Management of Potential Aortic Tears

1. Ensure an open airway.
2. Administer high-flow oxygen.
3. Rapidly transport to the appropriate hospital.
4. Establish IV access, but limit fluid administration.
5. Monitor the heart. The mechanism of injury is the same as for myocardial contusion.
6. If available, perform a 12-lead ECG (including V_{4R})
7. Notify medical direction early.

Tracheal or Bronchial Tree Injury

Tracheobronchial injuries may result in partial or complete disruption of the airway. Injury is localized within 2 cm of the carina in up to 80% of cases. These injuries usually cannot be diagnosed in the field but will present with dyspnea and pneumothorax.

Victims may suffer penetrating or blunt mechanism such as MVC or crush injury to the chest and exhibit dyspnea, subcutaneous emphysema associated hemo/pneumothorax, and deformed chest.

Diaphragmatic Tears

Tears in the diaphragm may result from a severe blow to the abdomen. A sudden increase in intra-abdominal pressure, such as a seat-belt injury or a kick to the abdomen, may tear the diaphragm and allow herniation of the abdominal organs into the thoracic cavity. This occurs more commonly on the left than the right because the liver protects the right hemidiaphragm. Blunt trauma produces large radial tears in the diaphragm. Penetrating trauma also may produce holes in the diaphragm, but these tend to be small.

Traumatic diaphragmatic hernia is difficult to diagnose even in the hospital. The herniation of abdominal contents into the thoracic cavity may cause marked respiratory distress. On examination, the breath sounds may be diminished, and infrequently, bowel sounds may be heard when the chest is auscultated. The abdomen may appear scaphoid if a large quantity of abdominal contents is in the chest.

PROCEDURE

Management of Diaphragmatic Rupture

1. Ensure an open airway.
2. Assist ventilation as necessary
3. Administer high-flow oxygen.
4. Transport the patient to the appropriate hospital.
5. Treat shock. Insert an IV en route. Associated injuries are common and hypovolemia may occur.
6. Notify medical direction early.

Pulmonary Contusion

Pulmonary contusion is a very common chest injury, caused by hemorrhage into lung parenchyma secondary to blunt force trauma or penetrating injury such as a missile. It occurs commonly with flail segment or multiple rib fractures. A pulmonary contusion takes hours to develop and rarely develops during prehospital care, unless very long transport or delayed discovery of the victim occurs. Children may have severe pulmonary contusions without rib fractures due to the flexibility of their chest wall. Contusion of the lung may produce marked hypoxemia. Management consists of intubation and/or assisted ventilation if indicated, oxygen administration, transport, and IV insertion.

Blast Injuries

With the increase in terrorism, understanding blast injury is important. The magnitude of the blast wave depends on the size of the explosion and the environment in which it occurs. Closed spaces, such as buses, produce highly lethal blast injury.

The mechanism of injury by explosions is due to three to five factors: (Also see Chapter 1.)

- *Primary*. This is the initial air blast. A primary blast injury is caused solely by the direct effect of blast overpressure on tissue. Air is easily compressible, unlike water. As a result, a primary blast injury almost always affects air-filled structures such as the lungs, ears, and gastrointestinal tract. Depending on the pressure wave, there may be pulmonary contusions, pneumothorax, or tension pneumothorax.
- *Secondary*. The patient is being struck by material (shrapnel) propelled by the blast force.
- *Tertiary*. The patient's body is being thrown by the pressure wave and impacting the ground or another object. These injuries, including crush injury, also are seen from structural collapse.
- *Quaternary*. This is the thermal burns from the explosion, radiation from radiological material that was dispersed by the explosion (dirty bomb), or respiratory injuries from inhalation of toxic dust or fumes.
- *Quinary*. This is reported as a hyperinflammatory state caused by chemicals used in making a bomb or added to the bomb (another form of dirty bomb).

PROCEDURE

Management of the Blast Injury Patient

1. Ensure an open airway.
2. Administer high-flow oxygen. Be aware that positive pressure ventilation may lead to or worsen pneumothorax or tension pneumothorax.
3. Load and go to appropriate level of care.
4. Manage the other injuries found.
5. Obtain venous access.
6. Notify online medical direction

Other Chest Injuries

Impaled Objects

Penetrating objects, such as a knife, may cause impalement injuries of the chest. As in other areas of the body, the object should not be removed in the field. Stabilize the object, ensure an airway, insert an IV, and transport the patient.

Traumatic Asphyxia

Traumatic asphyxia is an important set of physical findings (Figure 6-21). However, the term *traumatic asphyxia* is a misnomer because the condition is not caused by asphyxia. The syndrome results from a severe compression injury to the chest, such as from a steering wheel, conveyor belt, or heavy object. The sudden compression of the heart and mediastinum transmits this force to the capillaries of the neck and head. The patients appear similar to those of strangulation, with cyanosis and swelling of the head and neck. The tongue and lips are swollen, and conjunctival hemorrhage is evident. The skin below the level of the crush injury to the chest will be pink unless there are other problems.

Traumatic asphyxia indicates that the patient has suffered a severe blunt thoracic injury, and major thoracic injuries are likely to be present. Management includes airway maintenance, IV access, treating other injuries, and rapid transport.

Simple Pneumothorax

Simple pneumothorax may result from blunt or penetrating trauma. Fractured ribs are the usual cause in blunt trauma. Pneumothorax is caused by accumulation of air within the potential space between the visceral and parietal pleura. The lung may be totally or partially collapsed as the air continues to accrue in the thoracic cavity. In a healthy patient this should not acutely compromise ventilation, if a tension pneumothorax does not evolve. Patients with less respiratory reserve may not tolerate even a simple pneumothorax.

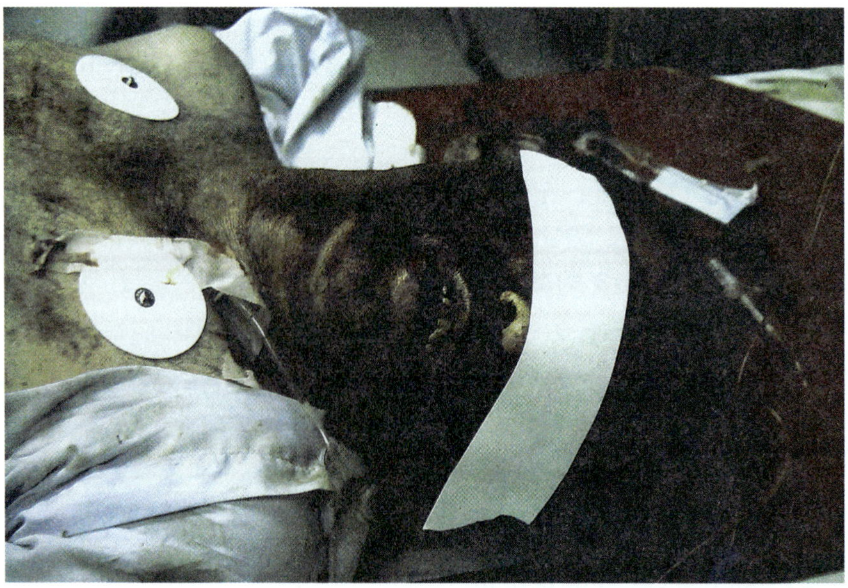

FIGURE 6-21 Traumatic asphyxia.

Diagnosis of a pneumothorax is based on pleuritic chest pain, dyspnea, decreased breath sounds on the affected side, and hypertympany to percussion. Close observation is required in anticipation of the patient developing a tension pneumothorax.

Sternal Fractures

Sternal fractures also indicate that the patient has suffered marked blunt trauma to the anterior chest. These patients should be presumed to have a myocardial contusion. Diagnosis of sternal fracture may be made by palpation.

Simple Rib Fracture

Simple rib fracture is the most frequent injury to the chest. If the patient does not have an associated pneumothorax or hemothorax, the major problem is pain. This pain will prohibit the patient from breathing adequately. On palpation, the area of rib fracture will be tender and may be unstable. Give oxygen and monitor for pneumothorax or hemothorax while encouraging the patient to breathe deeply. It is reasonable to give medication for pain management.

CASE PRESENTATION (continued)

An ALS ambulance has been called to a local bar where a patron has been stabbed. The scene size-up reveals that the police are on scene, have cleared the bar, and are questioning bystanders outside. There is a single male victim who is sitting in a chair and holding his right anterior chest. Because the scene is safe and the mechanism of injury (stab wound) is readily apparent, the team dons personal protective equipment and each carries their essential trauma care equipment as they approach the patient. The patient, a man in his 20s, states that during an argument his drinking buddy stabbed him once in the right chest before bystanders could take the knife away from him. The patient denies falling or any other injuries.

The team leader begins the initial assessment and her general impression is good. The patient is sitting in a chair and is awake and answering appropriately. He does not appear to be in any distress and there is no obvious external bleeding. Respiration appears to be of normal rate and depth and when his hand is removed from his right chest, there is a single small stab wound lateral to the sternum at about the fourth intercostal space. The wound is not bleeding. The radial pulse seems a little fast but is strong. The team leader asks rescuer 2 to apply a nonrebreather oxygen mask and then clean the chest wound and apply an occlusive dressing. Because of the nature of the injury she decides to do a focused exam. Exam of the airway is normal, with good movement of air and a normal speaking voice. The neck veins are flat, and the trachea is in the midline. The breath sounds are present and equal bilaterally. Heart sounds are normal but a little fast and irregular. The abdomen is soft and nontender. There are no other wounds. Vital signs are pulse 120–130, respiration 16/minute, and blood pressure 120/70. The patient is placed on a stretcher (no backboard or packaging) and moved to the ambulance.

He is treated with 100% oxygen by nonrebreather mask. A large-bore IV is started during transport, but because the blood pressure is normal, the flow rate is set just fast enough to keep the vein open. There is concern about causing worsening of any possible intrathoracic bleeding. The history reveals:

S —Slight pain in the wound site

A —None

M —None

P —No history of serious illness.

L —Just ate some chips and salsa; admits to drinking "three beers"

E —States he was drinking with his friend, who became upset when they got into an argument over football. In a snit, his friend stabbed him with a pocketknife. His friend is now outside talking to the police and is crying and protesting that he never meant to hurt the patient.

While rescuer 2 applies a cardiac monitor and a pulse oximeter (95% on 100% oxygen), the team leader performs an ITLS Ongoing Exam. The level of consciousness is normal, airway is still normal with normal breathing, but the pulse is now more rapid (around 140 with occasional PVCs on monitor) and thready. The pulse disappears when the patient takes a deep breath. The patient is a little diaphoretic. The neck veins are now distended and trachea is midline. Breath sounds are equal bilaterally, but heart sounds are not as easily heard as before. Rescuer 2 reports the blood pressure is now 80/60 mm Hg. The fluid rate is increased to raise the blood pressure to 90 mm Hg systolic, and while rescuer 2 starts a second IV, the team leader immediately notifies medical direction that they will be arriving in five minutes with a young male patient with a probable pericardial tamponade and shock. She is told to watch the vital signs and try to keep the blood pressure 80–90 mm Hg systolic.

The ITLS Secondary Survey was not performed because they arrived at the emergency department before she had time to do one. Immediately on arrival in the emergency department, an ultrasound confirmed blood in the pericardial sac but no hemothorax and no blood in the abdomen. The patient was taken directly to surgery, where the blood was evacuated from the pericardium and a small laceration of the heart repaired. The patient had an uneventful recovery.

This is one of the few examples of a focused exam being adequate for a trauma patient. Note that even a focused exam required that both the chest and the abdomen be examined because the diaphragm rises so high in the chest that a mid-chest stab wound may go through the diaphragm and cause abdominal injuries. Repeated exams are very important here because pericardial tamponade, tension pneumothorax, and massive hemothorax could all develop after a penetrating wound of the chest.

Studies have found that for penetrating wounds of the chest, the pneumatic antishock garment (PSAG) or IV fluids may significantly increase internal bleeding and worsen survival. (See Chapter 8.) Thus, the PASG is contraindicated, and IV fluids should only be used to maintain systolic pressure of 80–90 mm Hg systolic. ■

Summary

Chest injuries are common in multiple-trauma patients. Many of the injuries are life threatening. If you follow the ITLS Primary Survey, you will be able to identify most of them. These are often load-and-go patients. Primary goals in treating the patient with chest trauma are the following:

- Ensure an open airway while protecting the cervical spine.
- Administer high-flow oxygen and ventilate if necessary.
- Stabilize flail segments.
- Seal sucking chest wounds.
- Decompress the chest if needed.
- Load and go to appropriate level of care.
- Obtain venous access.
- Transport to appropriate level of care.
- Notify online medical direction.

The thoracic injuries discussed are life threatening, but treatable by prompt intervention and transport to the appropriate level of care. Early recognition along with appropriate interventions and rapid transport may be lifesaving.

Bibliography

1. American College of Surgeons Committee on Trauma. 2008. "Thoracic Trauma." In *Advanced Trauma Life Support.* 8th ed., 85–101. Chicago: American College of Surgeons.
2. Ball, C. G., et al. 2010, June. Thoracic needle decompression for tension pneumothorax: Clinical correlation with catheter length. *Can J Surg* 53(3): 184.
3. DePalma R. G., Burris D. G., Champion H. R., et al. 2005. Blast injuries. *New Engl J Med* 352: 1335–1342.
4. Livingston, D. H., Hauser, C. J. 2008. Chest Wall and Lung. In D. V. Feliciano, K. L. Mattox, E. E. Moore (Eds.), *Trauma.*6th ed., 525-552. New York: McGraw-Hill.
5. Harcke H. T. et al. 2007. Chest wall thickness in military personnel: implications of needle thoracentesis in tension pneumothorax. *Mil Med* 172: 1260–1263.
6. Netto, F. A. C. S., et al. 2008. Are needle decompressions for tension pneumothoraces being performed appropriately for appropriate indications? *American J Emerg Med* 26: 597.
7. DePalma, R. G., et al. 2005. Blast injuries. *N Engl J Med* 352: 1335–13428.
8. Peitzman, A. B., et al. 2008. Thoracic injury. In J. P. Pryon, J. A. Asensio (Eds.), *The Trauma Manual: Trauma and Acute Care Surgery.* 3rd ed., 209–229. Philadelphia: Lippincott Williams & Wilkins.

Explore Resource Central

For additional review and practice tests, visit www.bradybooks.com and click on Resource Central to access book-specific resources for this text. To access Resource Central, follow directions on the Student Access Card provided with this text. If there is no card, go to www.bradybooks.com and follow the Resource Central link to Buy Access from there.

Thoracic Trauma Skills

Donna Hastings, EMT-P
Arthur Proust, MD, FACEP

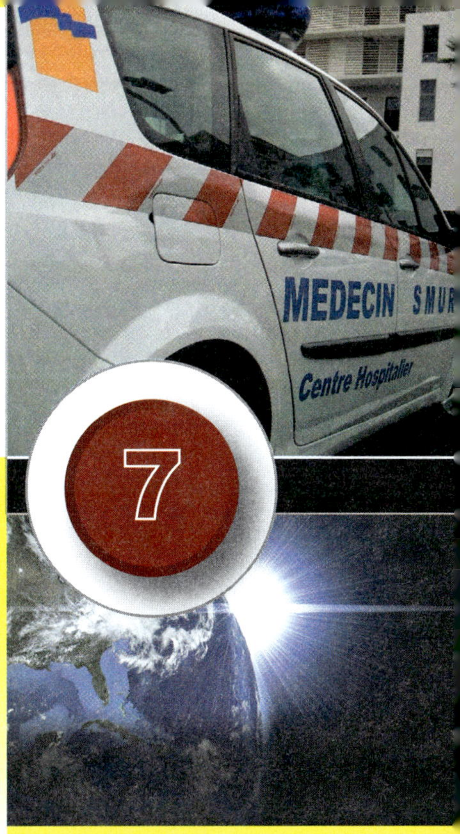

(© yannik LABBE, Fotolia, LLC)

Thoracic Trauma

Trauma Toracico

Traumatismo Torácico

Traumatisme Thoracique

Urazy klatki piersiowej

Thorax Trauma

Ozljeda prsnog koša

إصابات القفص الصدري

torakalna trauma

Poškodbe prsnega koša

Mellkasi sérülés (as Injury Pattern)

OBJECTIVES

Upon successful completion of this chapter, you should be able to:

1. Describe the indications for emergency decompression of a tension pneumothorax.
2. Explain the advantages, disadvantages, and complications of needle decompression of a tension pneumothorax by the anterior approach and the lateral approach.
3. Perform needle decompression of a tension pneumothorax by either the anterior or lateral approach.

Chest Decompression

For many years needle decompression of a tension pneumothorax has been advocated as a lifesaving procedure and the anterior approach (second or third intercostal space, midclavicular line) has been most commonly used by prehospital providers. In the last few years the lateral approach has become popular with the military, who favor it because it can be used to decompress the chest without removing a soldier's body armor. Multiple studies also have been published showing that the catheters being used were too short to decompress the chest in many patients. It is recommended that for the anterior approach the catheter needle needs to be large bore (8 French or about 14 gauge) and 6 to 9 cm long. Because there are advantages and disadvantages to each decompression site, this chapter will cover both of them. Follow your state protocol or consult your service medical director for guidance about which site to use routinely.

Indications to Perform Chest Decompression

As with all advanced procedures, this technique must be accepted local protocol or you must obtain medical direction before performing it. The conservative management of tension pneumothorax is oxygen, ventilatory assistance, and rapid transport. The indication for performing emergency decompression is the presence of a tension pneumothorax with decompensation as evidenced by *more than one* of the following:

- Respiratory distress and cyanosis
- Loss of the radial pulse (late shock)
- Decreasing level of consciousness

Performing a Chest Decompression by the Lateral Approach

Advantages

The lateral chest wall is thinner than the anterior chest wall (averages 2.6 cm), so you are more likely to decompress the pneumothorax with a shorter needle and less likely to inadvertently cause hemorrhage from vascular structures.

The military and tactical medics prefer the lateral approach because in a tactical situation it has the advantage of allowing decompression while keeping body armor in place.

Disadvantages and Complications

- The decompression catheter is more likely to be dislodged when moving the patient or if the patient moves his arm. Using the Asherman Chest Seal for a one-way valve also will provide some protection against dislodgement of the decompression catheter.
- It can be difficult to reach this area when the patient is in the ambulance (especially if the tension pneumothorax is on the right).
- Laceration of the intercostal vessels may cause hemorrhage. The intercostal artery and vein run around the inferior margin of each rib (Figure 7-1). Poor needle placement can lacerate one of these vessels.
- If performing the lateral approach, inserting the needle too low may lacerate the liver or spleen, and inserting the needle too high may lacerate the axillary artery, vein, or brachial plexus.

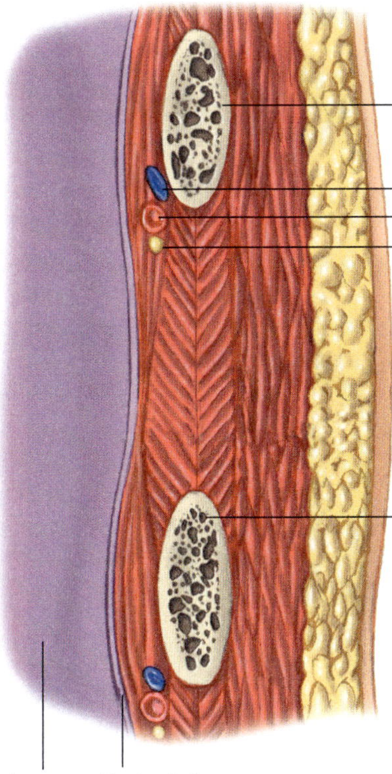

FIGURE 7-1 Rib with intercostal vessels and nerves.

- Creation of a pneumothorax may occur if not already present. If your assessment was incorrect, you may give the patient a pneumothorax when you insert the needle into the chest.
- Laceration of the lung is possible. Poor technique or inappropriate insertion (no pneumothorax present) can cause laceration of the lung, with subsequent bleeding and an air leak.
- Risk of infection is a consideration. Adequate skin preparation with an antiseptic will usually prevent this.

PROCEDURES

Performing a Chest Decompression by the Lateral Approach

1. Assess the patient to make sure that his condition is due to a tension pneumothorax. Signs of tension pneumothorax are
   a. Decreased level of consciousness (LOC)
   b. Open airway
   c. Rapid shallow respiration; respiratory distress
   d. Weak/thready pulses; possible absent radial pulse
   e. Skin cool, clammy, diaphoretic; pale or cyanotic
   f. Neck vein distention (may not be present if there is associated severe hemorrhage)
   g. Possible tracheal deviation away from the side of the injury (almost never present)
   h. Absent or decreased breath sounds on the affected side
   i. Tympany (hyperresonance) to percussion on the affected side

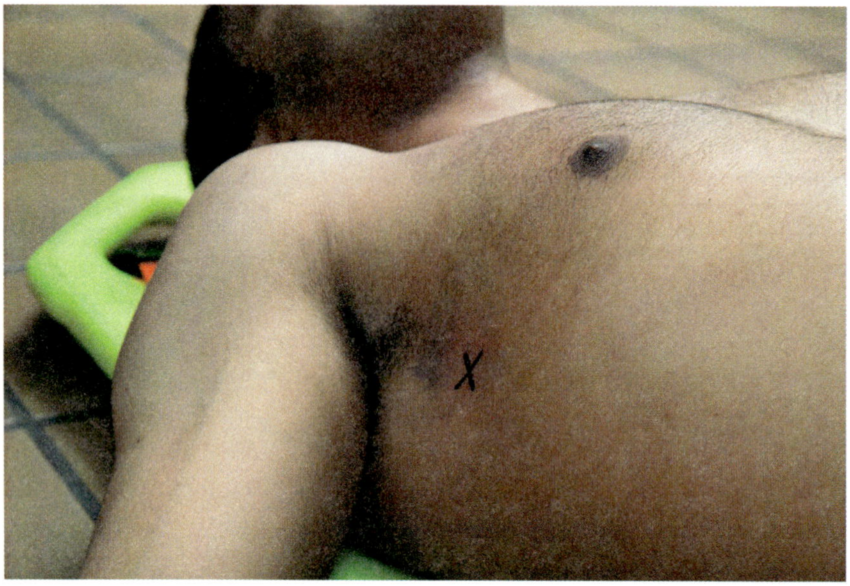

FIGURE 7-2 Determine the patient has a tension pneumothorax and mark the site for needle decompression using the lateral approach. *(Courtesy of Louis B. Mallory, MBA, REMT-P)*

2. Give the patient high-flow oxygen and ventilatory assistance.
3. Determine that indications for emergency decompression are present. Then, if required, obtain medical direction to perform the procedure.
4. Lateral site for decompression: Expose the side of the tension pneumothorax and identify the intersection of the nipple (fourth rib) and anterior axillary line on the same side as the pneumothorax (Figure 7-2).
5. Quickly prep the area.
6. Remove the plastic cap from a 14-gauge catheter needle at least 2 inches or 5 cm long and insert the needle into the intercostal space at a 90-degree angle to the superior border of the fourth rib to avoid the neurovascular bundle (Figure 7-3). If the patient is muscular or obese, you may need to use a 6- to

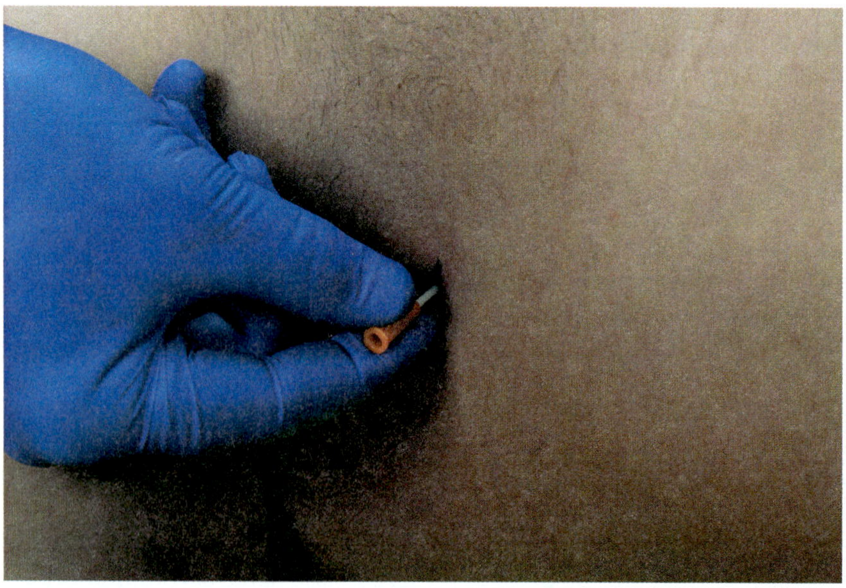

FIGURE 7-3 Needle decompression by the lateral (anterior axillary) approach. Advance the catheter into the chest and secure with tape. *(Courtesy of Louis B. Mallory, MBA, REMT-P)*

9-cm catheter needle. Direction of the bevel is irrelevant to successful results. As the needle enters the pleural space, there will be a "pop." If a tension pneumothorax is present, there will be a hiss of air as the pneumothorax is decompressed. If using an over-the-needle catheter, advance the catheter into the chest. Remove the needle and leave the catheter in place. *The catheter hub must be stabilized to the chest with tape.*

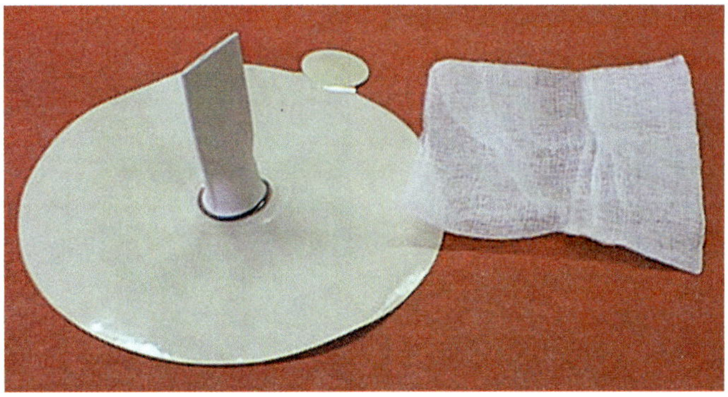

FIGURE 7-4 Asherman Chest Seal may be used to provide a one-way valve for the properly secured decompression needle. *(Photo courtesy of Teleflex Incorporated, all rights reserved. No other use shall be made of the image without the prior written consent of Teleflex Incorporated.)*

7. Place a one-way valve on or over the decompressing needle. The Asherman Chest Seal will go over the needle and provide a one-way valve (Figure 7-4) and will protect the needle from accidently being dislodged. Other one-way valves are available or can be made but should be tested before using. (A needle through the finger of a rubber glove will not work as a one-way valve.) Young healthy patients will tolerate having no valve at all on the decompressing needle.
8. Leave the plastic catheter in position until it is replaced by a chest tube at the hospital.
9. Intubate the patient if indicated. Monitor closely for recurrence of the tension pneumothorax. If available monitor with capnography. An increase in the CO_2 is an early sign the catheter is kinked or the tension pneumothorax is worsening. (A 13- or 14-gauge catheter may not be large enough to decompress a large air leak.)

Performing a Chest Decompression by the Anterior Approach

Advantages

- The anterior site is preferred by many because, in the supine patient, air in the pleural space tends to accumulate anteriorly. Thus, there is a better chance of having the air in the pleural space removed when decompressing at the midclavicular area.
- Monitoring of the site is easier if performed in the anterior site because the catheter is not as likely to be unintentionally dislodged when the patient is moved or if the patient moves his arm.

Disadvantages and Complications

- Unless a needle of proper length is used, it is likely that the needle will not reach the pleural space, and the tension pneumothorax will not be decompressed. The recommended catheter length is 6 to 9 cm (2.5 to 3.5 inches) (Figure 7-5).
- If the insertion of the needle is medial to the midclavicular line (nipple line), there is danger of cardiac puncture or great vessel laceration.
- Laceration of the intercostal vessels may cause hemorrhage. The intercostal artery and vein run around the inferior margin of each rib. Poor needle placement can lacerate one of these vessels.

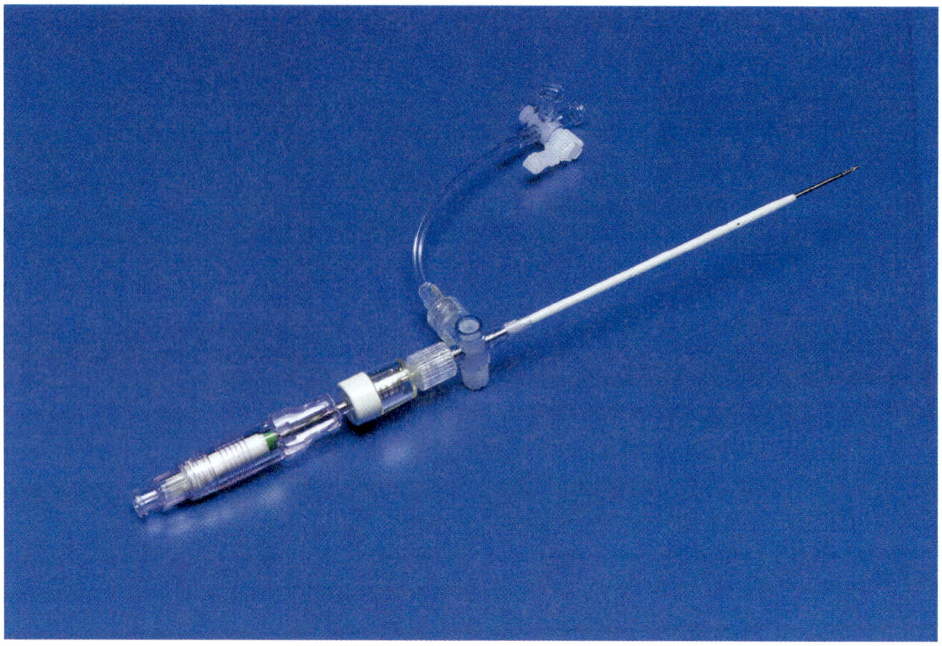

FIGURE 7-5a Examples of catheters long enough to decompress a tension pneumothorax: In this photo, a Turkel Safety needle. *(Courtesy of Covidien. Covidien and ™ marked brands are trademarks of Covidien AG)*

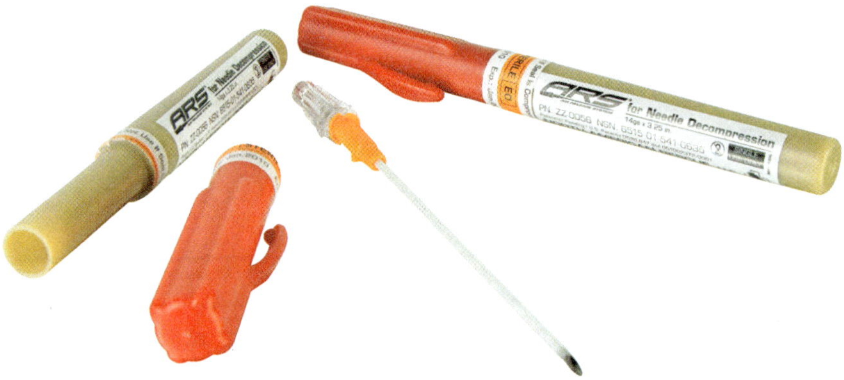

FIGURE 7-5b An ARS needle for decompression. *(Courtesy of © 2020 North American Rescue, LLC)*

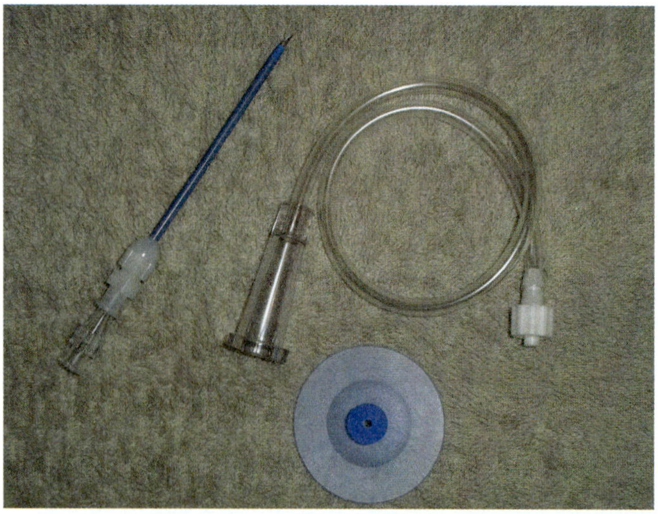

FIGURE 7-5c A Cook pneumothorax needle (has wire coil inside to prevent kinking).

- Creation of a pneumothorax may occur if not already present. If your assessment was incorrect, you may give the patient a pneumothorax when you insert the needle into the chest.
- Laceration of the lung is possible. Poor technique or inappropriate insertion (no pneumothorax present) can cause laceration of the lung, with subsequent bleeding and an air leak.
- Risk of infection is a consideration. Adequate skin preparation with an antiseptic will usually prevent this.

Decompression by the Anterior Approach

1. Assess the patient to make sure that his condition is due to a tension pneumothorax. Signs of tension pneumothorax are
   a. Decreased level of consciousness (LOC)
   b. Open airway
   c. Rapid shallow respiration; respiratory distress
   d. Weak/thready pulses; possible absent radial pulse
   e. Skin cool, clammy, diaphoretic; pale or cyanotic
   f. Neck vein distention (may not be present if there is associated severe hemorrhage)
   g. Possible tracheal deviation away from the side of the injury (almost never present)
   h. Absent or decreased breath sounds on the affected side
   i. Tympany (hyperresonance) to percussion on the affected side
2. Give the patient high-flow oxygen and ventilatory assistance.
3. Determine that indications for emergency decompression are present. Then, if required, obtain medical direction to perform the procedure.
4. Anterior site for decompression: Expose the side of the tension pneumothorax and identify the second or third intercostal space on the anterior chest at the midclavicular line on the same side as the pneumothorax. This may be done by feeling for "angle of Louis," the bump located on the sternum about a quarter of the way from the suprasternal notch (Figure 7-6). The insertion site should be slightly lateral to the midclavicular line (nipple line) to avoid cardiac or major vascular complications in the mediastinum.

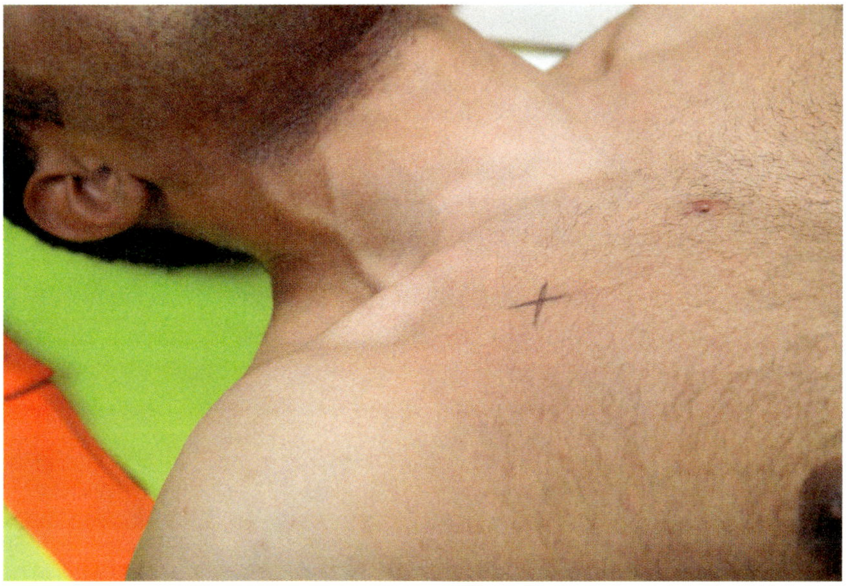

FIGURE 7-6 Determine the patient has a tension pneumothorax and mark the site for needle decompression using the anterior approach. Note the distended neck veins. *(Courtesy of Louis B. Mallory, MBA, REMT-P)*

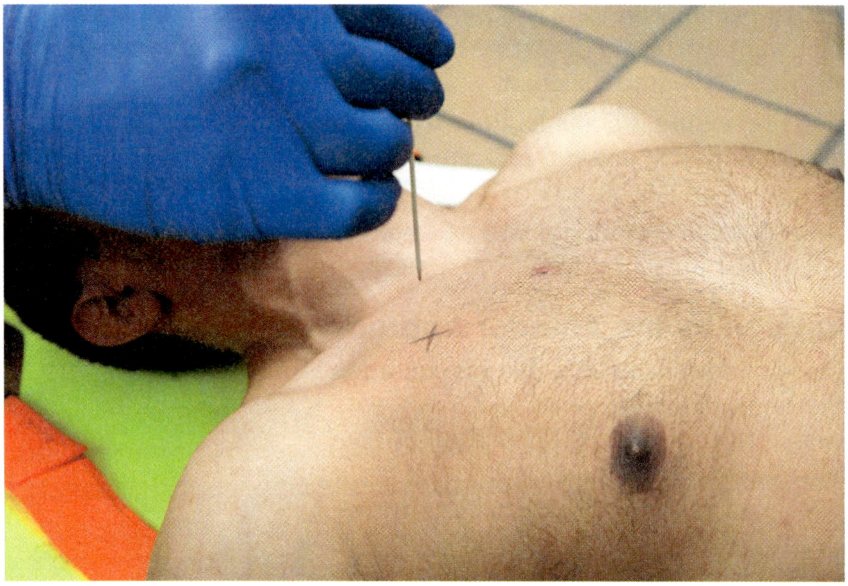

FIGURE 7-7 Insert the catheter at a 90-degree angle over the superior border of the second or third rib. *(Courtesy of Louis B. Mallory, MBA, REMT-P)*

5. Quickly prepare the area with an antiseptic.
6. Remove the plastic cap from a 14 gauge or larger catheter 6 to 9 cm long (8 French, 9-cm Turkel Safety Needle, 14-gauge, 8.25-cm ARS decompression needle, 8.5 French, 6-cm Cook pneumothorax needle, or 14-gauge, 8-cm angiocath) and insert the needle into the intercostal space at a 90-degree angle to the superior border of the third rib to avoid the neurovascular bundle (Figure 7-7). Direction of the bevel of the needle is irrelevant to successful results. Be very careful not to angle the needle toward the mediastinum. As the needle enters the pleural space, there will be a "pop." If a tension pneumothorax is present, there will be a hiss of air as the pneumothorax is decompressed. If using an over-the-needle catheter, advance the catheter into the chest (Figure 7-8). Remove the needle and leave the catheter in place. The catheter hub must be stabilized to the chest with tape.

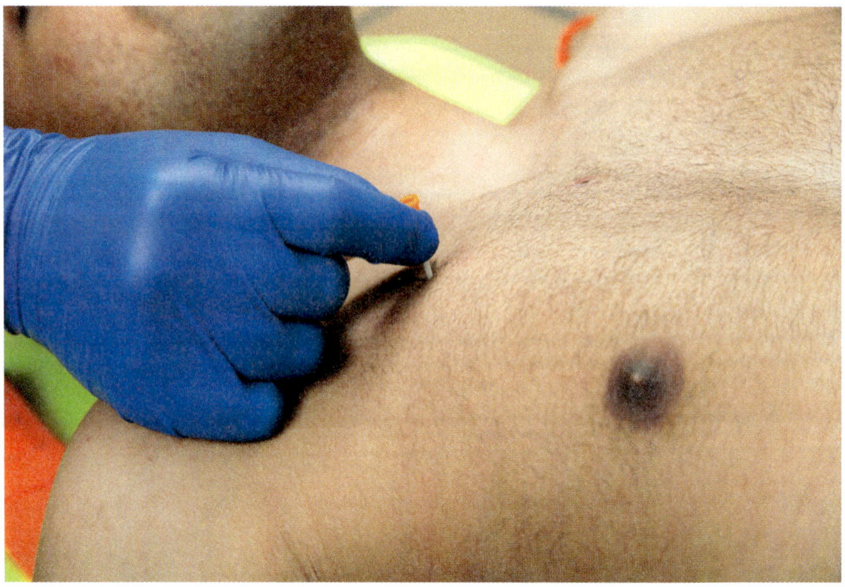

FIGURE 7-8 Advance the catheter into the chest. There should be a rush of air as the pressure is relieved. Secure the catheter with tape. *(Courtesy of Louis B. Mallory, MBA, REMT-P)*

7. Place a one-way valve on or over the decompressing needle. The Asherman Chest Seal will go over the needle to provide a one-way valve and to protect the needle from accidental dislodgment. Other one-way valves are available or can be made but should be tested before using. (A needle through the finger of a rubber glove will not work as a one-way valve.) Young healthy patients will tolerate having no valve at all on the decompressing needle.
8. Leave the plastic catheter in position until it is replaced by a chest tube at the hospital.
9. Intubate the patient if indicated. Monitor closely for recurrence of the tension pneumothorax.

Bibliography

1. American College of Surgeons Committee on Trauma. 2008. Chest trauma management. In *Advanced Trauma Life Support.* 8th ed., 107–108. Chicago: American College of Surgeons, 2008.
2. Ball C. G., et al. 2010, June. Thoracic needle decompression for tension pneumothorax: Clinical correlation with catheter length. *Can J Surg* 53(3): 184–188.
3. Butler, F. K. 2010, July Supplement. Tactical combat casualty care: Update 2009. *J Trauma* 69(1): s 10–13.
4. Netto, F. A. C. S., et al. 2008. Are needle decompressions for tension pneumothoraces being performed appropriately for appropriate indications? *American J Emerg Med* 26: 597–602.

Explore Resource Central

For additional review and practice tests, visit www.bradybooks.com and click on Resource Central to access book-specific resources for this text. To access Resource Central, follow directions on the Student Access Card provided with this text. If there is no card, go to www.bradybooks.com and follow the Resource Central link to Buy Access from there.

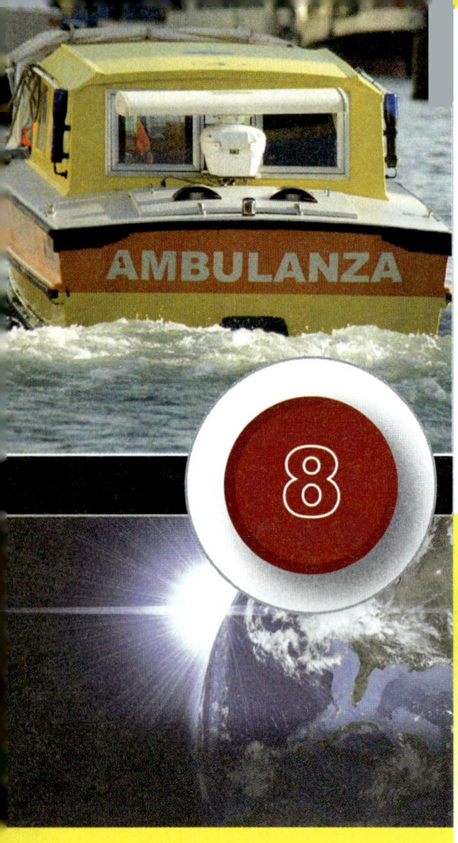

(© yannik LABBE, Fotolia, LLC)

8 Shock

Raymond L. Fowler, MD, FACEP
Paul E. Pepe, MD, MPH, FACEP, FCCM
John T. Stevens, EMT-P
Mario Luis Ramirez, MD, MPP

Shock Shock Shock Choc
Wstrząs Schock Šok الصدمة
šok Šok Sokk

KEY TERMS

capillary refill time (CRT), *p. 145*
hemorrhagic shock, *p. 147*
hemostatic agents, *p. 154*
hypovolemic shock, *p. 143*
mechanical shock, *p. 151*
neurogenic shock, *p. 142*
pulse pressure, *p. 144*
vasoconstriction, *p. 143*

OBJECTIVES

Upon successful completion of this chapter, you should be able to:

1. List the four components of the vascular system necessary for normal tissue perfusion.
2. Describe the symptoms and signs of shock in the order that they develop, from the very least to the very worst.
3. Describe the three common clinical shock syndromes.
4. Explain the pathophysiology of hemorrhagic shock, and compare it to the pathophysiology of mechanical and neurogenic shock.
5. Describe the management of the following:
   a. Hemorrhage that can be controlled
   b. Hemorrhage that cannot be controlled
   c. Nonhemorrhagic shock syndromes
6. Discuss the use of hemostatic agents for uncontrolled extremity hemorrhage.
7. Discuss the current indications for the use of IV fluids in the treatment of hemorrhagic shock.

Chapter Overview

The management of shock has been the subject of intensive research for decades. As a result, changes continue to be made in the recommendations for prehospital treatment of the patient with hemorrhagic shock. The experience of the U.S. military and its Coalition Partners in the Iraq and Afghanistan wars has led to new thinking in the management of life-threatening hemorrhage. This chapter will review present knowledge. It also offers the results of recent research about the pathophysiology and treatment of shock in the trauma patient and in patients with various other shock states.

CASE PRESENTATION

An ALS ambulance has been dispatched to a bar where a patron has been stabbed. The scene size-up reveals that the police are on scene, have cleared the bar, and are questioning bystanders outside. There is a single male victim who is sitting in a chair and holding his chest. Because the scene is safe and the mechanism of injury (stab wound) is readily apparent, the team dons personal protective equipment. As they approach the patient, each carries essential trauma care equipment. *How would you approach this patient? What type of assessment would you perform? What would you do first? Is this a load-and-go situation?* Keep these questions in mind as you read the chapter. Then, at the end of the chapter, find out how the rescuers completed this call. ■

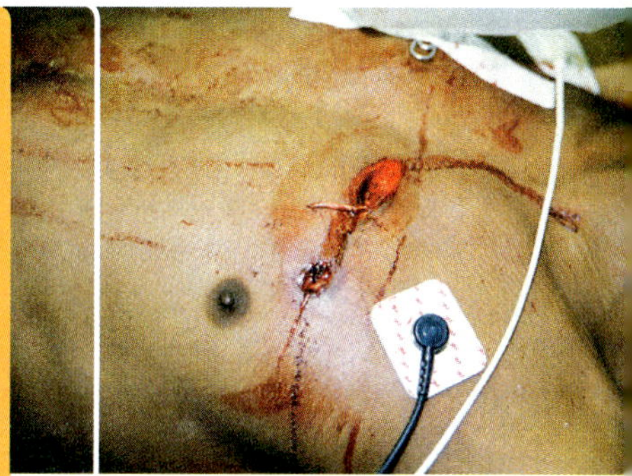

(©Edward T. Dickinson, MD)

Basic Pathophysiology

The normal perfusion of body tissues requires four intact components. They are as follows:

- Intact vascular system to deliver oxygenated blood throughout the body: the blood vessels
- Adequate air exchange in the lungs to allow oxygen to enter the blood: oxygenation
- Adequate volume of fluid in the vascular system: red blood cells and plasma
- Functioning pump: the heart

It is important to remember that blood pressure requires a "steady state" activity of all the preceding factors. The heart must be pumping, the blood volume must be adequate, the blood vessels must be intact, and the lungs must be oxygenating the blood. An important formula regarding the maintenance of blood pressure should be fresh in the mind of every emergency medical provider:

$$\text{Blood Pressure} = \text{Cardiac Output} \times \text{Peripheral Vascular Resistance}$$

In addition, the formula for cardiac output is written as follows:

$$\text{Cardiac Output} = \text{Heart Rate} \times \text{Stroke Volume}$$

neurogenic shock shock caused by spinal injury in which the spinal connections to the adrenal glands are interrupted and the vasoconstrictors, epinephrine and norepinephrine, are not produced. Without the vasoconstrictors the blood vessels dilate and redistribute blood flow to a larger vascular volume causing a relative hypovolemia.

PEARLS: Basic Rules

Shock kills. Look for early signs of shock, and manage it appropriately. The basic rules of shock management are

- Maintain the airway.
- Maintain oxygenation and ventilation.
- Control bleeding where possible.
- Maintain circulation through an adequate heart rate and intravascular volume.

Thus, if cardiac output falls (either due to falling heart rate or lowered stroke volume) or if peripheral vascular resistance falls (such as in the dilated arteries that occur in **neurogenic shock**), then blood pressure will fall.

The preservation of these components can be related to the basic rules of shock management, which are:

- Maintain the airway.
- Maintain oxygenation and ventilation.
- Control bleeding where possible.
- Maintain circulation through an adequate heart rate and intravascular volume.

An important point to remember is that the positive pressure breaths you give when you ventilate someone actually can decrease blood return to the heart, lowering cardiac output.

The term *shock* describes a condition that occurs when the perfusion of the body's tissues with oxygen, electrolytes, glucose, and fluid becomes inadequate to meet the body's needs. Several processes cause this drop in perfusion. For example, the loss of red blood cells in hemorrhaging patients results in less oxygen transport to the body tissues. Decreased circulating blood volume leads to lowered glucose, fluid volume, and electrolytes to the cells. Those circulatory disturbances result in the cells of the body becoming "shocked," and grave changes in body tissue begin to occur. Eventually, cell death follows.

Deprived of oxygen, cells begin to use "backup" processes, which use energy less efficiently and produce toxic by-products such as lactic acid. The backup (anaerobic) processes may postpone cellular death for a time. However, the lack of oxygen is compounded by those toxic by-products because they can poison certain cellular functions, such as the production of energy by mitochondria. Eventually, accumulating lactic acid in the blood and organs creates a systemic acidosis that further disrupts cellular activity. Respiratory muscle function also weakens, respiratory failure develops, and hypoxia worsens.

Inadequate oxygen delivery causes the body to respond with increased activity of the sympathetic nervous system (increased sympathetic tone), resulting in the increased release of circulating catecholamines (epinephrine and norepinephrine). Those hormones increase both the rate and strength of the heart's contractions and constrict peripheral arterial blood vessels. The midbrain responds to the progressive hypoxia and acidosis with an increase in the respiratory rate.

As you can see, shock begins with an injury. It then spreads through the body as a multisystem insult to major organs. Specific symptoms result, symptoms that you can detect at the bedside as the patient becomes progressively sicker. Thus, shock is a cellular process with clinical manifestations. The patient with shock may be pale, diaphoretic, and tachycardic. At the cellular level, the patient's cells are starving for oxygen and nutrients. Shock, therefore, is a condition in which poor tissue perfusion can severely and permanently damage the organs of the body, causing disability or death. The clinical signs and symptoms of shock imply that critical processes are threatening every vulnerable cell in the patient's body, particularly those in vital organs.

Finally, the part of shock that field personnel do not usually see occurs after the patient is admitted to the hospital. Days after hemorrhagic shock in the field, the patient may suffer multisystem organ failure in the ICU. So, discovering a patient in shock, treating him according to current standards, and rapidly delivering him to the appropriate hospital facility are essential aspects in saving the patient's life.

Assessment of Shock

Shock produces signs and symptoms that you can observe during patient assessment. The initial diagnosis of the shock state often can be made from the physical exam findings. Although blood pressure should be monitored frequently to help determine whether or not organ perfusion is adequate, remember that hypotension is a late sign. Assessment tools other than measuring the blood pressure must be used to recognize early shock in the trauma patient.

The blood pressure required to maintain adequate perfusion varies among people. The question, "How low can you go?" while maintaining adequate perfusion has not yet been answered. It is known that the healthy young patient often can maintain adequate perfusion in the face of hypotension. In contrast, older patients, hypertensive patients, and those with head injury often cannot tolerate hypotension for even short periods. It is vital that you work with your medical director to stay up to date on recommendations for shock management as new research is completed.

> **PEARLS:** Hypotension
>
> Shock is poor perfusion, not just hypotension. Hypotension is a late finding, after the compensatory mechanisms have failed.

Although this chapter is about trauma, shock is a clinical condition associated with medical problems as well. Following is a discussion of shock syndromes, many of which are caused by traumatic conditions. The take-home point, though, is that the shock state is one of low tissue perfusion. Although there are some similarities in the body's response to different kinds of shock, there also are some differences. For example, the stabbed and bleeding patient in hemorrhagic shock often shows many of the same signs as the burned or dehydrated patient with low blood volume *not* due to hemorrhage.

Compensated and Decompensated Shock

Generally, the onset of the symptoms and signs of **hypovolemic shock** (including hemorrhagic shock) occur in the following order: compensated shock and then decompensated shock.

hypovolemic shock shock caused by insufficient volume (blood or fluid) within the vascular system.

Compensated Shock

During compensated shock, the body is still able to maintain perfusion by compensatory mechanism and will present with the following signs and symptoms:

- *Weakness and lightheadedness*—caused by decreased blood volume
- *Thirst*—caused by hypovolemia (especially with relatively low fluid amounts in the blood vessels)
- *Pallor* (pale, white color of the skin)—caused by catecholamine-induced **vasoconstriction** and/or loss of circulating red blood cells
- *Tachycardia*—caused by the effect of catecholamines on the heart as the brain increases the activity of the sympathetic nervous system
- *Diaphoresis* (sweating)—caused by the effects of catecholamines on sweat glands
- *Tachypnea* (elevated respiratory rate)—caused by the brain elevating the respiratory rate under the influence of stress, catecholamines, acidosis, and hypoxia
- *Decreased urinary output*—caused by hypovolemia, hypoxia, and circulating catecholamines (important to remember in interfacility transfers)
- *Weakened peripheral pulses*—the "thready" pulse (meaning "threadlike"; arteries actually shrink in width as intravascular volume is lost); caused by vasoconstriction, tachycardia, and loss of blood volume

vasoconstriction the constriction (narrowing) of the arteries to maintain the blood pressure and perfusion of vital organs.

Note: The signs and symptoms listed here are in the order of progressive "compensation," as the body attempts to deal with the cause of shock. Beginning with the next sign, hypotension, the body is no longer able to maintain perfusion, and the shock condition is now "decompensated."

Decompensated Shock

- *Hypotension*—caused by hypovolemia, either absolute or relative (see later paragraphs for a discussion of relative hypovolemia), and/or by the diminished cardiac output seen in "obstructive" or "mechanical" shock
- *Altered mental status* (confusion, restlessness, combativeness, unconsciousness)—caused by decreased cerebral perfusion, acidosis, hypoxia, and catecholamine stimulation
- *Cardiac arrest*—caused by critical organ failure secondary to blood or fluid loss, hypoxia, and occasionally arrhythmia caused by catecholamine stimulation and/or low perfusion

To summarize, many of the symptoms of shock of any etiology including the classic hemorrhagic shock picture are caused by the release of catecholamines. When the brain senses that perfusion to the tissues is insufficient, chemical messages are sent down the spinal cord to the sympathetic nervous system and the adrenal glands, causing a release of catecholamines (epinephrine and norepinephrine) into the circulation. The circulating catecholamines cause the tachycardia, anxiety, diaphoresis, and vasoconstriction. This narrowing of the small arteries shunts blood away from the skin and intestines to the heart, lungs, and brain.

Close monitoring early in the shock syndrome may allow you to detect an initial rise in the blood pressure due to shunting, though this does not always happen. The **pulse pressure** is the pressure driving blood through the vascular system. It is calculated by subtracting the diastolic blood pressure from the systolic. It is usually about 40 mm Hg (blood pressure of 120/80 equals pulse pressure of 40). There will almost always be an initial narrowing of the pulse pressure because vasoconstriction raises the diastolic pressure more than the systolic. The shunting of blood from the skin and the loss of circulating red blood cells cause the pallor of shock.

pulse pressure the pressure driving blood through the vascular system. It is calculated by subtracting the diastolic from the systolic blood pressures.

Decreased perfusion causes weakness and thirst initially and then, later, an altered level of consciousness (confusion, restlessness, or combativeness) and worsening pallor. Development of confusion, restlessness, or combativeness always should alert you to possible hypoxia or shock. As shock continues, the prolonged tissue hypoxia leads to worsening acidosis. This acidosis can ultimately cause a loss of response to catecholamines, worsening the drop in blood pressure. This is often the point at which the patient in "compensated" shock suddenly "crashes." Eventually, the hypoxia and acidosis cause cardiac dysfunction, including cardiac arrest and, ultimately, death.

Although the individual response to post-traumatic hemorrhage may vary, many patients will have the following classic patterns of "early" and "late" shock:

- *Early shock.* This is the loss of approximately 15% to 25% of the blood volume. That is enough to stimulate slight to moderate tachycardia, pallor, narrowed pulse pressure, thirst, weakness, and possibly delayed capillary refill. In "early shock," the body is "compensating" for the physical insult that is causing the problem (hemorrhage, dehydration, tension pneumothorax, and so on).

- *Late shock.* Late shock is the loss of approximately 30% to 45% of the blood volume. It is enough to cause hypotension as well as the other symptoms of hypovolemic shock listed earlier. When "late shock" occurs, it means the body's ability to compensate for the physical insult has failed. As mentioned earlier, hypotension is the first sign of "late shock." The hypotensive patient, then, is near death. Aggressive assessment and management must be provided to prevent the death of the patient.

Note that during the initial assessment, early shock presents as a fast pulse with pallor and diaphoresis. In contrast, late shock may present as weak pulse or loss of the peripheral pulse. A useful tip is to remember that the lowest pressure at which the radial pulse can usually be felt by the examiner begins at a systolic pressure of about 80 mm Hg, the femoral pulse can initially be felt at a systolic pressure of about 70 mm Hg, and the carotid pulse can initially be felt at a systolic pressure of about 60 mm Hg. Thus, if you had a trauma victim with a carotid pulse but no radial pulse, you could estimate that the patient's systolic pressure was between 60 and 80 mm Hg. A scientific study suggests that those numbers are slightly high (Demetriades et al., 1998). Nevertheless, weakened pulses taken with other signs of shock should lead you quickly to suspect decompensated shock. The aggressiveness with which you treat the shock will depend on a number of factors. You will be guided by the patient's systolic blood pressure as well as respiratory rate, pulse rate, level of consciousness, and any obvious bleeding.

Prolonged **capillary refill time (CRT)** was previously thought to be very useful for detecting early shock. CRT is tested by pressing on the palm of the hand or the sides of the fingertips. For a small child, CRT may be checked squeezing the whole foot and looking to see how quickly color returns to the ball of the foot. The test is suspicious for shock if the blanched area remains pale for longer than 2 seconds. Scientific evaluation of this test has shown it to have a high correlation with late shock but to be of little value for detecting early shock. The test was associated with both frequent false-positive and false-negative results. Low blood volume, cold temperatures, and catecholamine-induced vasoconstriction can all cause decreased perfusion of the capillary bed in the skin and thus cause results that cannot be trusted. Measurement of capillary refill is useful for small children in whom it is difficult to get an accurate blood pressure, but it is of little use for detecting early shock in adults.

capillary refill time (CRT) a test for shock performed by pressing on the palm of the hand or sides of the fingertips and noting how quickly color returns to the blanched area. The test is suspicious for shock if the blanched area remains pale for longer than 2 seconds. It has been found to be unreliable for early shock and neurogenic shock.

Evaluation of Tachycardia

One of the first signs of illness, and arguably one of the most common, is that of tachycardia. You will frequently be confronted with the patient with an elevated pulse rate, and you must make some sort of distinction about the cause.

First, remember that you must always attempt to explain why a patient has tachycardia. An elevated pulse rate (generally considered to be above 100 in an adult and higher at younger ages) is never normal. Humans can transiently raise their pulses in the setting of anxiety, but such elevation quickly returns to normal or fluctuates in rate, depending on the waxing and waning of the anxiety state.

Second, remember that an elevated pulse rate is one of the first signs of shock. Any adult trauma patient with a sustained pulse rate above 100 must be suspected of having occult hemorrhage until proven otherwise. During the ITLS Primary Survey, a pulse rate greater than 120 should be a red flag for possible shock.

Finally, some patients who are in shock may not develop tachycardia. Patients with traumatic hypotension may develop a "relative bradycardia." As many as

PEARLS: Tachycardia

A persistently elevated pulse rate while at rest is *always* an indication of something medically wrong with the patient, including the possibility of occult hemorrhage. Absence of tachycardia does not rule out shock, however.

20% of patients with bleeding into the abdomen may not show tachycardia. Another point to consider is the injured patient's medications. Can they affect the intrinsic heart rate? Beta-blockers or calcium channel blocking medications would prevent them from developing a tachycardia even with excessive blood loss. Their presence should always alert the prehospital care provider to evaluate all hemodynamic parameters, not just heart rate alone. So, the absence of tachycardia in an injured patient does not always rule out shock. Children are unable to increase their stroke volume, so their cardiac output depends on their heart rate alone (cardiac output = stroke volume × heart rate). Children in decompensated shock may develop bradycardia, which can have a devastating effect on their ability to maintain blood flow to their vital organs.

Capnography

PEARLS: Capnography

Falling height of the capnography waveform may be one of the first indicators that a patient is going into a shock state.

The heart delivers oxygen and nutrients to the cells of the body by way of blood vessels. The cells "burn" the nutrients in the presence of oxygen to produce energy, water, and carbon dioxide (CO_2). The water and CO_2 move into the bloodstream, the CO_2 being carried to the lungs by the red blood cells for excretion during exhalation. CO_2, then, is the exhaled by-product of metabolism. Put another way, the level of exhaled CO_2 indicates how brightly the fire of metabolism is burning in the cells. When measured moment to moment at the airway, the level of CO_2 being excreted may be graphed as a waveform and can give some measure of the patient's underlying metabolic rate.

Devices are now commonly available, either separately or on ECG monitors, that measure CO_2 levels and display them as a waveform. The typical exhaled CO_2 is approximately 35 to 45 mm Hg. Falling measured CO_2 indicates either that the patient is hyperventilating (from anxiety or acidosis) or that the amount of oxygen being supplied to the cells is falling. You might say it this way: A falling exhaled CO_2 level suggests that the fire of metabolism in the patient may be burning low.

Patients in shock have decreased oxygen being supplied to their cells. This is either because they have lost blood through hemorrhage or the heart is not circulating it effectively. Thus, if you are monitoring a patient either in shock or at risk of going into shock, monitor the level of exhaled CO_2 as part of your overall care. A level of exhaled CO_2 that falls much under 35—especially if it falls into the 20s or below—may be an indication of circulatory collapse and thus can be an additional warning sign of worsening shock. (See Chapter 5, Figures 5-15 and 5-16.)

The Shock Syndromes

Although the most common shock state seen in trauma patients is associated with hemorrhage and the accompanying hypovolemia, there are actually three major classifications of shock. Those "types" of shock relate directly to the blood pressure equation discussed earlier in this chapter (Blood Pressure = Cardiac Output × Peripheral Vascular Resistance). These three shock states can be categorized according to their causes as follows:

- *Low-volume shock* (absolute hypovolemia) is caused by hemorrhage or other major body fluid loss (diarrhea, vomiting, and "third spacing" due to burns, peritonitis, and other causes).
- *High-space shock* (relative hypovolemia) is caused by spinal injury, vasovagal syncope, sepsis, and certain drug overdoses that dilate the blood vessels and redistribute blood flow to a larger vascular volume.

- *Mechanical shock* (cardiogenic or obstructive) is a "pump" problem either caused by a damaged heart (myocardial contusion or myocardial infarction) or by conditions preventing the filling of the heart (pericardial tamponade, tension pneumothorax), or something obstructing blood flow through the lungs (massive pulmonary embolism).

There are notable differences in the appearance of patients with these conditions, and it is critical that you be aware of the signs and symptoms that accompany each one.

Low-Volume Shock (Absolute Hypovolemia)

Loss of blood from injury is called *post-traumatic hemorrhage*. In addition to head injury, **hemorrhagic shock** is the number-one cause of preventable death from injury. The amount of volume that the blood vessels can hold is many liters more than what actually flows through the vasculature. The sympathetic nervous system keeps the vessels constricted. That reduces their volume and maintains blood pressure high enough to perfuse vital organs. If blood volume is lost, "sensors" in the major vessels signal the adrenal gland and the nerves of the sympathetic nervous system to secrete catecholamines. They cause vasoconstriction and thus further shrink the vascular space and maintain perfusion pressure to the brain and heart. If the blood loss is minor, the sympathetic system can shrink the space enough to maintain blood pressure. If the loss is severe, the vascular space cannot be shrunk down enough to maintain blood pressure, and hypotension occurs.

hemorrhagic shock shock caused by insufficient blood within the vascular system.

Normally, the blood vessels are elastic and are distended by the volume that is in them. This produces a radial artery pulse that is full and wide. Blood loss allows the artery to shrink in width, becoming more threadlike in size. The term *thready pulse* means that the actual width of the artery shrinks, becoming barely wider than a thread.

Hypovolemic shock victims usually have tachycardia, are pale, and have flat neck veins. So, if you find a trauma victim with a fast heart rate, who is pale, with weak radial pulses and flat neck veins, this patient is probably bleeding from some injury.

Absolute hypovolemic shock may be identified in your patient during the ITLS Primary Survey (Figure 8-1).

ABSOLUTE HYPOVOLEMIC SHOCK

SCENE SIZE-UP
Is the scene SAFE?

↓

INITIAL ASSESSMENT
LOC
Possibly decreased
Airway
Possibly snoring
Breathing
Rapid and shallow
Pulses
Rapid/thready
Skin cool/clammy and pale
Possibly uncontrolled hemorrhage

↓

RAPID TRAUMA SURVEY
Neck Veins
Flat
Trachea
Midline
Chest
May be normal
Possibly contusions or penetrating injury
Breath Sounds
Normal or unilaterally diminished with dullness to percussion
Abdomen
Possibly tender/rigid/distended
Pelvis
May be unstable or painful
Extremities
Possibly femur fractures

FIGURE 8-1 Absolute hypovolemic shock may be identified during the ITLS Primary Survey.

High-Space Shock (Relative Hypovolemia)

As mentioned earlier, the volume that the blood vessels can hold is many liters more than the blood volume in the blood vessels. The average-size adult has around 5 liters of blood in the vascular system. However, the vascular system could hold as many as 25 liters of blood, if the arterioles were to fully dilate. Again, it is the steady-state action of the sympathetic nervous system that keeps the arterioles of the vascular bed constricted in the normal state, keeping most of the blood in the arteries and maintaining perfusion to the heart and brain. Anything that interrupts the outflow from the sympathetic nervous system and causes the loss of this normal vasoconstriction allows the vascular space to dilate, becoming much "too large" for the amount of blood in the vascular system. If blood vessels dilate, the 5 liters or so of blood flowing through the normal adult's vascular space may not be sufficient to maintain blood pressure and vital tissue perfusion. The condition causing the vascular space to be too large for a normal amount of blood has been called "high-space shock," or relative hypovolemia (also known as "vasodilatory shock"). Although several causes of high-space shock exist (such as sepsis syndrome and drug overdose), neurogenic shock, commonly called *spinal shock*, is addressed here because it may be caused by trauma.

The nerves of the sympathetic nervous system come off the spinal cord in the thoracic (chest) and lumbar area. This is why the sympathetic nervous system is often called the "thoracolumbar autonomic nervous system." Neurogenic shock occurs most typically after an injury to the spinal cord. An injury to the spinal cord in the neck can prevent the brain from being able to send out the sympathetic nervous system signals. Thus, a cervical spinal-cord injury can prevent the brain from raising the pulse rate, from raising the strength of the heart's contraction, or from constricting the peripheral arterioles (the vessels that maintain blood pressure). Although circulating catecholamines already present in the bloodstream may preserve the blood pressure for a short time, the disruption of the sympathetic nervous system outflow from the spinal cord results in loss of the normal vascular tone and in the inability of the body to compensate for any accompanying hemorrhage.

The clinical presentation of neurogenic shock differs from hemorrhagic shock in that there is no catecholamine release and thus no pallor (vasoconstriction), tachycardia, or sweating. The patient will have a decreased blood pressure, but the heart rate will be normal or slow, and the skin is usually warm, dry, and pink. The patient also may have accompanying paralysis and/or sensory deficit corresponding to the spinal-cord injury. You also may see a lack of chest wall movement and only simple diaphragmatic movement when the patient is asked to take a deep breath. This diaphragmatic breathing is seen as protruding of the abdomen during inspiration. In males, priapism (erection of the shaft of the penis) may be present. The important point is that neurogenic shock does not have the typical picture of hemorrhagic shock, even when associated with severe bleeding. The neurologic assessment is therefore very important, and you should not rely on typical shock symptoms and signs to suspect internal bleeding or accompanying hemorrhage-associated shock. Neurogenic shock patients may "look better" than their actual condition really is and can be some of the most difficult patients to accurately assess.

Certain drug overdoses and chemical exposures also can result in shock from vasodilatation and relative hypovolemia. Very often injuries result after such overdoses, and their effect on typical clinical signs and symptoms (like neurogenic shock) should be considered. Examples of drug overdoses and chemical exposures that may produce the relative hypovolemia syndrome include nitroglycerin, calcium channel blockers, antihypertensive medications, cyanide, and even the ethyl alcohol found in legal alcoholic beverages.

Whereas the patient with neurogenic shock (due to spinal-cord injury) has a slow heart rate, is pink, and has flat neck veins, some of the persons with medical causes of high-space shock (some drug overdoses, cyanide, sepsis) may be pink and have flat neck veins but they usually have a fast heart rate. The physical evaluation of these patients may give signs difficult to interpret. Calcium channel blocker or beta-blocker poisonings often produce bradycardia, whereas nitroglycerin overdose might produce tachycardia. In these patients, taking a good history becomes very important. Be sure to get information from others who may know the patient, including what medication(s) the patient may be taking. This information may be lifesaving.

Relative hypovolemia due to neurogenic (spinal) shock may be identified in your patient during the ITLS Primary Survey (Figure 8-2).

Mechanical (Cardiogenic or Obstructive) Shock

The heart is a pump. Like any pump, it has a "power" stroke and a "filling" stroke, just like a piston moving up and down in the cylinder of a motor. In the normal adult's resting state, the heart pumps out about 5 liters of blood per minute. This means, of course, that the heart also must take in about 5 liters of blood per minute. Therefore, any traumatic or medical condition that slows or prevents the venous return of blood can cause shock by lowering cardiac output and thus oxygen delivery to the tissues. Likewise, anything that obstructs the flow of blood to or through the heart can cause shock.

The following are traumatic conditions that can cause mechanical shock:

- *Tension pneumothorax.* It is so named because of the high air tension (pressure) that may develop in the pleural space (between the lung and chest wall) due to a lung or chest wall injury. This very high positive pressure collapses the low-pressure superior and inferior vena cava, preventing the return of venous blood to the heart. The resulting "backup" of blood presents as distended neck veins. Shifting of mediastinal structures also may lower venous return by impinging on the superior and inferior vena cava, also causing a deviation of the trachea away from the affected side (rarely seen clinically). Decreased venous return results in lower cardiac output and the development of shock. (See Figure 8-3 and Chapters 6 and 7 for a complete description of the signs, symptoms, and treatment of tension pneumothorax.)
- *Cardiac tamponade.* Cardiac tamponade, or "pericardial tamponade," occurs when blood fills the "potential" space between the heart and the pericardium, squeezing the heart and preventing the heart from filling (Figure 8-4). Like the "squeezing" of the superior and inferior vena cava present as distended neck veins, the "squeezing" of the heart produces the same sign. This decreased filling of the heart causes cardiac output to fall, resulting in the development of shock.

  Pericardial tamponade may occur in more than 75% of cases of penetrating cardiac injury. The signs of tamponade have been labeled "Beck's triad," consisting of distended neck veins, mufflied heart tones, and pulsus paradoxus. On-scene interventions should be avoided if this diagnosis is suspected because any time wasted on scene could result in death of the patient. Definitive surgical care in the nearest appropriate facility for pericardial decompression may be the only lifesaving measure available. Using intravenous fluids to increase filling pressure of the heart may possibly be of some value, but IV fluids could also worsen the condition if there is an additional internal exsanguinating injury. Use of IV fluids in this situation should be during transport and only on the order of medical direction. (See Chapter 6 for a more complete discussion.)

RELATIVE HYPOVOLEMIA

SCENE SIZE-UP
Is the scene SAFE?

↓

INITIAL ASSESSMENT
LOC
Possibly decreased
Airway
Possibly snoring
Breathing
Possibly diaphragmatic only
Pulses
Normal or slow rate
Weak
Skin color normal without diaphoresis

↓

RAPID TRAUMA SURVEY
Neck Veins
Flat
Trachea
Midline
Chest
May be normal
Breath Sounds
Normal
Extremities
Absent motor/sensory (usually from neck or upper chest down)

FIGURE 8-2 Relative hypovolemia due to neurogenic (spinal) shock may be identified during the ITLS Primary Survey.

PEARLS: Mechanical or High-Space Shock

Look for signs of mechanical or high-space shock, especially if there is no bleeding.

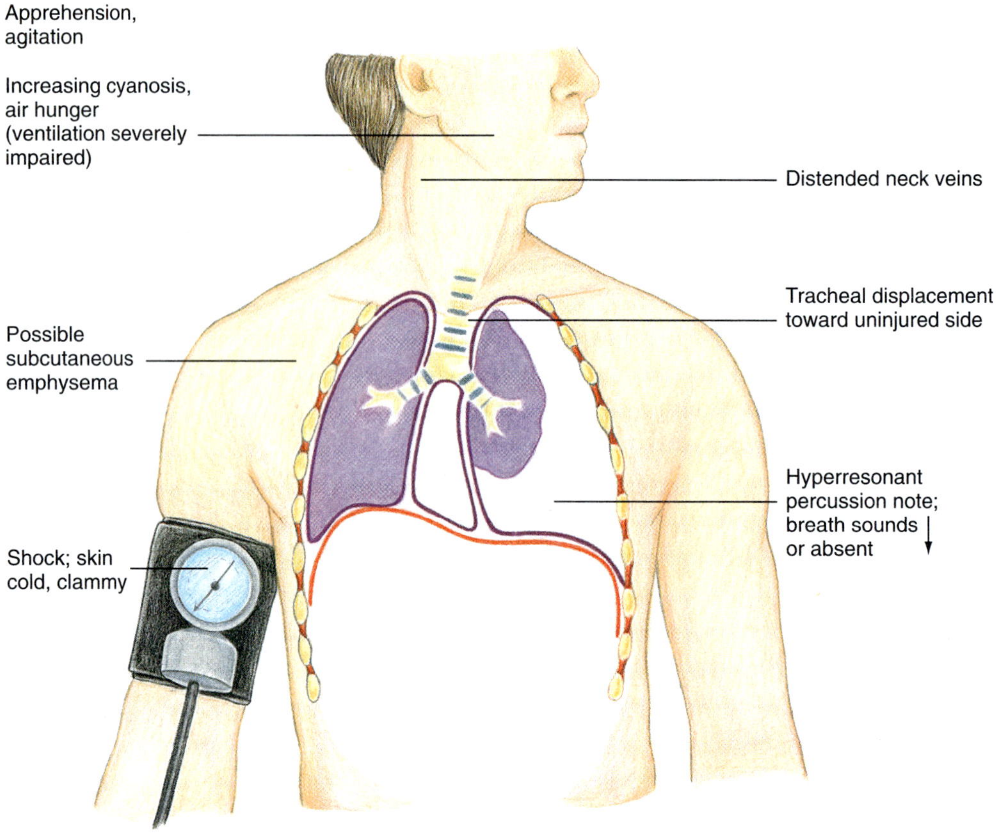

FIGURE 8-3 Physical findings of tension pneumothorax.

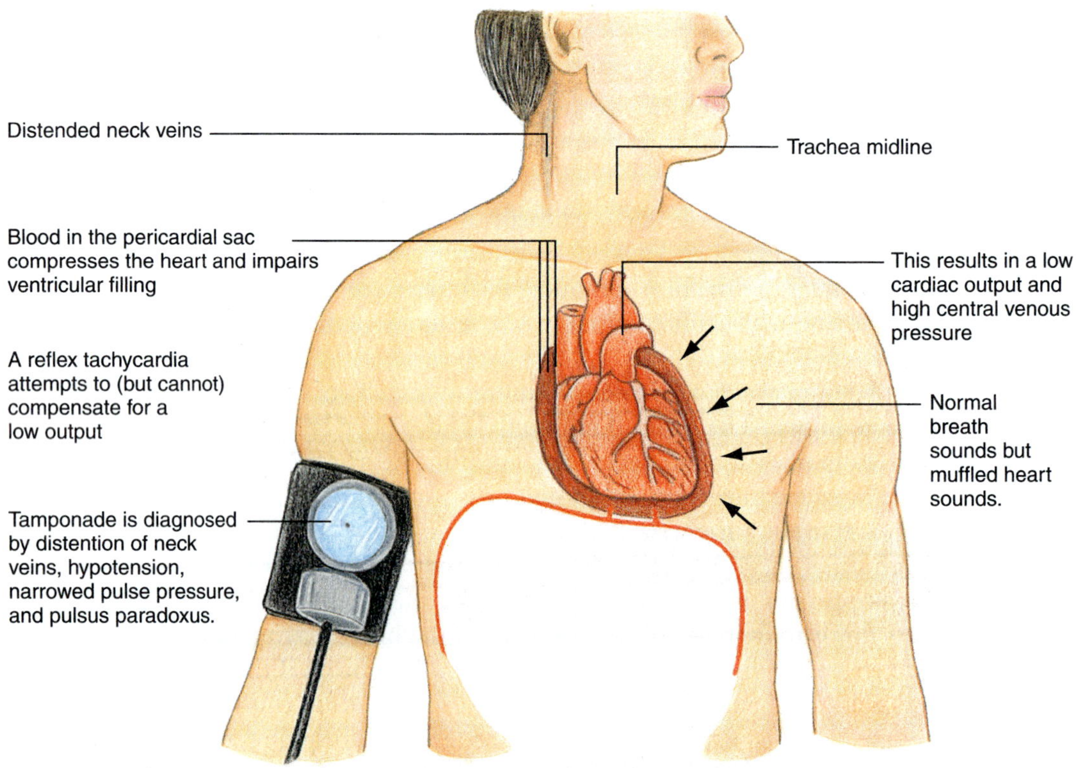

FIGURE 8-4 Pathophysiology and physical findings of cardiac tamponade.

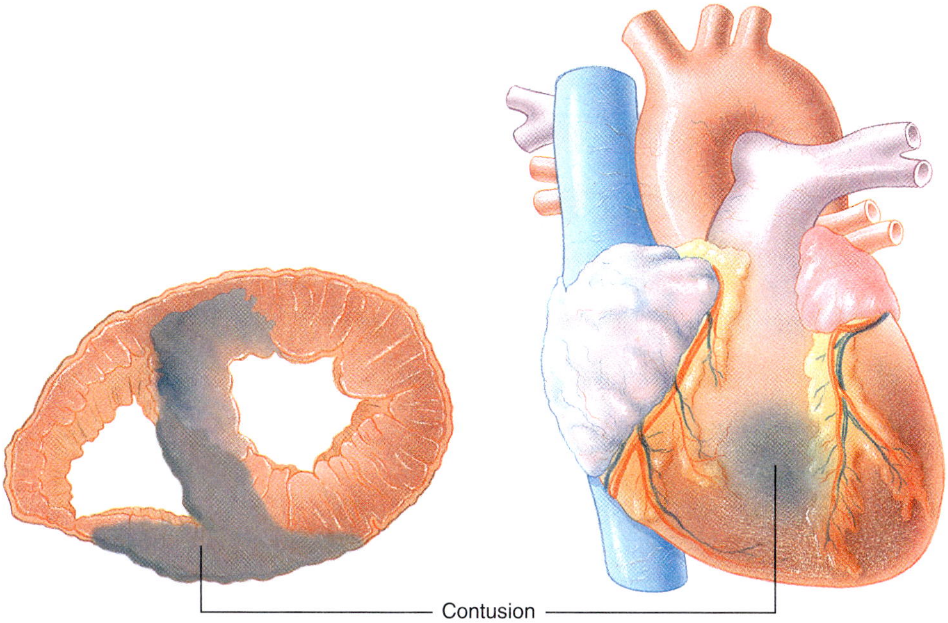

FIGURE 8-5 Myocardial contusion most frequently affects the right atrium and ventricle as they collide with the sternum.

- *Myocardial contusion.* Myocardial contusion can result in diminished cardiac output because the heart loses pumping strength due to direct injury to the heart muscle (Figure 8-5) and/or cardiac dysrhythmias (Figure 8-6). Myocardial contusion often cannot be differentiated from cardiac tamponade in the field. Therefore, rapid transport, supportive care, and cardiac monitoring are the mainstays of therapy.

A word of caution is important here. Patients with shock from mechanical causes can be very near death. Delay on the scene may prevent salvage of the patient. For example, one urban study has suggested that, in applicable cases, the time from development of a traumatic cardiac tamponade to circulatory arrest may be as little as 5 to 10 minutes. Another study (Haut, 2010) found that if the patient had penetrating trauma to the trunk, taking the time to package the patient on a backboard doubled the death rate (7.2% versus 14.7%). Survival following traumatic circulatory arrest, even in the best of trauma systems, is rarely achieved if pericardiocentesis and then surgery are not performed within 5 to 10 minutes.

Mechanical shock is caused by a diminished cardiac output rather than blood loss. Thus, these patients usually have a different appearance at the bedside than hemorrhagic shock patients. Because the cardiac output is diminished, the blood backs up into the venous system, resulting in distended neck veins. The lungs are not being perfused well, causing the patient to become cyanotic. Because the patient is in shock with an intact spinal cord, catecholamines are released, and the patient develops tachycardia and diaphoresis. Thus, mechanical shock patients are cyanotic with distended neck veins and tachycardia. A post-trauma patient with these signs is near death, requiring rapid transport to a trauma center. In the setting of a tension pneumothorax, needle decompression of the affected side of the thorax can be lifesaving.

mechanical shock shock produced by conditions that affect the ability of the heart to pump blood; caused by a damaged heart (myocardial contusion) or by conditions preventing the filling of the heart (pericardial tamponade, tension pneumothorax).

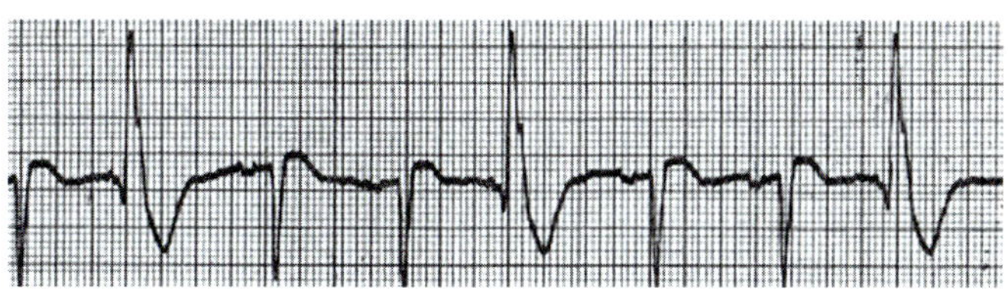

FIGURE 8-6 Myocardial contusion may cause ventricular ectopy.

FIGURE 8-7 Mechanical (obstructive) shock may be identified during the ITLS Primary Survey.

MECHANICAL (OBSTRUCTIVE) SHOCK

SCENE SIZE-UP
Seat belt? Steering wheel? Is the scene SAFE?

INITIAL ASSESSMENT
LOC
Possibly decreased
Breathing
Rapid and labored
Pulses
Weak/thready; possibly irregular; possibly absent radials
Skin
Pale/cool/diaphoretic; possibly cyanotic

RAPID TRAUMA SURVEY
Head/Neck
Neck vein distention; possible tracheal deviation
Chest
Contusions or penetrating wounds, possibly asymmetrical
Breath Sounds
Possibly diminished or absent on affected side
Possibly hyperresonant to percussion
Possibly wet rales
Heart Tones
Possibly muffled

Mechanical (obstructive) shock may be identified in your patient during the ITLS Primary Survey (Figure 8-7).

PEARLS: Hemorrhage

Control hemorrhage. If it cannot be done in the field, the patient needs to be in the operating room as soon as possible.

Management and Treatment

General Management of Post-Traumatic Shock States

Management of post-traumatic shock states includes the following:

1. *Control bleeding.* Red blood cells are necessary to carry oxygen. Control of bleeding must be obtained either by direct pressure, tourniquet, hemostatic agent, or rapid transport to surgery.
2. *Administer high-flow oxygen.* Patients in shock need oxygen supplementation. Evaluation of skin color in shock patients may not tell you what the patient's oxygen requirement is. Generally, patients in hemorrhagic shock are pale. Cyanosis (from mechanical shock states) is an extremely late sign of hypoxemia and may not occur at all if there has been extensive blood loss. Indeed, a patient has to have at least 5 grams of deoxygenated hemoglobin per 100 cc of blood (normal is 14 grams) for cyanosis to occur. Someone bleeding to death, literally, may not have enough hemoglobin around to manifest cyanosis. So, it is safe to say regardless of the patient's skin color, you should give high-flow oxygen to all patients at risk for shock. Try to maintain a pulse oximeter reading of about 95%.
3. *Load and go.* Trauma patients in shock from any cause are considered to be in the load-and-go category. Transport as soon as you finish the ITLS Primary Survey (initial assessment and rapid trauma survey). Almost all critical interventions should be done in the ambulance. (See Chapter 2.)

Treatment of Post-Traumatic Hemorrhage

Specific prehospital management of the patient in shock remains both controversial and the subject of ongoing research. There is no question of the need for control of hemorrhage, supplemental oxygen, and early transport, but the indications for most other therapies are still being debated. For example, the results of the National Institutes of Health Resuscitation Outcomes Consortium trial on the treatment of hemorrhagic shock due to trauma—reported in 2010—indicated that low-volume resuscitation with hypertonic saline in patients in severe hemorrhagic shock showed no benefit over conventional IV fluids. Further studies to find the "best" resuscitation fluid, including how much fluid should be administered, are ongoing at this time.

Since the early days of modern shock treatment (about the middle of the 20th century), intravenous crystalloid solutions (and sometimes colloid) have been tested and/or utilized to reverse the effects of hypovolemia. In addition, it has been previously proposed that intra-abdominal and pelvic bleeding may possibly be diminished by use of the pneumatic antishock garment (PASG; or military antishock trousers, MAST). Research showed that the PASG seemed to cause a worsening death rate when the garment was applied to patients with uncontrolled bleeding.

Patients in hypovolemic shock due to hemorrhage may be generally thought of as falling into one of the following two categories: those with bleeding that you can control (such as many extremity injuries) and those with bleeding that you cannot control (such as hemorrhage from internal injuries).

Hemorrhage That Can Be Controlled

A patient with controllable bleeding is fairly easy to manage. Most bleeding can be stopped with direct pressure. In some situations (usually blast or tactical injuries) there may be life-threatening hemorrhage that you cannot control with direct pressure. In these most extreme circumstances you should not hesitate to apply a tourniquet. A tourniquet is rarely needed, but when it is needed, it should be applied quickly.

If the patient has clinical evidence of shock that persists after direct control of the bleeding, you should take the following steps.

PEARLS: IV Access

Do not waste scene time to establish IV access. Consider the use of IO vascular access if the patient is critical and you cannot obtain IV access.

PROCEDURE

Managing Shock When Bleeding Has Been Controlled

1. Put the patient's body in a horizontal position.
2. Administer high-flow oxygen, preferably using a nonrebreather mask with a reservoir.
3. Transport immediately in a safe, rapid manner.
4. Obtain IV access with large-bore catheters (16 gauge or greater if possible). Consider intraosseous (IO) vascular access if the patient is critical and you are unable to quickly establish an intravenous line.
5. Give normal saline as a bolus of 20 mL/kg IV rapidly and then repeat the ITLS Ongoing Exam. When bleeding is controlled, it is permissible to attempt to normalize blood pressure, unlike the situation of uncontrolled bleeding. If shock symptoms persist, continue to administer fluid in boluses and reassess. In some cases of very severe hemorrhage—because of the substantial loss of red blood

cells and markedly impaired oxygen delivery to the tissues—shock symptoms and signs may persist despite hemorrhage control and IV volume infusion. These patients need the rapid transfusion of blood and blood products.

6. Place the patient on an ECG monitor early during evaluation and treatment.
7. Apply pulse oximetry and, if available, waveform capnography.
8. Perform Ongoing Exams, and observe closely, especially for any return of bleeding.

Hemorrhage That Cannot Be Controlled

External Hemorrhage. A patient with external hemorrhage that is not controlled by direct pressure must be rapidly transported to an appropriate facility where necessary procedures to gain surgical hemostasis can be performed. Although most physicians advocate fluid resuscitation to treat hemorrhagic shock, you also must remember that elevating blood pressure can increase uncontrolled hemorrhage. To manage this patient, you should take the following steps.

hemostatic agents chemical or physical agents that help stop hemorrhage by facilitating clotting of the blood at the bleeding site.

PROCEDURE

Managing Shock Due to Exsanguinating External Hemorrhage That You Cannot Control

1. Apply direct pressure on the bleeding site (e.g., femoral artery, facial hemorrhage). Substantial pressure may be required. Releasing of direct pressure may result in the continuation of bleeding.
2. Put the patient's body in a horizontal position.
3. Do not hesitate to apply a tourniquet to a bleeding extremity to stop severe bleeding that cannot be otherwise controlled.
4. If you cannot stop severe bleeding with pressure and cannot use a tourniquet (groin, axilla, neck, face, scalp), you may use one of the **hemostatic agents** such as QuikClot® Combat Gauze, Hemcon Dressing, or Celox™, if available. (See Chapter 14.) Pack the hemostatic agent in the wound and hold firm pressure. Always remember that the hemostatic agent is an "adjunct" to assist in controlling hemorrhage, not a hemorrhage control by itself. The agents must be part of an overall "hemorrhage control protocol" authorized by the medical director or by state protocol.
5. Administer high-flow oxygen through a nonrebreather mask with a reservoir.
6. Transport immediately and in a rapid, safe manner.
7. Gain IV access when en route. Consider IO vascular access if patient is critical and you are unable to establish an intravenous line.
   a. Give only enough normal saline to maintain a blood pressure high enough for adequate peripheral perfusion. Maintaining peripheral perfusion may be defined as producing a peripheral pulse (such as a radial pulse), maintaining consciousness (assuming a traumatic brain injury is not also present), and maintaining an "adequate blood pressure." The definition of an adequate blood pressure ("How low can you go?") remains controversial and will continue to be subject to change based on ongoing research. Certainly most young patients can maintain adequate perfusion with a blood pressure of 80 to 90 mm Hg systolic, but some experts now advocate even lower pressures.

Keep in mind that a higher systolic pressure may be required in the setting of head injury with increased intracerebral pressure and in patients with a history of hypertension. (See Chapter 10.) Rely on local medical direction for guidelines in this area.

b. Early blood transfusion is the most important fluid replacement in severe cases.

c. Finally, as discussed earlier, research continues into trying to find the "best" resuscitation fluid. Also, early work at this time indicates a potential role in the future for artificial blood products that carry oxygen to the tissues. Again, you should rely on local medical direction for guidelines about using these products because they have not yet become the standard of care.

8. Monitor the heart, and apply pulse oximetry and waveform capnography (if available).
9. Perform ITLS Ongoing Exams, and observe closely.

NOTE: Hemorrhage control should remain the priority, when help is not available and when other procedures interrupt. In the case of wounds with exsanguinating hemorrhage, the military has changed the initial assessment from ABC (airway, breathing, and circulation) to CABC, making control of the hemorrhage the first priority. ITLS also has refined its approach to hemorrhage. It specifies that on approaching the patient, if the medic encounters life-threatening external hemorrhage, immediate efforts to control the bleeding are to be undertaken. (See Chapter 2.)

Internal Hemorrhage. The patient with uncontrolled internal hemorrhage is the classic critical trauma victim who will almost certainly die unless you promptly transport to an appropriate facility for rapid operative hemostasis (control of bleeding). The results of the most current medical research on the management of patients with exsanguinating internal hemorrhage is that there exists no substitute for gaining surgical control of bleeding. Research into the administration of IV fluids to patients with uncontrolled hemorrhage has indicated the following:

- The use of large amounts of IV fluids in the setting of uncontrolled internal hemorrhage may increase internal bleeding and mortality. IV fluids increase the blood pressure and may also dilute clotting factors. Furthermore, IV fluids carry almost no oxygen and are not a replacement for red blood cells. Early blood transfusion is very important in severe cases of hemorrhagic shock.
- Any delay in providing rapid transport of such patients should not occur unless absolutely unavoidable, as in the case of a patient requiring prolonged extrication or in a tactical setting where transport is delayed. Always document such circumstances carefully in the patient care report.
- Moribund trauma patients (ones in very deep shock with blood pressures under 50 mm Hg systolic, i.e., no pulses can be felt) often die, and fluid administration is indicated to maintain some degree of circulation, according to current understanding. Treatment of this extreme amount of hemorrhage may override the concerns for increased hemorrhage secondary to the use of these interventions. However, this approach is still controversial. Local medical direction should guide such therapy pending further research.

The recommendations, therefore, for a patient with probable exsanguinating internal hemorrhage are described as follows.

PROCEDURE

Managing Shock Due to Internal Hemorrhage

1. Transport immediately and in a rapid, safe manner.
2. Place the patient in a horizontal position.
3. Administer high-flow oxygen.
4. Gain IV access with large-bore catheters. Consider IO vascular access if unable to quickly establish an intravenous line.
5. Administer sufficient normal saline to maintain peripheral perfusion. Local medical direction should guide what is acceptable practice in this setting. Maintaining peripheral perfusion is generally defined as giving enough fluid—usually in boluses—to return a peripheral pulse, such as a radial pulse. However, most research experts now recommend that fluid resuscitation be kept to a minimum until hemorrhage control is obtained (operative intervention). Hemostatic agents are not indicated for internal hemorrhage.
6. Monitor the heart, and apply pulse oximetry and waveform capnography (where available).
7. Perform ITLS Ongoing Exams, and observe closely.

Patients with blunt injuries can lose a significant amount of blood and fluid from the intravascular space, including into the sites of large-bone fractures (hematoma and edema). This loss can be enough to cause shock, though the blood loss from these fractures tends to be self-limited. Pelvic fractures, though, are a very important exception. Pelvic fractures can result in exsanguination and death, so any suspicion for a pelvic fracture (especially one that appears severe or even unstable) is a sign that this patient may become unstable very quickly.

However, if the blunt injury patient has a tear of a large internal blood vessel or a laceration or avulsion of an internal organ, raising the blood pressure prior to surgical intervention also may result in accelerated bleeding or a secondary hemorrhage. Therefore, if an internal hemorrhage is not suspected (patient is alert and oriented and has no apparent chest, abdominal, or pelvic injuries), fluids may be used judiciously for fractures and externally controlled hemorrhage.

In the case of a severe mechanism of injury or inability to assess the patient, use fluids with caution. As indicated earlier, administer enough fluids to maintain peripheral perfusion, remembering that early blood transfusion, when available, is the most appropriate fluid replacement of severe blood loss. Frequent patient assessments and local EMS medical direction should guide therapy.

Special Situations in Hypovolemic Shock

Head Injury

The patient with severe head injury (Glasgow Coma Scale score of 8 or less) and shock is a special situation. (See Chapter 10.) These patients do not tolerate hypotension. Therefore, if necessary, adults with suspected hemorrhagic shock in addition to head injury should be fluid resuscitated to a blood pressure of 120 mm Hg systolic to maintain a cerebral perfusion pressure of at least 60 mm Hg. (See Chapter 10.)

Nonhemorrhagic Hypovolemic Shock

The patient who has low-volume shock syndrome not due to hemorrhage can generally be managed in the same manner as a patient with shock due to bleeding that can be controlled. An example of this type of patient would be one with shock due to fluid loss from burns or severe diarrhea. Low-volume shock is a common cause of death in these patients. Because the loss of volume in this case is not from an injured vascular system, it is reasonable to treat such patients with aggressive volume replacement to restore vital signs toward normal. Just beware. Hemorrhagic shock due to a bleeding internal organ (such as a bleeding ulcer or a ruptured ectopic pregnancy) may be rapidly lethal. The bleeding may not be at all apparent from the physical exam. So, if you see signs of shock present, follow the basic rules of shock management until you have explained the cause. For example, an unconscious, pale young woman of childbearing age with no obvious cause for her abnormal signs, is bleeding to death from a ruptured ectopic pregnancy until proved otherwise.

Treatment of Nonhemorrhagic Shock Syndromes

Treatments for the other shock syndromes, namely, mechanical (cardiogenic) and high-space (relative hypovolemia) are somewhat different. All patients require high-flow oxygen, rapid transport, shock positioning, and IV line placement (usually en route).

Mechanical Shock

The patient with mechanical shock must first be accurately assessed to determine the cause of the problem. The patient with tension pneumothorax needs prompt decompression of the elevated pleural pressure. (See Chapter 7 for indications and procedure for decompression.)

The patient with suspected pericardial tamponade must be rapidly transported to an appropriate facility, because the time from onset of tamponade to the time of cardiac arrest can be a matter of minutes (the ultimate load-and-go situation). Although anecdotal support exists for use of an intravenous volume challenge as a temporizing measure, no clear evidence exists that such treatment will improve survival. Use of IV fluids in this situation should be during transport and only on the order of medical direction. Obtaining IV access certainly should not delay direct transport or airway/oxygen interventions. Consider IO vascular access if you are unable to quickly establish an intravenous line. Bear in mind that trauma is not the only cause of tamponade. Metastatic cancer and other diseases such as pericarditis resulting in pericardial effusion also may cause tamponade.

Myocardial contusion rarely causes shock. Recent reports indicate that most contusions cause little or no clinical findings. However, severe contusion may cause acute heart failure, manifested by distended neck veins, tachycardia, cyanosis, and possibly arrhythmias. These are the same signs seen with pericardial tamponade. These patients require rapid transport for proper care. Give high-flow oxygen and perform cardiac monitoring on the patient with suspected myocardial contusion. IV fluids may cause worsening of the patient's condition.

High-Space Shock

High-space shock, in theory, resembles controlled hemorrhage, in that there is relative hypovolemia with an "intact" vascular system (no "leaks"). Therefore, initial management includes IV fluid boluses. Consider IO vascular access if the patient is critical and you are unable to establish an intravenous line.

In the absence of a head injury, the patient's level of consciousness is a useful monitor of the success or failure of resuscitation. Be alert for possible occult internal injuries, and keep in mind that raising the blood pressure may increase internal bleeding in that situation. An argument can be made for the use of vasopressors in patients with vasodilatory shock due to causes such as calcium channel blocker overdose or sepsis. Consult with medical direction in those cases.

Areas of Current Study

Much work continues into finding the "ideal resuscitation fluid." Even after decades of research, it is not at all clear at this time what the best initial resuscitation fluid is. It remains quite reasonable to begin with normal saline as a resuscitation fluid for trauma, with the understanding that patients in shock due to hemorrhagic causes need blood and blood products.

Current research is examining what the ratio of "blood administration" to "blood product" administration should be. Although beyond the scope of this chapter, this is an important area that will continue to guide emergency medicine and surgery in the resuscitation of these patients.

It was mentioned earlier that hypertonic saline resuscitation was not found to be beneficial by the Resuscitation Outcomes Consortium (ROC) in patients with severe hemorrhagic shock. This treatment seems to work by mobilizing internal, interstitial fluid (fluid found *between* the cells but outside the vascular space) into the vascular system. The ROC trial found that some hemorrhagic shock patients receiving hypertonic saline appeared to be clinically better on arrival to the emergency department. Overall, though, the mortality rate of the patients was not changed from those receiving conventional fluid therapy.

Methods of evaluating and monitoring patients in traumatic shock continue to appear. One important method that is being evaluated is in the use of "lactate levels" in the prehospital arena to monitor patients in shock. Early work at this time suggests that increasing lactate levels may be predictive of worsening outcome for the patient. Elevated lactate in a prehospital trauma patient could be a marker to triage the patient to a level I trauma center. Indeed, a large international trial may soon evaluate this technique.

It should be stressed that hemostatic agents should only be used in the setting of an overall hemorrhage control protocol and not as agents that control bleeding by themselves. This is an area in which the recommended agent to use seems to change frequently, so consult your medical director or state protocols for current recommendations.

Tourniquets are lifesaving devices and should be part of all EMS education. The rapid control of massive external bleeding—by tourniquets if necessary—is a critical part of patient care.

The role of hypothermia in the care of critically ill patients is being evaluated. In the setting of the return of spontaneous circulation after nontraumatic cardiac arrest, therapeutic hypothermia appears to be beneficial. The trauma patient, however, appears to suffer from being cold. Trauma resuscitation rooms are often kept at body temperature (to the discomfort of some members of the resuscitation team, who are in gowns). IV fluids may be warmed to try to help maintain the patient's body temperature. The benefit at this time of warming IV fluids in the first few minutes of resuscitation in the field are unknown as far as actually improving survival. This remains an important area of study.

The use of waveform capnography is important in managing the critically ill patient. However, in patients with both hemorrhagic shock and traumatic brain injury, waveform capnography may not be reliable for managing ventilator rate settings. Presumably the reason for that is, in shock, the amount of carbon dioxide being produced and being returned to the lungs is unpredictable. So, on these particular patients, decisions about ventilator settings are apparently best made using conventional arterial blood gas analyses. This has very little application to prehospital care but might be important in hospital transfers.

CASE PRESENTATION (continued)

An ALS ambulance has been called to a local bar where a patron has been stabbed. The scene size-up reveals that the police are on scene and have cleared the bar and are questioning bystanders outside. There is a single male victim who is sitting in a chair and holding his right anterior chest. Because the scene is safe and the mechanism of injury (stab wound) is readily apparent, the team dons personal protective equipment, and each carries their essential trauma care equipment as they approach the patient. The patient, a male in his 20s, states that during an argument his drinking buddy stabbed him once in the right chest before bystanders could take the knife away from him. The patient denies falling or any other injuries.

The team leader begins the initial assessment, and her general impression is not good. The patient is sitting in a chair and is awake and answering appropriately. He is pale and diaphoretic but there is no obvious external bleeding. Respiration appears to be slightly fast but depth appears normal. When his hand is removed from his right chest, there is a single small stab wound about the fourth intercostal space and anterior axillary line. The wound is not open or bleeding. The radial pulse seems a little fast but strong. The team leader asks rescuer 2 to apply a nonrebreather oxygen mask and then apply an occlusive dressing over the chest wound. Because of the nature of the injury she decides to do a focused exam. Exam of the airway is normal, with good movement of air and a normal speaking voice. The neck veins are flat, and the trachea is in the midline. The breath sounds are decreased on the right and dull to percussion. Heart sounds are normal but fast. The abdomen is soft and nontender. There are no other wounds. The patient is placed on a stretcher (no backboard or packaging) and immediately moved to the ambulance.

Vital signs are pulse 120–130, respiration 24/minute, and blood pressure is 104/84. He is treated with 100% oxygen by nonrebreather mask. Two large-bore IVs are started during transport, but because the blood pressure is greater than 90 mm Hg, the flow rate is set just fast enough to keep the vein open. There is concern about causing worsening of the intrathoracic bleeding. The history reveals

S —Slight pain in the wound site.

A —None.

M —None.

P —No history of serious illness.

L —Just ate some chips and salsa; admits to drinking "three beers."

E —States he was drinking with his friend, who became upset when they got into an argument over football. In a snit, his friend stabbed him with a pocketknife. His friend is now outside talking to the police and is crying and protesting that he never meant to hurt the patient.

While rescuer 2 applies a cardiac monitor and a pulse oximeter (95% on 100% oxygen), the team leader performs an ongoing exam. The patient is becoming restless but is still oriented and cooperative, airway is still normal with slight tachypnea, but the pulse is now thready and more rapid (around 140 beats/minute on monitor). The patient is still diaphoretic and is noticeably pale. The neck veins are flat and trachea is midline. Breath sounds are normal on the left and still decreased on the right with dullness to percussion. Heart sounds are rapid and not muffled. Rescuer 2 reports the blood pressure is now 80/60 mm Hg. The fluid rate is increased to maintain the blood pressure above 80 mm Hg systolic, and the team leader immediately notifies medical direction that they will be arriving in 5 minutes with a young male with shock from a massive hemothorax. She is told to watch the vital signs and hold fluids unless the systolic blood pressure is less than 80 mm Hg.

The ITLS Secondary Survey was not performed because they arrived at the emergency department before she had time to do one. Immediately on arrival in the emergency department, a chest tube was inserted and 1,600 cc of blood obtained. There was only slight bleeding after this, so the blood was autotransfused and the patient observed. Imaging of the chest and abdomen failed to show other injuries, and the patient's bleeding stopped without surgery. He had an uneventful recovery.

This is one of the few examples of a focused exam being adequate for a trauma patient. Note that even a focused exam required that both the chest and the abdomen be examined because the diaphragm rises so high in the chest that a midchest stab wound may go through the diaphragm and cause abdominal injuries. Note also that this case and the case in Chapter 6 had the same mechanism of injury and the same initial presentation but very different injuries and treatments. The case in Chapter 6 had mechanical shock, whereas this patient had hypovolemic shock.

Studies have found that for penetrating wounds of the chest, the pneumatic antishock garment (PASG) and/or IV fluids may significantly increase internal bleeding and worsen survival. Thus, the PASG is contraindicated, and IV fluids should only be used to maintain systolic pressure of 80 to 90 mm Hg systolic. ■

Summary

A patient with shock must be diagnosed early. The early signs and symptoms of shock may be subtle, and when the later signs such as hypotension develop, the patient may be near death. The importance of careful assessment and reassessment cannot be overemphasized. You must understand the risk of any of the shock states to your patient. Further, you need to study and memorize the shock syndromes, especially in regard to the rapid provision of the proper treatment for such conditions as internal hemorrhage, pericardial tamponade, and tension pneumothorax. Finally, you should be aware of the controversy on the use of IV fluid resuscitation for cases of uncontrolled hemorrhage. Rely on your local medical direction to help keep you current on the standard of care in these areas.

Bibliography

1. Bickell, W. H., M. J. Wall, P. E. Pepe, et al. 1994. Immediate versus delayed fluid resuscitation for hypotensive patients with penetrating torso injury. *New England Journal of Medicine* 331 (October): 1105–1109.
2. Champion, H. 2003. Combat fluid resuscitation. *Supplement to the Journal of Trauma* 54.
3. Chiara, O., P. Pelosi, L. Brazzi, et al. 2003. Resuscitation from hemorrhagic shock: Experimental model comparing normal saline, dextran, and hypertonic saline solutions. *Critical Care Medicine* 31: 1915–1922.
4. Demetriades, D., L. S. Chan, P. Bhasin, et al. 1998. Relative bradycardia in patients with traumatic hypotension. *Journal of Trauma* 45(3): 534–539.
5. Haut, E. R., B. Kalish, et al. 2010. Spine immobilization in penetrating trauma: More harm than good? *Journal of Trauma* 68(1): 115–121.
6. Kowalenko, T., S. Stern, S. Dronen, X. Wang. 1992. Improved outcome with hypotensive resuscitation of uncontrolled hemorrhagic shock in a swine model. *Journal of Trauma* 33: 349–353.
7. Mapstone, J., I. Roberts, P. Evans. 2003. Fluid resuscitation strategies: A systematic review of animal trials. *Journal of Trauma* 55: 571–591.
8. Mattox, K. L., W. H. Bickell, P. Pepe, et al. 1989. Prospective MAST study in 911 patients. *Journal of Trauma* 29: 1104–1112.
9. Moore, E. 2003. Blood substitutes: The future is now. *Journal of the American College of Surgeons* 196: 1–16.
10. Schriger, D. L., L. J. Baraff. 1991. Capillary refill—Is it a useful predictor of hypovolemic states? *Annals of Emergency Medicine* 20: 601–5.
11. Warner, K., J. Cuschieri, B. Garland, D. Carlbom, B. Baker, M. Copass, et al. 2009. The utility of early end-tidal capnography in monitoring ventilation status after severe injury. *Journal of Trauma* 66: 26–31.

Explore Resource Central

For additional review and practice tests, visit **www.bradybooks.com** and click on Resource Central to access book-specific resources for this text. To access Resource Central, follow directions on the Student Access Card provided with this text. If there is no card, go to www.bradybooks.com and follow the Resource Central link to Buy Access from there.

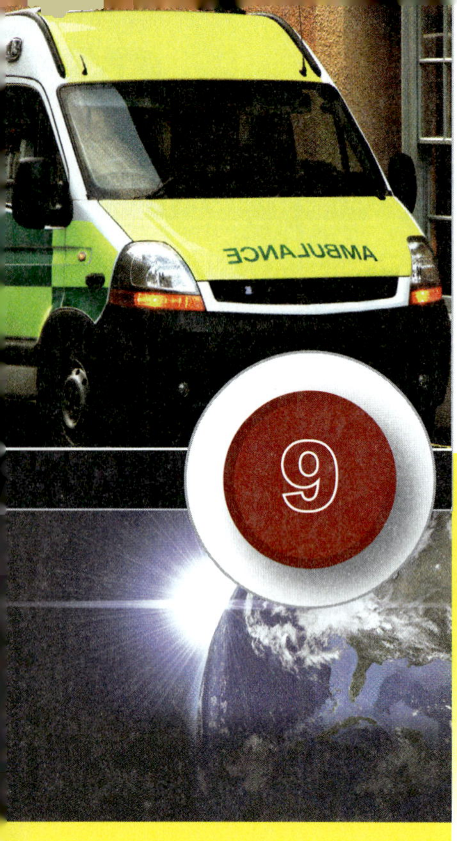

(© TA Craft Photography, Fotolia, LLC)

Vascular Access Skills

Donna Hastings, EMT-P
Kyee Han, MD

Fluid Resuscitation

Infusione di Liquidi

Reanimación con Líquidos

Réanimation fluide

Płynoterapia (Resuscytacja płynowa)

Volumentherapie

Nadoknada tekućine

الإنعاش بالسوائل

nadoknada tečnosti

Tekočinska reanimacija

Folyadék reszuszcitáció

OBJECTIVES

Upon successful completion of this chapter, you should be able to:

1. Perform the technique of cannulation of the external jugular vein.
2. Recite indications for the use of intraosseous infusion.
3. Perform intraosseous infusion using the EZ-IO Drill.
4. Use length-based resuscitation tape to estimate the weight of a child.

All advanced students of this course are expected to be familiar with the technique of inserting an IV cannula in the veins of the lower arm or antecubital space; thus, these sites will not be discussed here.

Cannulation of the External Jugular Vein

The external jugular vein runs in a line from the angle of the jaw to the junction of the medial and middle third of the clavicle (Figure 9-1). This vein is usually easily visible through the skin. Pressing on it just above the clavicle will make it more prominent. It runs into the subclavian vein.

Indication for cannulation of the external jugular vein is the pediatric or adult patient who needs IV access and in whom no suitable peripheral vein is found.

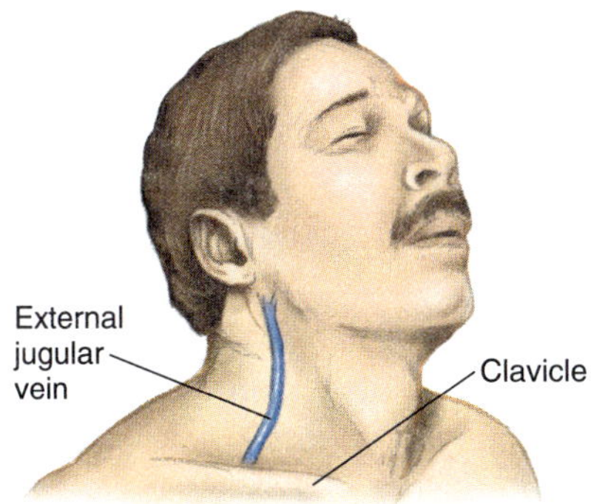

FIGURE 9-1 Anatomy of the external jugular vein.

PROCEDURE

Performing External Jugular Cannulation

1. The patient must be in the supine position, preferably head down, to distend the vein and to prevent air embolism.
2. If no suspicion of cervical-spine injury exists, turn the patient's head to the opposite side. If there is a danger of cervical-spine injury, one rescuer must stabilize the head (it must not be turned) while the IV is being started. The cervical collar should be opened or the front removed during the procedure.
3. Quickly prepare the skin with an antiseptic and then align the cannula with the vein. The needle will be pointing at the clavicle at the junction of the middle and medial thirds.
4. With one finger, press on the vein just above the clavicle. This should make the vein more prominent.
5. Insert the needle into the vein at about the midportion and cannulate in the usual way.
6. If not already done, draw a 30-cc sample of blood and store it in the appropriate tubes (if the hospital will accept blood drawn in the field).
7. Tape down the line securely. If there is danger of cervical-spine injury, a cervical collar can be applied over the IV site.

Intraosseous Infusion

The technique of bone marrow infusion of fluid and drugs is not new. It was first described in 1922 and was used commonly in the 1930s and 1940s as an alternative to IV infusion of crystalloids, drugs, and blood. The technique was "rediscovered" in 1985 by James Orlowski, MD, on a trip to India. Studies have confirmed it to be a fast, safe, and effective route to infuse medications, fluids, and blood. It is an established standard of care in Pediatric Advanced Life Support and more recently adopted standard of care in cardiac arrest by the AHA and European Resuscitation Council Guidelines revisions.

Intraosseous (IO) infusion can be used for giving medications in both adults and children. It is now an early second-line choice for venous vascular access following two attempts at peripheral venous cannulation in adults as well. With pressures of 300 mm Hg applied to the infusion bag or pump, adequate flow rates of 150 mL/minute can be achieved for crystalloids. IO infusion has the advantage of being quick and simple to perform while providing a stable (anchored in bone) access that is not easily dislodged during transport.

PEARLS: Lo Infusion

- If infiltration occurs (rare), do not reuse the same bone. Another site must be selected because fluid will leak out of the original hole made in the bone. If this occurs, apply a pressure dressing and secure it with an elastic bandage.
- Never place an IO line in a fractured extremity. If the femur is fractured, use the other leg.

Indications

Indications for the use of IO infusion include the pediatric or adult patient who is in cardiac arrest and in whom you cannot quickly obtain peripheral venous access, or the patient with hypovolemic shock and difficult intravenous placement.

It is indicated for any patient who needs drugs or fluids within five minutes, when a peripheral intravenous cannula cannot be placed in two attempts or 90 seconds.

Contraindications

- Local infection at selected site for insertion
- Fractures in the selected limb
- Prosthesis
- Recent (24 hours) IO access in same extremity
- Absence of anatomical landmarks or excessive tissue at site of insertion

Recommended Sites

- Proximal tibia, one finger breadth medial to the tibial tuberosity
- Proximal humerus, laterally over prominence of the greater tubercle
- Distal tibia, two finger breadths above the medial malleolus

Potential Complications

Studies have shown that the following complications are rare. However, good aseptic technique is important, just as it is with IV therapy. Potential complications of IO infusion include the following:

- Extravasation
- Compartment syndrome
- Dislodgment
- Fracture
- Failure (device or user in origin)
- Pain
- Infection; adult infection rates < 0.6 % (retrospective analysis)

PROCEDURE

Performing IO by Use of EZ-IO Device (Adult or Child)

The equipment needed to perform IO by use of EZ-IO device is as follows:

- EZ-IO® driver
- EZ-IO AD® or EZ-IO PD® needle set
- Alcohol or Betadine swab
- EZ-Connect® or standard extension set
- Two 10 mL syringes
- Normal saline (or suitable sterile fluid)
- Pressure bag or infusion pump
- 2% lidocaine for IV/IO use (preservative free, epinephrine free)

PROCEDURE

Insertion of IO Needle by Use of the EZ-IO System

Determine the need for this procedure. Obtain permission from medical direction if required. If the patient is conscious, advise him of emergent need for this procedure and obtain informed consent. To perform the insertion (Scan 9-1):

1. Wear approved body substance isolation (BSI) equipment.
2. Determine EZ-IO AD or EZ-IO PD indications.
3. Rule out contraindications.
4. Locate appropriate insertion site.
5. Prepare insertion site, using aseptic technique, and then allow to dry.
6. Prepare the EZ-IO driver (power or manual) and appropriate needle set.
   a. EZ-IO 15 mm for 3–39 kg
   b. EZ-IO 25 mm for 40 kg and greater
   c. EZ-IO 45 mm for 40 kg and greater with excessive tissue
7. Stabilize site to insert appropriate needle set.
8. Remove needle cap. Insert the EZ-IO needle into the selected site. (Keep your hand and fingers away from the needle.) Position the driver at the insertion site with the needle set at a 90-degree angle to the bone surface.
9. Gently pierce the skin with the needle until the needle touches the bone. The black line on the needle should be visible. Penetrate the bone cortex by squeezing driver's trigger and applying gentle, consistent, steady downward pressure. (Allow the driver to do the work.) *Do not use excessive force.* In some patients insertion may take 10 seconds. If the driver sounds like it is slowing down during insertion, reduce pressure on the driver to allow the RPMs of the needle tip to do the work. If the battery fails, you may manually finish inserting the needle just as you would a manual IO needle.
10. Release the driver's trigger and stop the insertion process when a sudden "give or pop" is felt on entry into the medullary space or when desired depth is obtained.
11. Remove EZ-IO driver from the needle set while stabilizing the catheter hub.
12. Remove the stylet from the catheter by turning counterclockwise. Place the stylet in the shuttle or approved sharps container.
13. Confirm placement. Connect the primed EZ-Connect. Syringe bolus (flush) the EZ-IO catheter with the appropriate amount of normal saline (10 cc for adults and 5 cc for children). Remember: no flush = no flow!
14. If the patient is responsive to pain or complains of pain when you flush the marrow cavity, slowly (0.2 cc increments), administer the appropriate dose of preservative-free (for IV/IO use) Lidocaine 2% (20 mg/cc) IO to anesthetize the IO space. (IO infusion causes severe pain in alert patients.)
   a. 2–4 cc (20–40 mg) for adults
   b. 0.5 mg/kg (0.025 mL per kg) for children.

   Then wait 15–30 seconds for the Lidocaine to take effect.
15. Begin the infusion. Utilize pressure—300 mm Hg (pressure bag or infusion pump)—for continuous infusions.
16. Dress the site, secure the tubing, and apply the wristband (document time and date) as directed.
17. Monitor the EZ-IO site and the patient's condition.

SCAN 9-1 Insertion of IO Needle by Use of Easy-IO System

1

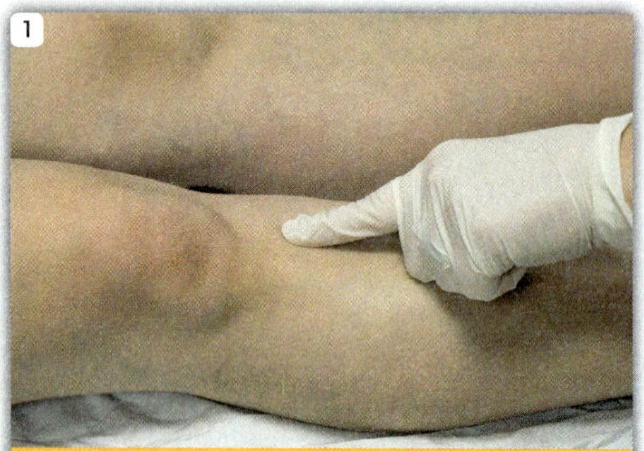

Identify insertion site. *(Photo courtesy of Vidacare Corp)*

2

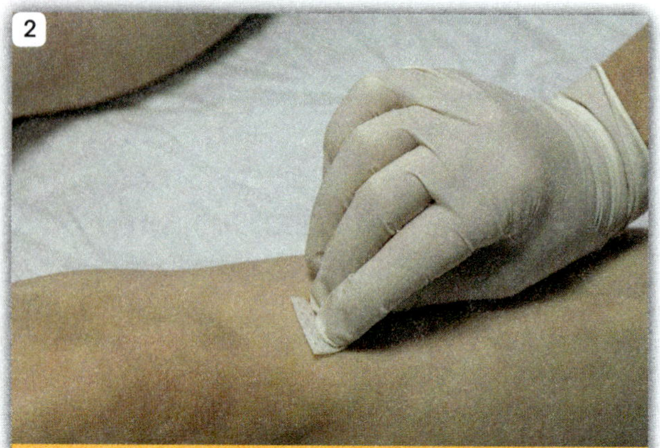

Prepare site using aseptic technique and allow to dry. *(Photo courtesy of Vidacare Corp)*

3

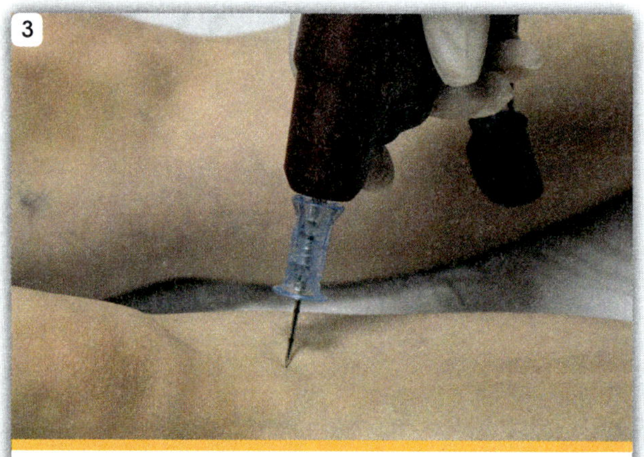

Insert the needle at a 90-degree angle to the bone surface. Keep your hand and fingers away from the needle. *(Photo courtesy of Vidacare Corp)*

4

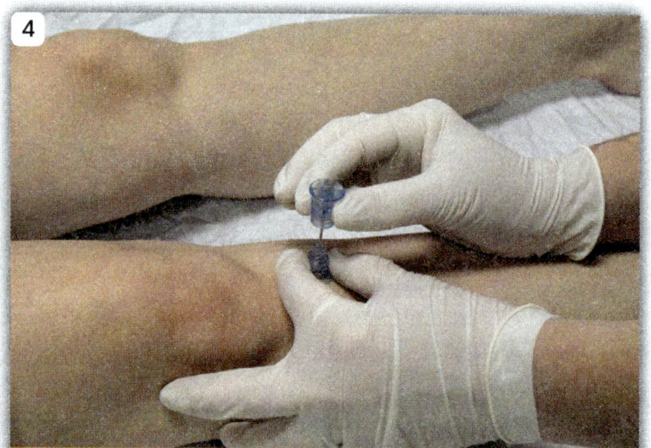

While stabilizing the catheter hub, remove the stylet from the catheter by turning counterclockwise. *(Photo courtesy of Vidacare Corp)*

5

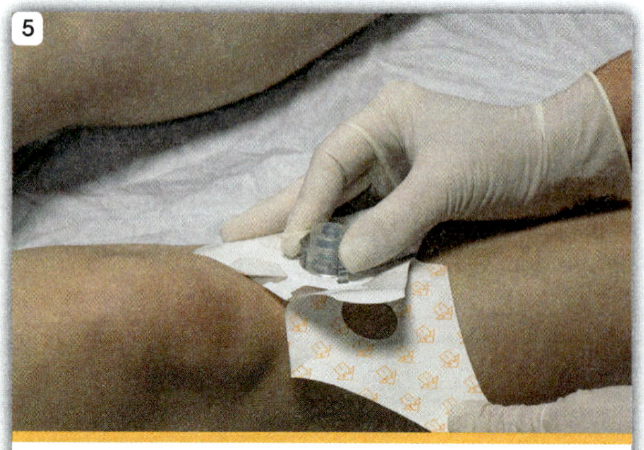

Attach the EZ-connect and secure the needle. *(Photo courtesy of Vidacare Corp)*

6

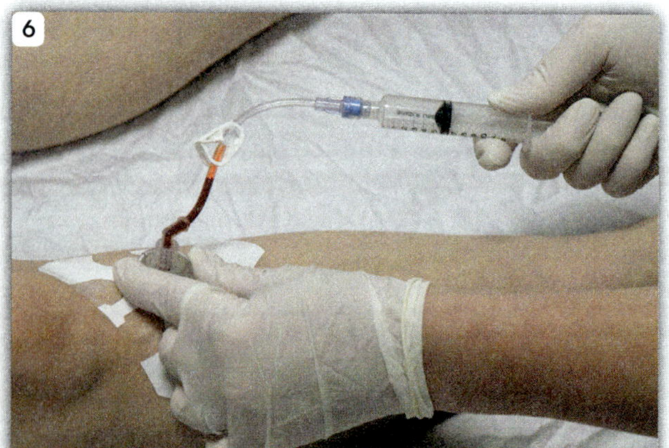

Confirm the placement of the needle by aspirating blood from the marrow cavity. *(Photo courtesy of Vidacare Corp)*

7

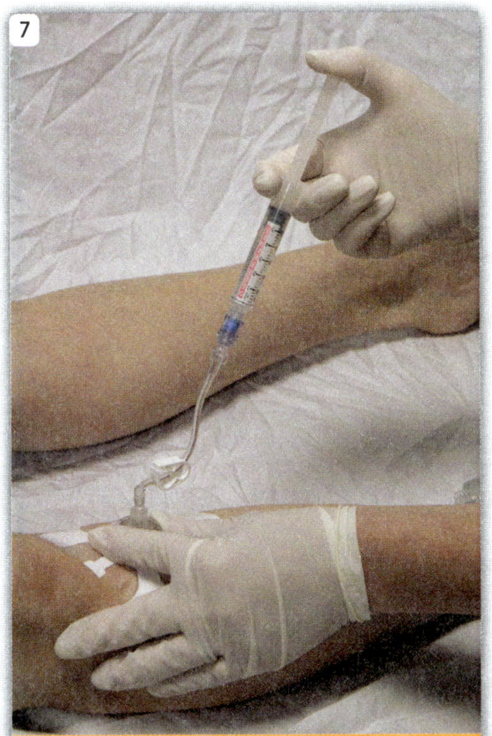

Flush the catheter with saline (10 cc adults, 5 cc children). No flush, no flow. *(Photo courtesy of Vidacare Corp)*

8

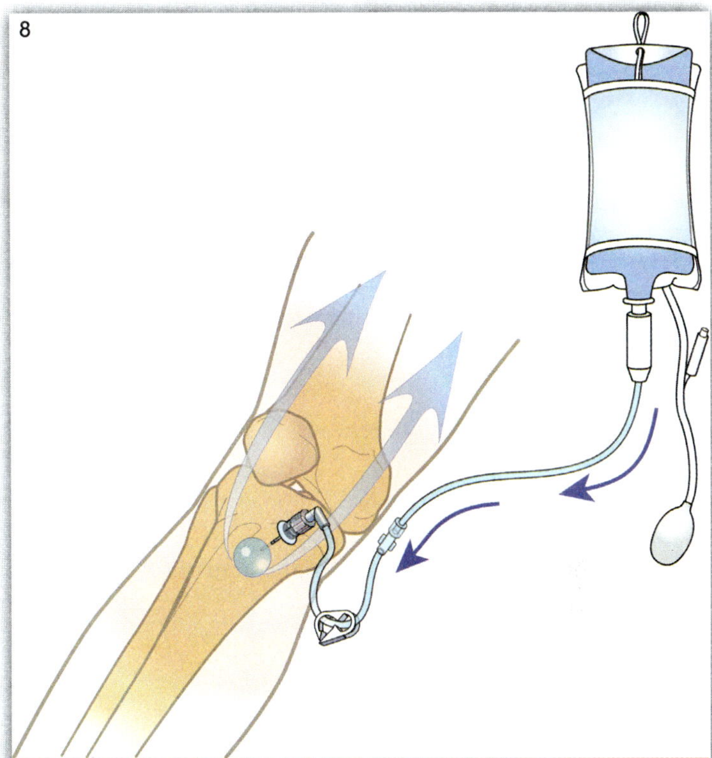

Connect IV infusion. *(Image courtesy of Vidacare Corp)*

9

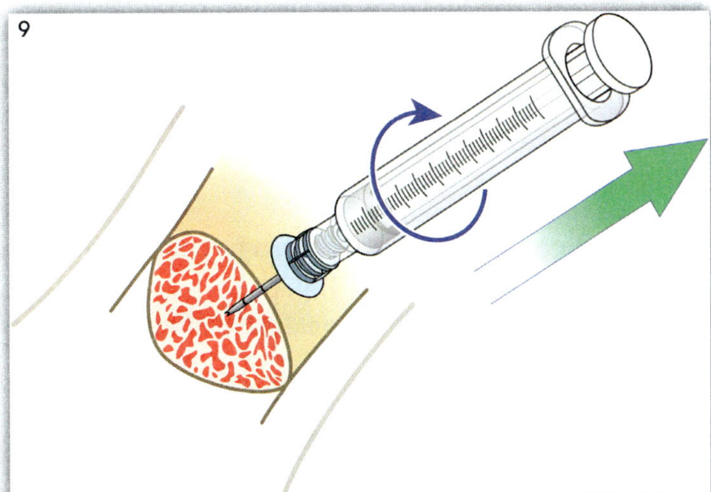

To remove the catheter, support the leg while simultaneously connecting a sterile Luer-Lok syringe to the hub of the catheter. Rotate the syringe and catheter clockwise while gently pulling. *(Image courtesy of Vidacare Corp)*

To remove the catheter, start by supporting the patient's leg. Simultaneously, connect a sterile Luer-Lok syringe to the hub of the catheter. Once connected, rotate the syringe and catheter clockwise while gently pulling. When the catheter has been removed, immediately place it in an appropriate biohazard container. *Do not leave the EX-IO catheter in place for more than 24 hours.*

PROCEDURE

Performing Manual IO Infusion in a Child

1. Determine the need for this procedure. Obtain permission from medical direction if required.
2. Have all needed equipment ready prior to bone penetration.
   a. 16–18 gauge IO needles
   b. 5-cc and 10-cc syringes
   c. Antiseptic solution to prep the skin
   d. IV tubing and IV fluids
   e. Tape and dressing material to secure the IO needle
   f. Blood pressure cuff or commercial pressure device to infuse fluid under pressure

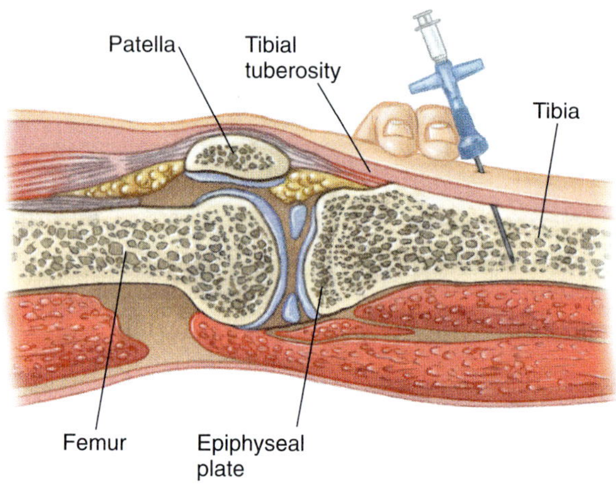

FIGURE 9-2 Insertion site for intraosseous infusion needle in the proximal tibia.

3. Identify the site, which is the proximal tibia, one finger breadth below the tibial tuberosity, either midline or slightly medial to the midline (Figure 9-2).
4. Prep the skin with an appropriate antiseptic (very important).
5. Obtain the proper needle. The needle must have a stylet so that it does not become plugged with bone. Although 13-, 18-, and 20-gauge spine needles will work, they are difficult and uncomfortable to grip during the insertion process. Long spine needles tend to bend easily, so if you use spine needles, try to obtain the short ones. The preferred needle is a 14- to 18-gauge IO needle, but bone marrow needles also can be used.
6. Using aseptic technique, insert the needle into the bone marrow cavity perpendicular to the skin, directed away from the epiphyseal plate (Figure 9-2). Advance it to the periosteum. Penetrate the bone with a slow boring or twisting motion until you feel a sudden "give or pop" (decrease in resistance) as the needle enters the marrow cavity. This can be confirmed by removing the stylet and aspirating blood and bone marrow (Figures 9-3 and 9-4).
7. Syringe bolus (flush) the IO catheter with 5 cc of normal saline. Remember: no flush = no flow!
8. If the child is responsive to pain or complains of pain when you flush, slowly (0.2 cc increments) administer a 0.5 mg/kg (0.025 mL per kg) dose of preservative-free (for IV/IO use) Lidocaine 2% (20 mg/cc) IO to anesthetize the IO space. A 10-kg child would get 0.25 cc (5 mg of 2% Lidocaine). Wait 15–30 seconds for the Lidocaine to take effect. Assess for potential IO complications.
9. Attach standard IV tubing and infuse the fluid and/or medications (Figure 9-5). You may have to infuse fluid under pressure (blood pressure cuff blown up around IV bag) to obtain an adequate infusion rate.
10. Tape the tubing to the skin and secure the bone marrow needles as if to secure an impaled object. (Use gauze pads taped around the insertion site.)

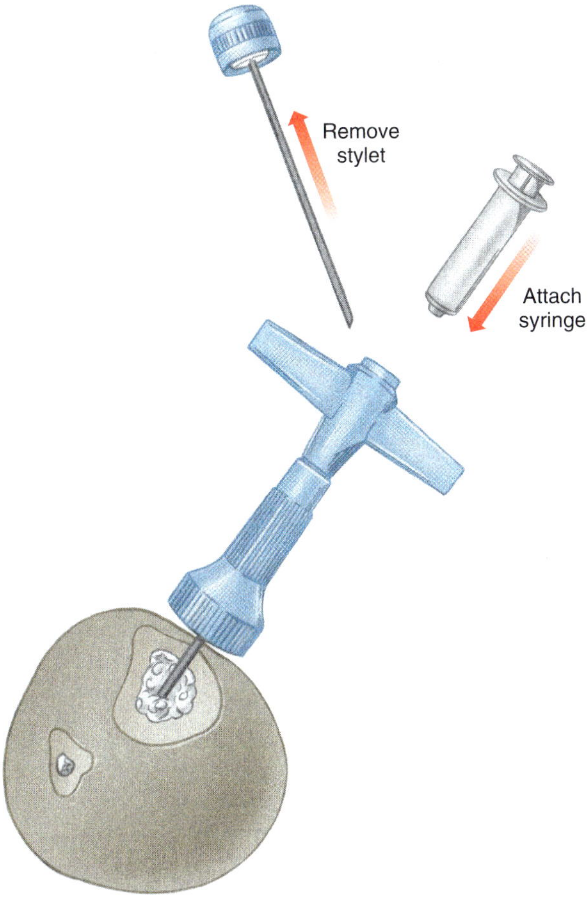

FIGURE 9-3 Remove stylet from the needle and attach syringe.

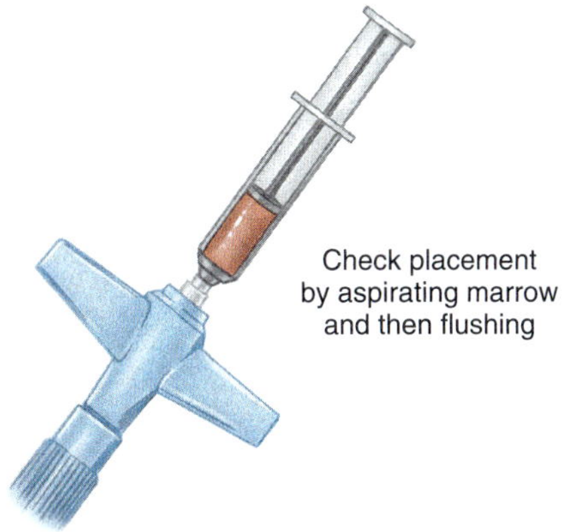

FIGURE 9-4 To check needle placement, aspirate approximately 1 cc of bone marrow.

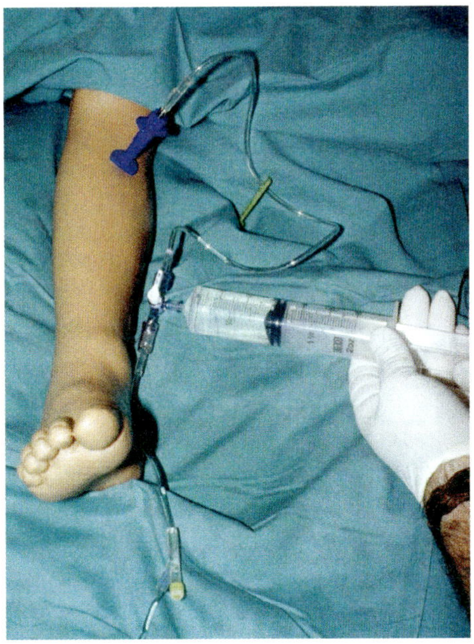

FIGURE 9-5 Intraosseous needle in child's tibia being used for fluid infusion. *(Courtesy of Bob Page, NREMT-P)*

Length-Based Resuscitation Tapes

Calculation of the volume of fluid resuscitation or the dose of an IV medication for the pediatric patient depends on the patient's weight. In an emergency situation the age and weight of a child may not be known. The weight of a child is directly related to his length, and resuscitation tapes (Broselow tape or SPARC system) have been developed that estimate a child's weight by measuring his length. The tapes contain precalculated doses of IV fluids and emergency drugs for each weight range (Figure 9-6). They also include the correct sizes of emergency equipment and supplies for each weight range.

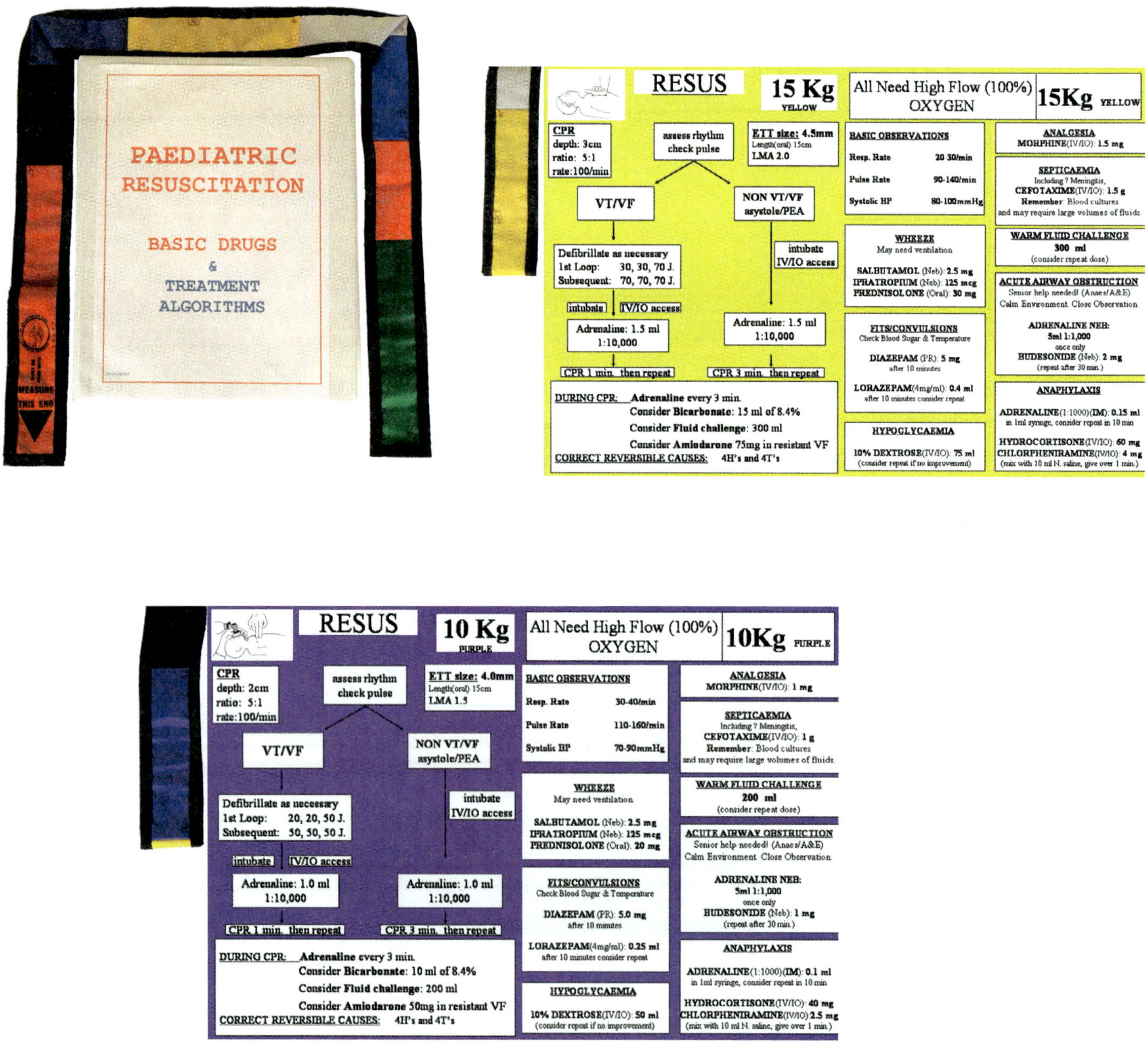

FIGURE 9-6 SPARC system has color-coded tape and booklet of precalculated doses of fluids and medications. *(Photos courtesy of Kyee Han, MD)*

PROCEDURE

Estimating a Child's Weight with a Length-Based Resuscitation Tape

1. Place the patient in the supine position.
2. Using the tape, measure the patient from the crown to the heel. The red end with an arrow goes at the child's head. (See Figure 9-7.)
3. Note the box on the tape at which the child's heel falls. With the SPARC system, match the color of the tape at which the child's heel falls with the same colored area of the booklet.
4. If the measurement falls on a line, the box or colored panel proximal to the line is used to generate the fluid and drug doses and the size of equipment needed for resuscitation.
5. The tape may be disinfected if it becomes contaminated.

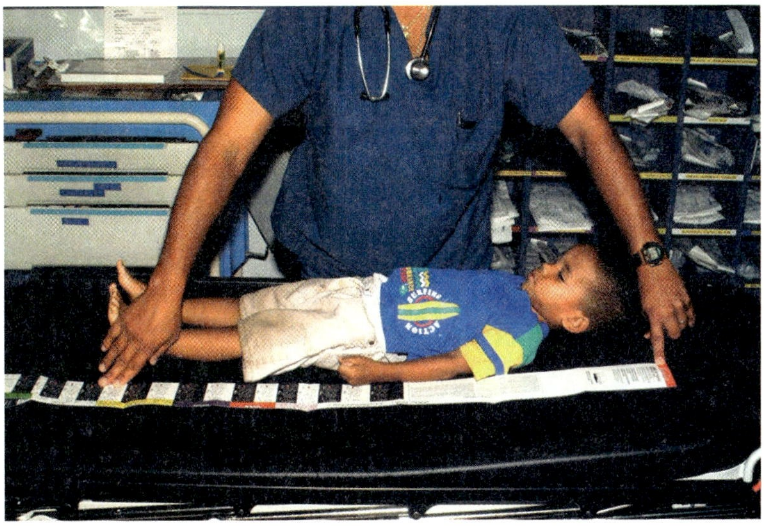

FIGURE 9-7 Measure the patient from crown to heel to read precalculated doses of fluids and medications. *(Courtesy of James Broselow, MD)*

American Heart Association. 2010. Guidelines for Cardiopulmonary Care Resuscitation (CPR) and Emergency Cardiovascular Care (ECC) *Science* 122 (18)Supplement 3.

Explore Resource Central

For additional review and practice tests, visit www.bradybooks.com and click on Resource Central to access book-specific resources for this text. To access Resource Central, follow directions on the Student Access Card provided with this text. If there is no card, go to www.bradybooks.com and follow the Resource Central link to Buy Access from there.

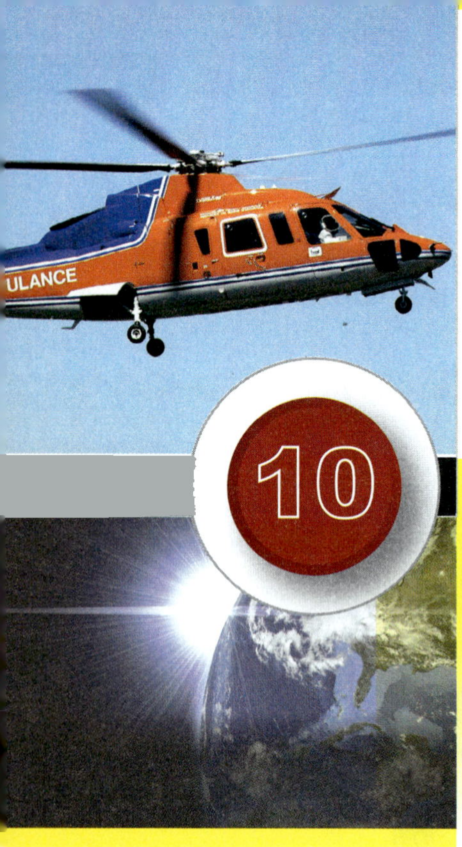

(© Pierre Landry, Fotolia, LLC)

10

Head Trauma

Roy L. Alson, PhD, MD, FACEP

Head Trauma

Trauma Cranico

Traumatismo Craneal

Traumatisme Crânien

Urazy czaszkowo-mózgowe

Schädel Hirn Trauma

Ozljede glave

إصابات الرأس

trauma glave

Poškodbe glave

Koponya-Agy-sérülés (Skull-Brain Trauma)

KEY TERMS

cerebral herniation syndrome, *p. 177*
cerebral perfusion pressure (CPP), *p. 176*
contracoup, *p. 175*
coup, *p. 175*
Cushing's reflex, *p. 176*
drug-assisted intubation (DAI), *p. 184*
intracranial pressure (ICP), *p. 176*
mean arterial blood pressure (MAP), *p. 176*
no-reflow phenomenon, *p. 180*
primary brain injury, *p. 175*
secondary brain injury, *p. 175*

OBJECTIVES

Upon successful completion of this chapter, you should be able to:

1. Describe the anatomy of the head and brain.
2. Describe the pathophysiology of traumatic brain injury.
3. Explain the difference between primary and secondary brain injury.
4. Describe the mechanisms for the development of secondary brain injury.
5. Describe the assessment of the patient with a head injury.
6. Describe the prehospital management of the patient with a head injury.
7. Recognize and describe the management of the cerebral herniation syndrome.
8. Identify potential problems in the management of the patient with a head injury.

Chapter Overview

Head injury or, more specifically, traumatic brain injury (TBI), is a major cause of death and disability in multiple-trauma patients. Of all multisystem trauma patients, 40% have a central nervous system (CNS) injury. Those patients have a death rate twice as high (35% versus 17%) as that of patients with no CNS injuries. Head injuries account for an estimated 25% of all trauma deaths and up to one-half of all motor-vehicle fatalities. Worldwide, the cost of TBI is staggering in terms of lives lost, families destroyed, and money spent for care. Prevention remains the most effective treatment. EMS personnel can help reduce this major epidemic by encouraging the use of helmets in sports and work and restraint devices in vehicles.

As an emergency responder you may encounter head injuries that can range from the trivial to the immediately life threatening. By recognizing injuries that need immediate intervention and providing transport to the appropriate facility, you can significantly improve the chances for a patient to have a good outcome. Because it is not possible to perform a field clearance of the cervical spine in a patient with altered mental status and because head injury often results in the alteration of consciousness, you must always assume that a serious head injury is accompanied by an injury to the cervical spine and spinal cord and provide appropriate spinal motion restriction, as described elsewhere in this text. (See Chapter 12.)

Beginning with the third edition of this text, material included in this chapter has been based on the recommendations of the Brain Trauma Foundation (a multidisciplinary organization dedicated to improving care of TBI victims by use of evidence-based treatment).

CASE PRESENTATION

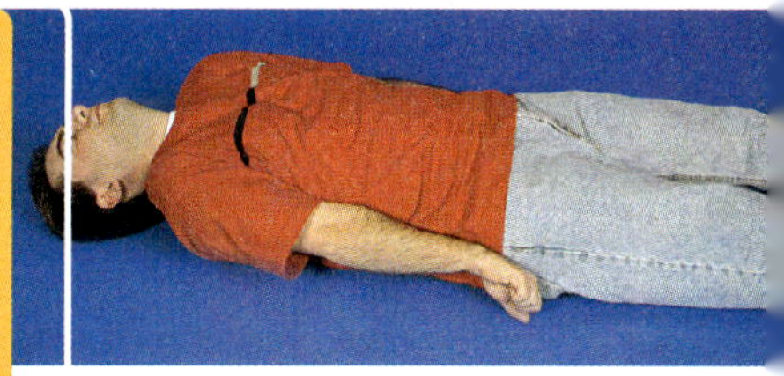

An ALS ambulance has been dispatched to a private home where a man has fallen. When they arrive, a woman who appears to be in her 60s meets them at the door. She states that her husband fell in the shower and hit his head on the tile floor. He was unconscious for a few minutes, during which time she called 911. He is better now but he cannot remember what happened other than he awakened in the shower with his wife shaking him. He complains of a headache and nausea and says his neck hurts but denies any other pain. *What injuries would you suspect from a mechanism such as this?* Keep this question in mind as you read the chapter. Then, at the end of the chapter, find out how the rescuers completed this call. ■

Anatomy of the Head

To most effectively manage the head-injured patient, one must understand the basic anatomy and physiology of the head and brain. The head (excluding the face and facial structures) includes the following (Figure 10-1):

PEARLS: Cervical-Spine Injury

Always anticipate a cervical-spine injury in the head-injured patient.

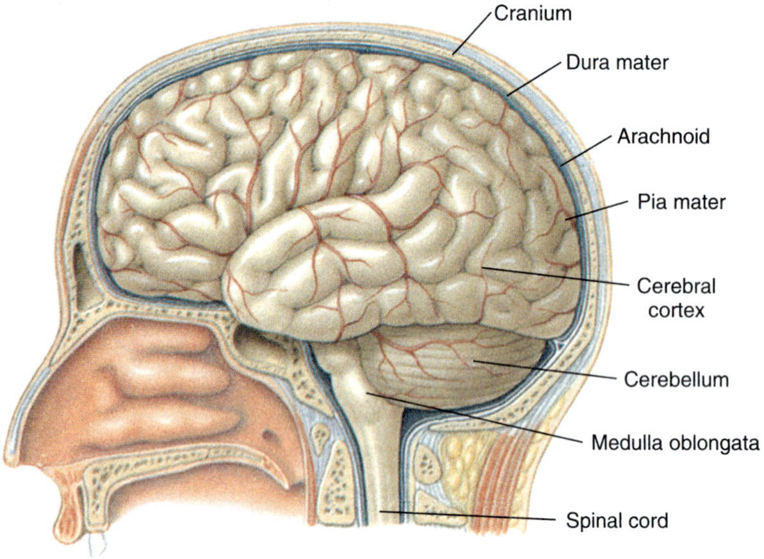

FIGURE 10-1 Anatomy of the head.

- Scalp
- Skull
- Fibrous coverings of the brain (meninges: dura mater, arachnoid mater, pia mater)
- Brain tissue
- Cerebrospinal fluid
- Vascular compartments

The scalp is a protective covering for the skull, but it is very vascular and bleeds freely when lacerated. The skull is a closed box. The rigid and unyielding bony skull protects the brain from injury. It also contributes to several injury mechanisms in head trauma. The temporal bone (temple) is quite thin and easily fractured, as are portions of the base of the skull. The fibrous coverings of the brain are inside the skull and include the dura mater ("tough mother"), which covers the entire brain; the thinner pia arachnoid (called simply the *arachnoid*), which lies underneath the dura and in which are suspended both arteries and veins; and the very thin pia mater ("soft mother"), which lies underneath the arachnoid and is adherent to the surface of the brain. The cerebrospinal fluid (CSF) is found beneath the arachnoid and pia mater.

Because the brain "floats" inside the cerebrospinal fluid and is anchored at its base, there is greater movement at the top of the brain than at the base. On impact, the brain is able to move within the skull and can strike bony prominences within the cranial cavity. (This is the "third collision" described in mechanisms of injury in Chapter 1.)

The intracranial volume is composed of the brain, the CSF, and the blood in the blood vessels. The three completely fill the cranial cavity. Thus, the increase of any one is at the expense of the other two. This is of great importance in the pathophysiology of head trauma. Following injury, the brain, like an ankle that is twisted, will swell. Because of the fixed space of the rigid skull, as the brain tissue swells and the volume of fluid inside the skull increases, so does the pressure inside the skull. The only significant opening through which the pressure can be released is the foramen magnum at the base, where the brain stem becomes the spinal cord. This rise in pressure can cause the brain to herniate through the foramen magnum with devastating effects.

Cerebrospinal fluid (also called *spinal fluid*) is a nutrient fluid that bathes the brain and spinal cord. Spinal fluid is continually created within the ventricles of the brain at a rate of 0.33 mL/minute. The arachnoid membrane that covers the brain and spinal cord reabsorbs it. Anything obstructing the flow of spinal fluid will cause an accumulation of spinal fluid within the brain (hydrocephalus) and an increase in intracerebral pressure (ICP).

Pathophysiology of Head Trauma

Head injuries are either open or closed, depending on whether the object responsible for the injury compromised the skull and exposed the brain. Brain injury also can be divided into two components, primary and secondary.

Primary and Secondary Brain Injuries

Primary brain injury is the immediate damage to the brain tissue that is the direct result of the injury force and is essentially fixed at the time of injury. Little can be done to change the injury after it has occurred. Primary brain injury is better managed by prevention with such measures as use of occupant restraint systems in autos; the use of helmets in sports, work, and cycling; firearms education; and so forth.

Whereas penetrating wounds to the brain always cause primary injury, most primary injuries occur either as a result of external forces applied against the exterior of the skull or from movement of the brain inside the skull. In deceleration injuries, the head usually strikes an object such as the windshield of an automobile, which causes a sudden deceleration of the skull. The brain continues to move forward, impacting first against the skull in the original direction of motion ("third" collision) and then rebounding to hit the opposite side of the inner surface of the skull (a "fourth" collision). Thus, injuries may occur to the brain in the area of original impact ("**coup**") or on the opposite side ("**contracoup**"). The interior base of the skull is rough (Figure 10-2), and movement of the brain over this area may cause various degrees of injury to the brain tissue or to blood vessels supporting the brain.

Secondary brain injury is the result of hypoxia or decreased perfusion of brain tissue. Good prehospital care can help prevent the development of secondary brain injury. In response to the primary insult, swelling can cause a decrease in perfusion. As a consequence of other injuries, hypoxia or hypotension may occur, and both are damaging to brain tissue. The initial response of the injured brain is to swell. Bruising or injury causes vasodilatation with increased blood flow to the injured area, and thus an accumulation of blood that takes up space and exerts pressure on surrounding brain tissue. Because there is no extra space inside the

primary brain injury the immediate damage to the brain tissue that is the direct result of an injury force.

coup an injury to the brain in the area of original impact.

contracoup an injury to the brain on the opposite side of the original impact.

secondary brain injury an injury to the brain that is the result of hypoxia or decreased perfusion of brain tissue after a primary injury.

PEARLS: Hypoxia and Hypotension

- Patients with serious head injuries cannot tolerate hypoxia or hypotension. Give high-flow oxygen and monitor oxygenation with a pulse oximeter.
- Usually pediatric patients have a better recovery from TBI. If an adult and a child have the same injury, the child has a much better chance of recovery. However, hypoxia and hypotension appear to eliminate any neuroprotective mechanism normally afforded by age. If the child with a serious brain injury is allowed to become hypoxic or hypotensive, the chance of recovery is even worse than an adult with the same injury.

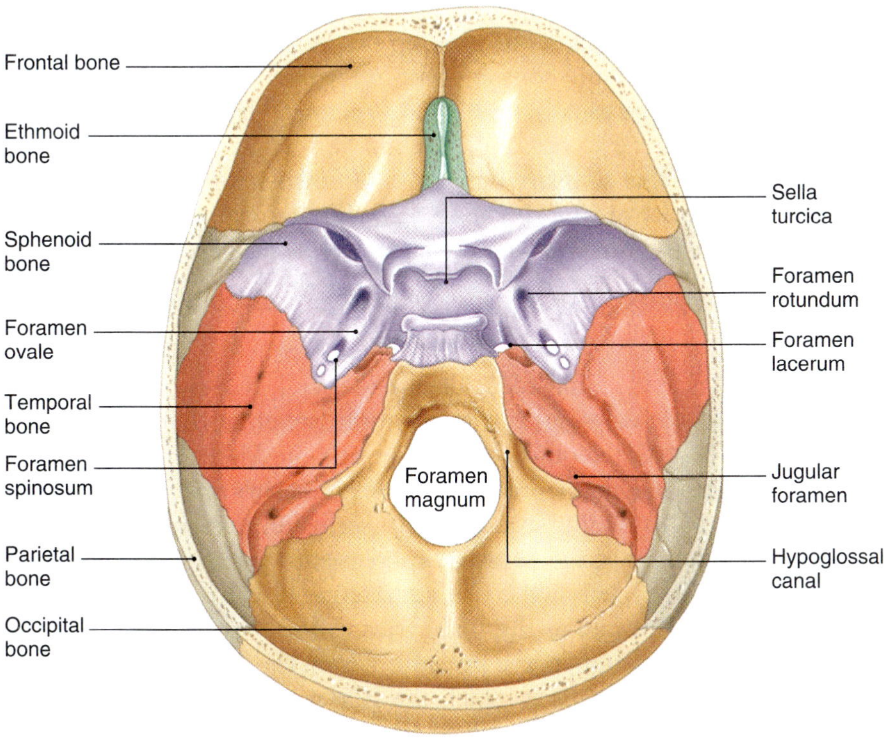

FIGURE 10-2 The rough inner base of the skull.

skull, swelling of the injured area increases intracerebral pressure, and this leads to a decreased cerebral blood flow that causes further brain injury. The increase in cerebral water (edema) does not occur immediately, but develops over hours. Early efforts to maintain perfusion of the brain can be lifesaving.

The brain normally adjusts its own blood flow in response to metabolic needs. The autoregulation of blood flow is adjusted based on the level of carbon dioxide (CO_2) in the blood. The normal level of CO_2 is 35 to 45 mm Hg. An increase in the level of CO_2 (hypoventilation) promotes cerebral vasodilatation and increases ICP. Lowering the level of CO_2 (hyperventilation) causes vasoconstriction and decreases blood flow. In the past, it was thought that hyperventilation (lowering of CO_2) in the head-injured patient would decrease brain swelling and thus improve cerebral blood flow. Research has shown that hyperventilation actually has only a slight effect on brain swelling, but causes a significant decrease in cerebral perfusion from vasoconstriction, which results in cerebral hypoxia. The injured brain does not tolerate hypoxia. Thus, both hyperventilation and hypoventilation can cause cerebral ischemia and increased mortality in the TBI patient. Maintaining good ventilation (not hyperventilation) with high-flow oxygen at a rate of about one breath every 6 to 8 seconds (8 to 10 per minute) to maintain an end-tidal CO_2 ($ETCO_2$) of 35–45 is very important. Prophylactic hyperventilation for head injury is no longer recommended.

Intracranial Pressure

Within the skull and fibrous coverings of the brain are the brain tissue, cerebrospinal fluid, and blood. An increase in the volume of any one of those components must be at the expense of the other two because the adult skull (a rigid box) cannot expand. Although there is some give to the volume of cerebrospinal fluid, it accounts for little space and cannot offset rapid brain swelling. Blood supply cannot be compromised, for the brain requires a constant supply of blood (oxygen and glucose) to survive. Thus, because none of the supporting components of the brain can be compromised, brain swelling can be rapidly catastrophic.

intracranial pressure (ICP) the pressure of the brain and contents within the skull.

cerebral perfusion pressure (CPP) the pressure of the blood flowing through the brain.

mean arterial blood pressure (MAP) the sum of the diastolic blood pressure plus one-third (systolic blood pressure minus the diastolic blood pressure).

Cushing's reflex a reflex whereby the body reacts to increased intracerebral pressure by raising the blood pressure. Also called Cushing's response.

The pressure of the brain and contents within the skull is termed **intracranial pressure (ICP)**. This pressure is usually very low. Intracranial pressure is considered dangerous when it rises above 15 mm Hg; cerebral herniation may occur at pressures above 25 mm Hg. The pressure of the blood flowing through the brain is termed the **cerebral perfusion pressure (CPP)**. Its value is obtained by subtracting the intracranial (intracerebral) pressure from the **mean arterial blood pressure** (MAP).

$$\text{MAP} = \text{Diastolic BP} + 1/3\,(\text{Systolic BP} - \text{Diastolic BP})$$
$$\text{CPP} = \text{MAP} - \text{ICP}$$

If the brain swells or if bleeding occurs inside the skull, ICP increases and the perfusion pressure decreases, resulting in cerebral ischemia (hypoxia). If the swelling of the brain is severe enough, the ICP equals the MAP, and blood flow to the brain ceases. The body has a protective reflex (**Cushing's reflex** or Cushing's response) that attempts to maintain a constant perfusion pressure. When the ICP increases, the systemic blood pressure increases to try to preserve blood flow to the brain. The body senses the rise in systemic blood pressure, and this triggers a drop in the pulse rate as the body tries to lower the blood pressure. With severe injury and/or ischemia, the pressure within the skull continues in an upward spiral until a critical point at which the ICP approaches the MAP, and there is no cerebral perfusion. All vital signs deteriorate, and the patient dies. Because CPP depends on both the arterial pressure and the ICP, hypotension also will have a devastating effect if the ICP is high.

As stated earlier, the injured brain loses the ability to autoregulate blood flow. In this situation perfusion of the brain is directly dependent on the CPP. You must maintain a cerebral perfusion pressure of at least 60 mm Hg (see earlier formula), which requires maintaining a systolic blood pressure of at least 110 to 120 mm Hg in the patient with a severe head injury. This will rarely be a problem, because hypotension only occurs in about 5% of patients with isolated severe TBI (GCS of < 9). Aggressive attempts to maintain CPP above 70 mm Hg with fluids and pressors (dopamine, epinephrine) should be avoided because of the risk of adult respiratory distress syndrome (ARDS).

PEARLS: Cerebral Herniation Syndrome

A patient who, after correction of hypoxia and hypotension, shows rapid progression of brain injury (e.g., unresponsive with dilated pupil; decerebrate posturing; or drop in GCS score of > 2 with an initial GCS score of < 9) should be transported rapidly to a trauma center capable of managing severe TBI patients. This is the only situation in which hyperventilation is still indicated. Hyperventilation, although known to cause ischemia, may decrease brain swelling temporarily. Although a desperate measure, this might buy enough time to get the patient to surgery that might be lifesaving. Call ahead so that a neurosurgeon can be available and the operating room prepared by the time you arrive at the hospital.

Cerebral Herniation Syndrome

When the brain swells, particularly after a blow to the head, a sudden rise in ICP may occur. This may force portions of the brain downward, obstructing the flow of cerebrospinal fluid and applying great pressure to the brain stem resulting in **cerebral herniation syndrome**. The classic findings on exam in this life-threatening situation are a decreasing level of consciousness (LOC) that rapidly progresses to coma, dilation of the pupil and an outward–downward deviation of the eye on the side of the injury, paralysis of the arm and leg on the side opposite the injury, or decerebrate posturing (arms and legs extended). As the cerebral herniation is occurring, the vital signs frequently reveal increased blood pressure and bradycardia (Cushing's response). The patient may soon cease all movement, stop breathing, and die. This syndrome often follows an acute epidural or subdural hemorrhage.

cerebral herniation syndrome a critical syndrome in which swelling of the brain forces portions of the brain tissue down through the opening at the base of the skull squeezing the brain stem and causing coma, dilatation of pupils, contralateral paralysis, elevated blood pressure, and bradycardia.

If these signs are developing in a TBI patient, cerebral herniation is imminent, and aggressive therapy is needed. As noted earlier, hyperventilation will decrease the size of the blood vessels in the brain and briefly decrease ICP. In this situation the danger of immediate herniation outweighs the risk of cerebral ischemia that can follow hyperventilation. *The cerebral herniation syndrome is the only situation in which hyperventilation is still indicated.* (You must ventilate every three seconds [20/minute] for adults, every two and one-half seconds [25/minute] for children, and every two seconds [30/minute] for infants.) If you have waveform capnography, attempt to keep the $ETCO_2$ at about 30 to 35 mm Hg.

To simplify knowing when to hyperventilate in the field, the clinical signs of cerebral herniation in the patient who has had hypoxemia and hypotension corrected are any one (or more) of the following:

- TBI patient with a Glasgow Coma Scale (GCS) score < 9 with extensor posturing (decerebrate posturing)
- TBI patient with a GCS score < 9 with asymmetric (or bilateral), dilated, or nonreactive pupils
- TBI patient with an initial GCS score < 9, who then drops his or her GCS by more than two points

For the preceding, "asymmetric pupils" means 1 mm (or more) difference in the size of one pupil, "fixed" means no response (<1 mm) to bright light. Bilateral dilated and fixed pupils usually are a sign of brain-stem injury and are associated with 91% mortality. A unilateral dilated and fixed pupil has been associated with good recovery in up to 54% of patients. Remember that hypoxemia, orbital trauma, drugs, lightning strike, and hypothermia also affect pupillary reaction, so take this into account before beginning hyperventilation. Flaccid paralysis usually means spinal cord injury. If the patient has signs of herniation (as listed earlier) and the signs resolve with hyperventilation, you should discontinue the hyperventilation. (See Table 10-1.)

Table 10-1 Normal Ventilation Rates and Hyperventilation Rates

Age Group	Normal Ventilation Rate	Hyperventilation Rate
Adult	8–10 breaths/minute ($ETCO_2$ 35–45)	20 breaths/minute ($ETCO_2$ about 30–35)
Children	15 breaths/minute ($ETCO_2$ 35–45)	25 breaths/minute ($ETCO_2$ about 30–35)
Infants	20 breaths/minute ($ETCO_2$ 35–45)	30 breaths/minute ($ETCO_2$ about 30–35)

Head Injuries

The head is made up of the face, scalp, skull, and brain, and serious injuries can occur to any one or all of them. The head is the heaviest part of a young child's body, so children involved in falls or other deceleration trauma frequently have head injuries.

Facial Injuries

The soft tissue of the face is very vascular, and the wounds can range from minor contusions, abrasions, and lacerations, to wounds that can be fatal, such as airway compromise or hemorrhagic shock. Most bleeding can be controlled by direct pressure, but some hemorrhage from the nose or pharynx can be life threatening and impossible to control in the prehospital setting. Nasal fractures are the most common fractures of facial bones, and rarely are they associated with severe hemorrhage. Fractures of the bones of the face and jaw are common, and the greatest danger is swelling and bleeding compromising the airway. Injuries to the eyes are not life threatening but can be severely disabling. Treatment of eye trauma in the field should be gentle irrigation with normal saline if needed and then application of an eye shield. Do not allow any pressure on the globe itself.

Scalp Wounds

PEARLS: Shock

Any unexplained shock in a patient with head injury is hypovolemic until proven otherwise. Treat hypotension.

The scalp is highly vascular and often bleeds briskly when lacerated. Because many of the small blood vessels are suspended in an inelastic matrix of supporting tissue, the normal protective vasospasm that would limit bleeding is inhibited, which may lead to prolonged bleeding and significant blood loss. This is more likely to occur in children because they have a smaller blood volume than an adult. Though an uncommon cause of shock in an adult, a child may develop shock from a briskly bleeding scalp wound.

As a general rule, if you have an adult patient with a scalp injury who is in shock, look for another cause for the shock (such as internal bleeding). However, do not underestimate the blood loss from a scalp wound. Most bleeding from the scalp can be easily controlled in the field with direct pressure if your exam reveals no unstable fractures under the wound.

Skull Injuries

Skull injuries can be linear nondisplaced fractures, depressed fractures, or compound fractures (Figure 10-3). Suspect an underlying skull fracture in adults who have a large contusion or darkened swelling of the scalp. There is very little that can be done for skull fractures in the field except to avoid placing direct pressure on an obvious depressed or compound skull fracture. The real concern is the amount of force that can cause a skull fracture also can cause a brain injury. Treat the brain injury with adequate oxygenation and maintain perfusion. Open skull

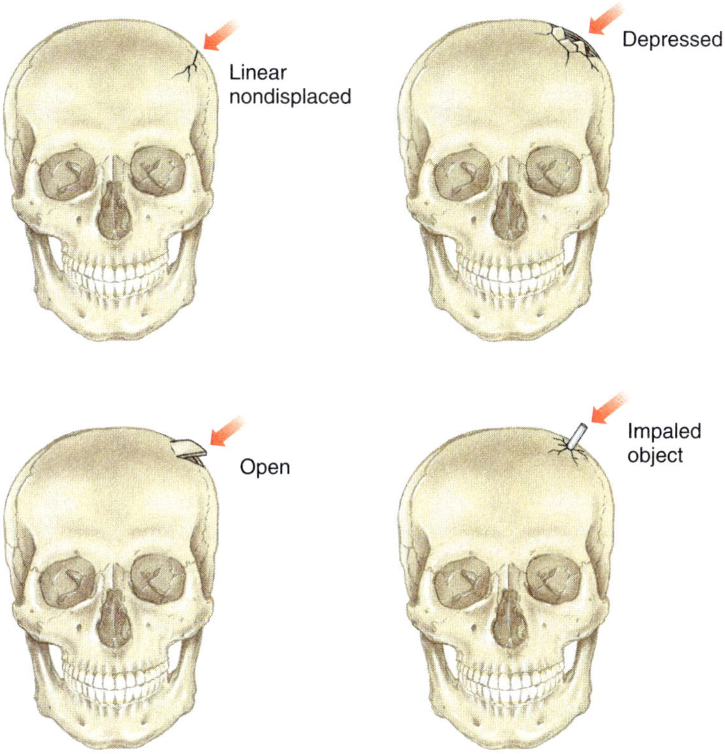

FIGURE 10-3 Types of skull fractures.

fractures should have the wound dressed, but avoid excess pressure when controlling bleeding. Penetrating objects in the skull should be secured in place (not removed) and the patient transported immediately. If your patient has a gunshot wound to the head, unless there is a clear entrance and exit wound in a perfectly linear path, assume that the bullet may have ricocheted and is lodged in the neck near the spinal cord.

Consider child abuse when you find a child with a head injury and no clear explanation of the cause. Suspect possible abuse if the story about the injury is inconsistent with the injury or the responsible adult suggests the child performed an activity that a child of this age is not physically capable of performing. Pay particular attention to the setting from which you rescued the child. Request police or social service assistance if the circumstances are suspicious for child abuse.

Brain Injuries

There are multiple types of injuries to the brain and associated blood vessels. They are discussed in this section, beginning with the least severe and progressing through to life-threatening injuries.

Concussion

A concussion implies no structural injury to the brain that can be demonstrated by current imaging techniques. There is a brief disruption of neural function that often results in loss of consciousness, but many people will have a concussion without a loss of consciousness.

Classically, there is a history of trauma to the head with a variable period of unconsciousness or confusion and then a return to normal consciousness. There may be amnesia following the injury. The amnesia usually extends to some point before the injury (retrograde short-term amnesia), so often the patient will not remember the events leading to the injury. Short-term memory is often affected, and the patient may repeat questions over and over as if he has not been paying attention to your answers. Patients also may report dizziness, headache, ringing in the ears, and/or nausea.

Long-term effects of concussion can vary, especially if a patient has had multiple episodes, such as is seen in athletes, especially boxers and American football players, rugby players, or those involved in contact sports. Any person who sustains a concussion while playing sports or other activities should not be allowed to return to that activity that day and not until cleared by a physician.

Cerebral Contusion

A patient with cerebral contusion (bruised brain tissue) will have a history of prolonged unconsciousness or serious alteration in level of consciousness (e.g., profound confusion, persistent amnesia, abnormal behavior). Brain swelling may be rapid and severe. The patient may have focal neurological signs (weakness, speech problems) and appear to have suffered a cerebrovascular accident (stroke). Depending on the location of the cerebral contusion, the patient may have personality changes such as inappropriately rude behavior or agitation.

Subarachnoid Hemorrhage

Blood can enter the subarachnoid space as a result either of trauma or a spontaneous hemorrhage. The subarachnoid blood causes irritation that results in intravascular fluid "leaking" into the brain and causing more edema. Severe headache, coma, and vomiting from the irritation are common. The patients may have so much brain swelling that they develop cerebral herniation syndrome.

Diffuse Axonal Injury

A diffuse axonal injury is the most common type of injury as a result of severe blunt head trauma. The brain is injured so diffusely that there is generalized edema. Usually, there is no evidence of a structural lesion such as a hematoma. In most cases the patient presents unconscious, with no focal motor deficits.

Anoxic Brain Injury

Injuries to the brain from lack of oxygen (e.g., cardiac arrest, airway obstruction, near-drowning) affect the brain in a serious fashion. Following an anoxic episode, perfusion of the cortex is interrupted because of spasm that develops in the small cerebral arteries. After 4 to 6 minutes of anoxia, restoring oxygenation and blood pressure will not restore perfusion of the cortex (**no-reflow phenomenon**), and there will be continuing anoxic injury to the brain cells. If the brain is without oxygen for a period greater than 4 to 6 minutes, irreversible damage almost always occurs.

no-reflow phenomenon the inability of restoring oxygenation and blood pressure to restore perfusion to the cortex after an anoxic episode of 4 to 6 minutes or more.

Hypothermia seems to protect against this phenomenon, and there have been reported cases of hypothermic patients being resuscitated after almost an hour of anoxia. Recent research post medical cardiac arrest shows improved neurological outcome when resuscitated patients are treated with controlled hypothermia. This has yet to be established in the head-injured trauma patient. Current research is directed toward finding medications that either reverse the persistent postanoxic arterial spasm or protect against the anoxic injury to the cells.

Intracranial Hemorrhage

Hemorrhage can occur between the skull and dura (the fibrous covering of the brain), between the dura and the arachnoid, or directly in the brain tissue.

Acute Epidural Hematoma. An acute epidural hematoma is most often caused by a tear in the middle meningeal artery that runs along the inside of the skull in the temporal region. The arterial injury is often caused by a linear skull fracture in the temporal or parietal region (Figure 10-4). Because the bleeding is usually arterial (although it may be venous from one of the dural sinuses), the bleeding and rise in ICP can occur rapidly, and death may occur quickly.

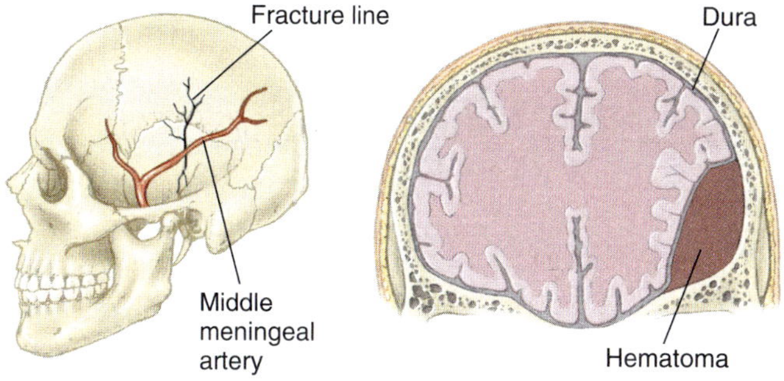

FIGURE 10-4 Acute epidural hematoma. This hemorrhage may follow injury to the extradural arteries. The blood collects between the fibrous dura and the periosteum.

Symptoms of an acute epidural hematoma include a history of head trauma with initial loss of consciousness often followed by a period during which the patient is conscious and coherent (the "lucid interval"). After a period of a few minutes to several hours, the patient will develop signs of increasing ICP (vomiting, headache, altered mental status), lapse into unconsciousness, and develop body paralysis on the side opposite of the head injury (see the earlier section on cerebral herniation syndrome). There is often a dilated and fixed (no response to bright light) pupil on the side of the head injury. The signs are usually followed rapidly by death. The classic example is the boxer who is knocked unconscious, wakes up, and is allowed to go home, only to be found dead in bed the next morning. If the underlying brain tissue is not injured, surgical removal of the blood and ligation of the ruptured blood vessel before herniation occurs often allows for full neurological recovery.

> **PEARLS: Altered Mental Status**
>
> Remember that hypoglycemia, hypoxia, cardiac dysrhythmias, and drugs can cause altered mental status. When narcotic abuse is a possibility, administer naloxone (Narcan) to any patient with altered mental status. Monitor the heart and oxygenation and check the blood glucose level on all patients with altered mental status. If you cannot perform a glucose determination but suspect hypoglycemia (diabetics and alcoholics), give glucose or thiamine and glucose.

Acute Subdural Hematoma. This is the result of bleeding between the dura and the arachnoid and is associated with injury to the underlying brain tissue (Figure 10-5). Because the bleeding is venous, intracranial pressure increases more slowly, and the diagnosis often is not apparent until hours or days after the injury.

The signs and symptoms include headache, fluctuations in the level of consciousness, and focal neurological signs (e.g., weakness of one extremity or one side of the body, altered deep tendon reflexes, and slurred speech). Because of underlying brain tissue injury, prognosis is often poor. Mortality is very high (60% to 90%) in patients who are comatose when found.

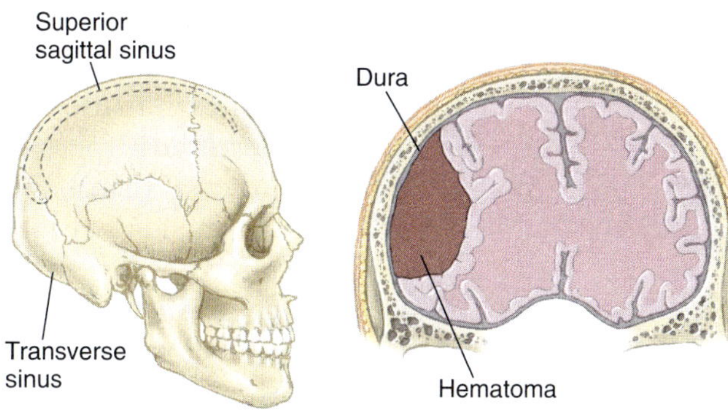

FIGURE 10-5 Acute subdural hematoma. This usually occurs following the rupture of dural veins. Blood collects and often severely compresses the brain.

Always suspect a subdural hematoma in an alcoholic with any degree of altered mental status following a fall. Elderly patients and those taking anticoagulants are also at high risk for this injury.

Intracerebral Hemorrhage. Intracerebral hemorrhage is bleeding within the brain tissue (Figure 10-6). Traumatic intracerebral hemorrhage may result from blunt or penetrating injuries of the head. Unfortunately, surgery often is not helpful. The signs and symptoms depend on the regions involved and the degree of injury. They occur in patterns similar to those that accompany a stroke. Spontaneous hemorrhages of this type may be seen in patients with severe hypertension. Alteration in the level of consciousness is commonly seen, though awake patients may complain of headache and vomiting.

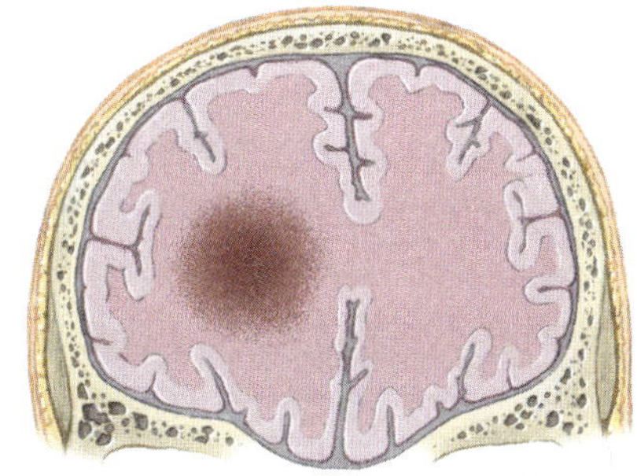

FIGURE 10-6 Intracerebral hemorrhage.

Evaluation of the Head Trauma Patient

Determining the exact type of TBI or hemorrhage cannot be done in the field, because it requires imaging techniques such as a CAT scan. It is more important that you recognize the presence of a brain injury and be ready to provide supportive measures while transporting the patient. TBI patients can be difficult to manage because they often are uncooperative and may be under the influence of alcohol or drugs. As a rescuer, you must pay extraordinary attention to detail and never lose your patience with an uncooperative patient.

ITLS Primary Survey

Remember that every trauma patient is initially evaluated in the same sequence (Figure 10-7).

Scene Size-up

The results of the scene size-up will begin to determine if you have a load-and-go patient. Dangerous generalized mechanisms (motor-vehicle collision, fall from a height) will require a complete examination (rapid trauma survey). Dangerous focused mechanisms (hit in the head with a baseball bat) will allow you to "focus" your exam (ABCs, with head, neck, and neurological exams) rather than having to perform a complete exam.

Initial Assessment

The goals of the initial assessment are to determine if this is a priority patient and to find immediate life-threats. The initial assessment in the head-trauma patient is used to determine quickly if the patient is brain injured and, if so, if the patient's condition is deteriorating. Obviously, a patient with a history and physical examination that indicate a loss of consciousness following a lucid period postinjury (possible epidural hematoma) should be transported with more urgency than one who is alert and oriented after being knocked out (possible concussion). It is very important that all observations be recorded (but do not interrupt patient care to do this) because later treatment is often dictated by detection of the deterioration of clinical stability.

All patients with head or facial trauma and an altered level of consciousness should be assumed to have a cervical-spine injury until proven otherwise. Because of the alteration of LOC, it is often not possible to clear the cervical spine until after arrival at the hospital. Restriction of cervical-spine movement should accompany airway and breathing management. Evaluation for head injury is begun as you obtain your initial level of consciousness by speaking to the patient.

During the initial assessment your neurological exam is limited to level of consciousness and any obvious paralysis. Level of consciousness is the most sensitive indicator of brain function. Initially, the AVPU method is adequate. (See Chapter 2.) If there is a history of head trauma, or if the initial exam reveals an altered mental status, then the rapid trauma survey will include a more complete neurological exam. A decrease in the level of consciousness is the first indicator of a brain injury or rising ICP.

Control of the airway cannot be overemphasized. The supine, restrained, and unconscious patient is prone to airway obstruction from the tongue, blood, vomit, or other secretions. Vomiting is very common within the first hour following a head injury.

PEARLS: Vomiting

Patients with head trauma frequently vomit. You must remain alert to prevent aspiration. If the patient is unconscious, with loss of protective reflexes, you should insert an endotracheal tube. Otherwise, keep mechanical suction available and be prepared to logroll the patient onto his side (maintaining motion restriction of the spine).

ITLS PRIMARY SURVEY

SCENE SIZE-UP

Standard Precautions Hazards, Number of Patients, Need for additional resources, **Mechanism of Injury**

INITIAL ASSESSMENT

GENERAL IMPRESSION

Age, Sex, Weight, General Appearance, Position, Purposeful Movement, Obvious Injuries, Skin Color

Life-threatening Bleeding

LOC

A-V-P-U

Chief Complaint/Symptoms

AIRWAY
(WITH C-SPINE CONTROL)

Snoring, Gurgling, Stridor; Silence

BREATHING

Present? Rate, Depth, Effort

CIRCULATION

Radial/Carotid Present? Rate, Rhythm, Quality

Skin Color, Temperature, Moisture; Capillary Refill

Has bleeding been controlled?

RAPID TRAUMA SURVEY

HEAD and NECK

Wounds?

Neck Vein distention? Tracheal Deviation?

CHEST

Asymmetry (Paradoxical Motion?), Contusions, Penetrations, Tenderness, Instability, Crepitation

Breath Sounds

Present? Equal? (If unequal: percussion)

Heart Tones

ABDOMEN

Contusions, Penetration/Evisceration; Tenderness, Rigidity, Distension

PELVIS

Tenderness, Instability, Crepitation

LOWER/UPPER EXTREMITIES

Obvious Swelling, Deformity

Motor and Sensory

POSTERIOR

Obvious wounds, Tenderness, Deformity

If radial pulse present:

VITAL SIGNS

Measured Pulse, Breathing, Blood Pressure

If altered mental status: Brief Neurological exam

PUPILS

Size? Reactive? **Equal?**

GLASGOW COMA SCALE

Eyes, Voice, Motor

FIGURE 10-7 The ITLS Primary Survey.

Protect the airway of the unconscious patient with no gag reflex by endotracheal intubation or by placement of an oral or nasal airway and frequent suctioning. Perform endotracheal intubation of the unconscious head-injured patient as rapidly and smoothly as possible to avoid patient agitation, straining, and breath-holding that may contribute to elevated intracranial pressure. Use of intravenous lidocaine when intubating head-injured patients is no longer recommended. Head-injured patients may seize from their injury (if hypoxic) or have their teeth and jaws clenched, making intubation difficult. Attempting to force an artificial airway into such a patient may cause additional injury.

drug-assisted intubation (DAI) the administration of a sedative and paralytic agent to improve the ability to intubate a patient. This is also called rapid sequence intubation (RSI).

Nasotracheal intubation or use of **drug-assisted intubation (DAI)** should be considered in this situation, if permitted under local protocols. Before beginning intubation, ventilate (do not hyperventilate) with high-flow oxygen. Do not allow the head-injured patient to become hypoxic. Even one brief episode of hypoxia can increase mortality. As stated earlier, it is important to note the patient's basic neurological status prior to DAI because the medications given can prevent a complete neurological assessment in the hospital.

Rapid Trauma Survey

All patients with an abnormal level of consciousness get a rapid trauma survey. (See Chapter 2.)

Head. Once the initial assessment is completed, continue with the exam guided by the mechanism of injury. Begin with the scalp and quickly, but carefully, examine for obvious injuries such as lacerations or depressed or open skull fractures. The size of a laceration is often misjudged because of the difficulty in assessment through hair matted with blood. Feel the scalp gently for obvious unstable areas of the skull. If none are present, you may safely apply a pressure dressing or hold direct pressure on a bandage to stop scalp bleeding.

A basilar skull fracture may be indicated by any of the following: bleeding from the ear or nose, clear or serosanguineous fluid running from the nose or ear, swelling and/or discoloration behind the ear (Battle's sign), and swelling and discoloration around both eyes (raccoon eyes) (Figure 10-8). Raccoon eyes are a sign of anterior basilar skull fracture that may go through the thin cribriform plate in the upper nasal cavity and allow spinal fluid and blood to leak out. Raccoon eyes with or without drainage from the nose are an absolute

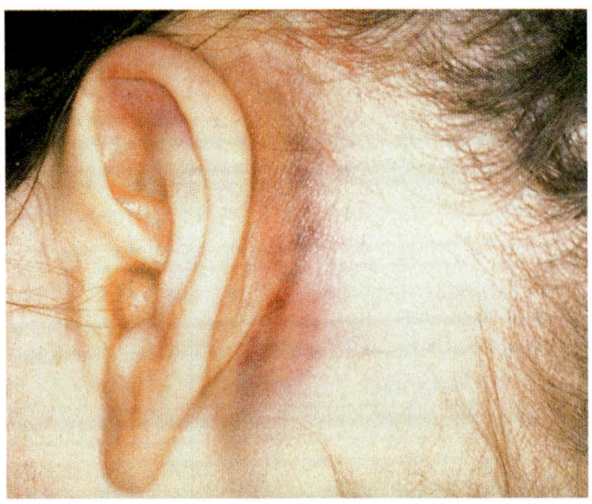

FIGURE 10-8a Battle's sign—evidence of a posterior basilar skull fracture. *(Courtesy of David Effron, MD, FACEP)*

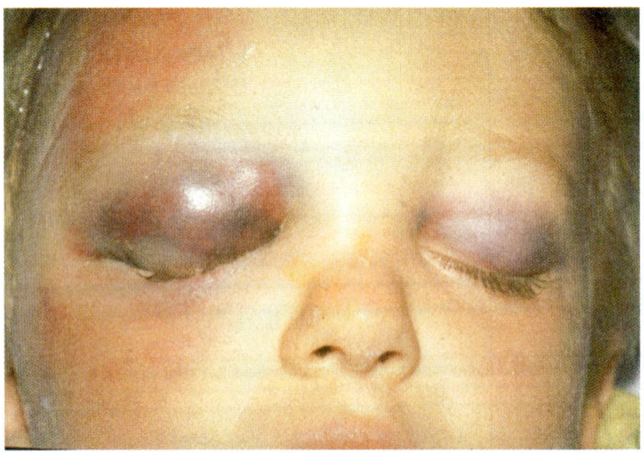

FIGURE 10-8b Raccoon eyes—evidence of an anterior basilar skull fracture. *(Courtesy of David Effron, MD, FACEP)*

contraindication to inserting a nasogastric tube or nasotracheal intubation. The tube can go through the fractured cribriform plate and into the brain.

Pupils. The pupils (Figure 10-9) are controlled in part by the third cranial nerve. This nerve takes a long course through the skull and is easily compressed by brain swelling, and thus may be affected by increasing ICP. Following a head injury, if both pupils are dilated and do not react to light, the patient probably has a brain stem injury, and the prognosis is grim. If the pupils are dilated but still react to light, the injury is often still reversible, so every effort should be made to transport the patient quickly to a facility capable of treating a head injury. A unilaterally dilated pupil that remains reactive to light may be the earliest sign of increasing ICP. The development of a unilaterally dilated, nonreactive pupil ("blown pupil") while you are observing the comatose patient is an extreme emergency and mandates rapid transport and hyperventilation. Other causes of dilated pupils that may or may not react to light include hypothermia, lightning strike, anoxia, optic nerve injury, drug effect (e.g., atropine), or direct trauma to the eye. Fixed and dilated pupils signify increased intracranial pressure only in patients with a decreased level of consciousness. If the patient has a normal level of consciousness, the dilated pupil is not from head injury (more likely due to eye trauma or drugs such as atropine).

Fluttering eyelids are often seen with emotional disorders. Slow lid closure (like a curtain falling) is usually caused by brain injury or effect of toxins (such as alcohol or other sedatives). Testing for a blink response (corneal reflex) by touching the cornea with the edge of a gauze pad or cotton swab, or by applying overly noxious stimuli to a patient to test for response to pain, are techniques that are unreliable and do not contribute to prehospital assessment.

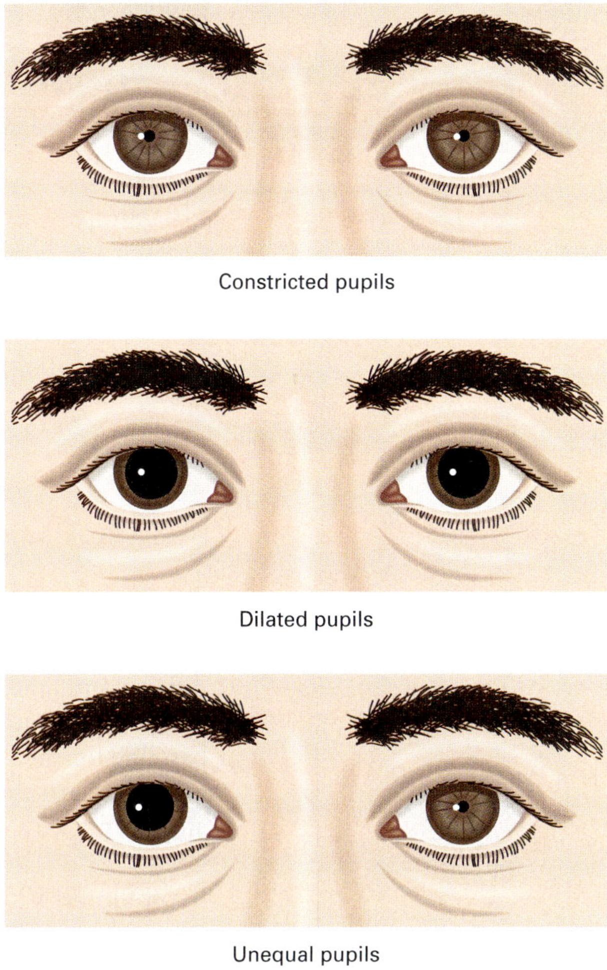

FIGURE 10-9 Examination of pupils.

Extremities. Note sensation and motor function in the extremities. Can the patient feel you touch her hands and feet? Can she wiggle her fingers and toes? If the patient is unconscious, note her response to pain. If she withdraws or localizes to the pinching of her fingers and toes, she has grossly intact sensation and motor function. This usually indicates that there is normal or only minimally impaired cortical function.

Both decorticate posturing or rigidity (arms flexed, legs extended) and decerebrate posturing or rigidity (arms and legs extended) are ominous signs of deep cerebral hemispheric or upper brain stem injury (Figure 10-10). Decerebrate posturing is worse and usually signifies cerebral herniation. It is one of the indications for hyperventilation. Flaccid paralysis usually denotes spinal-cord injury.

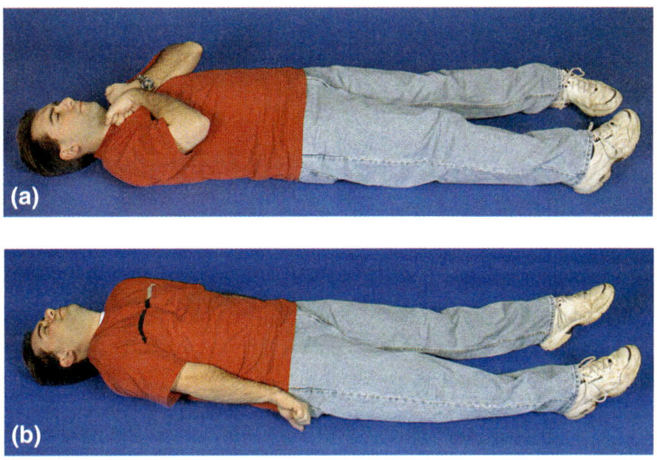

FIGURE 10-10 Decerebrate (a) and decorticate (b) posturing.

Neurological Exam. To apply the revised trauma score and other field triage scoring systems, you should be

Table 10-2 Glasgow Coma Scale

Eye Opening	Points	Verbal Response	Points	Motor Response	Points
Spontaneous	4	Oriented	5	Obeys commands	6
To voice	3	Confused	4	Localizes pain	5
To pain	2	Inappropriate words	3	Withdraws	4
None	1	Incomprehensible sounds	2	Abnormal flexion	3*
		Silent	1	Abnormal extension	2**
				No movement	1

* Decorticate posturing to pain
** Decerebrate posturing to pain

familiar with the Glasgow Coma Scale score (GCS), which is simple, is easy to use, and has good prognostic value for eventual outcome (Table 10-2). In the TBI patient, a Glasgow Coma Scale score of 8 or less is considered evidence of a severe brain injury. The GCS score that is determined in the field serves as the baseline for the patient; be sure to record it. Record the score for each part of the GCS, not just the total score. You also should perform a finger-stick glucose on all patients with altered mental status.

Vital Signs. Vital signs should be obtained by another team member while you are performing the exam. Vital signs are extremely important in following the course of a patient with head trauma. Most important, they can indicate changes in ICP (Table 10-3). Observe and record vital signs at the end of the ITLS Primary Survey, during the detailed exam, and each time you perform the ITLS Ongoing Exam.

- *Respiration.* Increasing intracranial pressure causes the respiratory rate to increase, decrease, and/or become irregular. Unusual respiratory patterns may reflect the level of brain or brain stem injury. Just before death, the patient may develop a rapid, noisy respiratory pattern called *central neurogenic hyperventilation.* Because respiration is affected by so many factors (e.g., fear, emotional disorders, chest injuries, spinal-cord injuries, diabetes), it is not as useful an indicator as are the other vital signs in monitoring the

Table 10-3 Comparison of Vital Signs in Shock and Head Injury

	Shock	Head Injury with Increased Intracranial Pressure
Level of consciousness	Decreased	Decreased
Respiration	Increased	Varies but frequently decreased
Pulse	Increased	Decreased
Blood pressure	Decreased	Increased
Pulse pressure	Narrows	Widens

course of head injury. Abnormal respiratory patterns may indicate a chest injury or other problem that could lead to hypoxia if untreated.

- *Pulse.* Increasing ICP causes the pulse rate to decrease.
- *Blood pressure.* Increasing ICP causes increased blood pressure. This hypertension is usually associated with a widening of the pulse pressure (systolic minus diastolic pressure). Other causes of hypertension include fear and pain. Hypotension in the presence of a head injury is usually caused by hemorrhagic or neurogenic shock and should be treated as if caused by hemorrhage. It is a rare (5%) finding in the patient with a severe TBI. The injured brain does not tolerate hypotension. A single instance of hypotension (90 mm Hg systolic) in an adult with a brain injury may increase the mortality rate by 150%. The increase in mortality rate for hypotension and a severe TBI is even worse in children. Give IV fluids to maintain a blood pressure of at least 110 to 120 mm Hg systolic in the adult patient with a severe head injury (GCS 8 or less) even if the patient has associated penetrating trauma with hemorrhage. As noted earlier, the goal is to maintain cerebral perfusion pressure (CPP) above 60 mm Hg. Children with severe TBI should have their blood pressure maintained at the normal range for their age.

History. Begin obtaining the history before and continue during the exam. It is essential to obtain as thorough a history about the event as possible. The circumstances of the head injury may be extremely important for patient management and may be of prognostic importance to the ultimate outcome. Pay particular attention to reports of near-drowning, electrocution, lightning strike, drug abuse, smoke inhalation, hypothermia, and seizures. Always inquire about the patient's behavior from the time of the head injury until the time of your arrival. Try to obtain the past medical history. Nontraumatic events also can cause an alteration in the LOC.

PEARLS: Seizures

Seizures in TBI patients are usually caused by hypoxia. If the patient has an open airway and you are already ventilating with 100% oxygen, you may be ordered to administer IV medication to control the seizures. Seizures should always cause you to recheck the airway, ventilation, and oxygenation of your patient.

ITLS Secondary Survey

Head-trauma patients with altered mental status are load-and-go situations. The ITLS Secondary Survey will be done during transport (or not at all, if a short transport). (See Chapter 2.)

ITLS Ongoing Exam

Each time you perform the ITLS Ongoing Exam, record the level of consciousness, the pupil size and reaction to light, the Glasgow Coma Scale score, and the development (or improvement) of focal weakness or paralysis. This, along with the vital signs, provides enough information to monitor the condition of the head-injured patient. Decisions on the management of the head-trauma patient are based on the changes in all the parameters of the physical and neurological examination. You are establishing the baseline from which later judgments must be made. Record your observations.

Management of the Head Trauma Patient

Your job is to prevent secondary brain injury. It is extremely important to make a rapid assessment and then transport the patient to a facility capable of managing head trauma. Appropriate triage of the patient to facilities capable of managing

TBI can have a significant impact on the outcome of the patient. The important points of management in the prehospital phase are listed here.

Brain Trauma Foundation guidelines are classified as follows:

- Level I recommendations, supported by Class I scientific evidence (formerly called Standards)
- Level II recommendations, supported by Class II scientific evidence (formerly called Guidelines)
- Level III recommendations, supported by Class III scientific evidence (formerly called Options)

PEARLS: Hyperventilation

Providers tend to assist respiration at too fast a rate. Use of an $ETCO_2$ monitor can prevent this.

PROCEDURE

Managing the Head Trauma Patient

1. Secure the airway and provide good oxygenation. The injured brain does not tolerate hypoxia, so every TBI patient should receive 100% oxygen. If possible, monitor the oxygen saturation with a pulse oximeter. Do not allow the SaO_2 to become less than 90% (Level II). It is best to maintain a level about 95%.

   Maintain good ventilation (not hyperventilation) with high-flow oxygen at a rate of about one breath every 6 to 8 seconds (8 to 10 breaths per minute). Studies have found that providers tend to hyperventilate the critical patient without realizing it. You can prevent this if you have an $ETCO_2$ monitor. Try to keep the CO_2 between 35 and 45 mm Hg.

   Endotracheal intubation is still recommended for adults if the airway cannot be maintained or if you cannot maintain adequate oxygenation with supplemental oxygen. There is no reason to routinely intubate patients who are maintaining their airway and have normal oxygen saturation. Some studies have found a decreased survival rate for TBI patients who have been intubated in the field. Possible causes of this are unrecognized hyperventilation and/or unrecognized esophageal intubation. Use of capnography will prevent both of those problems. (See Chapter 5.) Brain Trauma Foundation guidelines recommend capnography, pulse oximetry, and blood pressure monitoring as critical monitoring procedures for all intubated TBI patients (Level III).

   There is no evidence to support out-of-hospital endotracheal intubation over bag-mask ventilation of pediatric patients with TBI (Level II).

   Because head-injured patients are prone to vomiting, be prepared to logroll the motion-restricted patient and to suction the oropharynx, particularly if an endotracheal tube has not been placed. Try to avoid use of antiemetics because some may decrease the level of consciousness.
2. Stabilize the patient on a backboard. Restrict motion of the neck in a rigid collar and a padded head motion-restriction device.
3. Agitated and combative patients fighting against restraints or ventilations can raise their ICP, as well as place themselves at risk for further cervical-spine injury. Consider sedation in this situation, though be aware that sedation will complicate the neurological evaluation of your patient.

   Careful use of benzodiazepines can decrease agitation without dropping blood pressure. An added benefit to the use of benzodiazepines is that they prevent seizures. Seizure prophylaxis in the head-injured patient should be initiated on the recommendation of medical direction. Other agents suitable for use include phenytoin. Do not use barbiturates, as they can cause hypotension.

4. Record baseline observations. Record vital signs (describe rate and pattern of breathing), the level of consciousness, the pupils (size and reaction to light), the Glasgow Coma Scale score, and the development (or improvement) of focal weakness or paralysis. If the patient develops hypotension, suspect hemorrhage or spinal-cord injury. Every patient with altered mental status should have a finger-stick glucose checked and recorded.
5. Continuously monitor the observations listed in step 4. Record them every five minutes.
6. Insert two large-bore IV catheters. Fluid resuscitation (crystalloid) in patients with TBI should be administered to avoid hypotension and/or limit hypotension to the shortest duration possible (Level II). In the past it was thought that fluids should be limited in head-injured patients. It has been found that the danger of increasing brain swelling by giving fluids is much less than the danger of allowing the patient to be hypotensive.

   Hyperventilation is recommended for use in treating the patient with signs of cerebral herniation after correcting hypotension and/or hypoxia (Level III).

   If you have capnography available, try to maintain the CO_2 level at about 30 to 35 mm Hg during hyperventilation. Further research is needed on the utility of hypertonic saline solutions over current crystalloids for treatment of hypotension in TBI patients. Routine administration of steroids for TBI has not been shown to improve outcomes.

CASE PRESENTATION (continued)

The team leader introduces the team and asks the patient not to move during the examination. The team leader's initial impression is cautiously good because the patient, who appears to be in his late 60s or early 70s, is alert, oriented, and moving all extremities. The team leader explains that because he might have a neck injury, they need to check his neck and put a cervical collar on him. While rescuer 2 stabilizes the patient's neck, the leader continues the initial assessment. They know the patient's airway is open because he can speak normally. He responds appropriately to questions but has amnesia for the event. He has a strong, but irregular pulse, his skin color is good, and his respiration is normal.

Because of the mechanism, the leader performs a rapid trauma survey and finds a hematoma on the right side of the head in the occipital area. There is no bleeding from the ears or nose. No Battle's sign or raccoon eyes. The face feels stable. There is tenderness and spasm of the neck but no palpable deformity. The neck veins are flat and the trachea is in the midline. The chest is normal to inspection with no tenderness, and breath sounds are present and equal. Heart sounds are easily heard but the rate is irregular. The abdomen is nontender. The pelvis is stable and nontender. The extremities are nontender with normal PMS. There is some edema of the ankles. A cervical collar is placed on the patient, and he is carefully moved onto the backboard (the back is normal), packaged, and taken to the ambulance.

While rescuer 2 obtains the vital signs, the leader does a neurological exam. The patient is awake and oriented with a retrograde amnesia. He has a GCS of 15 (E-4, V-5, M-6). His pupils are 5 mm and react equally. He has good sensation and movement in his fingers and toes bilaterally.

The vital signs are pulse 95 and irregular, respiration 12, BP 140/80, and pulse oximeter 100% on oxygen by nasal cannula at 3 liters per minute.

The history reveals

S —Neck pain with occipital headache and mild nausea

A —None

M —Digitalis, furosemide, baby aspirin, and Coumadin

P —Chronic atrial fibrillation, coronary artery disease and one "mini" stroke from which he recovered

L —Had breakfast of cold cereal and coffee an hour ago

E —Was showering and woke on the tile floor of the shower

Because of the head trauma and history of taking Coumadin, the leader decides to immediately transport to the local Level I trauma center (also a stroke and cardiac center) and notifies medical direction that they have a patient with head trauma, neck pain, and history of taking anticoagulants. The leader starts a saline lock IV while rescuer 2 attaches a cardiac monitor and pulse oximeter. The patient begins to get restless and becomes confused. He tries to pull out his IV and then has a brief seizure followed by decerebrate posturing.

The leader immediately performs an ITLS Ongoing Exam. Exam of the head reveals no change in the occipital hematoma, but both pupils are now 8 mm and poorly reactive. The neck, chest, and abdomen are unchanged. The vital signs are pulse: atrial fibrillation at rate of 100 to 110, respiration 8, BP 170/80, and pulse oximeter 85% on oxygen by nasal cannula at three liters per minute. GCS: E1, V1, M2. The leader immediately intubates with a #7 endotracheal tube, attaches capnography and begins to hyperventilate to an $ETCO_2$ of 30 to 35.

Rescuer 2 notifies medical direction of the change, and she has the hospital trauma team meet them at the ambulance. The patient is taken straight to a CAT scan, where a large subdural hematoma is revealed. He is then taken directly to surgery. After a long and stormy course he eventually recovers.

The mechanism of injury, coupled with anticoagulant medication, alerted the team that the patient was likely to develop a subdural or intracerebral hemorrhage. The mechanism was also suspicious for spinal injury. The patient was packaged for transport. As is common with an injury of this type, the patient initially appeared to be stable but deteriorated soon afterward. He developed symptoms of cerebral herniation syndrome and required hyperventilation. They were wise in bypassing lower levels of care to go to a trauma center where he would receive immediate evaluation and lifesaving surgery before he reached the point of cerebral herniation. ■

Summary

Head injury is a serious complication of trauma. To give your patient the best chance of recovery, you should be familiar with the important anatomy of the head and central nervous system and understand how trauma to the various areas presents clinically. The most important steps in the management of the head-injured patient are rapid assessment, good airway management, prevention of hypotension, rapid transport to a trauma center, and frequent ITLS Ongoing Exams. In no other area of trauma care is the recording of repeated assessments so important to future management decisions.

Bibliography

1. The Brain Trauma Foundation. 2007. *Guidelines for prehospital management of traumatic brain injury*. 2nd ed. Published Jan 2007, *Prehospital Emergency* 12, Suppl 1.
2. Brain Trauma Foundation, American Association of Neurological Surgeons/ College of Neurological Surgeons, Joint Section on Neurotrauma and Critical Care. 2007. Guidelines for the management of severe head injury. *J Neurotrauma*, 3rd ed.
3. Chestnut, R. M., L. F. Marshall, M. R. Klauber, et al. 1993. The role of secondary brain injury in determining outcome from severe head injury. *Journal of Trauma* 34: 216–222.
4. Davis, D., D. Hoyt, M. Ochs, et al. 2003. The effect of paramedic rapid sequence intubation on outcome in patients with severe traumatic brain injury. *Journal of Trauma—Injury Infection & Critical Care* 54(3): 444–453.
5. Davis, D., J. Dunford, J. Poste, et al. 2004. The impact of hypoxia and hyperventilation on outcome after paramedic rapid sequence intubation of severely head-injured patients. *Journal of Trauma* 57(1): 1–8.
6. Davis, D., J. Dunford, M. Ochs, et al. 2004. The use of quantitative end-tidal capnometry to avoid inadvertent severe hyperventilation in patients with head injury after paramedic rapid sequence intubation. *Journal of Trauma—Injury Infection & Critical Care* 56(4): 808–814.
7. Franschman, G., S. Peerdeman, et al. 2009. Prehospital endotracheal intubation in patients with severe traumatic brain injury: Guidelines versus reality. *Resuscitation*, 80(10): 1147–1151.
8. Langlois, J. A., W. Rutland-Brown, M. A. Wald. 2006. The epidemiology and impact of traumatic brain injury: A brief overview. *Journal of Head Trauma Rehabilitation* 21(5): 375–378.
9. Pigula, F. A., S. L. Wald, S. R. Shackford, et al. 1993. The effect of hypotension and hypoxia on children with severe head injuries. *Journal of Pediatric Surgery* 28: 310–316.
10. Wang, H., A. Peitzman, et al. 2004. Out-of-hospital endotracheal intubation and outcome after traumatic brain injury. *Annals of Emergency Medicine* 44: 439–450.

11. McCrory, P., W Meeuwisse, et al. 2009. Consensus statement on concussion in sport: The 3rd International Conference on Concussion in Sports. *Br J Sports Med* 43: 176–184.

Explore Resource Central

For additional review and practice tests, visit www.bradybooks.com and click on Resource Central to access book-specific resources for this text. To access Resource Central, follow directions on the Student Access Card provided with this text. If there is no card, go to www.bradybooks.com and follow the Resource Central link to Buy Access from there.

Spinal Trauma

James J. Augustine, MD, FACEP

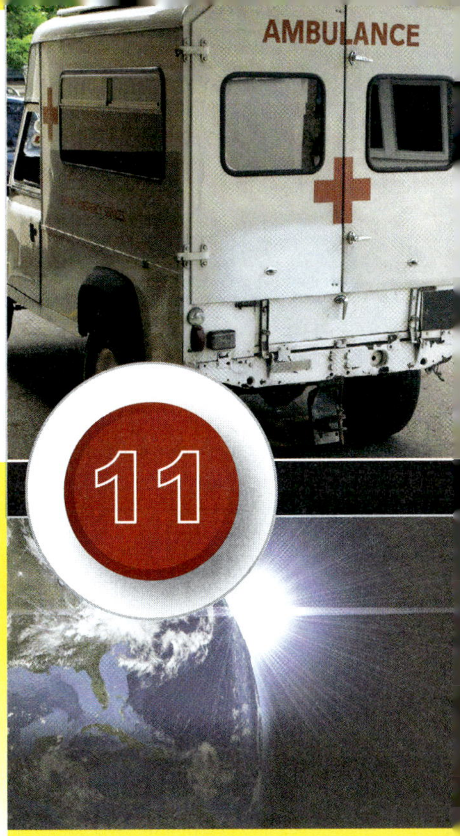

(Photo courtesy of Paul Cowan, Shutterstock.com)

Spinal Trauma

Trauma Spinale

Traumatismo Raquídeo

Traumatisme Médullaire

Urazy kręgosłupa

Wirbelsäulentrauma

Ozljede kralježnice

إصابات العمود الفقري

trauma kičme

Poškodbe hrbtenjače

Gerincsérülés

OBJECTIVES

Upon successful completion of this chapter, you should be able to:

1. Explain the normal anatomy and physiology of the spinal column and spinal cord.
2. Define spinal motion restriction (SMR) and explain why this term is more accurate than "spinal immobilization."
3. Describe mechanisms of injury for which SMR may be beneficial.
4. Describe one mechanism of injury for which SMR can cause a significant decrease in survival.
5. Explain the difference between Emergency Rescue and Rapid Extrication techniques, and give examples of when each would be appropriate.
6. Describe history and assessment criteria that identify patients who do not need SMR.
7. Give examples of special situations for which SMR techniques may need to be altered.
8. Using the clinical evaluation, differentiate neurogenic shock from hemorrhagic shock.

KEY TERMS

Emergency Rescue, *p. 201*
neutral alignment, *p. 202*
paresthesia, *p. 199*
primary spinal-cord injury, *p. 199*
Rapid Extrication, *p. 201*
secondary spinal-cord injury, *p. 199*
spinal column, *p. 195*
spinal cord, *p. 195*
spinal motion restriction (SMR), *p. 194*

Chapter Overview

Spinal-cord injury is a devastating and life-threatening result of modern trauma. In the United States there are about 250,000 persons with spinal-cord injuries. About half are paraplegic (paralyzed from the waist down) and half are quadriplegic (paralyzed from the neck down). Motor-vehicle collisions account for 44% of spinal-cord injuries, acts of violence cause 24%, falls cause 22%, and sports injuries cause 8%. Diving accidents cause over half of sports-related spinal-cord injuries. Spinal-cord injuries caused by acts of violence have increased over 50% in the past 15 years, surpassing the number of injuries caused by falls. If a patient with a spinal-cord injury survives, he could lose his independence. The cost of supporting a paraplegic over a lifetime is about $428,000. The cost of supporting a quadriplegic over a lifetime is about $1.35 million. The management of trauma patients requires continuous vigilance for injuries to the spinal canal and to the spinal cord.

Various terms have been used through the years to describe the process by which emergency personnel attempt to prevent spinal-cord injuries. It has been called spinal *traction* and then spinal *immobilization*. Now the preferred term is **spinal motion restriction (SMR)**. It most accurately defines the process used in the field because in certain patients, especially in the prehospital environment, the spine cannot be completely immobilized.

spinal motion restriction (SMR) techniques and equipment used to minimize movement of the spine and attempt to prevent further spinal column or cord injury.

There have been no large clinical trials that compare methods of spinal motion restriction. Thus, there is no Class I evidence and no formal standards of care. A growing number of studies raise concerns about the complications of SMR, particularly in victims of penetrating trauma to the trunk. The complications with the most potential danger are those related to the patient's ability to maintain an airway and breathe effectively. Therefore, recommendations in this chapter are guidelines. Remember, some patients require SMR, but this procedure is associated with potential complications for the patient and EMS providers.

Rescue personnel must skillfully assess the mechanism of injury and the patient to provide safe and appropriate SMR to trauma patients. This chapter reviews the process of evaluating the mechanism of injury, providing a structured assessment, and packaging, treating, and transporting patients with known or potential spinal-cord injuries.

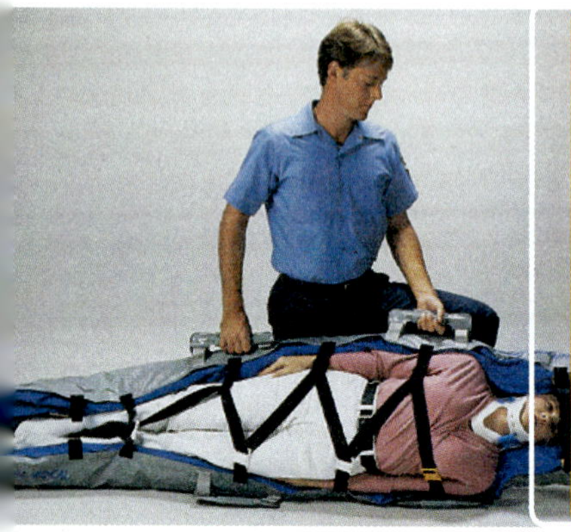

CASE PRESENTATION

An ALS ambulance has been dispatched at 2 a.m. to a motor-vehicle crash in which a single auto has left the road and hit a tree. *What injuries should they expect with a mechanism of this type? Is a spinal injury likely? Why or why not?* Keep these questions in mind as you read the chapter. Then, at the end of the chapter, find out how the rescuers completed this call. ■

The Normal Spinal Column and Cord

Spinal Column

It is important to differentiate the **spinal column** from the spinal cord. The spinal column is a bony tube composed of 33 vertebrae (Figure 11-1). It supports the body in an upright position, allows the use of our extremities, and protects the delicate spinal cord. The column's 33 vertebrae are identified by their location: 7 cervical (the C-spine), 12 thoracic (the T-spine), 5 lumbar (the L-spine), and the remainder fused together as the posterior portion of the pelvis (5 sacral and 4 coccygeal). The vertebrae are numbered in each section, from the head down to the pelvis. The third cervical vertebra from the head is designated C3, the sixth is called C6, and so forth. The thoracic vertebrae are T1 through T12, and each attaches to one of the 12 pairs of ribs. The lumbar vertebrae are numbered L1 through L5, with L5 being the last vertebra above the pelvis.

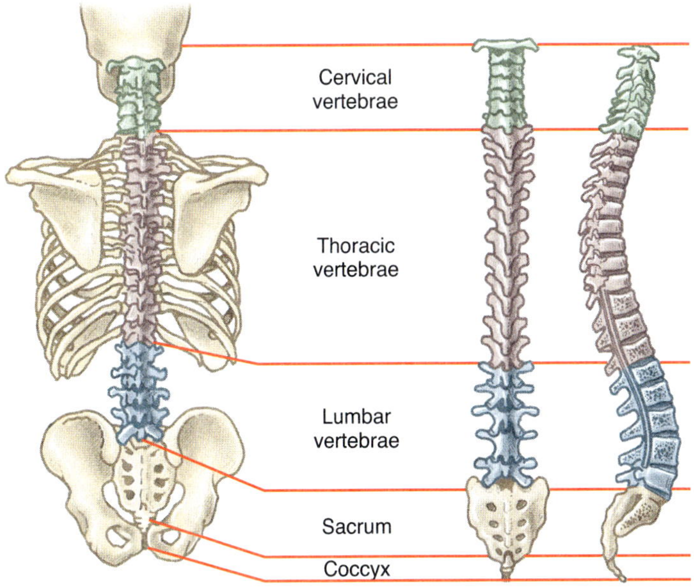

FIGURE 11-1 Anatomy of the spinal column.

spinal column the 33 vertebrae that house and protect the spinal cord.

The vertebrae are each separated by a fibrous disc that acts as a shock absorber. The alignment is maintained by strong ligaments between the vertebrae and by muscles that run along the length of the bony column from head to pelvis. (Those are the muscles strained when one lifts improperly.) The spinal column is aligned in a gentle S-curve that is most prominent at the C5–C6 and T12–L1 levels in adults, making those areas the most susceptible to injury.

Spinal Cord

The **spinal cord** is an electrical conduit that serves as an extension of the brain stem. It is continuous down to the level of the first lumbar vertebra and at that point separates into nerves. The cord is 10 to 13 mm in diameter and is suspended in the middle of the vertebral foramen (Figure 11-2). The cord is soft

spinal cord the spinal cord is an electrical conduit composed of specific bundles of nerve tracts. It connects the brain to the muscles and organs of the body.

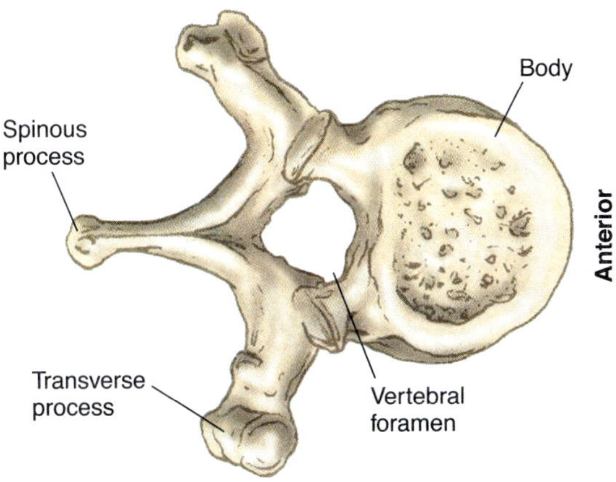

FIGURE 11-2a Vertebra viewed from above. The spinal cord passes through the vertebral foramen.

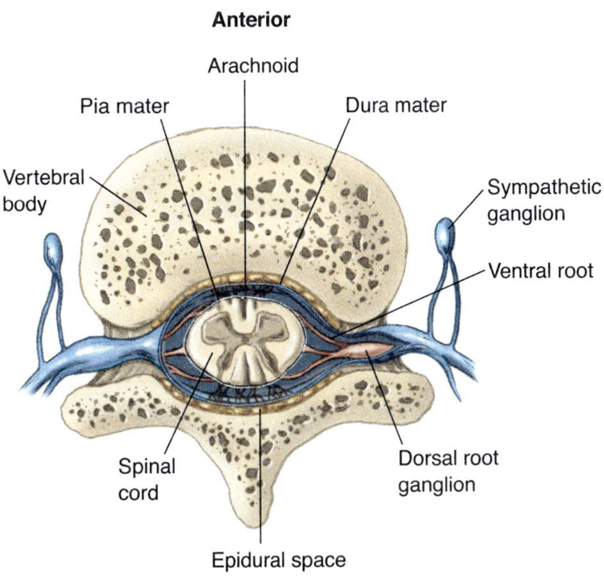

FIGURE 11-2b Vertebra with spinal cord in place.

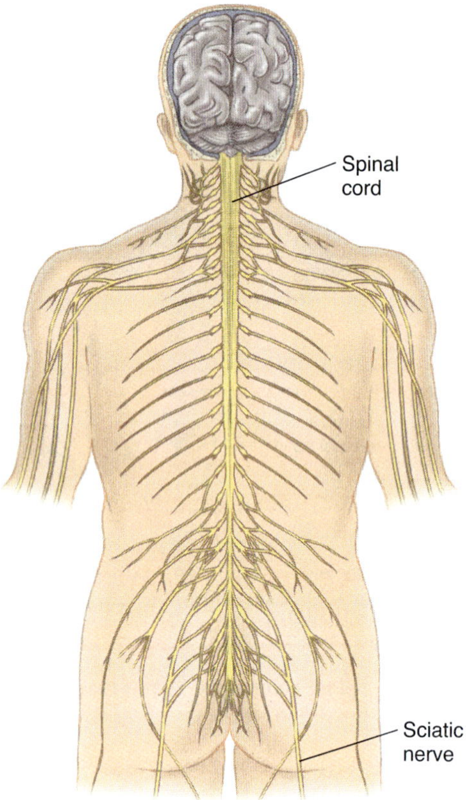

FIGURE 11-3 The spinal cord is a continuation of the central nervous system outside the skull.

and flexible like a cotton rope and is surrounded and bathed by cerebrospinal fluid along its entire length. The fluid and the flexibility provide some protection to the cord from injury.

The cord is composed of specific bundles of nerve tracts that are arranged in a predictable manner, much as a rope is composed of individual strands of fiber. The spinal cord passes down the vertebral canal and gives off pairs of nerve roots that exit at each vertebral level (Figure 11-3). The roots lie next to the intervertebral discs and the lateral part of the vertebrae, making the nerve roots susceptible to injury when trauma occurs in these areas (Figure 11-4). The nerve roots carry sensory signals from the body to the spinal cord and then to the brain.

The roots also carry signals from the brain to specific muscles, causing them to move. Those signals pass back and forth rapidly, and some are strong enough to cause actions on their own, called *reflexes*. This reflex system can be demonstrated by tapping the patella tendon below the knee, causing the lower leg to jerk. If you accidentally put your finger on a hot burner, your reflex system causes your hand to move even before your brain receives the warning message. Strong signals also can overwhelm the spinal cord's ability to keep signals moving separately to the brain. This is why a trauma patient with a fractured hip may complain of knee pain or a patient with a ruptured spleen may complain of shoulder pain.

The integrity of spinal-cord function is tested by motor, sensory, and reflex functions. The level of sensory loss is most accurate for predicting the level of spinal-cord injury. Muscle strength is another function that is easy to assess in the conscious patient. Reflexes are helpful

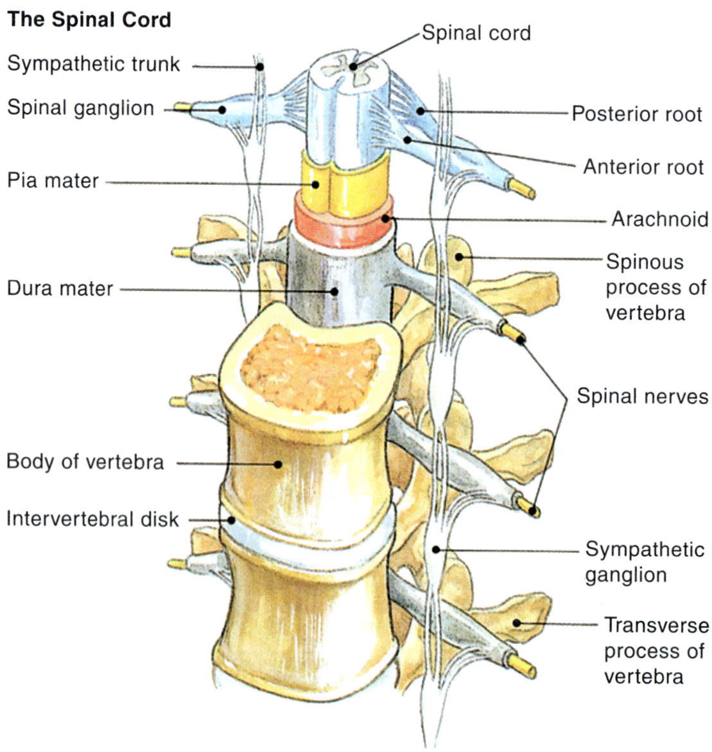

FIGURE 11-4 Relationship of the spinal cord to the vertebrae. Note how the nerve roots exit between the vertebrae.

for distinguishing complete from partial spinal-cord injuries, but are best left for hospital assessment. The spinal cord is also an integrating center for the autonomic nervous system, which assists in controlling heart rate, blood vessel tone, and blood flow to the skin. Injury to this component of the spinal cord results in neurogenic shock (commonly called *spinal shock*), which is discussed later.

Spinal Injury

A normal healthy spinal column can be severely stressed and maintain its integrity without damage to the spinal cord. However, certain mechanisms of trauma can overcome the protective defenses, injuring the spinal column and cord. The most common mechanisms are hyperextension, hyperflexion, compression, and rotation. Less commonly, lateral stress or distraction will injure the cord. Those mechanisms and their subsequent injuries are illustrated in Table 11-1.

Incidence of Spinal Injury

Spinal-cord injury occurs throughout the world with an annual incidence of 15 to 40 cases per million. The majority of demographic and epidemiological data related to traumatic spinal-cord injury has been collected in North America and Europe. Data collected by the Model Spinal Cord Care Systems and published by the National Spinal Cord Injury Statistical Center show that in the United States, the incidence of spinal injury is about 40 per million persons per year, with approximately 250,000 living survivors of spinal-cord injury in the United States in 2010.

The male-to-female ratio of individuals with spinal-cord injury in the United States is 4:1. More than 50% of all cases of spinal-cord injuries occur in persons aged 16 to 30 years. Greater mortality is reported in older patients with spinal injury.

Spinal injuries do occur in children, and it is estimated that about 1,500 children are admitted to U.S. hospitals annually. The major causes of pediatric spinal injury are slightly different from adults in that motor-vehicle crashes account for 56% of them. This includes a growing number of injuries related to all-terrain vehicle crashes. Other causes are:

- Accidental falls (14%)
- Firearm injuries (9%)
- Sports injuries (7%)

Among children so injured, 67% of those injured in a motor-vehicle collision were not wearing a seatbelt. Under age 8, the relatively large size of the head makes the upper end of the cervical cord the most common site of injury, which can be devastating.

Mechanisms of Blunt Spinal-Column Injury

The head is a relatively large ball perched on top of the neck. Sudden movement of the head or trunk will produce stresses that may damage the bony or connective tissue components of the spinal column. Injury to the spinal column is like injury to any other bone in the body. It requires a significant amount of force, unless there is a preexisting weakness or defect in the bone. For that reason, the elderly and those with severe arthritis are at higher risk for spinal injuries.

Like other bone injuries, pain is the most common symptom, but it may be unnoticed by the patient. This is especially true if the patient has other painful

Table 11-1 Mechanisms of Blunt Spinal injury

Description		Examples
Hyperextension (excessive posterior movement of the head or neck)	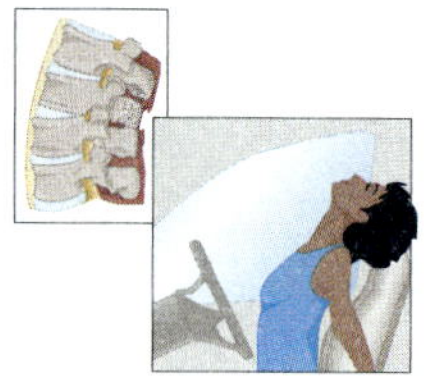	Face into windshield in MVC Elderly person falling to the floor Football tackler Dive into shallow water
Hyperflexion (excessive anterior movement of head onto chest)	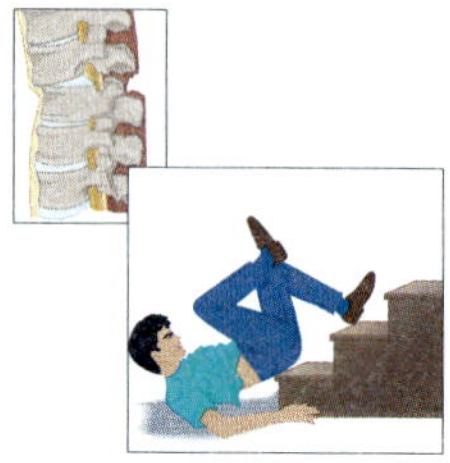	Rider thrown off horse or motorcycle Dive into shallow water
Compression (weight of head or pelvis driven into stationary neck or torso)	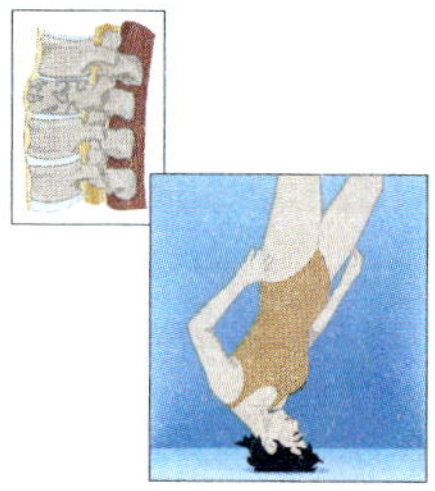	Dive into shallow water Fall of greater than 10 to 20 feet onto head or legs
Rotation (excessive rotation of the torso or head and neck, moving one side of the spinal column against the other)	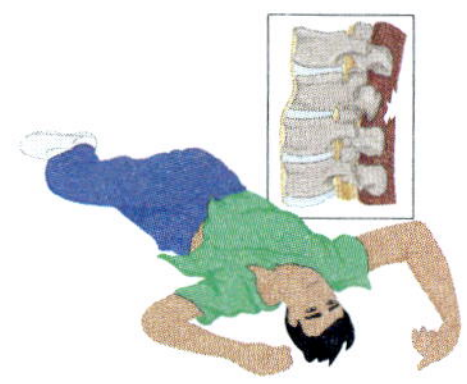	Rollover MVC Motorcycle crash
Lateral Stress (direct lateral force on spinal column, typically shearing one level of cord from another)	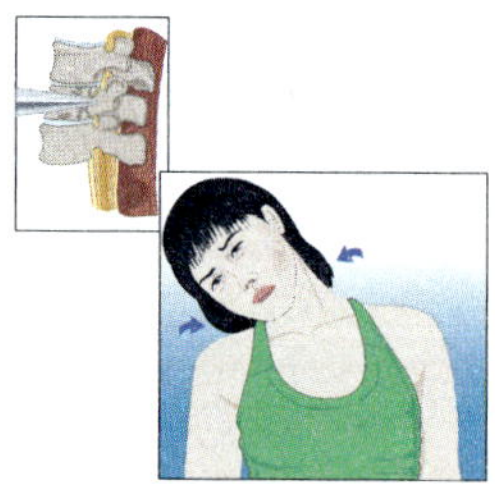	"T-bone" MVC Fall
Distraction (excessive stretching of column and cord)	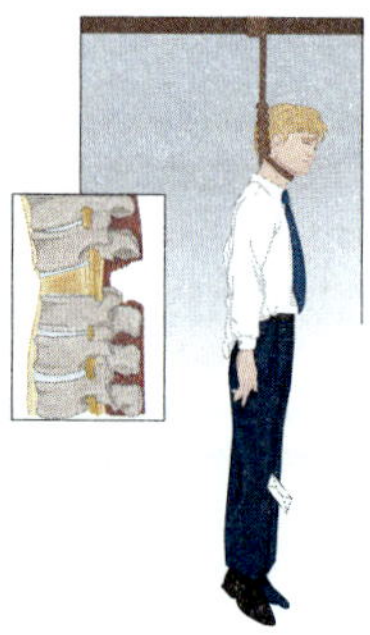	Hanging Child inappropriately wearing shoulder belt around neck Snowmobile or motorcycle under rope or wire

injuries. At the site of a bone injury, local muscle spasm may occur. Injury to individual nerve roots can result from bony spinal-column injury, with resulting localized pain, paralysis, or sensory loss. Therefore, signs that indicate spinal injury include back pain, tenderness along the spinal column, pain with movement of the back, obvious deformity or wounds of the back, paralysis, weakness, or **paresthesia** (tingling or burning feeling to the skin).

paresthesia abnormal sensation; a "tingling" or "burning" sensation.

Fortunately, spinal-column injury can occur without injuring the spinal cord. In the cervical-spine region it is much more common to have cord injury associated with column injury, with almost 40% of column injuries also having cord damage. The converse is also possible, in that cord injuries can occur in the absence of obvious spinal-column damage. This is particularly true in children. The unconscious trauma patient carries a high risk (15% to 20%) of spinal-column injury. The injuries are frequently in more than one place, and therefore SMR should be performed immediately on the unconscious trauma patient.

Pathophysiology of Spinal-Cord Injury

Spinal-cord injury results in a defective signal-conducting function, presenting as a loss of motor function and reflexes, loss or change in sensation, or neurogenic shock. The delicate structure of the spinal cord's nerve tracts makes it very sensitive to any form of trauma. What is termed **primary spinal-cord injury** occurs at the time of the trauma itself. Primary spinal-cord injury results from the cord being cut, torn, or crushed or by its blood supply being cut off. The damage is usually irreversible despite the best trauma care. **Secondary spinal-cord injury** occurs from hypotension, generalized hypoxia, injury to blood vessels, swelling, compression of the cord from surrounding hemorrhage or injury to the cord from movement of a damaged and unstable spinal column. Emergency efforts are directed at preventing secondary spinal-cord injury through attention to the ABCs, medications, and careful packaging of the patient.

primary spinal-cord injury injury to the spinal cord that occurs at the time of the trauma itself. This injury results from the cord being cut, torn, or crushed, or by its blood supply being cut off.

secondary spinal-cord injury injury to the spinal cord that occurs from hypotension, generalized hypoxia, injury to blood vessels, swelling, compression of the cord from surrounding hemorrhage, or injury to the cord from movement of a damaged and unstable spinal column.

Neurogenic Shock

Injury to the cervical or thoracic spinal cord can produce high-space shock. (See Chapter 8.) Neurogenic shock results from the malfunction of the autonomic nervous system in regulating blood vessel tone and cardiac output. Classically, neurogenic shock in the injured patient results in hypotension, with normal skin color and temperature and an inappropriately slow heart rate in contrast to the tachycardia normally seen with hypovolemic shock.

PEARLS: High-Space Shock

Injury to the spinal cord can produce high-space shock, with the patient experiencing hypotension, normal skin color and temperature, and an inappropriately slow heart rate.

In the healthy patient, blood pressure is maintained by the controlled release of catecholamines (epinephrine and norepinephrine) from the adrenal glands. Sensors in the aortic and carotid arteries monitor the blood pressure. Catecholamines cause constriction of the blood vessels, increase the heart rate, increase the strength of heart contractions, and stimulate sweat glands. The brain and spinal cord signal the adrenal glands to release catecholamines to keep the blood pressure in the normal range. In pure hemorrhagic shock, those sensors detect the hypovolemic state and compensate by constricting the blood vessels and speeding the heart rate. The high levels of catecholamines cause pale skin, tachycardia, and sweating.

The mechanism of shock from spinal-cord injury is just the opposite. There is no significant blood loss, but the injury to the spinal cord destroys the ability of the brain to regulate the release of catecholamines from the adrenals (no messages reach the adrenals), so no catecholamines are released. When the levels of catecholamines drop, the blood vessels dilate causing the blood to pool. This drop in preload causes the blood pressure to fall. The brain cannot correct this because it cannot get the message to the adrenal glands.

The patient with neurogenic shock cannot show the signs of pale skin, tachycardia, and sweating because the cord injury prevents release of catecholamines. Intra-abdominal injury is difficult to evaluate because the patient with neurogenic shock usually has a spinal-cord injury above the level of the abdomen so there is no sensation in the abdomen. The multiple-trauma patient may have both neurogenic shock and hemorrhagic shock. Neurogenic shock is a diagnosis of exclusion, after all other potential causes of shock have been ruled out. In the prehospital setting, neurogenic shock is treated in the same way as hemorrhagic shock. (See Chapter 8.)

Assessment and Management of the Trauma Patient

PEARLS: Motor and Sensory Function

Perform brief motor and sensory checks in the upper and lower extremities before and after moving any patient.

Assessing for Possible Spinal Injury

All trauma patients are evaluated in the same manner using the ITLS Primary Survey, of which evaluation of spinal-cord function is a part. Clues to spinal-cord injury are given in Table 11-2. Parts of the neurological exam are performed during the ITLS Primary Survey, and the remainder of the neurological exam is performed during the ITLS Secondary Survey. This is frequently done after the patient is loaded into the ambulance.

Table 11-2 Clues to Spinal-Cord Injury Revealed during Patient Assessment

Mechanism of Injury

- Blunt trauma above the clavicle
- Diving accident
- Motor-vehicle or bicycle crash
- Fall
- Stabbing or impalement anywhere near the spinal column
- Shooting or blast injury to the torso
- Any violent injury with forces that could act on the spinal column or cord

Patient Complaints

- Neck or back pain
- Numbness or tingling
- Loss of movement or weakness

Signs Revealed during Assessment

- Pain on movement of back or spinal column
- Obvious deformity of back or spinal column
- Guarding against movement of back
- Loss of sensation
- Weak or flaccid muscles
- Loss of bladder or bowel control
- Erection of the penis (priapism)
- Neurogenic shock

The patient who requires extrication is a special situation. Before beginning extrication, you should check sensory and motor function in the hands and feet and document the findings later in the written report. Not only does this preextrication neurological exam alert you to any spinal injury, but it also provides documentation on whether or not there was loss of function before extrication was begun. Sadly, there are a few reports of patients who have claimed that their spinal injuries were caused by their rescuers. You will not have time to perform the preextrication neurological exam on the patient who requires **Emergency Rescue**, and you may not have time on those requiring **Rapid Extrication**.

Emergency Rescue the immediate removal, without use of SMR, of a patient from an immediately life-threatening situation.

Rapid Extrication the rapid removal of a patient from a dangerous position or situation using modified SMR.

The ITLS Primary Survey must be time efficient. If the conscious patient can move his fingers and toes, the motor nerves are intact. Anything less than normal sensation (tingling or decreased sensation) is suspicious for cord injury. The unconscious patient may withdraw if you pinch his fingers and toes. If so, you have demonstrated intact motor and sensory nerves and thus an intact cord. However, this does not mean SMR is not needed. All unconscious trauma patients should have SMR. Flaccid paralysis and no reflexes or withdrawal, even in the unconscious head-injury patient, usually means spinal-cord injury. Document those important findings. (The neurological exam is described in more detail in Chapters 2 and 10.)

Managing the Trauma Patient

Minimizing Spinal Movement

Based on the mechanism of injury, it is appropriate to place the head and neck in a neutral position when you first evaluate the patient. The purpose of SMR is to minimize movement of the spine to avoid aggravating any spinal-cord or column injury. Preparation for managing spinal-cord or column injury can begin when you are dispatched to the scene of a motor-vehicle collision, fall, explosion, head injury, or neck injury.

Two types of situations require modification of the usual SMR. The patient who is in immediate danger of death in a hostile environment or in an immediate life-threatening position in a structure or vehicle may require Emergency Rescue. An example would be the patient who is in a motor-vehicle collision and, when you arrive, the auto is on fire. In some cases even a few seconds can mean the difference between life and death, you are justified in saving the patient in any way possible. This is called *Emergency Rescue*. Anytime this manner of rescue is used, you should document the reason and notify the staff at the emergency department where the patient is transported.

Some examples of situations that might require Emergency Rescue are when scene size-up identifies a condition that could immediately endanger you or the patient, such as:

- Fire or immediate danger of fire or explosion
- Hostile environment, gunfire, or other weapons
- Danger of being carried away by rapidly moving water
- Structure in immediate danger of collapse
- Continuing immediately life-threatening toxic exposure

The second situation that requires modification of usual SMR is for patients whose ITLS Primary Survey indicates a critical degree of ongoing danger that

PEARLS: Emergency Rescue

- Emergency Rescue is reserved for those situations in which there is immediate (within seconds) environmental threat to the life of the victim and/or rescuer. Patients should be moved to a safe area in a manner that places the rescuer at the least risk.
- Rapid Extrication should be considered for patients whose medical conditions or situations require fast intervention (1 or 2 minutes—but not seconds) to prevent death.

requires an intervention within 1 or 2 minutes. Indications for Rapid Extrication are the following:

- Airway obstruction that cannot be relieved by a modified jaw-thrust maneuver or a finger sweep
- Cardiac or respiratory arrest
- Chest or airway injuries requiring ventilation or assisted ventilation
- Deep shock or bleeding that cannot be controlled

Rapid Extrication requires multiple rescuers who remove the patient along the long axis of the body, using their hands to minimize movement of the spine. (See skills in Chapter 12.) When the Rapid Extrication technique is used, the written report should be carefully reviewed to ensure appropriate documentation of the technique and its indication.

PEARLS: Traction

Do not apply traction to the head and neck. Maintain in-line stabilization of the head, neck, and spine.

neutral alignment aligning the patient according to the baseline physiologic spinal position.

The most easily applied and readily available method of cervical-motion restriction is with your hands or knees. Your hands should be placed to stabilize the neck in **neutral alignment** to the long axis of the spinal column (Figure 11-5). "Pulling traction" is not a prehospital option, and the term *traction* is not an appropriate description for motion restriction of the spine. Traction usually results in further instability of any spinal-column injury. The correct approach is stabilization, with no pulling on the neck. When packaging the body on a backboard, the neutral in-line position allows the most room for the spinal cord, so that is the optimal position for SMR.

You can place an appropriately sized cervical-spine extrication collar on the patient as airway assessment is being done. Commercial cervical motion-restriction devices may be left in place on the backboard. The one- or two-piece collars are not definitive devices for restricting cervical-spine motion, but should be used only as a reminder that SMR is necessary and to prevent gross neck movement. The rescuer's hands can be removed only when the patient (head and body) has been strapped on a backboard with an attached head-motion-restriction device.

For the conscious patient, having the head and neck in a position of comfort is a good guideline. Adequate strapping must secure the head, torso, and upper legs to the backboard. Inadequate strapping will torque the neck against the body if the patient moves, rolls or is dropped or rotated.

PEARLS: Protecting the Airway

A patient in spinal motion restriction is at risk for aspiration and other problems. You are responsible for checking and maintaining the airway.

Placing and strapping a patient on the board effectively eliminates the patient's ability to protect the airway; therefore, the rescuer is responsible. Once the patient is secured to the board, a rescuer must be present and capable of rolling the board if the patient begins to vomit or loses his airway. This rule continues in effect in the emergency department, where an emergency department staff person must assume responsibility for airway protection.

Definitive SMR occurs when the body is strapped securely to the board with cushions, blanket, or towel rolls, maintaining the head, cervical spine, torso, and pelvis in line. In the past, sandbags have been used for motion restriction of the head and perform well when the patient is kept supine. However, if the board is tilted or the patient and the board are rotated (to prevent aspiration when the patient vomits), the weight of the sandbags can cause a dangerous amount of head movement. Therefore sandbags are an extremely poor option for prehospital SMR. Lighter-weight bulky objects, such as towel rolls, blanket rolls, or head cushions are better tools for this job. When applied properly, those devices allow removal of the front portion of the cervical collar and observation of the neck, as in the patient with open neck wounds.

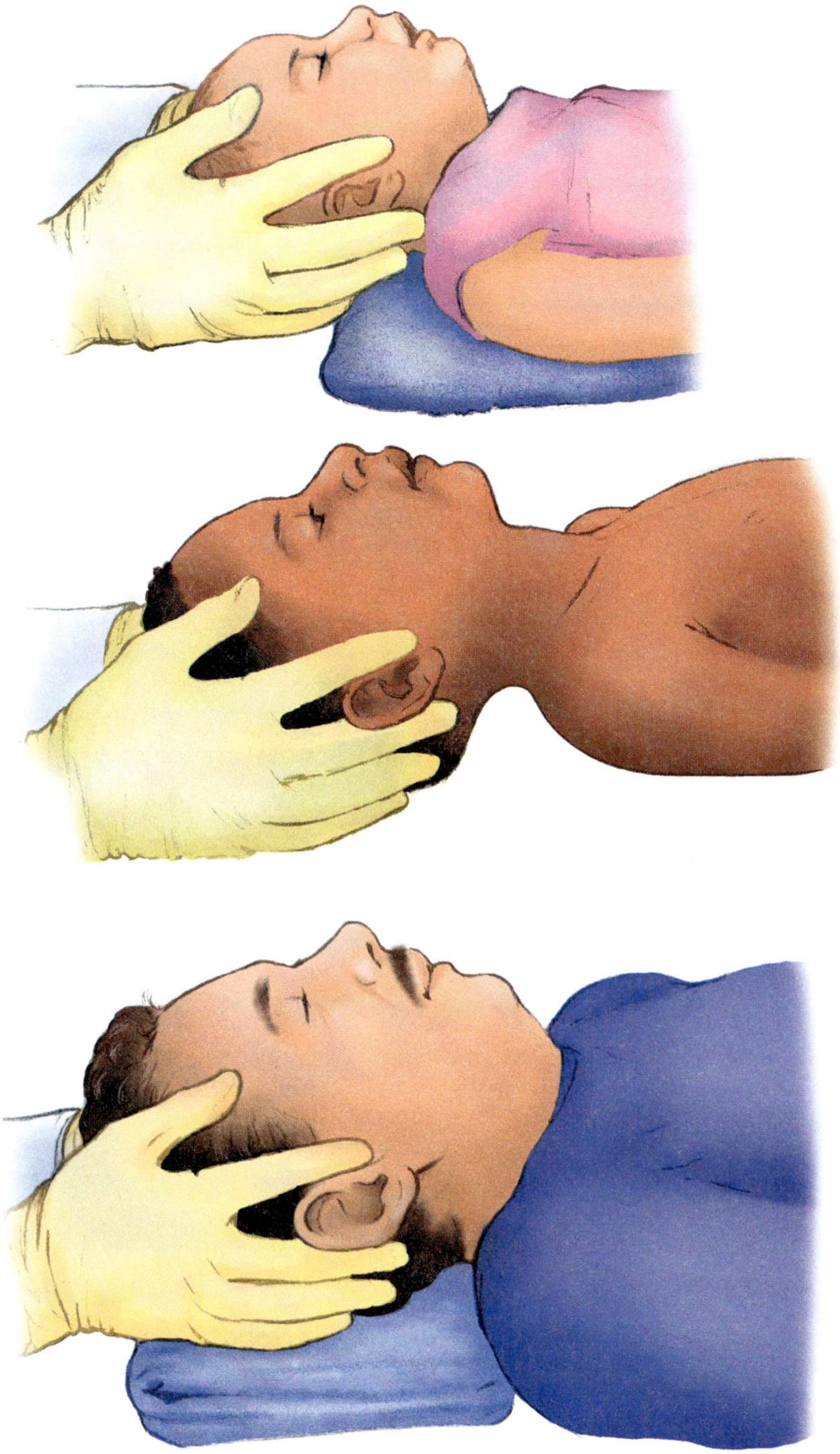

a.

b.

c.

FIGURE 11-5 Neutral spinal positioning for infant, child, and adult patients. (a) Due to the large heads of younger children, you may need to raise the shoulders with padding. (b) In older children, obtain neutral positioning with shoulders and head on a flat surface. (c) With adults, elevate the head 1 to 2 inches.

Some patients (frightened children and patients with altered mental status) will struggle so violently that they defeat your attempts to eliminate movement of the spine. There may be no good solution to this. The Reeves sleeve (Figure 11-6) may be the best device to restrict spinal motion in the combative adult patient. Always carefully document those situations in which the patient refuses to cooperate with SMR.

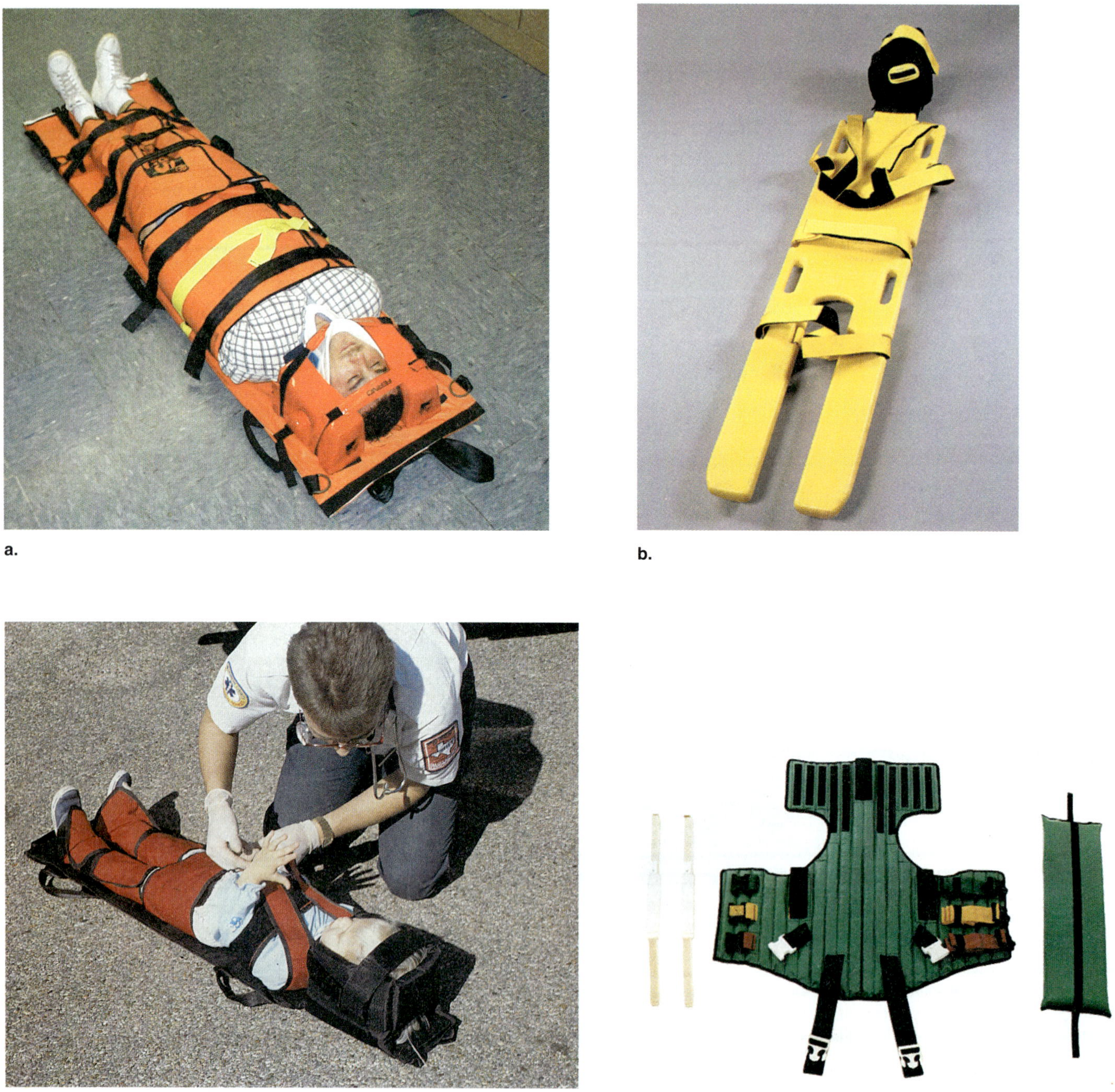

a. b. c. d.

FIGURE 11-6 (a) Reeves sleeve; (b) Miller body splint; (c) pediatric SMR device; (d) Kendrick extrication device; (e) short backboard; (f) short backboard applied to seated patient.

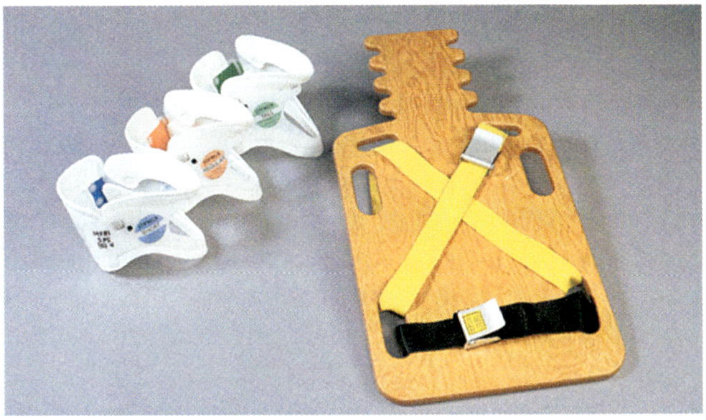

e.

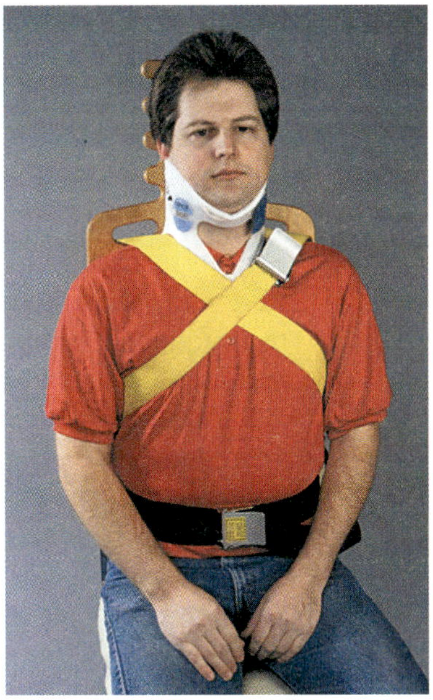

f.

FIGURE 11-6 (Continued)

A truly neutral cervical-spine position for an adult is usually obtained with the use of 1 to 2 inches of occipital padding on a long backboard. This slightly elevates the head and brings the neck into a neutral position, which tends to make the patient more comfortable and also makes endotracheal intubation easier if needed. This is accomplished with the head pad on a cervical motion-restriction device or the padding that is used with many backboard devices. Elderly patients whose necks have a natural flexed posture will require more padding. Children, because their heads are proportionately larger, usually require padding under the shoulders to prevent neck flexion on the backboard.

PEARLS: Neutral Alignment

Proper padding is often required to obtain and maintain neutral alignment of the patient's cervical spine when you perform spinal motion restriction.

Research points out that crews should *not* apply any neck traction or allow the cervical device to purposely, accidentally, or unintentionally extend the neck upward during application, adjustment, or tightening a cervical collar or device. This is particularly true for severe multiple-trauma patients, who could have very unstable injuries to the spinal column. In those patients, the traction would pull the spinal cord apart or worsen an existing injury.

In certain situations, once the patient is packaged onto the backboard, the board and patient might have to be rolled up onto the side (Figure 11-7). Careful strapping can prevent lateral movement of the spine in this situation, but use of the vacuum backboard is far superior. Women who are more than 20 weeks pregnant should always be transported with the backboard tilted 20 to 30 degrees to the patient's left side to keep the uterus off the inferior vena cava.

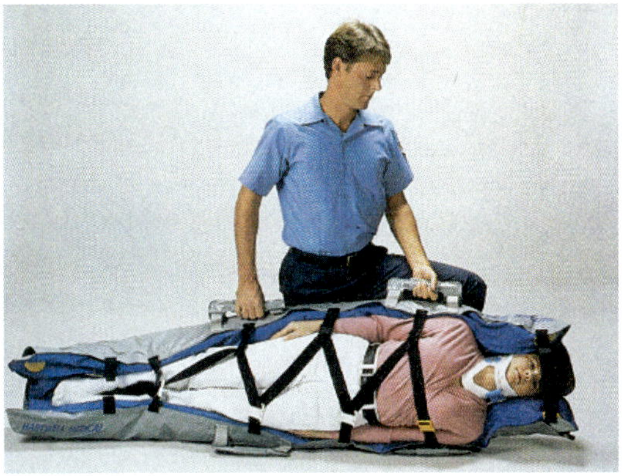

FIGURE 11-7 Patient in vacuum backboard turned on side. Notice that the body is maintained in a straight line.

Patients with airway problems who are not intubated are better transported on their side. This is especially critical when there is uncontrolled bleeding into the airway or if there is massive face or neck trauma. In those situations gravity helps drain fluids out of the airway and could prevent aspiration if the patient vomits. Because of the danger of vomiting and aspiration, unconscious patients who are not intubated should be transported tilted to the side. Once patients are placed on a backboard in SMR, they might not be able to clear their airway should they begin to vomit; therefore a rescuer should remain with them at all times.

The Log Roll

The log-roll technique is used for moving a patient onto a backboard. It is commonly used because it is easy to perform with a minimum number of rescuers. As yet, no technique has been devised that maintains complete spinal immobilization while moving a patient onto a backboard. Properly performed, the log-roll technique will minimize movement of the spinal column as safely and efficiently as any other technique for moving a patient onto the backboard.

The log-roll technique moves the spinal column as a single unit with the head and pelvis. It can be performed on patients lying prone or supine. Using three or more rescuers—controlled by the rescuer at the patient's head—the patient (with her arms at her side) is rolled onto her uninjured side, a board is slid underneath her, and the patient is rolled faceup onto the board. The log-roll technique is then completed when the patient's chest, pelvis, and head are secured to the board.

The log-roll may be modified for patients with painful arm, leg, and chest wounds who need to be rolled onto their uninjured side. The side to which you turn the patient during the log-roll procedure is not critical and can be changed in situations in which you can only place the backboard on one side of the patient.

The log-roll technique is useful for most trauma patients, but for patients with an unstable fractured pelvis, rolling their weight onto the pelvis could aggravate the injury. If the pelvic fracture appears stable, the log-roll should be carefully performed, turning the patient onto the uninjured side (if it can be identified). Patients with obviously unstable pelvic fractures should not be log-rolled, but should be lifted carefully onto a board by four or more rescuers. The scoop stretcher also could be used to move patients with unstable pelvic fractures onto the backboard. At least one model of scoop stretcher can be used in place of a backboard (Kleiner, Pollack, & McAdam, 2001).

Spinal Motion-Restriction Devices

A wide range of devices that provide SMR for injured patients is available in the marketplace (Figure 11-6). No device has yet been proven to excel over all others, and no device will ever be produced that can be used to provide SMR for all patients. No device is better than the crew using it. Training with the available tools is the most critical factor in providing good patient care.

Complications of Spinal Motion Restriction

There are complications of strapping a patient to a board. The patient will be uncomfortable and will often complain of head and low back pain that is directly related to being strapped onto the hard backboard. The head and airway are in a fixed position, which can produce airway compromise and aspiration if the patient vomits. Obese patients and those with congestive heart failure can suffer life-threatening hypoxia. On a rigid board there is uneven skin pressure that can result in pressure sores. Lifting the patient and the board can cause injuries to rescue personnel. SMR should be applied appropriately to those who will most likely benefit, and it should be avoided if not necessary.

A recent study found that patients with penetrating trauma to the trunk were twice as likely to die if they were spinal packaged in the field. Because patients with penetrating trauma to the chest or abdomen are critical load-and-go patients, the extra time it takes to perform SMR can have a devastating effect on survival. When you have a patient with a gunshot or stab wound of the trunk that is not in proximity to the spine and no symptoms of spinal injury, you should carefully but quickly load the patient on the stretcher and transport immediately.

Similarly, isolated gunshot wounds to the head may not require SMR.

Indications for Spinal Motion Restriction

Worldwide controversy exists regarding when and how to stabilize the spine. The widely held belief is that injured patients must have SMR performed until an injury can be ruled out. However, as mentioned earlier, there are no Class I studies to confirm this, and some countries do not perform SMR. They report no difference in spinal injury occurrence or outcome. At least one study has been done comparing the EMS systems of a country that performs no SMR (Malaysia) and one that consistently performs SMR (the United States). The study concluded that prehospital SMR had little or no effect on neurological outcome in patients with blunt spinal trauma. This is not to condemn SMR, but to remind us that what we are doing is based on logic and not actually based on scientific evidence.

In circumstances under which spinal-column or spinal-cord injury is very unlikely, the patient may be managed without SMR. Studies have resulted in a clinical pathway referred to as the *Maine Protocol for Spinal Motion Restriction*, which was published in 1994 by Peter Goth, MD (Figure 11-8). This protocol is supported by the National Association of EMS Physicians. (See Table 11-3 for NAEMSP's position paper on spinal motion restriction.) You must assess the mechanism of injury, interview and examine the patient, then use this information to determine which patients need SMR. From the scene size-up, history, and assessment come the clues that identify the patients who do *not* need SMR.

Under the Maine protocol, the rescuer first assesses the mechanism of injury. SMR is not required if there is no mechanism of injury that would damage the spine (foot crushed by a car). If the mechanism is a high-risk event, SMR is performed regardless of other clinical findings. High-risk situations include high-speed motor-vehicle collisions, falls of greater than three times the patient's height, penetrating wounds into or near the spinal column, sports injuries to the head or neck, diving accidents, and any trauma situation in which the patient remains unconscious.

If the danger of spinal injury is uncertain (ground-level fall, low-speed "fender bender"), the rescuer should manually stabilize the spine and then assess

PEARLS: Spinal Motion Restriction

- Spinal clearance is not a priority in the patient suffering from multiple trauma. Spinal motion restriction is.
- Protocols have been developed to allow you to properly choose which trauma patients need SMR, using mechanism of injury and careful evaluation.

Table 11-3 Position Paper Statement on Spinal Motion Restriction by the National Association of EMS Physicians*

Spinal motion restriction is indicated in prehospital trauma patients who sustain an injury with a mechanism having the potential for causing spinal injury and who have at least one of the following clinical criteria:

- Altered mental status
- Evidence of intoxication
- A distracting, painful injury (e.g., long-bone extremity fracture)
- Neurologic deficit
- Spinal pain or tenderness

*www.naemsp.org

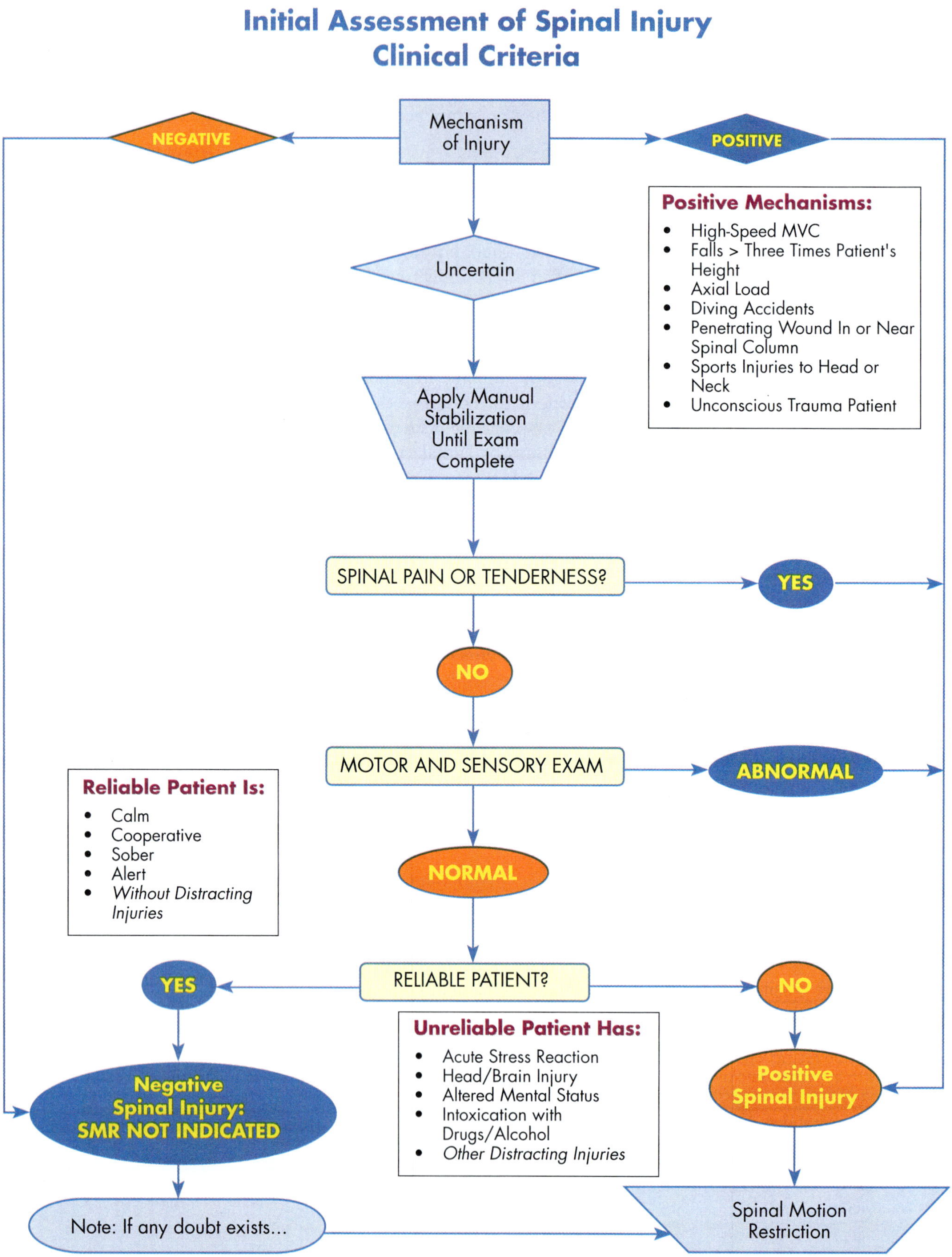

FIGURE 11-8 Decision tree for spinal motion restriction. *(Reprinted by permission of Peter Goth, MD)*

the patient for signs of spinal injury. The patient must be reliable enough to understand the EMS provider and answer the questions accurately, so children and patients with altered mental status or acute stress reactions are excluded. The patient is assessed for evidence of intoxication or distracting injuries that may not allow the patient to clearly feel the pain associated with a spinal injury. The patient is asked if he has pain in the area of the spinal column. If no pain is present in the neck or back, and no other injuries are so painful as to distract the patient from comprehending back or neck pain, the rescuer then carefully examines the spinal column and performs a neurological exam. If there is any tenderness on palpation of the spinal column area or if the patient complains of midline pain when asked to move his back, SMR is performed. SMR is also performed if there are alterations in the motor or sensory exam.

If the patient has no high-risk mechanism of injury, no alteration of mental status, no distracting injuries, is not intoxicated, has no pain or tenderness along the spine, and has no neurological deficits, the patient may be treated and transported without SMR. This protocol has proven effective in research studies but, like all medical protocols, must be approved for local use by medical direction and followed up with a quality assurance program.

Airway Intervention

When the rescuer performs SMR in any manner, the patient loses some of her ability to maintain her own airway. As mentioned earlier, the rescuer must then assume this responsibility until the patient has a controlled airway or has the spinal column cleared in the emergency department and is released from the motion-restricting equipment (Figure 11-9). This is particularly critical in children, who have a greater potential for vomiting and aspiration after a traumatic injury.

Airway manipulations in the trauma patient require careful application. Current research indicates that any airway intervention will cause some movement of the spinal column. In-line manual stabilization is the most effective manner for minimizing this movement. Nasotracheal, orotracheal, or cricothyroid intubations all induce some bony movement. Your ITLS Primary Survey should include manual stabilization, and then the use of the airway control method you are most skilled at performing. When weighing the risks and benefits of each airway procedure, recall that the risk of dying with an uncontrolled airway is greater than the risk of inducing spinal-cord damage using a careful approach to intubation.

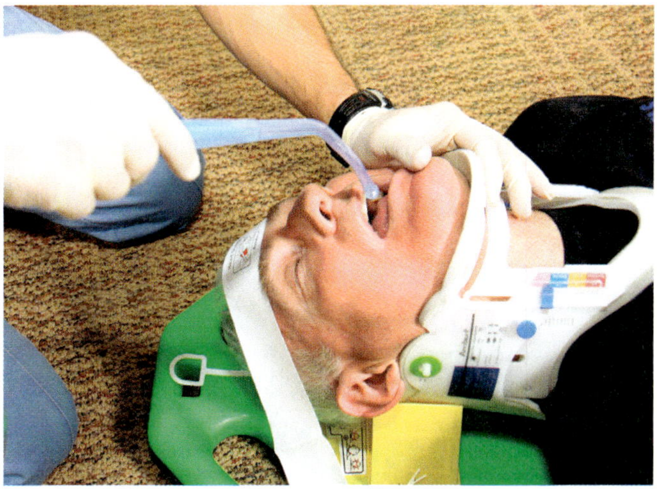

FIGURE 11-9 You are responsible for the patient's airway once the patient is strapped to a backboard. *(Courtesy of Stanley Cooper, EMT-P)*

Special Spinal Motion Restriction Situations

You must be prepared to stabilize the spinal column of all patients who sustain major trauma. In some patients (see following), traditional techniques must be modified to provide safe and effective SMR.

Closed-Space Rescues. Closed-space rescues are performed in a manner appropriate for the clinical condition of the patient. The only general rules that can be applied to these rescues are to prevent gross spinal movement and to move patients in line with the long axis of the body (Figure 11-10). Safety of the rescuer is of prime importance in all closed-space rescues. Asphyxia, toxic gases, and structure collapse are dangers of closed-space rescue

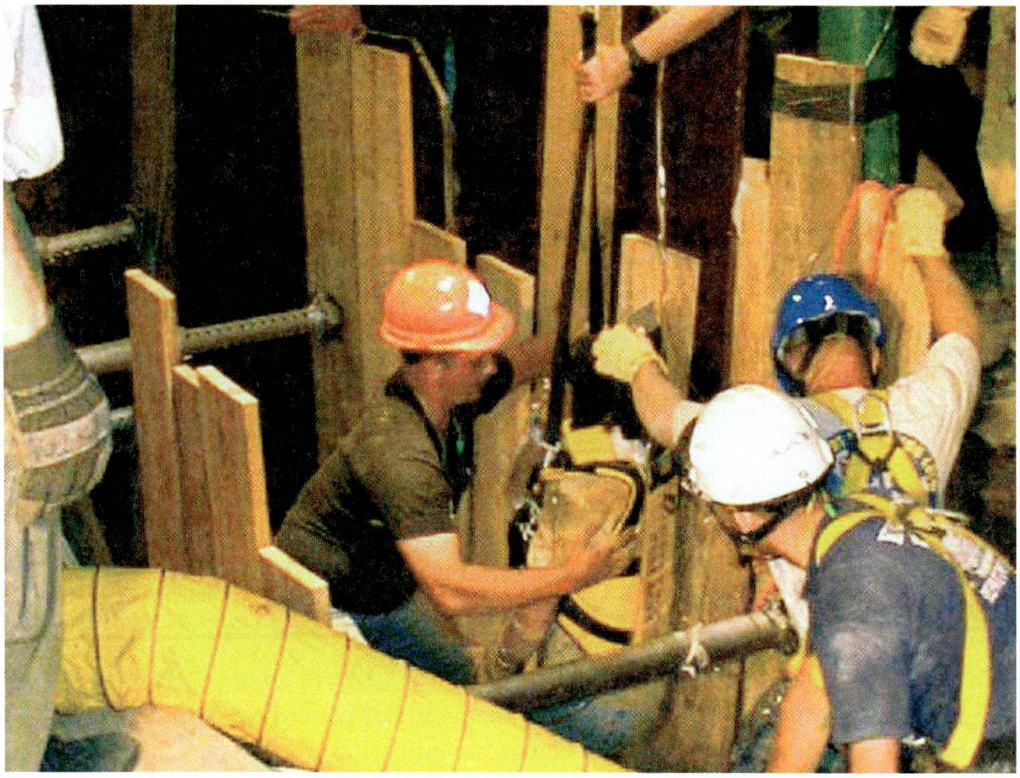

FIGURE 11-10 Patient entrapped in trench cave-in being lifted out along the long axis of the body. *(Courtesy of Roy Alson, MD)*

and may require the use of Emergency Rescue. Never enter a closed space unless you are properly trained, equipped (air pack, safety line, and so on), and sure of scene safety.

Water Emergencies. You can perform water rescues by moving the patient in line, thereby preventing gross cervical movement. When the rescuers are in a stable position for performing SMR, the backboard is floated under the patient, and the patient is then secured and removed from the water (Scan 11-1). Safety of both rescuers and patients is of paramount importance. If you are not trained in water rescue, do not attempt to rescue victims in hazardous situations such as deep or swift water.

Prone, Seated, and Standing Patients. Prone, seated, and standing patients are stabilized in a manner that minimizes spinal column movement, ending with the patient in the conventional supine position. (See Chapter 12 for techniques.)

- *Prone patients* are log-rolled onto a backboard, with the careful coordination of head and chest rescuers.
- *Seated patients* may be stabilized using short backboards or their commercial adaptations. Used appropriately, short backboards provide initial stabilization of the cervical and thoracic spine and then facilitate the movement of the patient onto a long backboard.
- *Standing patients* may be placed against the long board while upright. The board is then gently lowered to the supine position using either the two-person or three-person technique. (See Chapter 12.) The patient's body and then neck and head are secured to the backboard.

SCAN 11-1 Water Rescue

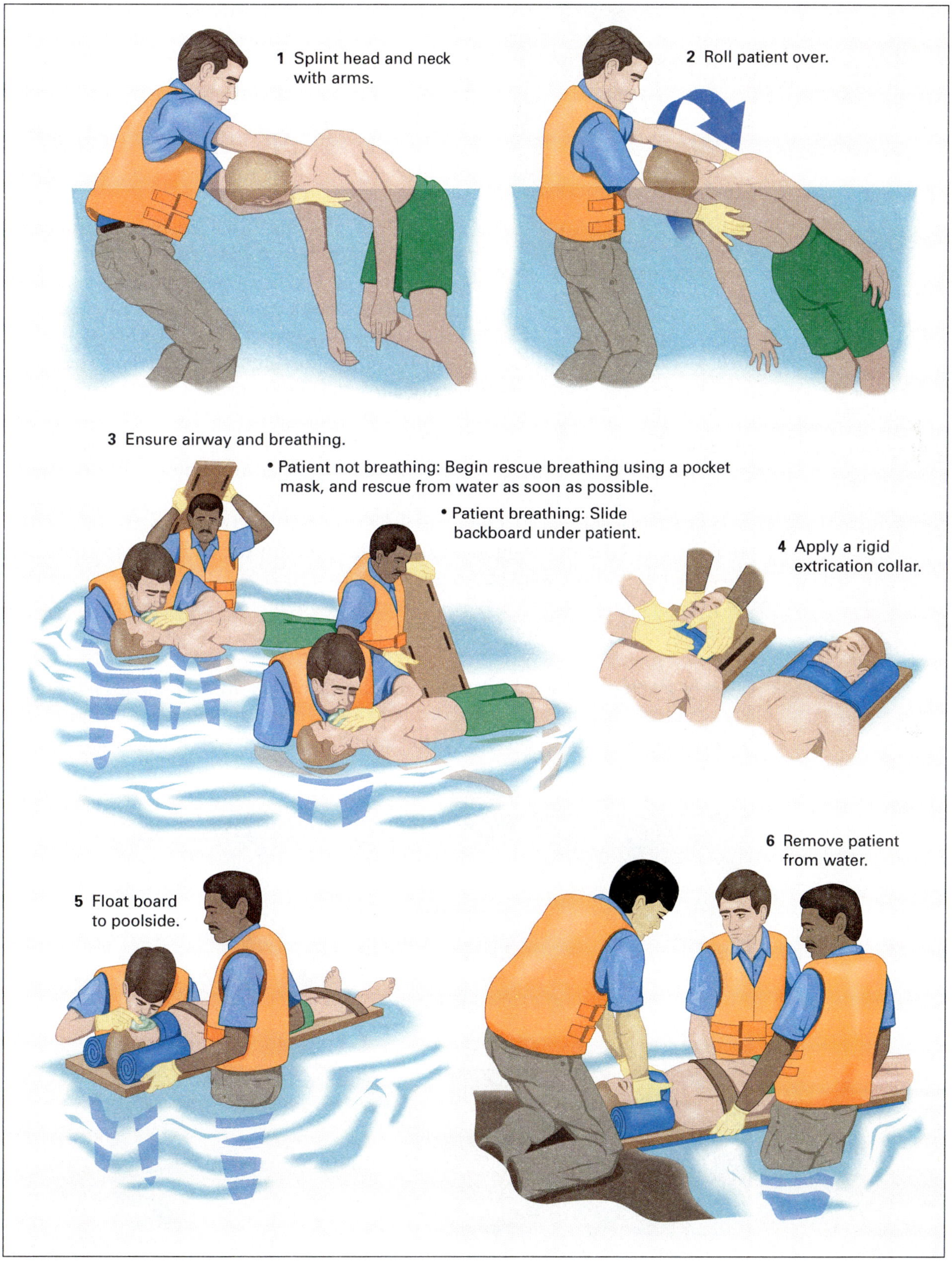

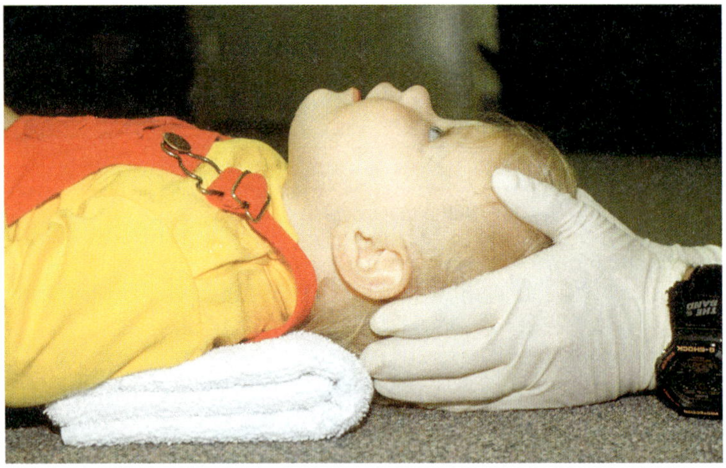

FIGURE 11-11 Most children require padding under back and shoulders to keep the cervical spine in a neutral position. *(Courtesy of Bob Page, NREMT-P)*

Pediatric Patients. It is best to provide initial SMR of the pediatric patient with your hands, and then use cushions or towel rolls to help secure the child on an appropriate board or device. Some pediatric trauma specialists suggest padding beneath the back and shoulders on the board in a child under the age of 3 years. (See Figures 11-5 and 11-11.) Those children normally have a relatively large head that flexes the neck when placed on a straight board. Padding under the back and shoulders will prevent this flexion and also make the child more comfortable.

Children who are involved in a motor-vehicle crash while restrained in a child safety seat but have no apparent injuries may be packaged in the safety seat for transport to the hospital. Using towel or blanket rolls, cloth tape, and a little reassurance, you can secure the child in the safety seat and then belt the seat into the ambulance (Figure 11-12). The technique minimizes movement of the child and provides a secure method for child transport in the ambulance.

> **PEARLS:** Car Seats
>
> Infants and small children involved in motor-vehicle crashes can be transported in their car seats as long as they have no apparent injury and the device is not damaged.

When the child is in a car seat that is damaged, or in a built-in child-restraint seat that cannot be removed, the child must be removed for SMR. Children in such situations will have to be carefully extricated onto a backboard or another pediatric SMR device, using manual stabilization. For the child who is frightened and struggling, there may be no good way to obtain SMR. Careful reassurance, the presence of a comforting family member, and gentle management will help prevent more complications and further struggling.

Elderly Patients. Elderly patients require flexibility in packaging techniques. Many elderly patients have arthritic changes of the spine and thin, frail skin. Such patients will be very uncomfortable when placed on a backboard. Some

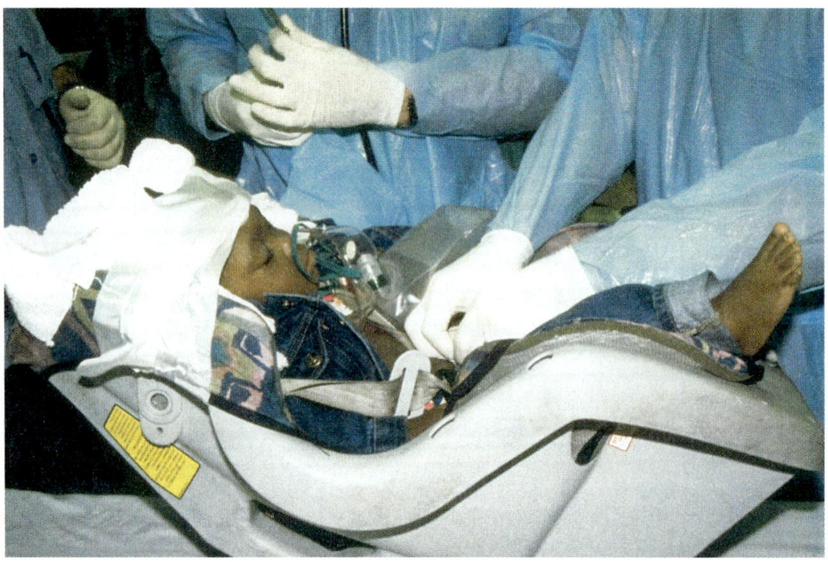

FIGURE 11-12 Infant secured in car seat. *(Courtesy of David Effron, MD, FACEP)*

arthritic spines are so rigid that the patient cannot be laid straight on the board, and some elderly patients have rigid flexion of the neck that will result in a large gap between the head and the board. You can make use of towels, blankets, and pillows to pad the elderly patient and prevent movement and discomfort on the backboard (Figure 11-13). This is a situation in which the vacuum backboard (which conforms to the shape of the patient) works very well. (See Figure 11-7.)

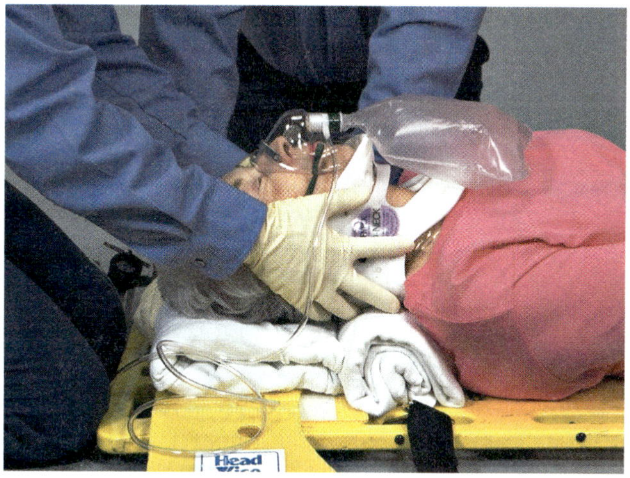

FIGURE 11-13 Additional padding, such as rolled blankets or towels behind the head, may be needed to keep the head in a neutral, in-line position.

Patients in Protective Gear. Large helmets used in sports and cycling must be removed at some point to permit complete assessment and care. Helmets used in different sports present different management problems for rescuers. Football and ice hockey helmets are custom fitted to the individual. Unless special circumstances exist, such as respiratory distress coupled with an inability to access the airway, the helmet should not be removed in the prehospital setting.

Athletic helmet design will generally allow easy airway access once the face guard is removed. The best way to remove a face guard is with a screwdriver. (A cordless screwdriver is best.) One should be on every response vehicle. However, sometimes the screw slot strips out, and the face guard will have to be cut off. There are commercial devices to do this (Trainer's Angel, Face Mask Extractor), but they cost 10 to 20 times as much as plain anvil pruning shears. The anvil pruning shears are just as satisfactory for removing a face guard (Figure 11-14). Pick one of those devices, train with it, and know how to use it appropriately when the time comes. Rescue scissors have been advocated in the past but studies have found them to be unsuitable for this task.

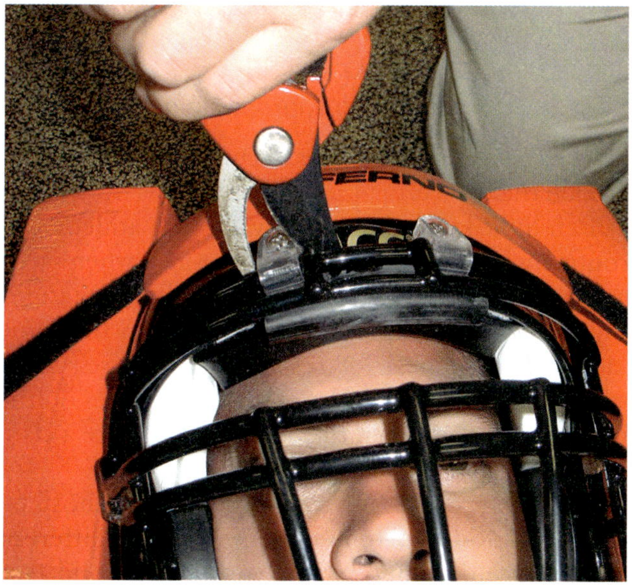

a.

FIGURE 11-14a The face guard of a football helmet can be removed with a screwdriver or pruning shears. *(Courtesy of Jeff Hinshaw, MS, PA-C, NREMT-P)*

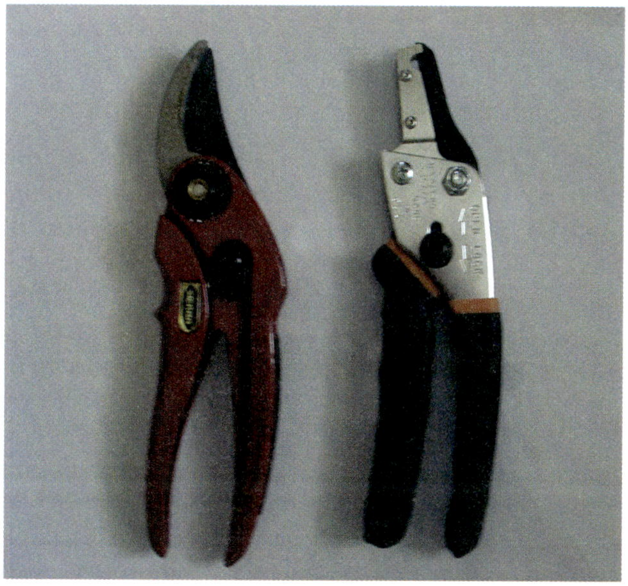

b.

FIGURE 11-14b Anvil pruning shears (left) or a face mask extractor (right) can be used to remove a football helmet face guard. *(Courtesy of Jeff Hinshaw, MS, PA-C, NREMT-P)*

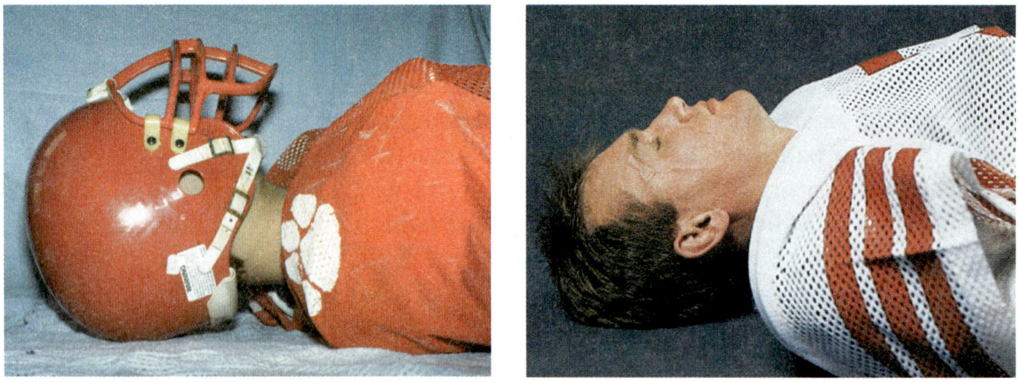

a. b.

FIGURE 11-15 (a) Patients with shoulder pads and helmets are usually best immobilized with the helmet in place. The spine is maintained in a neutral position with a minimum of movement. *(Courtesy of Bob Page, NREMT-P)* (b) Patients with shoulder pads must have padding under the head to maintain a neutral position if the helmet is removed.

The athlete wearing shoulder pads usually has his neck in a neutral position when on the backboard with the helmet in place. If the helmet is removed, padding must be inserted under the head to keep the neck from extending (Figure 11-15). After arrival at the emergency facility, the cervical spine can be x-rayed with the helmet in place. Once the spine is evaluated, the helmet can be removed by stabilizing the head and neck, removing the cheek pads, releasing the air inflation system, and then sliding the helmet off in the usual manner.

For prehospital providers, field removal of an athletic helmet is a last-ditch procedure, but it must be entertained in certain unique patient-care situations. The four main reasons to consider field helmet removal are as follows:

- Face mask cannot be removed in a timely fashion
- Airway cannot be controlled due to the design of the helmet and chin strap
- Helmet and chin straps do not hold the head securely
- Helmet prevents stabilization for transport in an appropriate position

When removing an athletic helmet, it is imperative to cut the chin strap and not attempt to unsnap or unbuckle the device.

Shoulder pad removal is often linked to helmet removal in the athletic setting. Not only is this done routinely with helmet removal, but also when faced with the inability to maintain neutral cervical-spine alignment (often due to ill-fitting shoulder pads), when you are unable to secure the athlete to the spine board, and when you need access to the chest for resuscitation efforts. Most shoulder pads can be removed by cutting the axillary straps and the laces on the front of the appliance, opening the appliance from the core outward (like a clam shell), and sliding the appliance out from under the athlete.

In contrast, motorcycle helmets often must be removed in the prehospital setting. The removal technique is modified to accommodate the different design. Motorcycle helmets often are designed with a continuous solid face guard that limits airway access. Those helmets are not custom designed and frequently are poorly fitted to the patient. Their large size will usually produce significant neck flexion if left in place when the patient is positioned on a backboard (Figure 11-16). The motorcycle helmet can make it difficult to stabilize

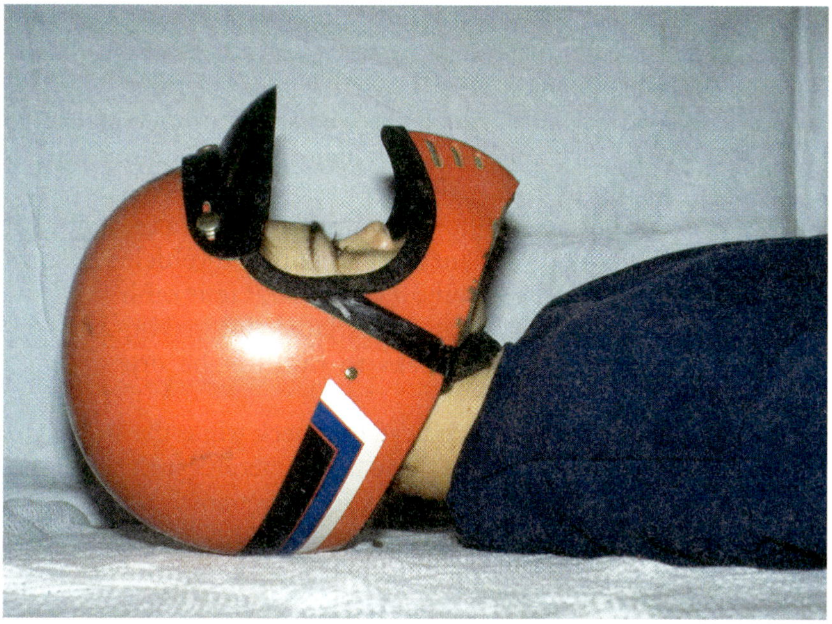

FIGURE 11-16 Full-face helmets obstruct access to the patient's airway. Notice that the helmet flexes the neck in a patient who is not wearing shoulder pads. *(Courtesy of Bob Page, NREMT-P)*

the neck in a neutral position, obstruct access to the airway, and hide injuries to the head or neck. It should be removed in the prehospital setting, using the techniques described in Chapter 12.

Very Large or Obese Patients. Very large or obese patients might not fit appropriately in standard equipment. You must be flexible, even using sheets of plywood and head cushions or towel rolls to stabilize the spine. In cold-weather climates, patients in bulky warm clothing will need to be snugly secured to prevent excessive movement.

Patients with Neck Wounds. Patients with penetrating or disfiguring wounds of the neck or lower face must be continually observed. Cervical collars will prevent continued examination of the wound site and could compromise the airway in wounds with expanding hematomas or subcutaneous air. If the mandible is fractured, the collar might again cause airway compromise. Therefore, for patients with such injuries, it may be wise to avoid collars and use instead manual stabilization and head cushion devices or blanket rolls for cervical motion restriction.

Trauma patients with paralysis or neurogenic shock have lost vascular control and thus cannot control blood flow to the skin. They can lose heat rapidly, so it is important for you to prevent hypothermia.

CASE PRESENTATION (continued)

An ALS ambulance has been dispatched at 2 a.m. to an MVC in which a single auto has left the road and hit a tree. When they arrive on scene, the local fire department is already there along with law enforcement (who reported the crash). The law officer says that he noticed the car was driving erratically and gave chase, but the driver of the auto refused to stop and sped away. The auto was traveling at a high rate of speed when it missed a turn, rolled over several times, and eventually struck a tree. The officer says the unrestrained driver was ejected through the windshield of the vehicle during one of the rollovers. The scene is secure, and the only victim is the driver of the auto.

The crew dons gloves and face shields, gathers essential equipment, and approaches the patient, who is about 20 feet from the vehicle. The patient is a man who appears to be about 30 years old. He is on his left side, bleeding from multiple lacerations of his face, and making gurgling respirations. The team leader speaks to him but he does not respond.

Team member 2 stabilizes the patient's head and neck while the leader does the assessment. The patient appears to have facial fractures including a broken jaw. There continues to be some bleeding from the mouth and gurgling respiration, so team member 3 suctions the airway, which improves the patient's breathing. They continue the assessment with the patient on his side to allow the blood to drain from his mouth.

The ITLS Primary Survey reveals facial and jaw injuries, and the patient has tenderness of his right ribs, but no deformity and no flail segment. Breath sounds are present and equal. The altered mental status suggests possible traumatic brain injury. There are no other obvious injuries, and the patient is moving all extremities and responds to pain by moaning louder. Pupils are mid position and respond equally to light. Blood pressure is 110/85, pulse 110, and respiration 16 breaths per minute. The patient is carefully log-rolled into a supine position and onto a vacuum backboard. It quickly molds around him, and he is secured. He is then immediately moved into the ambulance and rolled back on his left side to allow blood to drain from his mouth.

Because of the facial fractures, the rescuers are unable to perform endotracheal intubation but are able to maintain a pulse oximeter reading of 95% with use of a loosely fitting face mask with high-flow oxygen. The patient is taken to a local trauma center, where he is found to have facial and jaw fractures, nondisplaced right rib fractures, and a slight compression fracture of C4. The CT scan of his head reveals no intracranial injury. His blood alcohol is high, and his level of consciousness returns to normal within 12 hours. He eventually recovers from his injuries but continues to drink and drive. He is killed in another motor-vehicle collision a year after this incident.

This was a situation in which the patient had to be positioned to allow blood to drain and keep his airway open. If he had not been well packaged, he might have suffered a spinal-cord injury because of his spinal-column fracture. Careful strapping can hold a patient securely on a backboard while tilted up to allow drainage, but the vacuum backboard (Figure 11-7) is best for this situation. ■

Summary

Spinal-cord injury is a devastating consequence of modern-day trauma. Unstable or incomplete damage to the spinal column or cord is not completely predictable; therefore, trauma patients who are unconscious or have any dangerous mechanism of injury affecting the head, neck, or trunk should have SMR. Those trauma patients with uncertain mechanisms may not require SMR if they meet the criteria for the procedure in local protocols. Special trauma cases may require special SMR techniques. Once SMR is performed, the patient loses some ability to control his airway, so EMS providers must be prepared at all times to intervene should the patient vomit or have evidence of airway compromise.

Bibliography

1. Augustine, J. 2004. Failure on the board. *EMS* 33: 52–53.
2. Ben-Galim, P., et al. 2010. Extrication collars can result in abnormal separation between vertebrae in the presence of a dissociative injury. *Journal of Trauma* 88(1).
3. Ben-Galim P.J., T. A. Sibai, J. A. Hipp, M. H. Heggeness, C. A. Reitman. 2008. Internal decapitation: survival after head to neck dissociation injuries. *Spine* 33: 1744 –1749.
4. British Trauma Society. 2003. Guidelines for initial management and assessment of spinal injury. *Injury, International Journal of the Injured* 34: 405–425.
5. Cordell, W. H., J. Hollingsworth, et al. 1995. Pain and tissue-interface pressures during spine-board immobilization. *Annals of Emergency Medicine* 26: 31–36.
6. DeVivo, M. J. 2002. Epidemiology of traumatic spinal cord injury. In S. Kirshblum D. I. Campagnolo, & J. A. DeLisa (Eds.), *Spinal cord medicine* (pp. 69–81). Baltimore, MD: Lippincott Williams & Wilkins.
7. Dunham, C. M., B. P. Brocker, B. D. Collier, D. J. Gemmel. 2008. Risks associated with magnetic resonance imaging and cervical collar in comatose, blunt trauma patients with negative comprehensive cervical spine computed tomography and no apparent spinal deficit. *Crit Care* 12: R89.
8. Dunn, T. M., A. Dalton, T. Dorfman, W. Dunn. 2004. Are emergency medical technician-basics able to use a selective immobilization of the cervical spine protocol? A preliminary report. *Prehospital Emergency Care* 8: 207–211.
9. Goth, P. C. 1994. *Spine injury, clinical criteria for assessment and management.* Augusta, ME: Medical Care Development.
10. Haut, E. R, et al. 2010. Spine immobilization in penetrating trauma: More harm than good? *Journal of Trauma* 88(1): 115–121.
11. Kleiner, D. M., A. Pollak, C. McAdam. 2001. Helmet hazards. Do's and don'ts of football helmet removal. *JEMS* 26: 36–44, 46–48.
12. Knox, K. E, D. M. Kleiner, 1997. The efficiency of tools used to retract a football helmet face mask. *Journal of Athletic Trainers* 32(3): 211–215.
13. Krell, J. M., et al. 2006. Comparison of the Ferno scoop stretcher with the long backboard for spinal immobilization. *Prehospital Emergency Care* 10: 46–51.

14. Kwan, I., F. Bunn, I. Roberts. 2008. Spinal immobilisation for trauma patients (review). *Cochrane Library*:1–19.

15. Manoach, S., L. Paladino. 2007. Manual in-line stabilization for acute airway management of suspected cervical spine injury: historical review and current questions. *Annals of Emergency Medicine*. 50(3): 236–245.

16. Milby, A. H., C. H. Halpern,W. Guo, S. C. Stein. 2008. Prevalence of cervical spinal injury in trauma. *Neurosurg Focus* 25: E10.

17. Rhee, P., et al. 2006. Cervical spine injury is highly dependent on the mechanism of injury following blunt and penetrating assault. *The Journal of Trauma* 61(5): 1166–1170.

18. Sekhon, L. H., M. G. Fehlings. 2001. Epidemiology, demographics, and pathophysiology of acute spinal cord injury. *Spine* 26: S2–S12.

19. Vitale, M. G., J. M. Goss, H. Matsumoto, et al. 2006. Epidemiology of pediatric spinal cord injury in the United States: Years 1997 and 2000. *J Pediatr Orthop* 26(6): 745–749.

Explore Resource Central

For additional review and practice tests, visit www.bradybooks.com and click on Resource Central to access book-specific resources for this text. To access Resource Central, follow directions on the Student Access Card provided with this text. If there is no card, go to www.bradybooks.com and follow the Resource Central link to Buy Access from there.

Spine Management Skills

Donna Hastings, EMT-P
David Maatman, NREMT-P/IC

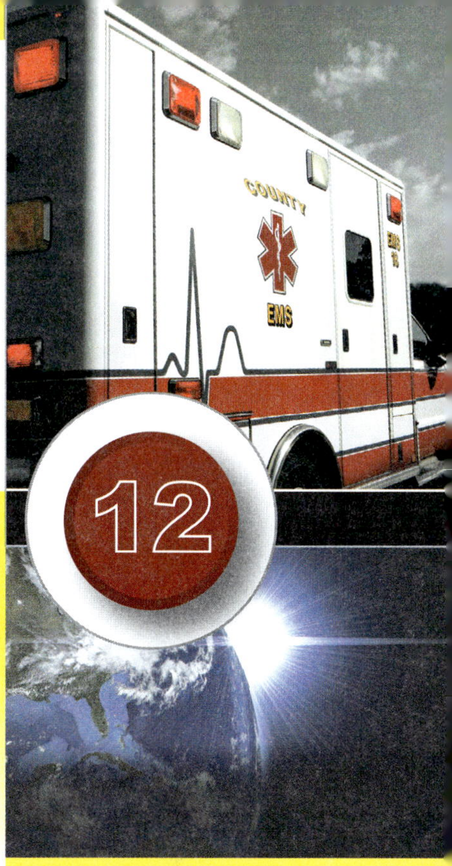

(Photo courtesy of Cheryl Casey, Shutterstock.com)

Spinal Trauma

Trauma Spinale

Traumatismo Raquídeo

Traumatisme Médullaire

Urazy kręgosłupa

Wirbelsäulentrauma

Ozljede kralježnice

إصابات العمود الفقري

trauma kičme

Poškodbe hrbtenjače

Gerincsérülés

OBJECTIVES

Upon successful completion of this chapter, you should be able to:

1. Describe the essential components of a spinal motion-restriction (SMR) system.
2. Describe the goals and principles of SMR.
3. Explain when to use SMR.
4. Explain when to use Emergency Rescue and Rapid Extrication.
5. Perform SMR with a short extrication device
6. Perform log-rolling of a patient onto a long backboard.
7. Properly secure a patient to a long backboard.
8. Perform SMR on a patient who is in a standing position.
9. Stabilize the head and neck when a neutral position cannot be safely attained.
10. Perform Rapid Extrication.
11. Explain when helmets should and should not be removed from injured patients.
12. Properly remove a motorcycle helmet.
13. Demonstrate proper stabilization of the neck in patients who are wearing shoulder pads and helmets.

Essential Components of a Spinal Motion-Restriction System

The five essential components of a full spinal motion-restriction (SMR) system are

- *Backboard.* The purpose of the backboard is to keep the spinal column from moving. Several types of backboards are available.
- *Cervical collar.* Though cervical collars do not immobilize the neck, they provide some support and can serve to remind the patient to keep the neck still. Several types are available.
- *Straps.* Strapping systems are used to bind the patient's body to the backboard to restrict movement of the spinal column. The straps should be positioned to decrease patient movement from side to side and from sliding up and down on the backboard. Several different systems are available.
- *Head motion-restriction device.* These devices attach to the backboard and are used to restrict movement of the patient's head after the patient's body has been strapped to the backboard. When the head motion-restriction device has been applied, the cervical collar may be removed if necessary. There are several different types of the devices.
- *Airway management kit.* When you strap someone's body and head to a board, you must assume responsibility for his or her airway. You must have the airway kit immediately available, and you must have the skills to use it. Airway management is a priority consideration with SMR. So, airway management skills and equipment are necessary components.

Goals and Principles of SMR

The SMR system aims at limiting the movement of the spine, and thus preventing secondary injury during extrication and transport. It also is meant to provide rescuers with a device to assist in the extrication, movement, and transport of the patient.

Principles of the SMR system include the following:

- Stabilization of the spine must be done so the patient is in the anatomical (neutral) position. Padding is frequently required to achieve this.
- Straps should be placed over stable bony structures. Avoid placing straps over the neck, navel, and knees.

Applying those goals and principles help the rescuer adapt to the various situations in which patients are found. Understand that SMR precautions are taken to minimize the potential of secondary trauma during the prehospital phase of a patient encounter. Though SMR substantially decreases the patient's risk for such injury, prolonged time strapped to a backboard can cause discomfort and pressure sores, so it has become common practice for emergency department personnel to perform a quick screening of the patient within five minutes of arrival. If appropriate, the patient is then moved off the backboard.

> **PEARLS:** The Short Extrication Device
>
> - When placing the straps around the legs on a male patient, do not catch the genitals in the straps.
> - Do not use the device as a "handle" to move the patient. Move patient and device as a unit. Many short extrication devices come with built-in handles. These are not to be used *alone* to move a patient.
> - You may need to modify your strapping techniques, depending on injuries.

Applying SMR

Patients Requiring SMR

Indications for SMR are listed in Figure 12-1. Patients requiring SMR must have it done before they are moved in any way. In the case of an automobile collision,

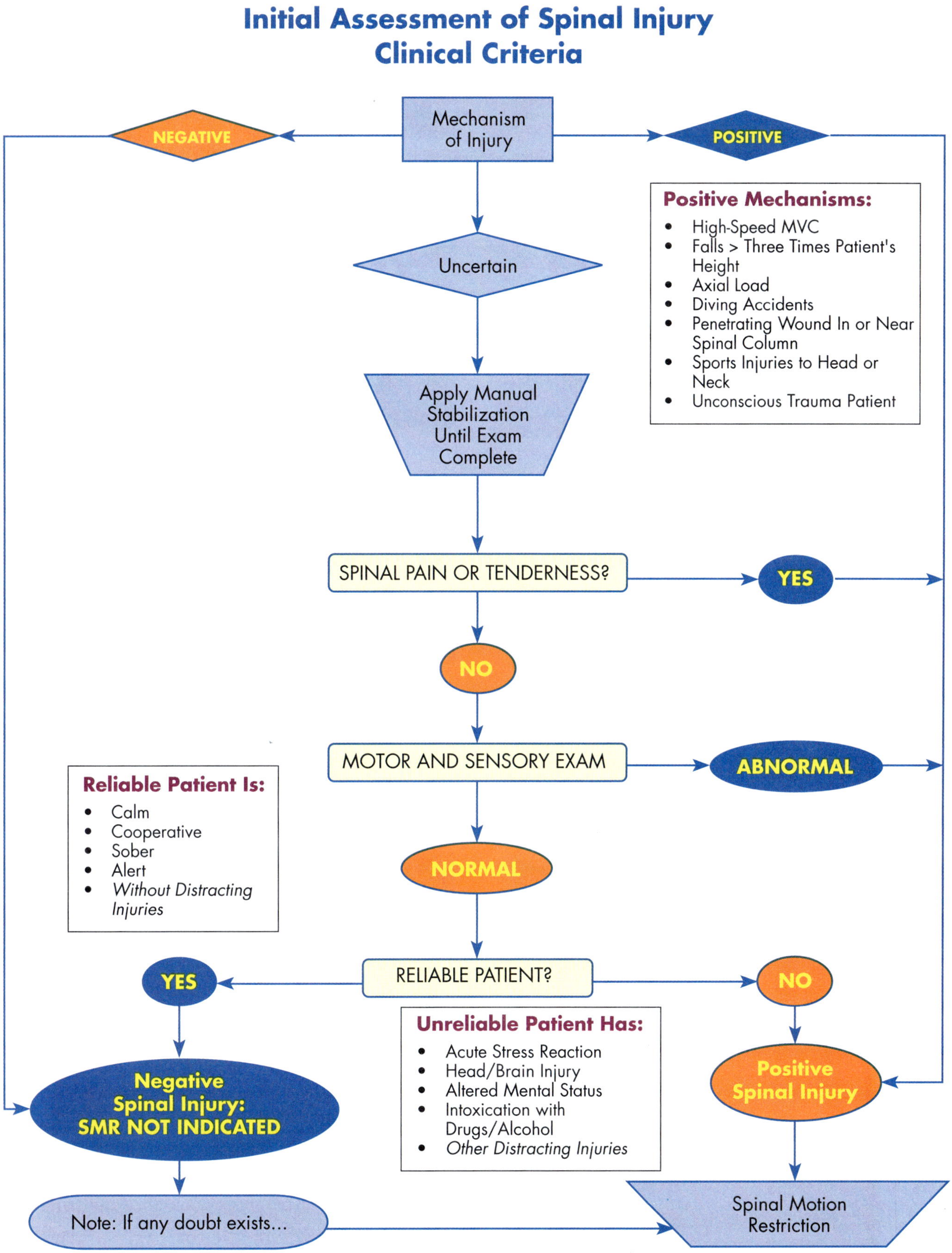

FIGURE 12-1 Decision tree for spinal motion restriction. *(Reprinted by permission of Peter Goth, MD)*

SCAN 12-1 Applying a Kendrick Extrication Device

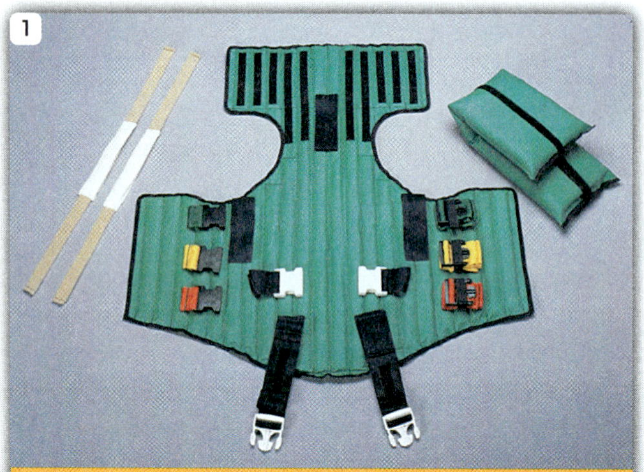

1 The Ferno Kendrick Extrication Device (KED). *(©Ferno Corporation)*

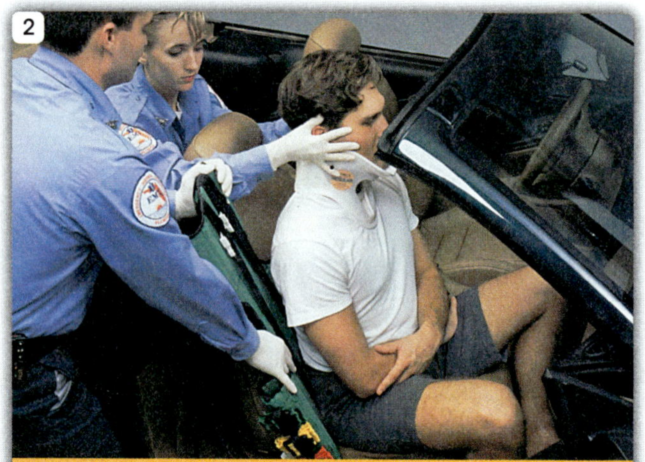

2 After a cervical-spine immobilization collar has been applied, slip the KED behind the patient and center it.

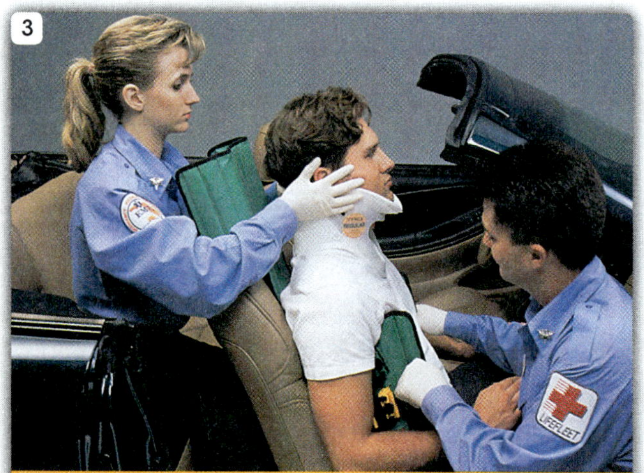

3 Properly align the device. Then wrap the vest around the patient's torso.

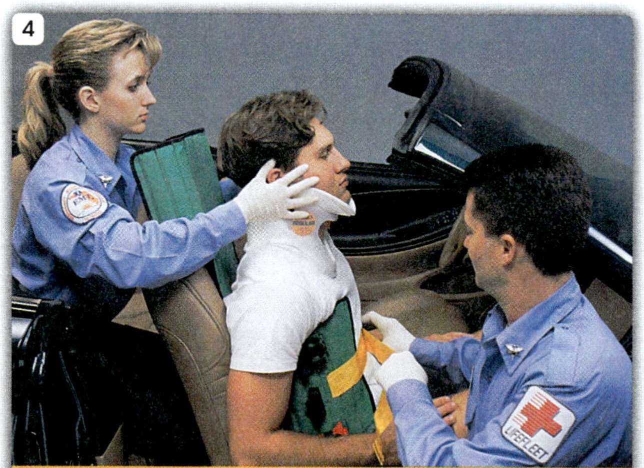

4 When the device is tucked well up into the armpits, secure the chest straps.

you must stabilize the spine before removing the patient from the wreckage. More patient movement is involved in extrication than at any other time, so you must carefully stabilize the neck and spine before beginning extrication. Remember that traction can cause permanent paralysis. You are stabilizing the spine, not pulling on it. Except in situations requiring Emergency Rescue or Rapid Extrication, always try to document sensation and motor function in the extremities before you move the patient.

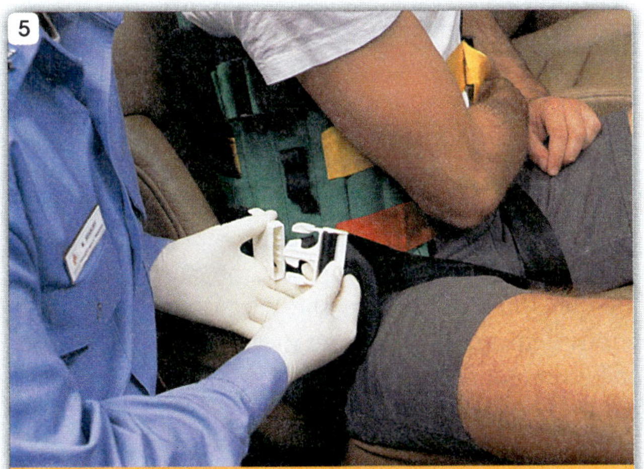

5 Bring each leg strap around the ipsilateral (same side) leg and back to the buckle on the same side. Fasten snugly.

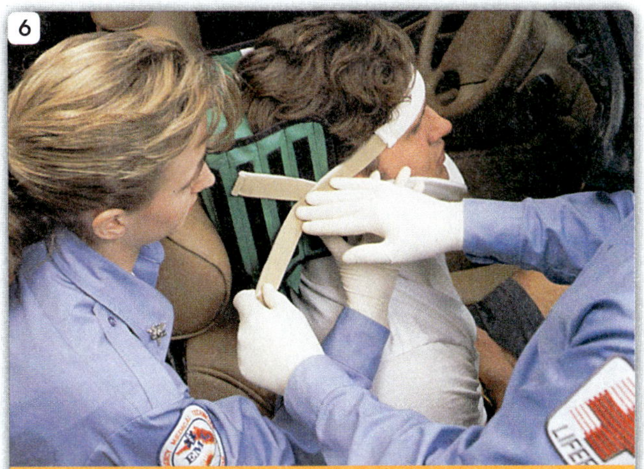

6 Secure the patient's head with the Velcro head straps. Apply padding as needed to maintain a neutral position.

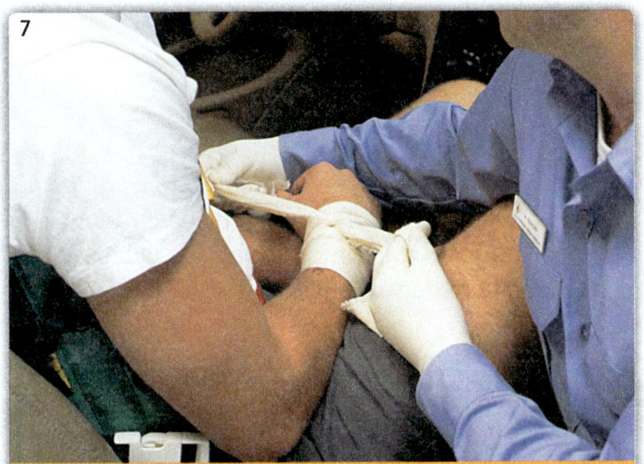

7 Tie the hands together.

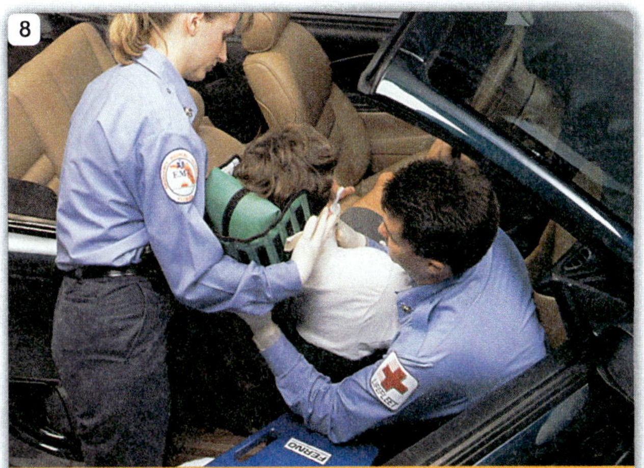

8 Turn the patient and device as a unit then lower the patient onto a long backboard. Loosen the leg straps and allow the legs to extend out flat. Finally secure the patient and device to the backboard.

SMR with a Short Extrication Device

A short extrication device is used for patients who are in a position that does not permit use of the long backboard (such as in a motor vehicle). There are several different devices of this type. Some have strapping mechanisms different from the one explained here. Become familiar with your equipment before employing it in an emergency. (See Scan 12-1 for directions on how to apply one type of short extrication device.)

Resource Central

See Optional Skills for use of a short backboard.

Emergency Rescue and Rapid Extrication

Patients left inside vehicles following a collision are usually stabilized on a short extrication device and then transferred onto a long backboard. Although this is the best way to extricate anyone with a possible spinal injury, there are certain situations in which a more rapid method must be used. Note: International Trauma Life Support (ITLS) offers a one-day course called "Access" on basic extrication from motor vehicles using basic hand tools. Call 888-495-4857 for information (international calls: 630-495-6442).

Situations Requiring Emergency Rescue

Emergency Rescue is used only in situations in which the patient's life is in immediate danger because of environmental hazards. In some of those situations you may not have time to use any technique other than pulling the patient to safety. This is an example of "desperate situations demanding desperate measures." Use good judgment. Do not sacrifice your life in a dangerous situation. Whenever you use this procedure, it should be noted in the written report, and you should be prepared to defend your actions at a review by your medical director.

Perform an Emergency Rescue if the scene size-up identifies a condition that could immediately (within seconds) endanger you or the patient, such as (Figure 12-2):

- Fire or immediate danger of fire or explosion
- Hostile environment, gunfire, or other weapons
- Danger of being carried away by rapidly moving water
- Structure in immediate danger of collapse
- Continuing and immediate life-threatening toxic exposure

Situations Requiring Rapid Extrication

You should perform a Rapid Extrication if your ITLS Primary Survey of a patient identifies a critical degree of ongoing danger that requires an intervention within 1 to 2 minutes. (See Scan 12-2 Performing a Rapid Extrication.) In such a situation, you must act immediately and rapidly, but you still can stabilize the patient to some

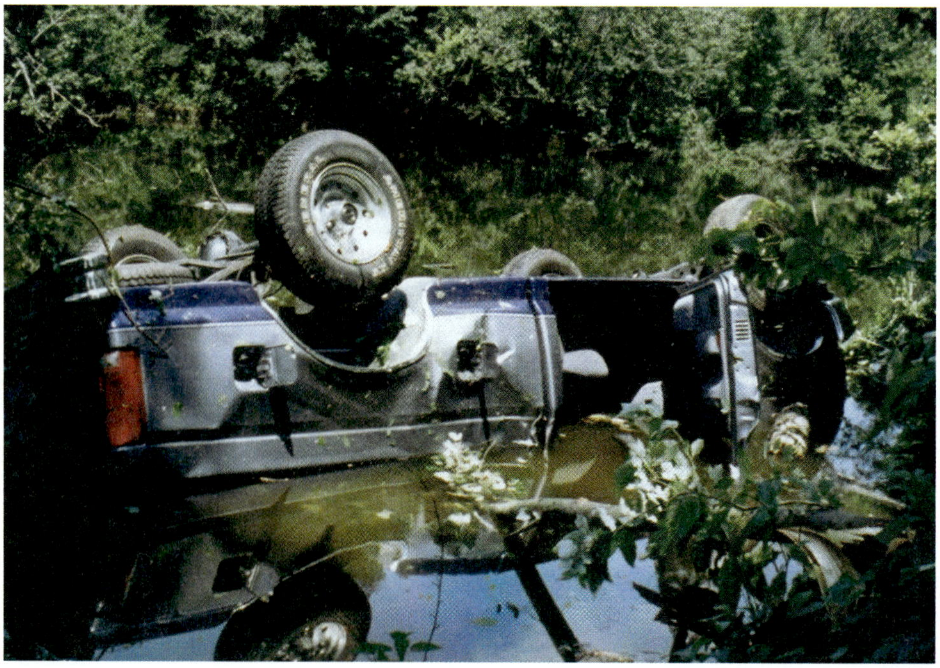

FIGURE 12-2 Example of a situation in which you may have to perform Emergency Rescue. *(Courtesy of Bonnie Meneely, EMT-P)*

SCAN 12-2 Rapid Extrication

1

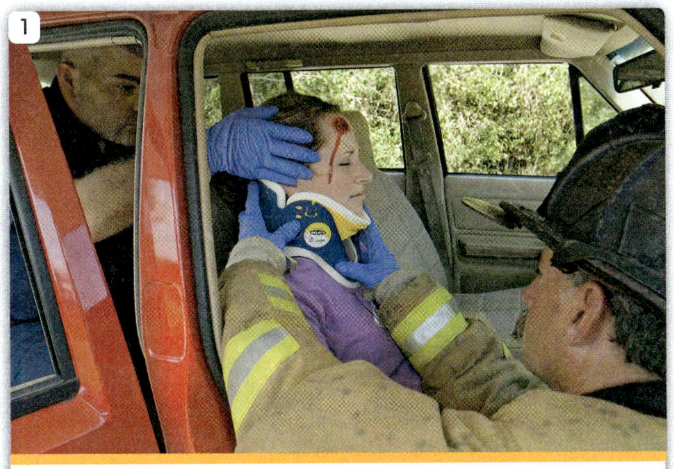

Stabilize the neck and perform the initial assessment. Apply a semirigid extrication collar.

2

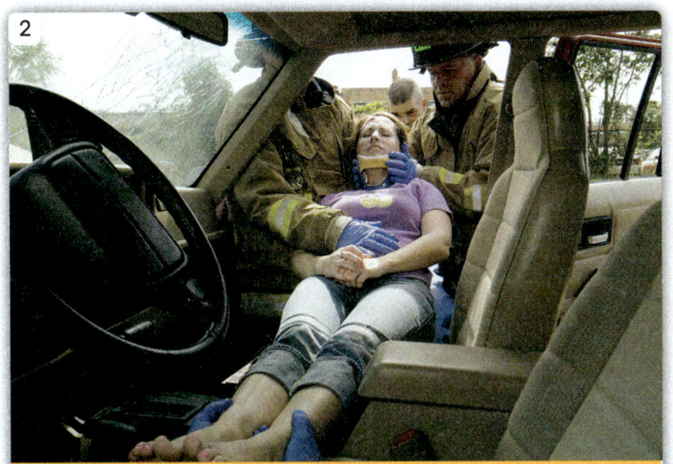

A second rescuer stands beside the open door of the vehicle and takes over control of the cervical spine. Slide the long backboard onto the seat and slightly under the patient. Carefully supporting the neck, torso, and legs, the rescuers turn the patient.

3

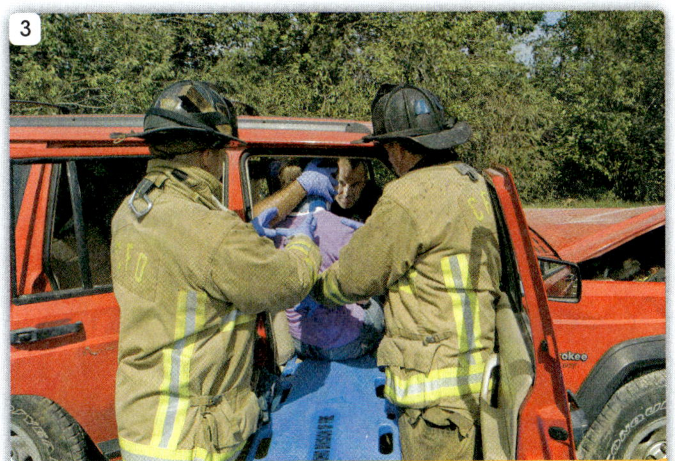

Stabilize the cot under the board. Begin to lower the patient onto the board.

4

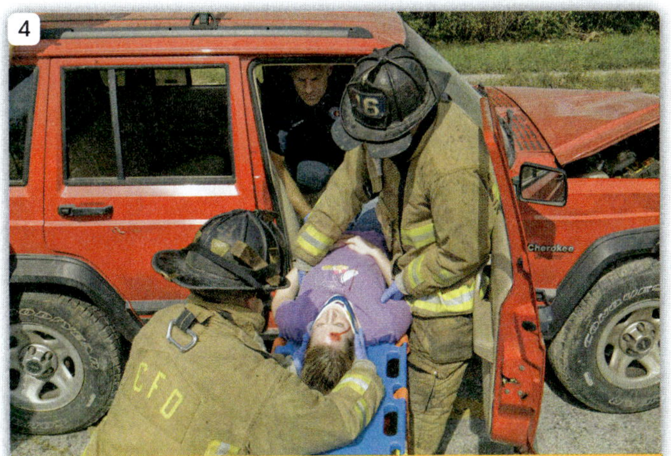

The legs are lifted, and the back is lowered to the backboard. Carefully slide the patient to the full length of the backboard. The patient is immediately moved away from the vehicle and into the ambulance, if available. Secure the patient to the backboard as soon as possible.

degree as you extricate him. Example situations that may require Rapid Extrication are as follows:

- Airway obstruction that you cannot relieve by a jaw-thrust maneuver or a finger sweep
- Cardiac or respiratory arrest
- Chest or airway injuries requiring ventilation or assisted ventilation
- Late shock or bleeding that you cannot control

SCAN 12-3 Log-Rolling a Supine Patient onto a Long Backboard

1

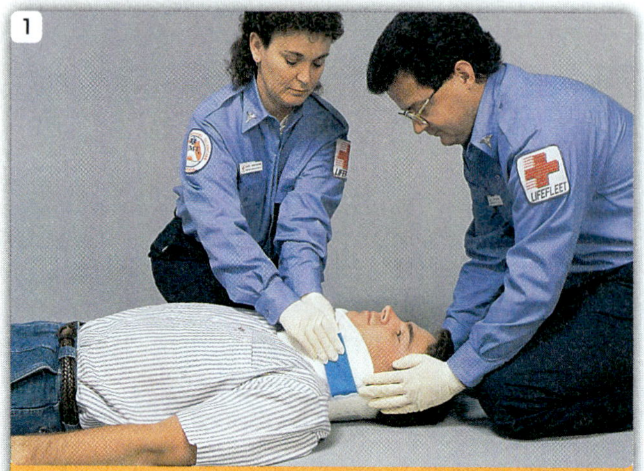

Establish and maintain in-line stabilization. Apply a semirigid cervical collar.

2

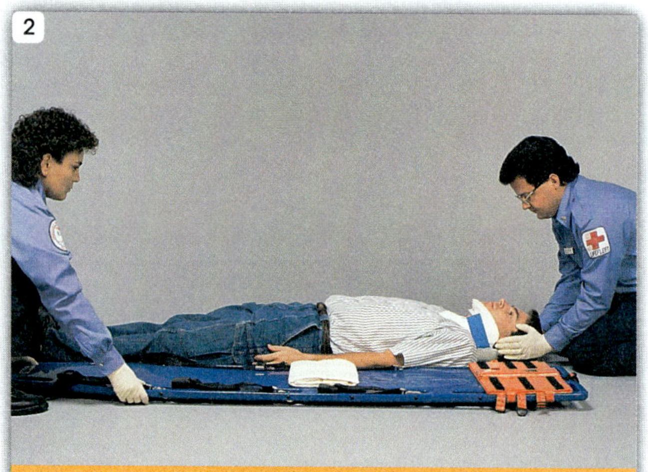

The long board is positioned beside the patient. Rescuer 1 maintains the neck stabilized in a neutral position.

3

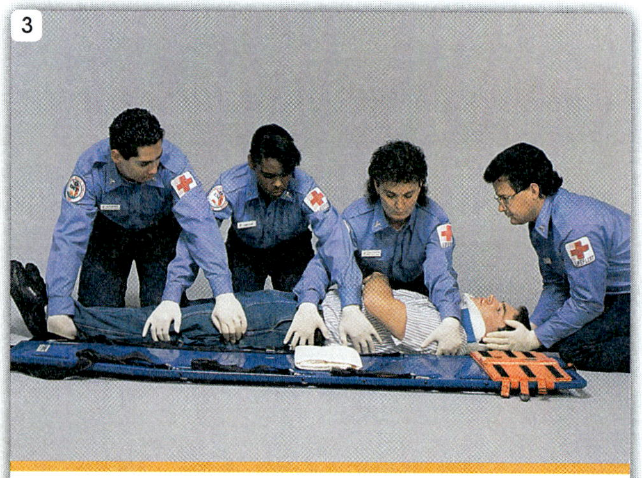

Rescuers 2, 3, and 4 assume their positions at the patient's side opposite the board, leaving space to roll the patient toward them.

4

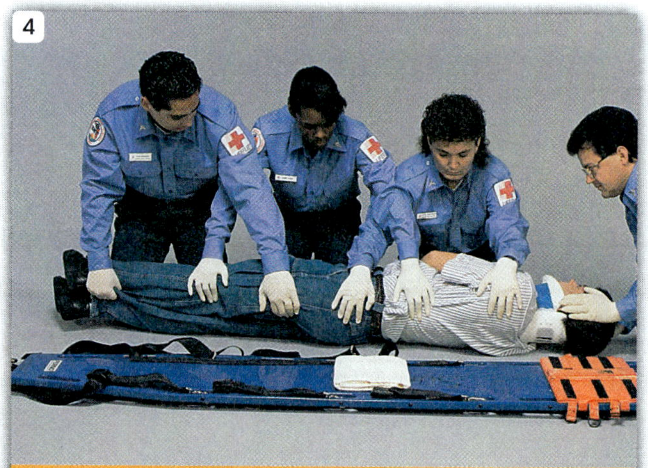

The rescuer at the head directs the others to roll the patient as a unit onto his side. Assess the patient's posterior side.

PEARLS: The Long Backboard

- When you are applying the upper horizontal strap around a woman, place the upper strap above her breasts and under her arms, not across the breasts.
- When you are applying the lower horizontal strap on a pregnant woman, place it across the pelvis and not across the uterus.

(*Continued on page* 227)

SMR with the Long Backboard

One of the most important ways to apply SMR to a patient with a suspected spinal injury is to secure him from head to toe to a long backboard. But moving the patient onto the backboard must be accomplished in a careful, coordinated way that protects him from any further injury. That procedure is called a *log-roll*.

See Scan 12-3 for log-rolling a supine patient onto a long backboard. In contrast, the prone patient most commonly has his head turned to one side. In this

5

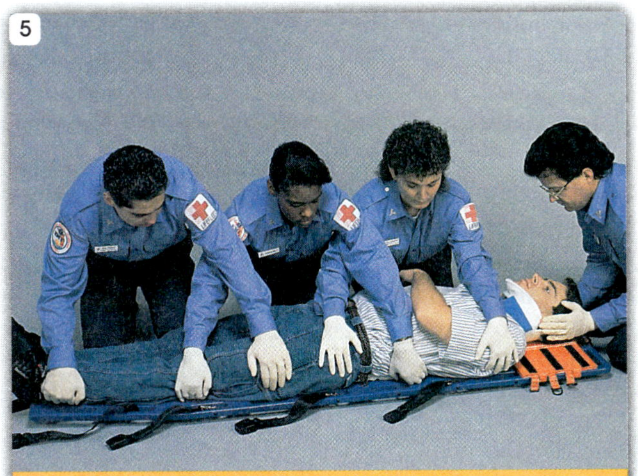

The rescuer at the waist reaches over, grasps the spine board, and pulls it into position against the patient. This also can be done by a fifth rescuer. The rescuer at the head instructs the rescuer to roll the patient onto the spine board.

6

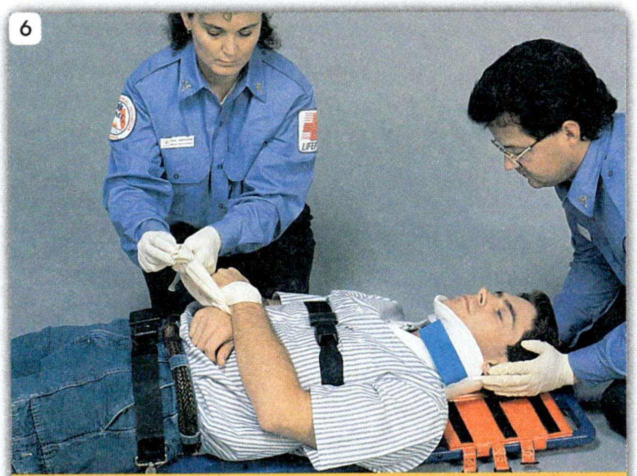

Secure the patient's body to the board with straps. Loosely tie the wrists together.

7

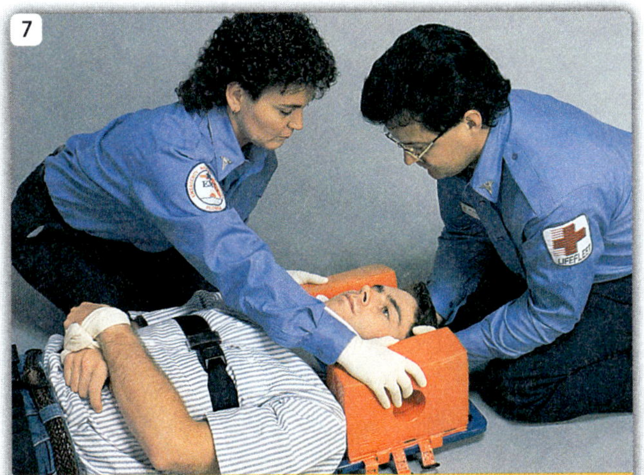

Using a head/cervical immobilizer, secure the patient's head to the spine board.

8

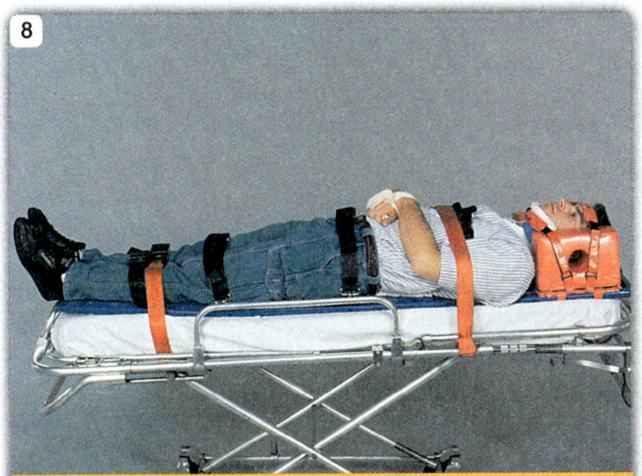

Transfer the patient and the spine board as a unit. Secure the patient and the spine board to the cot.

case, the rescuers will need to bring the head into neutral alignment. This can be done in one of three ways:

- Just before the log-roll , bring the patient's head into the neutral position (nose down).
- During the log-roll , gradually bring the patient's head into a neutral position.
- Keep the head turned in the direction the body is moving during the log-roll. Upon completion of the log-roll, bring the head into a neutral position.

PEARLS: The Long Backboard (*Continued*)

- You may need to modify your strapping techniques, depending on injuries.
- Secure the patient well enough so that little or no motion of the spine will occur if the board is turned on its side. Do not make straps so tight that they interfere with breathing.

The status of the airway in a prone patient is critical for decisions about the order in which a log-roll is performed. There are three clinical situations that dictate how to proceed. The first is for the patient who is not breathing or who is in severe respiratory difficulty. He must be log-rolled immediately so that you can manage the airway. Unless the backboard is already positioned, you must log-roll the patient, manage the airway, and then transfer him to the backboard (in a second log-rolling step) when ready to transport.

The second clinical situation occurs when a patient with profuse bleeding of the mouth or nose must not be turned to the supine position. Profuse upper airway bleeding in a supine patient is a guarantee of aspiration. This patient will have to have careful SMR and be transported prone or on his side, allowing gravity to help keep the airway clear. The vacuum backboard could be very useful in this situation. (See Chapter 11, Figure 11-7.)

The third clinical situation occurs when the patient with an adequate airway and respiration must be log-rolled directly onto a backboard.

PROCEDURE

Log-Rolling the Prone Patient with an Adequate Airway onto a Long Backboard

1. Rescuer 1 stabilizes the neck. When placing his hands on the patient's head and neck, the rescuer's thumbs always point toward the patient's face (Figure 12-3). This prevents having the rescuer's arms crossed when the patient is log-rolled. An initial assessment and exam of the backside is done. Then a semirigid extrication collar should be applied.
2. The patient is placed with his legs extended in the normal manner and his arms (palms inward) extended by his sides. The patient will be rolled up on one arm, with that arm acting as a splint for the body.

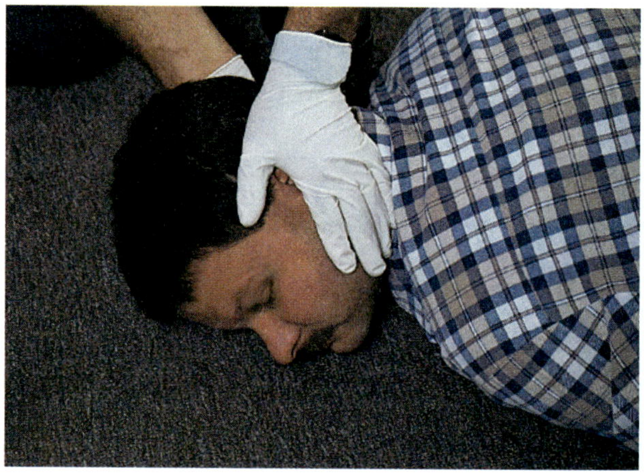

FIGURE 12-3 When stabilizing the neck of the prone (or supine) patient, your thumbs always point toward the face (not the occiput). This prevents having your arms crossed when the patient is rolled over.

3. The long backboard is positioned next to the patient's body on the side of the first rescuer's lower hand. (If the first rescuer's lower hand is on the patient's right side, the backboard is placed on the patient's right side.) If the patient's arm next to the backboard is the one injured, carefully raise it above the patient's head so he does not roll on the injured arm.
4. Rescuers 2 and 3 kneel at the patient's side opposite the board.
5. Rescuer 2 is positioned at the midchest area. Rescuer 3 should be beside the patient's upper legs.
6. Rescuer 2 grasps the shoulder and the hip. Usually, it is possible to grasp the patient's clothing (if not too loose) to help with the roll.
7. Rescuer 3 grasps the hip (holding the near arm in place) and the lower legs (holding them together).
8. When everyone is ready, Rescuer 1 gives the order to log-roll the patient.

9. Rescuers 2 and 3 roll the patient up onto his side away from them. The patient's arms are kept locked to his side to maintain a splinting effect. The head, shoulders, and pelvis are kept in line during the roll.
10. The backboard is now positioned next to the patient and held at a 30- to 45-degree angle by Rescuer 4. If there are only three rescuers, the board is pulled into place by Rescuer 2 or 3. The board is left flat in this case.
11. When everyone is ready, Rescuer 1 gives the order to roll the patient onto the backboard. This is accomplished by keeping the head, shoulders, and pelvis in line.
12. Now, complete the ITLS Primary Survey.

Special Considerations

The patient with chest or abdominal injuries should be log-rolled onto his uninjured side. Do it quickly so lung expansion is not compromised. In the case of a patient with injuries to the lower extremities, position Rescuer 2 at the feet of the patient, so he can provide in-line support to the injured leg during the log-roll. Again try to roll the patient onto the uninjured side. In general, the side to which you turn a patient during a log-roll is not critical and can be changed in situations where you can only place the backboard on one side of the patient.

The log-roll technique is useful for most trauma patients. However, it could aggravate a fractured pelvis. If the pelvic fracture appears stable, the log-roll should be carefully performed, turning the patient onto the uninjured side (if it can be identified). Patients with obviously unstable pelvic fractures should not be log-rolled but instead should be lifted carefully onto a board using four or more rescuers.

The scoop stretcher is a supplemental device that could help move the patient onto the backboard when specific injuries complicate log-rolling. (See Chapter 2, Figure 2-6.) Some newer scoop stretchers have been found to provide equal or superior stabilization when compared to the long backboard (Krell et al., 2006). Such scoop stretchers can be used in place of a long backboard.

Securing the Patient to the Backboard

There are several different methods of securing the patient to the long backboard using straps. As with all equipment, you should become familiar with your strapping system before using it in an emergency situation.

Two examples of commercial devices for full-body immobilization are the Reeves sleeve and the Miller body splint. The Reeves sleeve is a heavy-duty sleeve into which a standard backboard will slide. Attached to this sleeve are the following:

- Head motion-restriction device
- Heavy vinyl-coated nylon panels that go over the chest and abdomen and are secured with seat-belt-type straps and quick-release connectors
- Two full-length leg panels to secure the lower extremities
- Straps to hold the arms in place
- Six handles for carrying the patient
- Metal rings (2,500-pound strength) for lifting the patient by rope

When the patient is in the Reeves sleeve, he remains immobilized when lifted horizontally, vertically, or even carried on his side (like a suitcase). This device is

PEARLS: Protective Equipment

- Patients wearing both helmets and shoulder pads usually can have their spines maintained in a more neutral position by leaving the helmet in place and padding and taping the helmet to the backboard.
- Patients wearing helmets but no shoulder pads usually can have their spines maintained in a more neutral position by removing the helmet.
- Face guards on helmets can be removed with screwdrivers or pruning shears.
- Full-face motorcycle-type helmets must be removed to evaluate and manage the airway.

SCAN 12-4 Immobilizing a Standing Patient with Three Rescuers

1

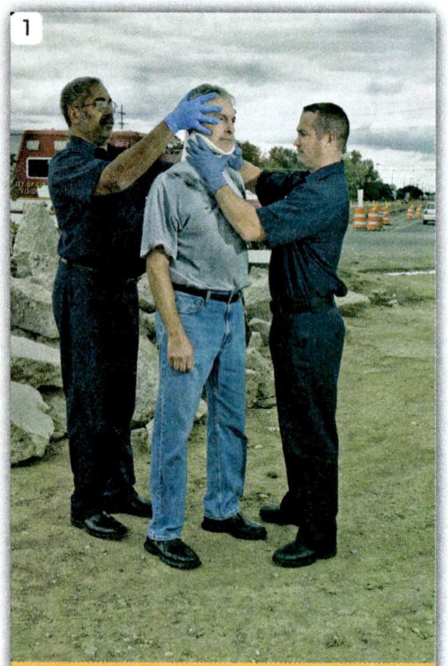

Apply a cervical collar while in-line stabilization is being held.

2

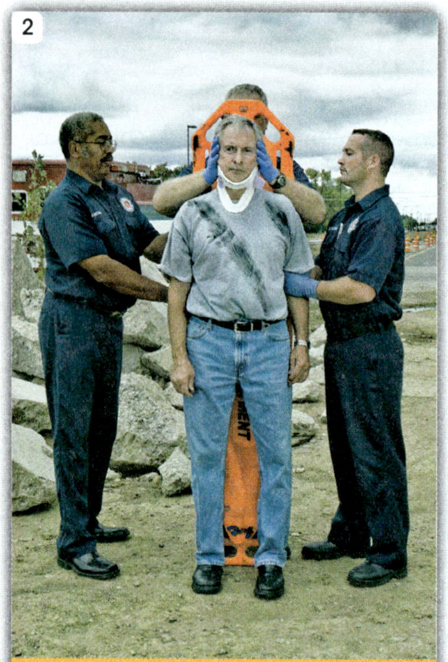

Position the backboard behind the patient and align it properly. Check the position of the board from the front of the patient.

excellent for the confused, combative patient who must be restrained for his safety (Figure 12-4).

The Miller body splint is a combination backboard, head immobilizer, and body immobilizer (see Chapter 11, Figure 11-6b). Like the Reeves sleeve, it does an excellent job of SMR with a minimum of time and effort.

The steps for immobilizing a standing patient are shown in Scans 12-4 and 12-5.

Special Considerations for the Head and Neck

Stabilizing the head and neck in a neutral position sometimes cannot be accomplished safely. If the head or neck is held in an angulated position and the patient complains of pain on any attempt to straighten it, you should stabilize it in the position found. The same is true of the unconscious patient whose neck is held to one side and does not easily straighten with a gentle attempt. You cannot use a cervical collar or commercial head motion-restriction device in this situation. You must use pads or a blanket roll, carefully taping to stabilize the head and neck in the position found.

Helmet Management

The procedure for motorcycle helmet management on a trauma patient is shown in Scans 12-6 and 12-7.

3

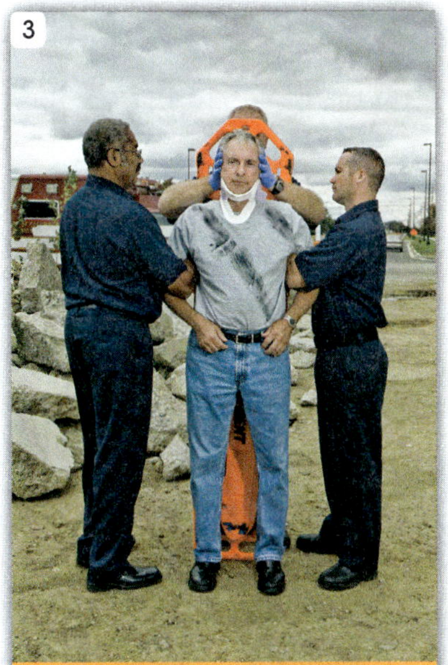

The rescuers at the sides of the patient place their hands under each arm and grasp the next highest handhold. Their other hands grasp the elbows of the patient to provide additional stabilization on the board.

4

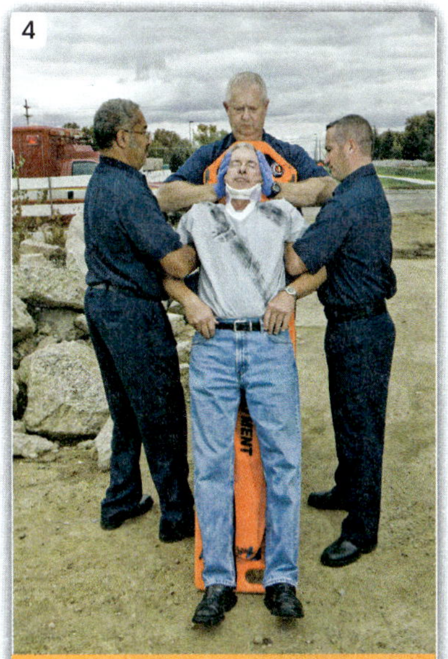

Lower the patient to the ground. Communicate your intentions before lowering the patient so that he is not startled, causing him to move or grab the rescuers. Continue holding in-line stabilization until the patient is completely immobilized to the backboard with straps and then a head/cervical stabilization device.

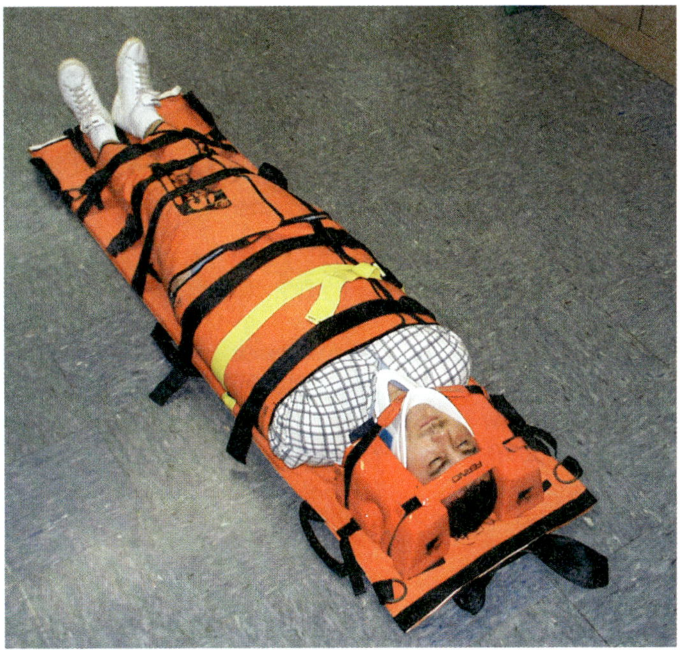

FIGURE 12-4 Patient restrained in a Reeves sleeve. Combative patients can have their arms enclosed within the panels and the straps.

SCAN 12-5 Immobilizing a Standing Patient with Two Rescuers

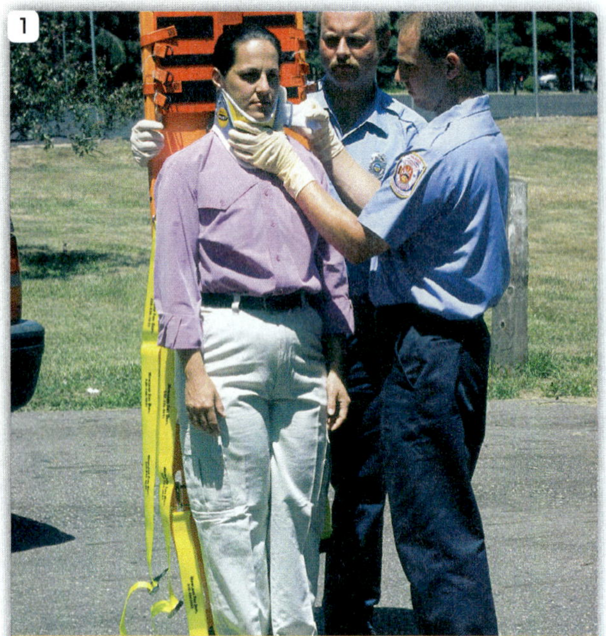

1 Apply a cervical collar and position the long backboard behind the patient.

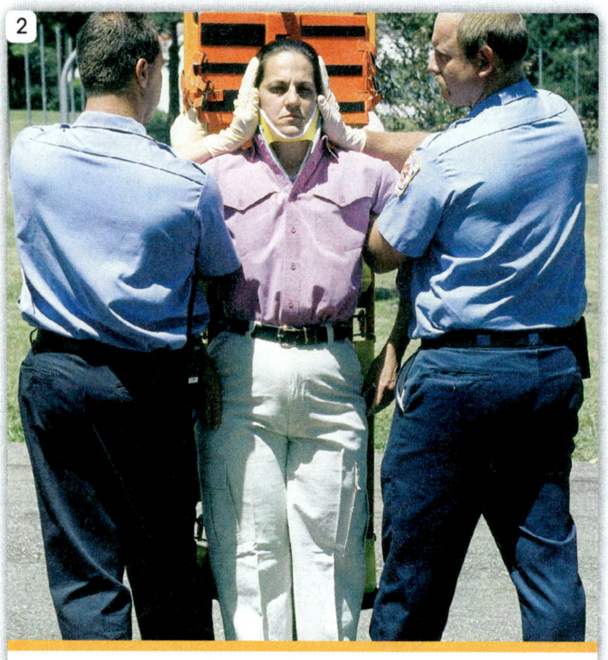

2 The rescuers on each side of the patient hold the long board in place and hold the patient's head in a neutral in-line position.

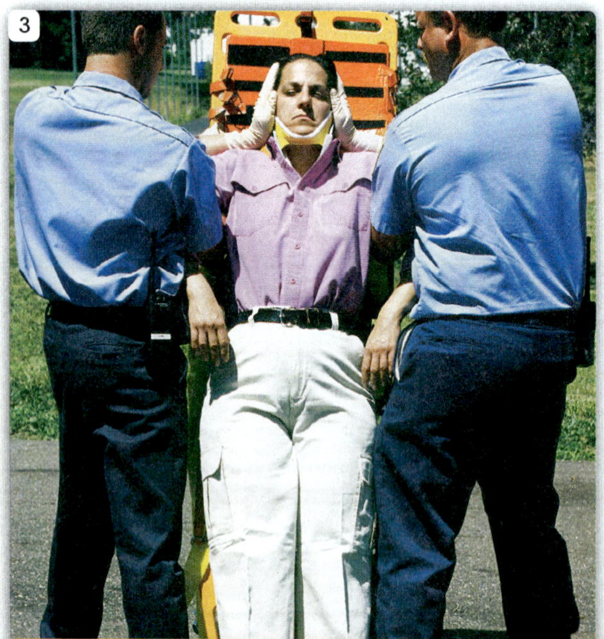

3 Each rescuer then place the leg closest to the board behind it and then lowers the board to the ground. Communicate your intentions before lowering the patient so that she is not startled, which could cause her to move or grab the rescuers.

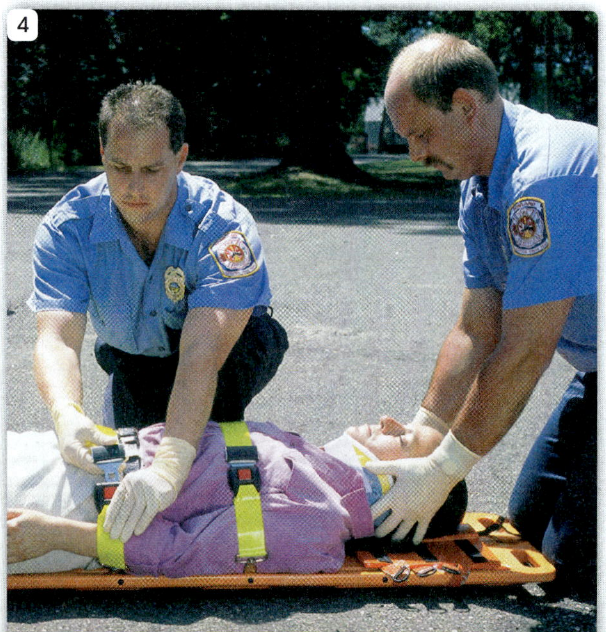

4 Once the patient is horizontal on the ground, one rescuer takes over in-line stabilization until SMR is completed.

SCAN 12-6 Removing a Motorcycle Helmet

1

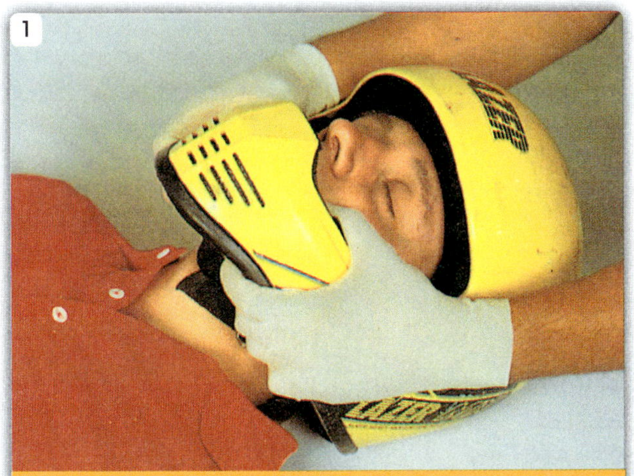

One rescuer applies stabilization by placing hands on each side of the helmet with fingers on the patient's mandible. This prevents slippage if the strap is loose.

2

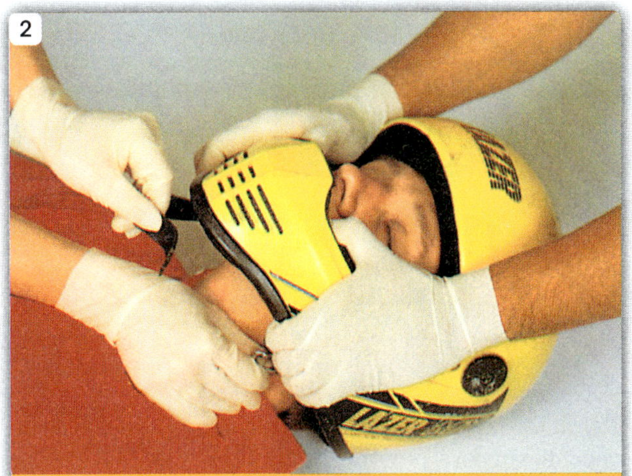

A second rescuer loosens the strap at the D-rings while stabilization is maintained.

3

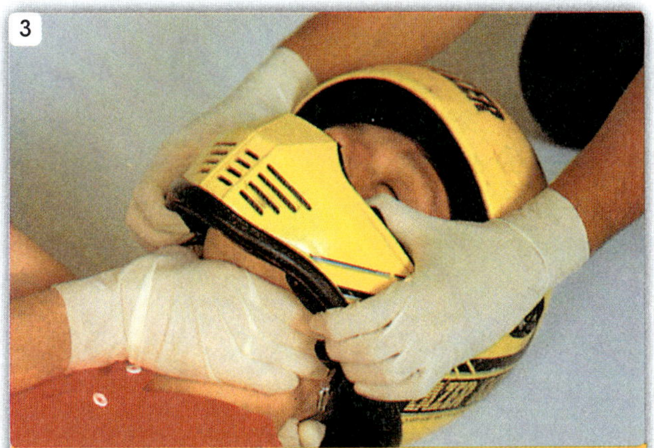

The second rescuer places one hand on the mandible at the angle, thumb on one side, long and index fingers on the other.

4

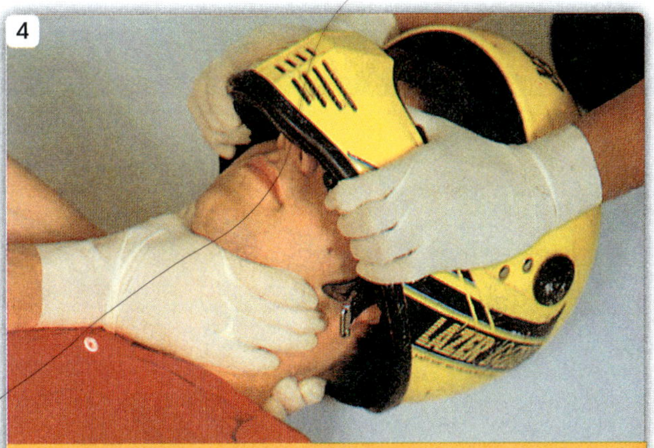

With the other hand, the second rescuer holds the occipital region. This maneuver transfers the stabilization responsibility to the second rescuer. The rescuer at the top removes the helmet in two steps, allowing the second rescuer to readjust his hand position under the occipital region. Three factors should be kept in mind: (a) The helmet is egg-shaped and therefore must be expanded laterally to clear the head. (b) If the helmet provides full facial coverage, glasses must be removed first. (c) If the helmet provides full facial coverage, the nose will prevent removal. To clear the nose, the helmet must be tilted back and raised over it.

(*Continued on next page*)

SCAN 12-6 Continued

5

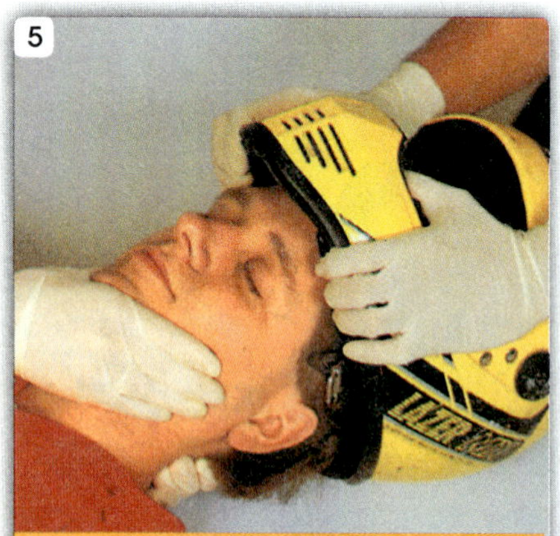

Throughout the removal process, the second rescuer maintains in-line stabilization from below to prevent head tilt.

6

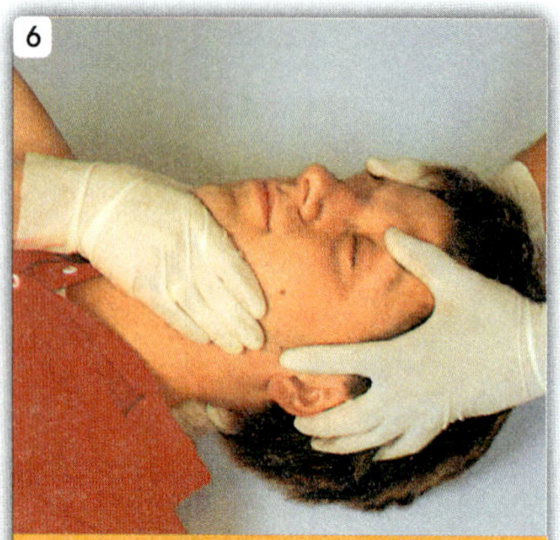

After the helmet has been removed, the rescuer at the top replaces his hands on either side of the patient's head with his palms over the ears, taking over stabilization.

7

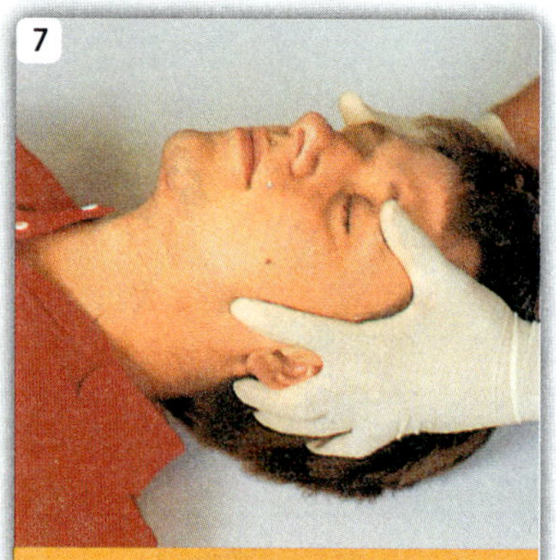

Stabilization is maintained from above until SMR is completed.

SCAN 12-7 Alternate Procedure for Removing a Motorcycle Helmet

1

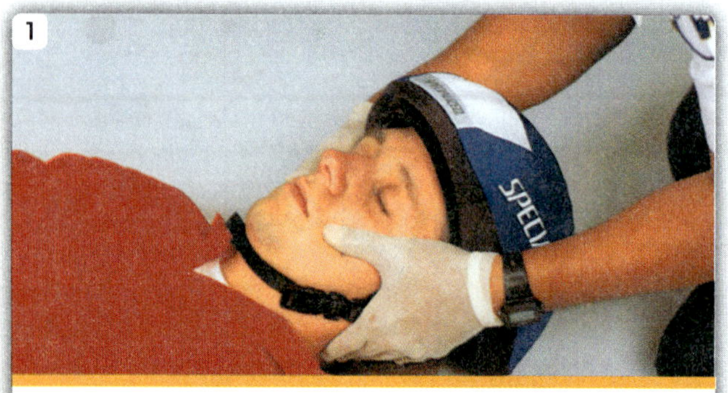

Apply steady stabilization in neutral position.

2

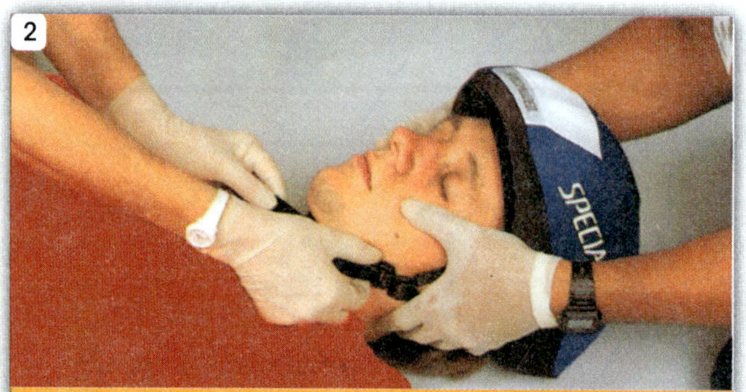

Remove the chin strap.

3

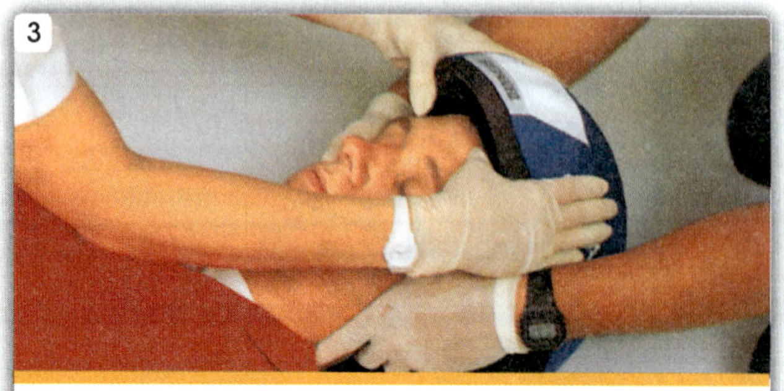

Remove the helmet by pulling gently on each side.

4

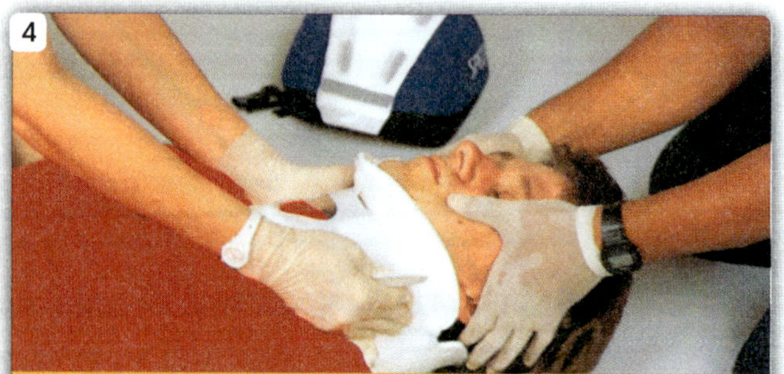

Apply a suitable cervical collar and secure the patient to a long backboard.

Bibliography

1. Johnson, D. R., M. Hauswald, C. Stockhoff. 1996. Comparison of a vacuum splint device to rigid backboard for spinal immobilization. *American Journal of Emergency Medicine* 14: 369–372.
2. Kleiner, D. M., A. Pollak, C. McAdam. 2001. Helmet hazards. Do's and don'ts of football helmet removal. *JEMS* 26: 36–44, 46–48.
3. Krell, J. M., et al. 2006. Comparison of the Ferno scoop stretcher with the long backboard for spinal immobilization. *Prehospital Emergency Care* Jan-Mar; 10(1): 46–51.

Explore Resource Central

For additional review and practice tests, visit www.bradybooks.com and click on Resource Central to access book-specific resources for this text. To access Resource Central, follow directions on the Student Access Card provided with this text. If there is no card, go to www.bradybooks.com and follow the Resource Central link to Buy Access from there.

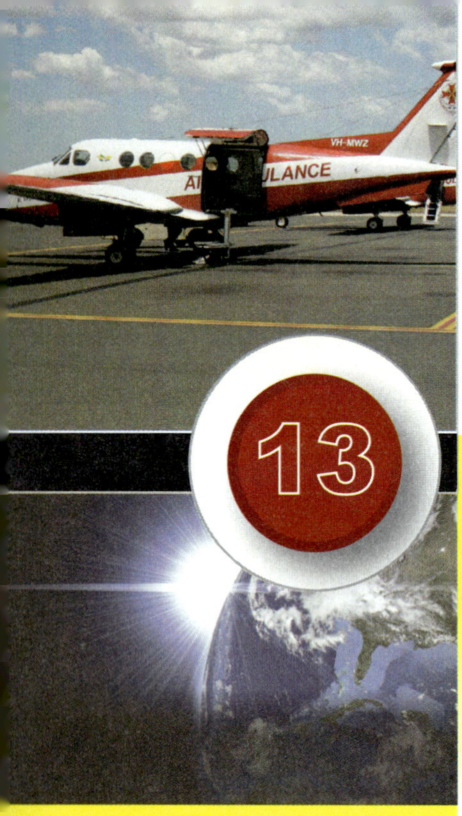

(Photo courtesy of J van der Wolf, Shutterstock.com)

13

Abdominal Trauma

Melissa White, MD, MPH
Arthur H. Yancey, II, MD, MPH, FACEP

Abdominal Trauma Trauma Addominale

Traumatismo Abdominal Traumatisme Abdominal

Urazy brzucha Abdominal Trauma

Ozljede trbuha إصابات البطن abdominalna trauma

Poškodbe trebuha Hasi sérülés

KEY TERMS

evisceration, *p. 240*
intrathoracic abdomen, *p. 238*
peritoneum, *p. 240*
retroperitoneal abdomen, *p. 238*
seat-belt sign, *p. 240*
true abdomen, *p. 238*

OBJECTIVES

Upon completion of this chapter, you should be able to:

1. Identify the basic anatomy of the abdomen and explain how abdominal and chest injuries may be related.
2. Differentiate between blunt and penetrating injuries and identify complications associated with each.
3. Describe the treatment required for the patient with protruding viscera.
4. Relate how injuries apparent on the exterior of the abdomen can damage underlying structures.
5. Describe possible intra-abdominal injuries based on findings of history, physical examination, and mechanism of injury.
6. List the advanced life support interventions for patients with abdominal injuries.

Chapter Overview

Injury to the abdomen can be a difficult condition to evaluate in the hospital setting. In the field it is usually even more so. Nevertheless, because intra-abdominal injury is one of the major causes of preventable traumatic death, the possibility of intra-abdominal injury must be recognized, addressed, and documented immediately. Penetrating abdominal injuries usually need immediate surgical attention. Blunt injuries (contact sports, motor-vehicle collisions, assault) may be more subtle, but potentially just as deadly.

Whether the result of blunt or penetrating trauma, an abdominal injury may present with two life-threatening dangers: hemorrhage and infection. Hemorrhage has immediate consequences, so you must be vigilant in assessing the signs and symptoms of shock in all patients with abdominal injury. Infection, which presents late, may be just as lethal, but does not require field intervention beyond prevention of gross contamination.

The role of prehospital providers in the management of abdominal trauma has been the subject of some controversy. Studies in the mid-1980s demonstrated that appropriate and timely intervention by well-trained paramedics could improve the hemodynamic status of critically injured patients with wounds to the abdomen. More recent studies have suggested that pneumatic antishock garment (PASG) application and/or vigorous IV fluid resuscitation in the prehospital setting may do more harm than good for patients with penetrating abdominal trauma. (See Chapter 8.) The effects of aggressive fluid resuscitation in blunt trauma are less well defined.

In the field, rapid patient assessment and early treatment of shock are critical aspects in the management of the patient with abdominal trauma.

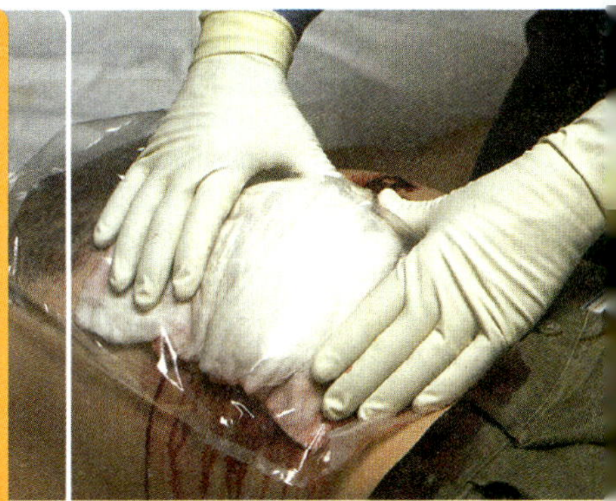

CASE PRESENTATION

An advanced life support (ALS) ambulance has been dispatched to a private home for a report of a person who has "passed out." When the team arrives at the house, they are met at the front door by a woman who says her husband had been taking a nap, and when he stood up he passed out for a few minutes. They find the man, who appears to be in his 40s, sitting in a chair. He says he is okay now, denies chest pain or history of heart disease, and is embarrassed that they were called. He appears a little pale.

They ask if they can examine him and he agrees. His pulse is 108 beats/minute, and his blood pressure is 114/90 mm Hg. When they stand him up, his pulse increases to 120 and his blood pressure drops to 90/70. He becomes lightheaded but does not lose consciousness. They have him recline on the stretcher, and his examination is normal except for mild generalized abdominal tenderness. When questioned about what he has done that day, he states the only thing out of the ordinary was earlier that morning when he sparred a few rounds with his teenage son, who is to be in a karate tournament soon. He denies any significant pain other than some aching in the back of his left shoulder. *What may be the cause of his syncope? What should be done to provide emergency care to this patient?* Keep these questions in mind as you read the chapter. Then, at the end of the chapter, find out how the rescuers completed this call. ■

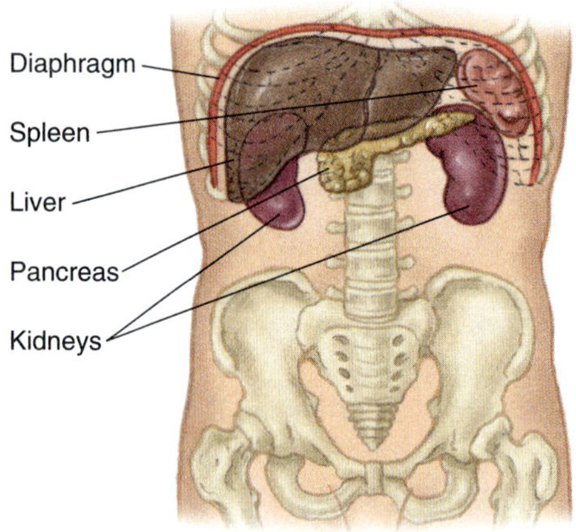

FIGURE 13-1 Intrathoracic abdomen.

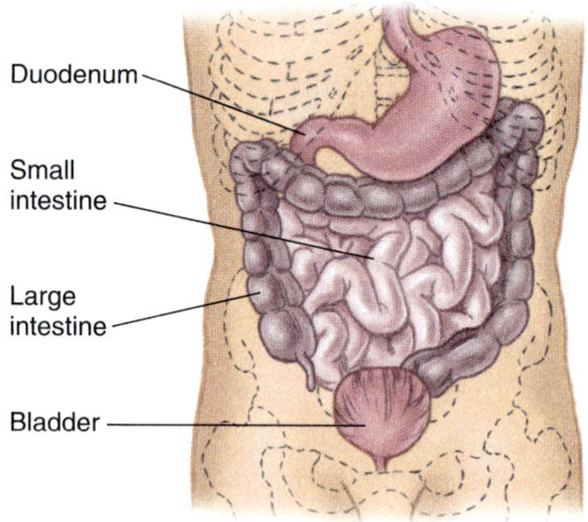

FIGURE 13-2 True abdomen.

intrathoracic abdomen that part of the abdomen that is enclosed by the lower ribs; contains the liver, gallbladder, spleen, stomach, and transverse colon.

true abdomen that part of the abdomen from the lower ribs and including the pelvis but anterior to the retroperitoneum; contains the large and small intestines, a portion of the liver, and the bladder. In a female, the uterus, fallopian tubes, and ovaries are also part of the true abdomen.

retroperitoneal abdomen that part of the abdomen behind the thoracic and true portions of the abdomen separated from the other abdominal regions by the thin retroperitoneal membrane; includes the kidneys, ureters, pancreas, posterior duodenum, ascending and descending colon, abdominal aorta, and the inferior vena cava.

Anatomy of the Abdomen

The abdomen is traditionally divided into three regions: the **intrathoracic abdomen**, the true abdomen, and the retroperitoneal abdomen. The thoracic portion of the abdomen is located underneath a thin sheet of muscle called the *diaphragm* and is enclosed by the lower ribs (Figure 13-1). It contains the liver, gallbladder, spleen, stomach, and transverse colon.

The **true abdomen** contains the large and small intestines, a portion of the liver, and the bladder (Figure 13-2). In females, the uterus, fallopian tubes, and ovaries are considered part of the pelvic portion of the true abdomen.

The **retroperitoneal abdomen** lies behind the thoracic and true portions of the abdomen (Figure 13-3). It is separated by the retroperitoneal membrane from the other abdominal regions. This area includes the kidneys, ureters, pancreas, posterior duodenum, ascending and descending colon, abdominal aorta, and the inferior vena cava. Because of its location away from the anterior body surface, injuries here are difficult to evaluate in the field.

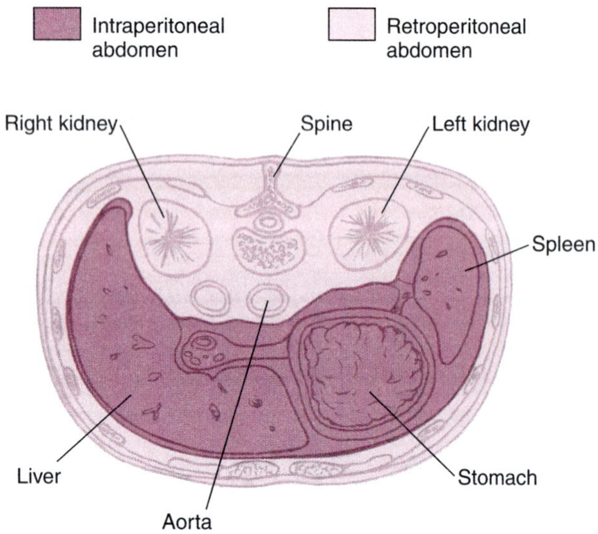

FIGURE 13-3 Retroperitoneal abdomen.

Although hemorrhage in the true abdomen may cause the anterior abdominal wall to become distended, hemorrhage severe enough to cause shock may occur in the retroperitoneal space without this dramatic sign. Furthermore, in the pelvic portion of the retroperitoneal abdomen are the iliac blood vessels. Those vessels and their branches may be damaged by abdominal trauma or pelvic fracture. Injury to this vasculature may cause serious hemorrhage with minimal localized symptoms.

Types of Injuries

Injuries to the abdomen are usually categorized as blunt or penetrating trauma, but a combination of the two also may occur. Blunt trauma is the most common mechanism of abdominal injury and has relatively high mortality rates of 10% to 30%. The reason for this is likely related to the frequency of accompanying injuries to the head, chest, pelvis, and/or an extremity in as many as 70% of motor-vehicle collision victims.

Blunt abdominal injury may be from direct compression of the abdomen against a fixed object with resulting tears or subcapsular hematomas involving the solid organ's associated viscera (spleen/liver). Injury also may arise from deceleration forces, with tearing of organs and their blood vessels at fixed areas within the abdominal region. This is particularly true of the liver and the renal arteries. Hollow organs (typically small intestine) may rupture due to increased intraluminal pressures.

The patient who has suffered blunt trauma may have no pain and little external evidence of injury, which may give a false sense of security. Patients with multiple lower rib fractures are notorious for having severe intra-abdominal injuries without significant abdominal pain. *The severe pain from the rib fractures becomes a distracting injury for the less noticeable abdominal pain.* As a result, the patient may have a poor outcome because abdominal injuries are not recognized.

Most penetrating injuries are caused by gunshot and stab wounds. Gunshot wounds to the abdomen may include direct trauma to an organ and vasculature through penetration from the bullet, its fragments, or the energy transmitted from the bullet's mass and velocity. This is known as a *blast effect.*

As a general rule, most patients with gunshot wounds to the abdomen will be definitively treated in the operating room. These patients have mortality rates of between 5% and 15% because of a greater incidence of injury to abdominal viscera from the higher energy imparted to the intra-abdominal organs. (See Chapter 1.)

The mortality rate from abdominal stab wounds is relatively low (1% to 2%). Unless the knife penetrates a major vessel or organ, such as the liver or spleen, the patient may not initially appear to be in shock at the scene. However, some patients can develop life-threatening peritonitis over the next few hours or days. Those wounds need to be carefully explored in the emergency department because approximately one-third of stab-wound patients require surgery for intra-abdominal bleeding.

Because the path of the penetrating object might not be readily apparent from the wound location, any penetrating wound of the chest may penetrate the abdomen, and vice versa. The course of a bullet may pass through numerous structures in different body locations. It is important to look at the patient's entire posterior surface because penetrating trauma in the gluteal area (iliac crests to the gluteal folds, including the rectum) is associated with up to a 50% incidence of significant intra-abdominal injuries.

PEARLS: Abdominal Injury

- When mechanisms of trauma or associated injuries such as lower rib fractures or gluteal penetrating wounds suggest possible intra-abdominal injury, do not be fooled by the patient's lack of abdominal pain or tenderness. Be prepared to treat hypovolemic shock from occult intra-abdominal bleeding.
- The patient who has had blunt trauma to the abdomen and has abdominal pain and/or tenderness probably has serious abdominal trauma and is likely to develop shock quickly (even if vital signs are initially normal). Load and go, preparing to treat the development of hemorrhagic shock en route to the hospital.

Assessment and Stabilization

Scene Size-up

You can glean important information from the scene by noting the circumstances surrounding the patient's injury. An accurate but rapid assessment of the scene will usually tip you off to the possibility of intra-abdominal trauma. Do circumstances on the scene suggest that the victim has fallen from a height or been hit by a passing vehicle? Has there been an explosion that could have hurled the victim against immobile objects or transmitted blast pressure to organs inside the abdomen? Has the victim of an automobile crash had the shoulder strap under the arm rather than over the shoulder? Or was the lap belt worn too high over the soft true abdomen instead of correctly across the pelvis? Any of those mechanisms can lead to abdominal injury.

If the patient was involved in a motor-vehicle crash, as you do your scene size-up, quickly observe the damage to the vehicle, such as passenger compartment intrusion, airbag deployment, broken windows, bent steering wheel/steering column, and location of occupants. If the patient needs to be extricated, note the location of the safety belts. Although they certainly save lives, safety belts incorrectly worn can cause blunt abdominal injuries by compressing the intra-abdominal organs against the spine. Remember that lap belts alone, especially in the young adolescent age group may, ironically, predispose an individual to intra-abdominal injuries.

The patient who is stabbed or shot may be able to give you some idea of the size of the instrument or trajectory of the bullet. With gunshot wounds, it is also important to know the caliber, the range from which it was fired, and the number of rounds that were fired. A bystander or the police may be able to provide such information. On arrival at the hospital (optimally, a trauma center), be sure to report any mechanism that suggests abdominal injury. However, while at the scene, it is important *not* to spend a great deal of time attempting to obtain a history. *The major cause of preventable mortality in abdominal trauma is delayed diagnosis and treatment.*

Patient Assessment

As in treating any other traumatic condition, the patient should first undergo the ITLS Primary Survey. During the rapid trauma survey the essence of the prehospital abdominal exam is rapid visualization and palpation of both the chest and abdomen. Quickly inspect the chest and abdomen for deformities, contusions, abrasions, and punctures (DCAP), **evisceration**, and distention. The chest is only one thin muscle sheet (the diaphragm) away from the abdominal cavity.

evisceration the protruding of intestinal organs through a wound.

Abdominal organs are enclosed within the lower ribs, thus injury to both chest and abdomen is not uncommon. Blunt or penetrating injuries to the chest from about the nipple line (fourth or fifth ribs) down should make you suspicious for both chest and abdominal injuries. Rib fractures may suggest hepatic, splenic, and diaphragmatic trauma. Splenic injury may present with referred left posterior shoulder pain, and a liver injury may present with referred right posterior shoulder pain. The presence of a **seat-belt sign**, a large bruise or abrasion across the abdomen, is indicative of intra-abdominal injury in approximately 25% of cases. Periumbilical bruising (Cullen's sign) may raise suspicion for retroperitoneal hemorrhage, but be mindful that this finding usually takes several hours to develop.

seat-belt sign a bruise or abrasion across the abdomen from an improperly positioned lap belt. It can be a clue to blunt intra-abdominal injury.

Palpate the patient's abdomen for distention, tenderness, or rigidity. Distention of the abdomen should be interpreted as a sign of severe intra-abdominal trauma with likely hemorrhage. Tenderness or guarding over the abdominal wall is also usually a sign of intra-abdominal injury. If tenderness or guarding is present in the prehospital setting, there is usually significant blood in the abdomen causing irritation of the **peritoneum**. This is an indication that shock may be imminent. (See Chapter 8.) Gentle palpation of the iliac crests (pelvic wings) and pubis of the pelvis may reveal the tenderness or bony crepitation associated with fractures. Pelvic fractures frequently result in hemorrhagic shock. The genitalia should be visualized for bruising or hemorrhage during the ITLS Secondary Survey.

peritoneum thin serous membrane that lines the abdominal cavity and encloses the organs of the intrathoracic and true abdomen.

Auscultation of the abdomen in the field usually does not offer further useful information. Abdominal wounds should never be probed with your finger or with an instrument. If clothing must be removed to visualize injury, try to preserve important potential legal evidence by cutting around (rather than through) areas that have signs of possible penetration.

Stabilization

Interventions should follow priorities established by the ITLS Primary Survey. They should proceed in the same order in which assessment occurred: (A) airway, (B) breathing, and (C) circulation. (This only changes to CABC if there is obvious severe uncontrolled external hemorrhage.) For the patient in whom you suspect only intra-abdominal injury, you would still give high-flow oxygen by the most appropriate method and be sure breathing was adequate before dealing with the circulatory issue of shock or potential shock.

The patient should be readied for immediate transport with appropriate spinal motion restriction (SMR). (Penetrating trauma to the abdomen or chest with no signs of neurological deficit should not have SMR because time is extremely critical.) Once en route to an appropriate facility, establish two large-bore IV lines of normal saline. If the patient's blood pressure drops below 90 mm Hg systolic with signs of shock, then the IV fluids should be given at a rate to maintain the systolic blood pressure at 80 to 90 mm Hg. (See Chapter 8.) It is thought that aggressive fluid resuscitation might dislodge protective clots and/or dilute clotting factors, both of which lead to worsening hemorrhage.

Gently cover any organ or viscera protruding from a wound with gauze moistened with saline or water. If you have a long transport time, you can apply a nonadherent material, such as plastic wrap or aluminum foil, to prevent drying of the gauze and intestines (Scan 13-1). If the intestines are allowed to dry, they may become irreversibly damaged. Do not push abdominal contents protruding from a wound back into the abdomen. Similarly, if a foreign body (such as a knife or glass shard) is impaled in the abdomen, do not attempt to remove or manipulate it because it may precipitate uncontrollable hemorrhage. Carefully stabilize the object in place without moving it. (Pregnant patients deserve the special considerations addressed in Chapter 19.)

Areas of Current Study

Deciding which patient should be taken to a local community hospital and which should be taken directly to a trauma center can be a difficult decision, with only a patient history, a scene size-up, and a patient assessment to guide it. Better tools are needed to distinguish between patients who have injuries that are either not severe or not time critical and will remain stable, and those with a significant mechanism of injury who appear stable initially, and then decompensate later, requiring emergent transfer to a trauma center. Tests performed quickly in the ambulance or on scene that could help predict which apparently stable patient might deteriorate would be very helpful. Current studies using finger-stick serum lactate levels and studies using abdominal ultrasound in the field (F.A.S.T. exam) show some promise. (See Chapter 2 for more about those studies.)

SCAN 13-1 Caring for an Evisceration

1
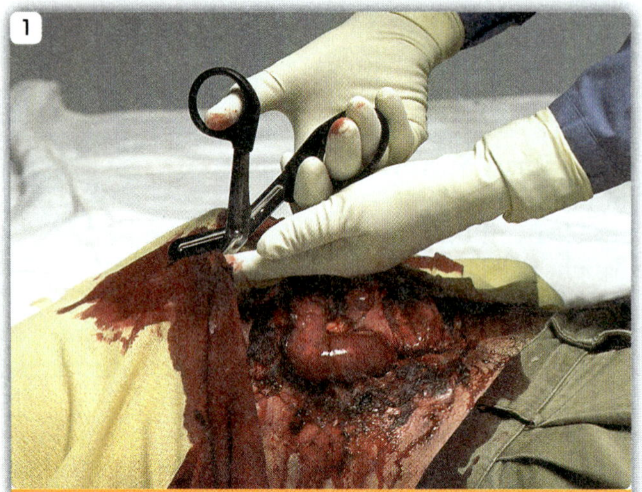
Remove clothing to fully expose the abdominal wound.

2
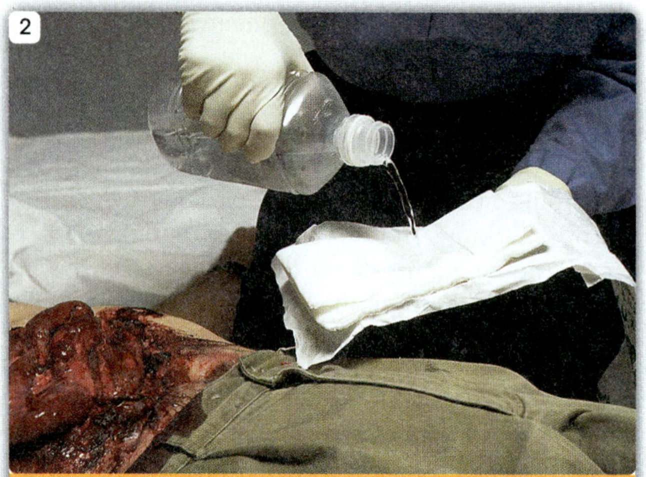
Cover the wound with a sterile dressing soaked with normal saline.

3
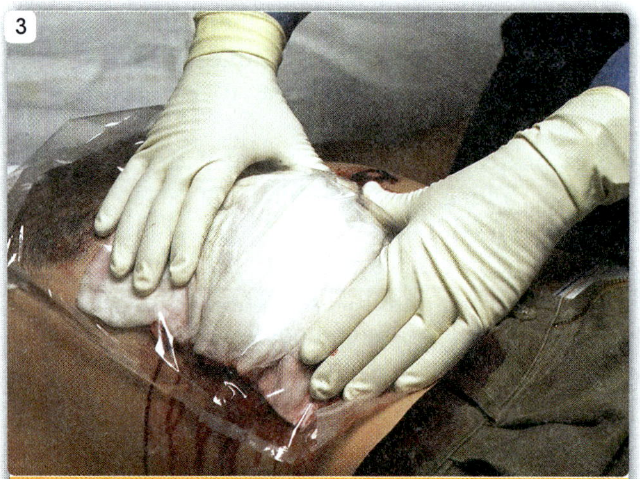
Cover the moistened dressing with a sterile occlusive dressing to prevent evaporative drying.

CASE PRESENTATION (continued)

An advanced life support (ALS) ambulance has been dispatched to a private home for a report of a person who has "passed out." They find a man who has postural hypotension (blood pressure drops and pulse rises when going from supine to standing position), a slightly tender abdomen, and some aching in the back of his left shoulder. His history is negative for any serious illnesses, and he takes no medications. He has not eaten since a light breakfast six hours ago. A 12-lead ECG shows slight tachycardia but is otherwise normal. He admits to getting "beat up a little" by his son when they practiced karate two hours before.

With the combination of postural hypotension post-trauma, slightly tender abdomen, and pain in posterior left shoulder (no tenderness), the team leader is suspicious of a traumatic splenic rupture. The team leader explains the danger to him, and he agrees to go to the hospital for evaluation. An IV line is started on the way to the trauma center, but fluids are kept at KVO rate because the supine blood pressure is 110/90 mm Hg. A CT scan at the trauma center revealed a tear of the spleen and blood in the abdomen. The patient has a complete recovery after surgery. ■

Summary

Effective prehospital management of the patient with abdominal trauma entails the following:

- Scene size-up for mechanisms of injury and pertinent history from the patient and/or witnesses
- Rapid patient assessment
- Rapid transport to the appropriate hospital (optimally, a trauma center)
- IV lines and other interventions as needed (usually performed en route)

The enemies of the abdominal trauma patient are bleeding and time elapsed from injury until optimal care. If you can minimize on-scene delays, you will help to maximize the patient's chance for survival.

Bibliography

1. Aprahamian, C., B. M. Thompson, J. B. Towne. 1983. The effect of a paramedic system on mortality of major open intra-abdominal vascular trauma. *Journal of Trauma* 23: 687–690.
2. Bickell, W. H., M. J. Wall, et al. 1994. Immediate versus delayed fluid resuscitation for hypotensive patients with penetrating torso injuries. *New England Journal of Medicine* 331 (October): 1105–1109.
3. Brooke, M., et al. 2010. Paramedic application of ultrasound in the management of patients in the prehospital setting: A review of the literature. *Emergency Medicine Journal* 27(9): 702–707.
4. Jansen, T. C., J. van Bommel, et al. 2008. The prognostic value of blood lactate levels relative to that of vital signs in the pre-hospital setting: A pilot study. *Critical Care* 12(6): 160–166.
5. Korner, M., M. Krotz, et al. 2008. Current role of emergency ultrasound in patients with major trauma. *Radiographics* 28(1): 225–242.

6. Newgard, C. D., et al. 2005. Steering wheel deformity and serious thoracic or abdominal injury among drivers and passengers involved in motor vehicle crashes. *Annals of Emergency Medicine* 45 (January): 43–50.
7. Pepe, P. E., et al. 2002. Prehospital fluid resuscitation of the patient with major trauma. *Prehospital Emergency Care* 6: 81.
8. Salomone, J. A., J. P. Salomone. *2009. Blunt abdominal trauma*. Retrieved October 2, 2009, from http://emedicine.medscape.com/article/821995-overview
9. Scalea, T. M., et al. 2004. Abdominal injuries. *Tintinalli's emergency medicine, A comprehensive study guide.* Sec. 22, chap. 260, 6th ed. New York: McGraw-Hill.
10. Rodriguiz, L. E., C. K. Gough. 2004. Immediate management of life-threatening injuries. In *Current emergency diagnosis and treatment*. 5th ed.; pp. 467–476. New York: McGraw-Hill.
11. Todd, S. R. 2004. Critical concepts in abdominal injury. *Critical Care Clinics* 20 (January): 119–34.
12. Townsend, C. M, et al. 2008. Abdominal trauma. In *Sabiston textbook of surgery*. 18th ed. Philadelphia: Saunders.
13. van Beest, P. A., J. Mulder, et al. 2009. Measurement of lactate in a prehospital setting is related to outcome. *European Journal of Emergency Medicine* 16(6): 318–322.

Explore Resource Central

For additional review and practice tests, visit www.bradybooks.com and click on Resource Central to access book-specific resources for this text. To access Resource Central, follow directions on the Student Access Card provided with this text. If there is no card, go to www.bradybooks.com and follow the Resource Central link to Buy Access from there.

Extremity Trauma

Sabina Braithwaite, MD, MPH, FACEP
S. Robert Seitz, M Ed, RN, NREMT-P

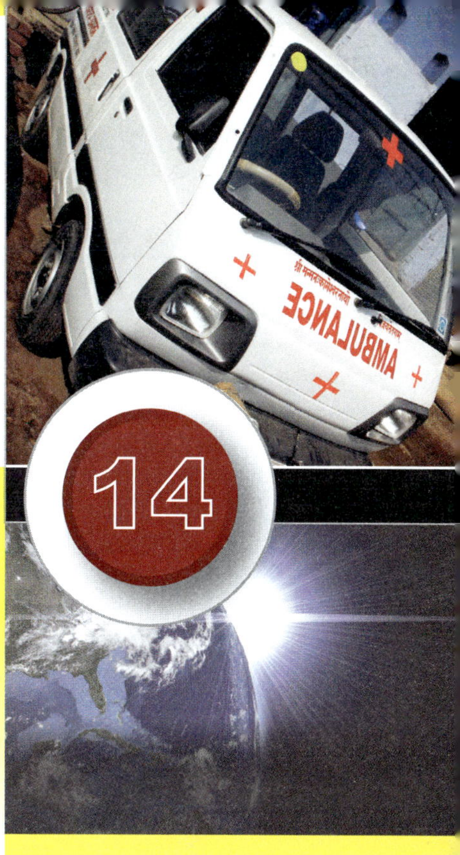

(Photo courtesy of Regien Paassen, Shutterstock.com)

Extremity Trauma Trauma alle Estremità

Traumatismo de Extremidades Traumatisme d'extrémité

Obrażenia kończyn Extremitäten Trauma Ozljede ekstremiteta

إصابات الأطراف trauma ekstremiteta Poškodbe okončin

Végtagsérülés

OBJECTIVES

Upon successful completion of this chapter, you should be able to:

1. Prioritize extremity trauma in the assessment and management of life-threatening injuries.
2. Discuss the major immediate and short-term complications and treatment of the following extremity injuries:
   a. Fractures
   b. Dislocations
   c. Open wounds
   d. Amputations
   e. Neurovascular injuries
   f. Sprains and strains
   g. Impaled objects
   h. Crush injuries
3. Discuss the pathophysiology of compartment syndrome and which extremity injuries are most likely to develop this complication.
4. Describe the potential amount of blood loss from pelvic and femur fractures.
5. Discuss major mechanisms of injury, associated injuries, potential complications, and management of injuries to the following:
   a. Pelvis
   b. Femur
   c. Hip
   d. Knee
   e. Tibia and fibula (including ankle)
   f. Clavicle and shoulder
   g. Elbow
   h. Forearm and wrist
   i. Hand or foot

KEY TERMS

amputation, *p. 249*
closed fracture, *p. 246*
compartment syndrome, *p. 251*
crepitation, *p. 253*
impaled object, *p. 251*
joint dislocation, *p. 248*
neurovascular injury, *p. 246*
open-book pelvic fracture, *p. 260*
open fracture, *p. 246*
sprain, *p. 251*
strain, *p. 251*

Chapter Overview

You must never let severely deformed or wounded extremities divert your attention from more life-threatening injuries that may also be present. Those dramatic injuries are easy to identify when you first encounter the patient. They may be disabling, but are rarely immediately life-threatening. It is important to remember that the movement of air through the airway, the mechanics of breathing, the maintenance of circulating blood volume, and the appropriate treatment of shock must always come before fracture or dislocation management.

Hemorrhagic shock is a potential danger of some musculoskeletal injuries. Only direct lacerations of arteries or fractures of the pelvis or femur are commonly associated with enough bleeding to cause shock. Unfortunately, that bleeding is often internal and may not be detectable on physical examination until a large amount of blood is lost, if then. Injuries to the nerves or blood vessels that serve the hands and feet are the most common complications of fractures and dislocations. Such injuries cause the loss of function that are included under the term *neurovascular compromise*, or **neurovascular injury**. Thus, evaluation of pulses, motor function, and sensation (PMS) distal to fractures is very important.

neurovascular injury an injury that involves nerves and blood vessels. Also called neurovascular compromise.

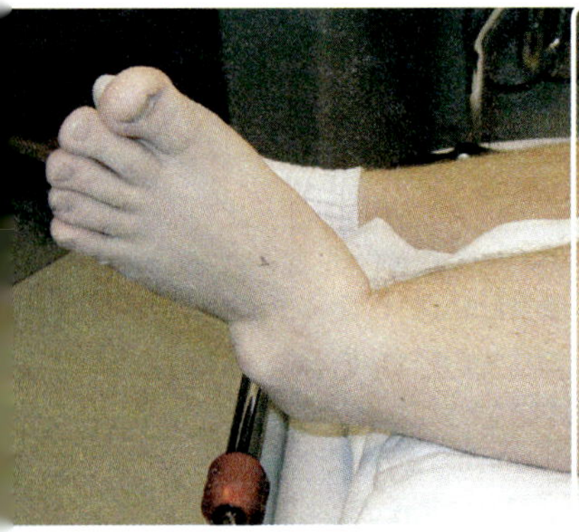

(Courtesy of Roy Alson, MD)

CASE PRESENTATION

An ALS ambulance has been called to the scene of a hiker who was injured when a rock fell on his leg. They are told that the patient is conscious. What injuries should they expect with a mechanism of this type? Are associated head and spinal injuries likely? Keep these questions in mind as you read the chapter. Then, at the end of the chapter, find out how the rescuers completed this call. ■

Injuries to Extremities

Fractures

A fracture may be open, with the broken end of the bone still protruding or having once protruded through the skin (Figure 14-1a), or it may be closed, with no communication to the outside (Figure 14-1b). Fractured bone ends are extremely sharp and are quite dangerous to all the tissues that surround the bone. Because nerves, veins, and arteries frequently travel either near the bone, generally across the flexor side of joints, or very near the skin (hands and feet), they are easily injured. Such neurovascular injuries may be due to direct injury from bone fragments, or the injuries may be indirect, from pressure due to swelling or hematoma.

A **closed fracture** can be just as dangerous as an **open fracture** because injured soft tissues often bleed profusely. It is important to remember that any break in the skin near a fractured bone may be considered an opening for contamination. A closed fracture of one femur can cause the loss of one to two liters of blood. Thus, bilateral femur fractures can cause life-threatening hemorrhage (Figure 14-2).

closed fracture a break in a bone in which there is no break in the continuity of the overlying skin.

open fracture a broken bone in which a piece of the bone is protruding or has protruded through the overlying skin.

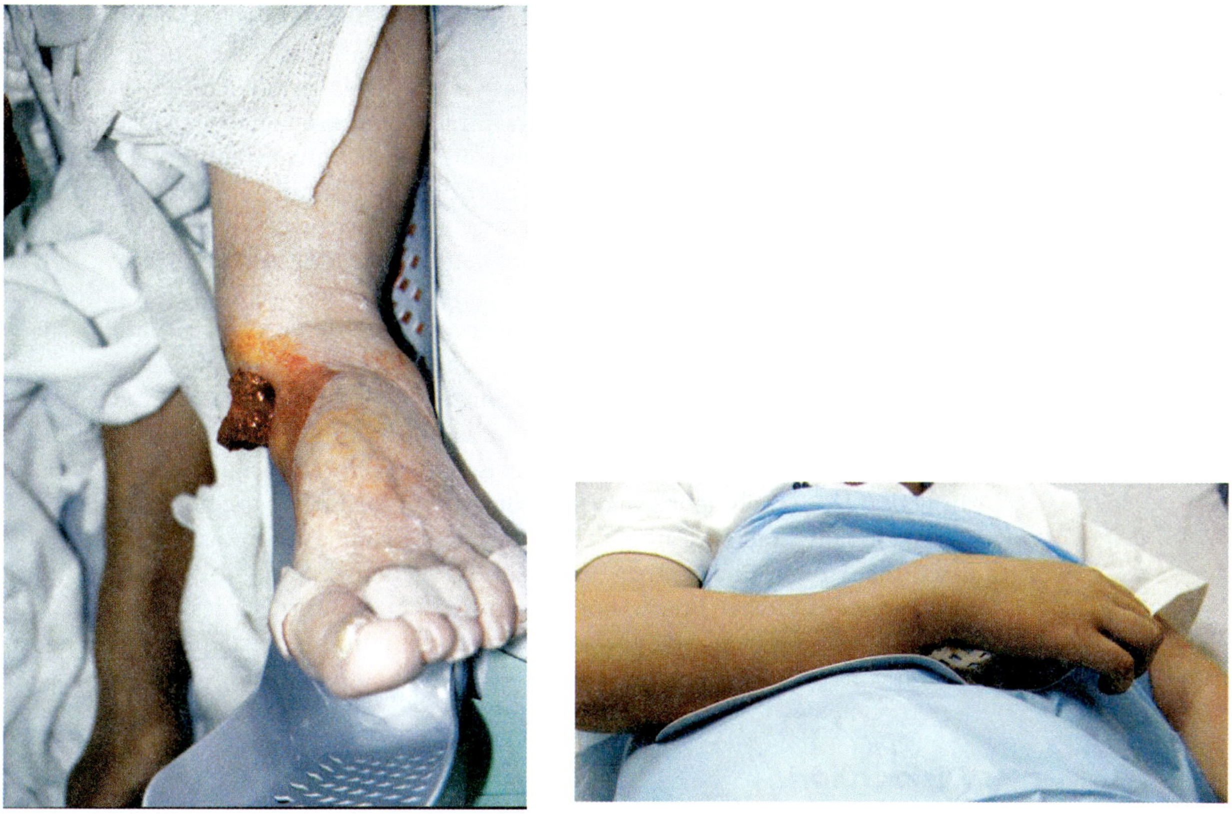

a. b.

FIGURE 14-1 (a) Open ankle fracture. (b) Closed forearm fracture. *(Photo courtesy of Roy Alson, MD)*

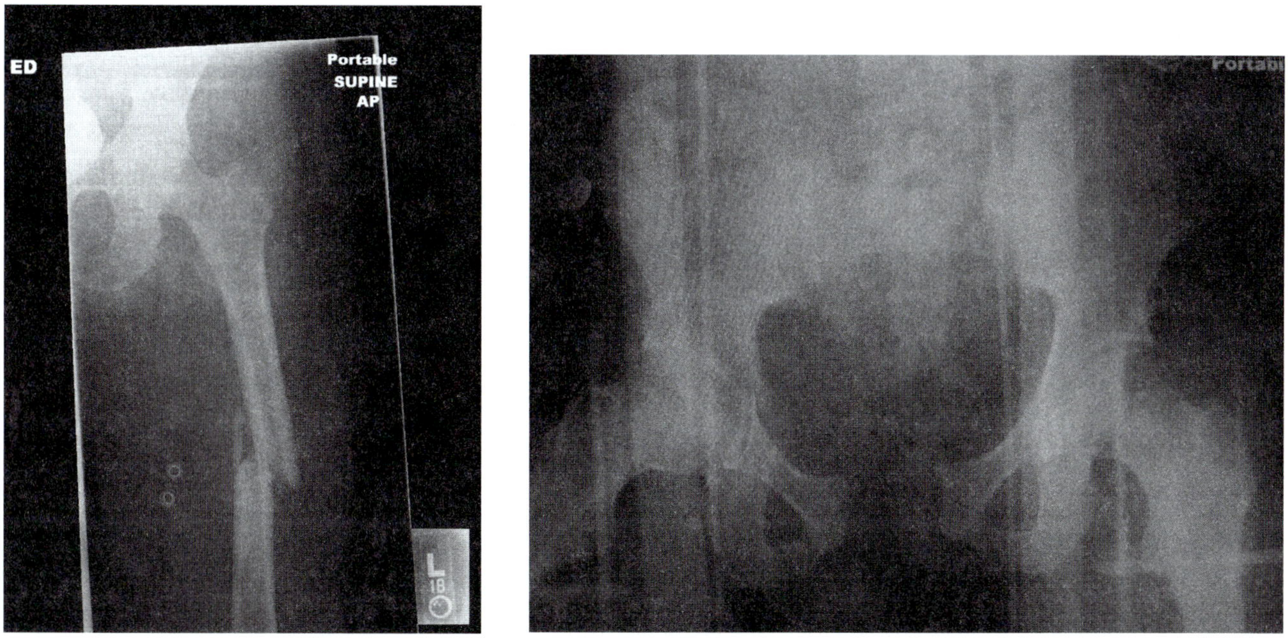

a. b.

FIGURE 14-2 Internal blood loss from fractures. (a) May lose up to two units of blood from closed femur fracture. *(Courtesy of ®E. M. Singletary, MD)* (b) May lose two units up to complete blood volume in closed pelvic fractures. This pelvic fracture, while usually a closed fracture, is called an "open-book" fracture because the pelvic symphysis is pulled apart like an open book. *(Courtesy of Sabina Braithwaite, MD)*

A fractured pelvis can cause extensive bleeding into the abdomen or the retroperitoneal space. An unstable pelvis is usually fractured in at least two places and may have caused more than one liter of associated blood loss. Depending on the location of the pelvic fracture, there may be associated injury to the urinary tract, bladder, or bowel. Posterior pelvic fractures or fracture-dislocations, which may include the sacroiliac joints, can damage the large pelvic blood vessels and result in massive retroperitoneal or intra-abdominal hemorrhage. Because of the significant force needed to fracture the pelvis, one-third of all patients with pelvic fractures have associated intra-abdominal injuries. Remember, multiple fractures can cause life-threatening hemorrhage without any external blood loss.

Open fractures add the dangers of contamination to the risk of external hemorrhage. If protruding bone ends are pulled back into the skin when the limb is splinted, bacteria-contaminated debris may be introduced into the wound. Infection from such debris may slow or prevent healing of the bone.

Generally, fractures are quite painful. Once you have fully assessed and stabilized the patient, your management should include splinting of the fracture not only to avoid further injury, but also for patient comfort. Unless there is a specific contraindication, you also should consider administering analgesic medication if your protocols and the patient's situation allow.

Dislocations

joint dislocation a complete disruption of a joint with total loss of contact between the joint's articular surfaces.

A **joint dislocation** is an extremely painful injury. It is generally easy to identify because normal anatomy is significantly distorted (Figure 14-3). Although major joint dislocations are not life threatening, they are still true emergencies because of the neurovascular compromise that can lead to significant disability and even amputation if not recognized and treated promptly. Because of this, it is critical to assess for pulses, motor function, and sensation (PMS) distal to major joint dislocations and to reassess following splinting, reduction, or movement.

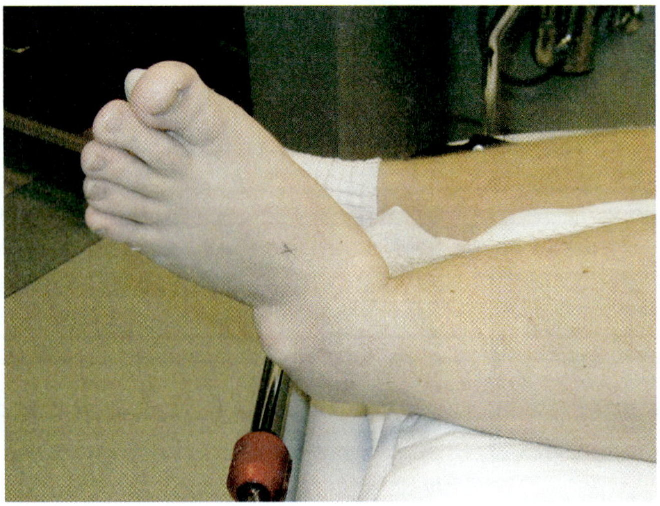

FIGURE 14-3 Ankle dislocation. *(Courtesy of Roy Alson, MD)*

Ordinarily, dislocations and fractures should be splinted in the position in which they are found with adequate padding and stabilization. Pain management should be considered for these patients if that option is available. There are certain exceptions to the general rule of splinting injuries in the position found, including when loss of distal pulse is noted. In that case, if you have a long transport time to the appropriate hospital, gentle traction should be applied in an effort to straighten it into a more anatomic position and restore the distal pulse. Ideally, this should occur with some pain control and/or sedation for the patient.

Open Wounds

Bleeding almost always can be stopped with direct pressure or pressure dressings. It is important to apply direct manual pressure to the source of the bleeding, not just the area of injury. If necessary, an appropriate tourniquet or blood pressure cuff may be appropriate. However, if the patient is exsanguinating from an extremity injury and you cannot stop the bleeding with pressure, you should not hesitate to use a tourniquet. If you have bleeding that cannot be stopped with pressure or with a tourniquet, such as injuries to the axilla, neck, or groin, you should use a hemostatic agent if available.

When used correctly, hemostatic agents in conjunction with direct pressure or tourniquets can be effective in stopping bleeding from penetration and laceration-type injuries. Note that the agents are not to be used in open abdominal or chest wounds, and some agents may require modification of the shape of the dressing to conform to the irregular shape of a wound. Patients with severe hemorrhage should be transported immediately after the ITLS Primary Survey. Obvious life-threatening hemorrhage is the only time you can change your ABC order to CABC (control bleeding, airway, breathing, and circulation). (See Chapter 2.)

For an open wound where bleeding is controlled, carefully cover it with a moist sterile dressing and bandage. Gross contamination such as leaves or gravel should be removed from the wound if possible. Smaller pieces of contamination can be irrigated from the wound with normal saline in the same manner you would irrigate a chemically contaminated eye.

Amputations

An **amputation** is a disabling and sometimes life-threatening injury that may present as partial or complete. Although it has the potential for massive hemorrhage, usually the bleeding from an amputation can be controlled with direct pressure applied to the stump. The stump should be covered with a damp sterile dressing and an elastic wrap that will apply uniform, reasonable pressure across the entire stump. If life-threatening bleeding cannot be controlled with direct pressure, a tourniquet should be applied (Figure 14-4). A tourniquet can be lifesaving with this type of injury.

amputation an open injury caused by the cutting or tearing away of a limb, body part, or organ.

Make an effort to find the amputated part and bring it with you, as long as the patient is stable, and there is no significant delay. That sometimes neglected detail can have serious future implications for the patient because it is impossible to determine in the field whether an amputated part can potentially be reimplanted, revascularized, or used for tissue grafting. It is important to bring amputated parts

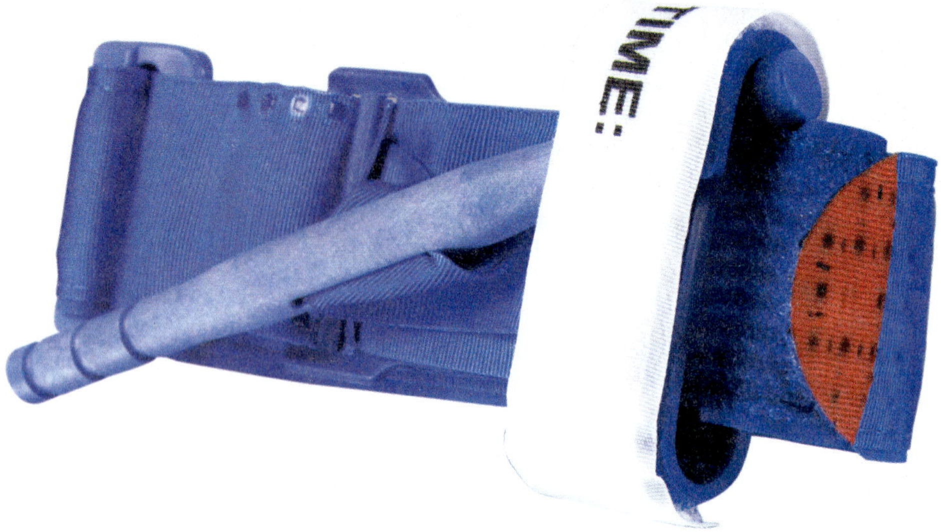

FIGURE 14-4 Combat application tourniquet (CAT). *(Courtesy of 2010 North American Rescue, LLC)*

even if reimplantation seems impossible. Note, for example, that digits have been successfully reimplanted over 24 hours following injury.

Small amputated parts should be rinsed off, wrapped in sterile gauze, and placed in a plastic bag (Figure 14-5). Label the bag with the patient's name, date, time the amputation happened, and time the part was wrapped and cooled. If ice is available, place the sealed bag in a larger bag or container containing ice and water. Do not use ice directly on the amputated part, alone, and never use dry ice. Cooling the part slows the chemical processes and will increase its viable time for reimplantation.

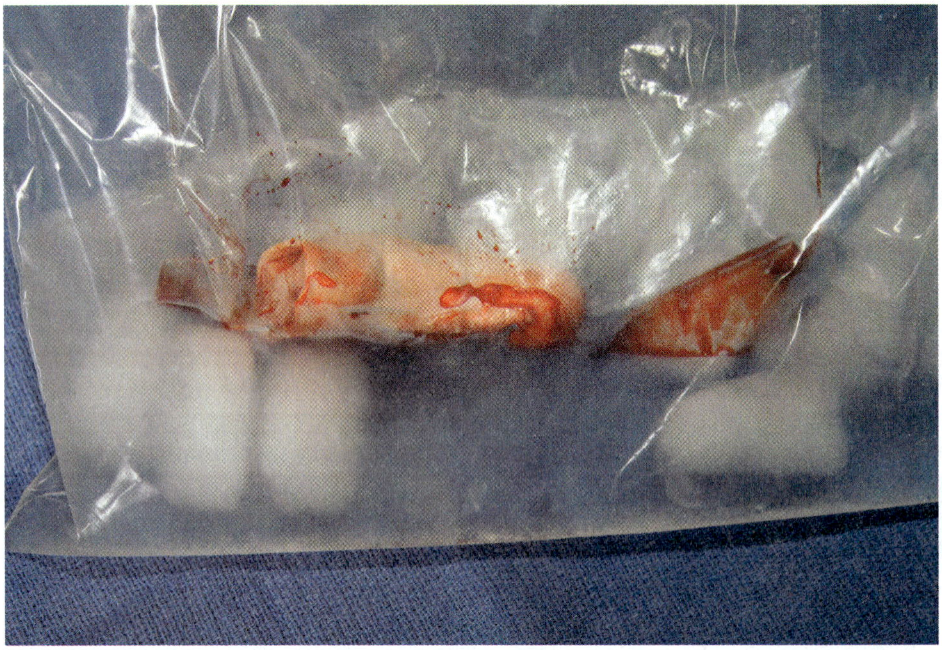

FIGURE 14-5 Amputated parts should be put in a dry bag, sealed, and placed in water that contains a few ice cubes. *(Courtesy of Stanley Cooper, EMT-P)*

Neurovascular Injuries

The nerves and major blood vessels generally run beside each other, usually in the flexor area of the major joints. They may be injured together, and loss of circulation or sensation can be due to disruption, swelling, or compression by bone fragments or hematomas. Foreign bodies or broken bone ends may well impinge on delicate structures and cause them to malfunction. Always check for PMS before and after any extremity manipulation, application of a splint, or traction.

If there is loss of sensation or circulation in an extremity, the patient must be immediately transported to a hospital with emergency orthopedic care available. If extremity position is causing the deficit, you may or may not be able to correct it in the field. Generally, it is best to splint the injured limb in the position found if transport time is not prolonged. If splinting or traction has caused the deficit, then either should be removed or repositioned.

PEARLS: Sprains and Strains

Sprains cannot be differentiated from fractures in the field. Treat them as though they were fractures. Strain injuries can usually be differentiated from factures but should be splinted for comfort.

Sprains and Strains

A **sprain** is a stretching or tearing of ligaments of a joint because of a sudden twist. It will cause pain and swelling. In the field, sprains cannot be differentiated from a fracture, so they should be splinted as if they were fractures. A **strain** is a stretching or tearing of a muscle or musculotendinous unit. It will cause pain, and often it will cause swelling. It should be splinted for comfort. Strains can usually (but not always) be differentiated from a fracture, but by splinting them you have protected the patient even if a fracture is present.

sprain a sudden twist of a joint with stretching or tearing of ligaments.

strain a stretching or partial tearing of a muscle or musculotendinous unit.

Impaled Objects

Do not remove objects impaled in extremities. **Impaled objects** in the neck that obstruct the airway or those in the cheek of the face are exceptions to this rule. Apply very bulky padding to hold the object securely in place and transport the patient. The skin is a pivot point in these exceptions, and any motion outside the body is translated or magnified within the tissues, where the end of the object may lacerate or cause additional harm to sensitive structures.

In the case of impaled objects in the neck that obstruct the airway, you must remove them or the patient will die from hypoxia. Removal could cause severe hemorrhage, and careful pressure plus hemostatic agents may be needed to control it. Impaled objects in the cheek can be safely removed because you can apply pressure from both inside and outside the wound.

impaled object an injury in which an object is embedded in the body tissue.

Compartment Syndrome

The extremities contain muscles and other structures surrounded by tough membranes, known as *fascia*, that do not stretch, creating multiple closed spaces known as *compartments*. Crush injuries, as well as closed (and some open) fractures can cause bleeding and swelling, which is contained within the closed space by the fascia. This condition is called **compartment syndrome**.

Lower leg injuries have the greatest risk of developing compartment syndrome, although it can occur in the forearm, thigh, hand, and foot as well. As the injured area swells, pressure compresses all the structures within the compartment, including arteries, veins, nerves, and muscle. At a certain point, the pressure prevents venous return. Then, as pressure continues to increase, it

compartment syndrome a condition in which increased tissue pressure in a confined space causes decreased blood flow, leading to hypoxia and possible muscle, nerve, and vessel impairment, which may be permanent if the cells die.

cuts off arterial circulation. The nerves also are compromised by the effect of the pressure and the lack of blood flow. Because these processes take some time, compartment syndrome does not present immediately, but several hours following the initial injury.

Late signs and symptoms of compartment syndrome are the five Ps: pain, pallor, pulselessness, paresthesia, and paralysis. The early symptoms are usually pain, typically described as pain out of proportion to injury, and paresthesia. Treatment requires emergent surgical compartment decompression with fasciotomy. As with shock, a high degree of suspicion is important to consider this diagnosis before the later symptoms develop and likely result in permanent damage.

Crush Injury

Following adequate addressing of the airway, breathing, and circulation, the anticipation and early detection of complications related to crush injuries is paramount for facilitating the best outcome for your patient. Pressure exerted on extremities due to a prolonged entrapment can disrupt blood flow, which promotes anaerobic metabolism within tissues. When extrication is complete and blood flow from the crushed tissue is reinstated to central circulation, hemorrhage from the crushed tissue and toxins produced in the crushed tissue being distributed throughout the body are potential complications. The toxins released include myoglobin, potassium, phosphorus, lactic acid, and uric acid, which may induce cardiac dysrhythmia and severe kidney damage. The systemic metabolic acidosis effects the toxins cause are described as *crush syndrome* or *compression syndrome*.

Assessment and Management

Scene Size-up and History

When assessing the patient with extremity trauma, it is especially important to get a history because the mechanism of injury may not be apparent in your scene size-up. The mechanism of injury and your assessment of the extremity may give you important clues to the potential severity of the injury. If there are enough rescuers, one rescuer can obtain the history while you are performing the ITLS Primary Survey. If not, you should *not* attempt to obtain a detailed verbal history until you have assessed the status of the airway, breathing, and circulation. In the conscious patient, you should obtain most of the history at the end of the ITLS Primary Survey.

Foot injuries from long jumps (falls landing on the feet) often have lumbar spinal injuries associated with them. Any injury to the knee when the patient is in the sitting position may have associated injuries to the hip. Similarly, hip injuries may refer pain to the knee, so the knee and the hip are intimately connected and must be evaluated together rather than separately. Falls onto the wrist frequently injure the elbow, and so the wrist and elbow must be evaluated together. The same is true of the ankle and the proximal fibula of the outside of the lower leg. Shoulder pain may be from the joint itself, or may be due to injury to the neck, chest, or even abdomen.

Fractures of the pelvis are often associated with very large amounts of blood loss. Whenever a fracture in the pelvis is identified, shock must be suspected and proper treatment begun immediately.

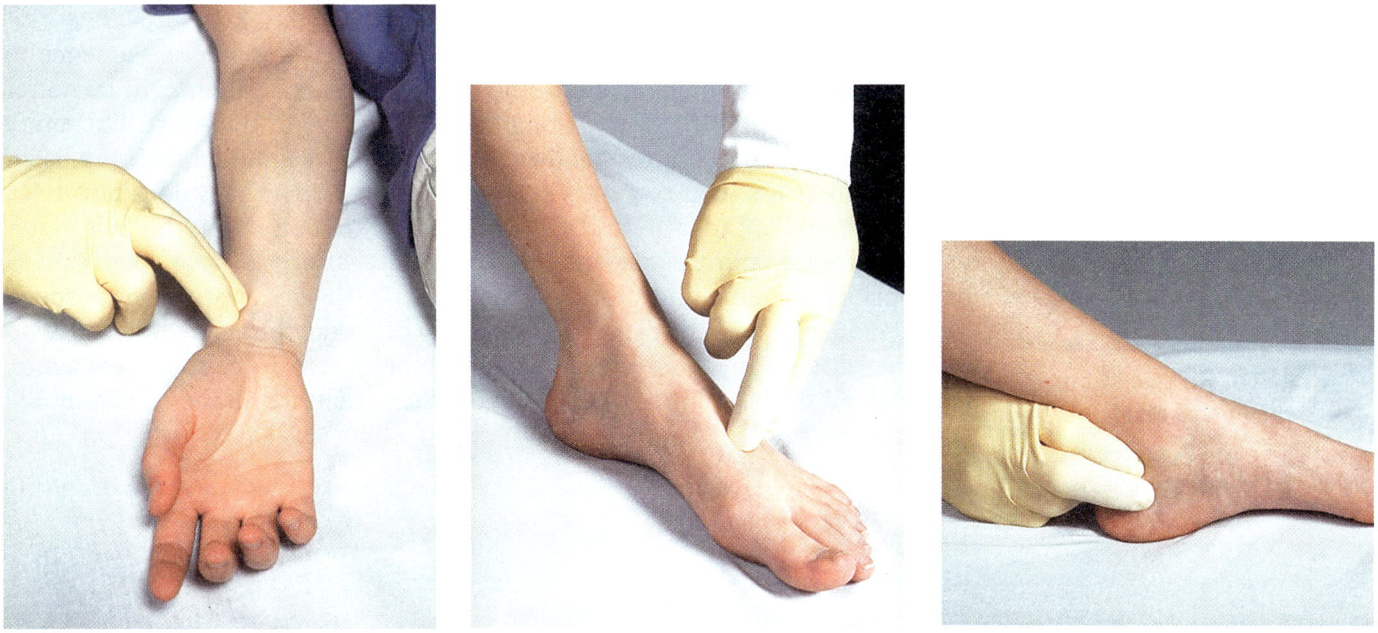

a. b. c.

FIGURE 14-6 Taking pulses distal to an injury: (a) Palpate the radial artery. (b) Palpate the dorsalis pedis pulse. (c) Palpate the posterior tibial pulse. *(Photos courtesy of Michal Heron)*

Assessment

During the ITLS Primary Survey, you are focused on obvious fractures to the pelvis and large bones of the extremities. You should also find and control major external bleeding from the extremities.

During the ITLS Secondary Survey, quickly assess the full length of each extremity, looking for deformity, contusions, abrasions, penetrations, burns, tenderness, lacerations, and swelling (DCAP-BTLS). Feel for instability and **crepitation**. (See Chapters 2 and 3.) Check the joints for pain and spontaneous movement if there is no obvious deformity or pain. Check and record distal PMS. Pulse location may be marked with pen to identify the area where the distal pulse is best felt (Figure 14-6). Crepitation or grating of bone ends is a definite sign of fracture, and once identified, the bone ends should be stabilized to prevent further soft-tissue injury. Checking for crepitation should be done very gently, especially when checking the pelvis, to avoid further injuries.

crepitation the sound or feel of broken fragments of bone grinding against each other.

Management of Extremity Injuries

Proper management of fractures and dislocations will decrease the incidence of pain, disability, and serious complications. Treatment in the prehospital setting is directed at proper immobilization of the injured part by the use of an appropriate splint and padding. Even with proper immobilization, patients may require analgesic medication to control their pain.

PEARLS: Priorities

- First assess and treat the ABCs and do not be distracted by obvious extremity trauma.
- Exsanguinating hemorrhage is the exception to the above (follow CABC rather than ABC), but you must not forget to assess airway and breathing.
- Be alert to the mechanism of injury so that you know what fractures to suspect and so that you can predict possible complications.

Purpose of Splinting

The objective of splinting is to prevent motion in the broken bone ends. The nerves that cause the most pain in a fractured extremity lie next to the bone. The broken bone can injure the nerves, causing a very deep, severe pain. Splinting not only decreases pain, but also limits further damage to muscles, nerves, and blood vessels by preventing further motion of the broken bone ends.

PEARLS: The Golden Period

- Do not waste the Golden Period. Be cautious but be rapid, and prioritize life over limb.
- Splint at an appropriate time. The axial skeleton is splinted after the ITLS Primary Survey. If a critical situation exists, extremities should be splinted en route if time allows.

PEARLS: Pulses, Motor Function, Sensation

Always assess and record PMS initially and after any manipulation, particularly splinting.

When to Splint

There is no simple rule for splinting that determines the precise sequence to follow in every patient. In general, the seriously injured patient will be better off if you splint only the spine (long backboard) before transport. Extremity fractures can be temporarily stabilized by careful packaging on the long backboard for patients who require a load-and-go approach. This does not mean that you should not identify and protect extremity fractures, but that it is better to do additional splinting en route to the hospital after you have taken care of other priorities, including shock management. It is never appropriate to spend time splinting a limb to prevent disability when that time may be needed to save the patient's life. Conversely, if the patient appears to be stable, extremity fractures should be splinted before moving the patient for all the reasons noted earlier.

PROCEDURE

Rules of Splinting

- You must adequately visualize the injured part. Clothing should be removed, preferably by cutting it off, to allow adequate assessment of the injury and proper immobilization.
- Check and record distal pulse, motor function, and sensation (PMS) before and after splinting. To check motor function distal to the fracture, ask the conscious patient to wiggle his fingers, or you can observe motion in an unconscious patient when a painful stimulus is applied. Pulses may be marked with a pen to identify where they were palpated.
- If the extremity is severely angulated, pulses are absent, and you have a long transport to the appropriate hospital, apply gentle traction in an attempt to straighten the extremity (Figure 14-7). If you encounter significant resistance, splint the extremity in the position found. When you are attempting to straighten an extremity, it is very important to be honest with yourself with regard to resistance. It takes very little force to lacerate the wall of a vessel or to interrupt the blood supply to a large nerve. If the appropriate hospital is near, it is probably best to splint in the position found.
- Open wounds should be covered with a moist sterile dressing before you apply the splint. Whenever possible, splints should be applied on the side of the extremity away from any open wounds.
- Use a splint that will immobilize one joint above and one below the injury.
- Pad the splint well. This is particularly true if there is any skin defect or if bony prominences might press against a hard splint and cause additional pain or injury to the skin.
- Do not attempt to push bone ends back under the skin. If you apply traction and the bone end retracts back into the wound, do not increase the amount of traction. You should not try to pull the bone ends back out. It is important to be sure to notify the receiving physician that the bone ends were visible. Carefully cover bone ends with moist sterile bandages. If transport is prolonged, this will help improve bone healing.
- In a life-threatening situation, injuries may be splinted while the patient is being transported. When the patient appears stable, splint fractures or deformities before movement.
- If in doubt, splint a possible injury.

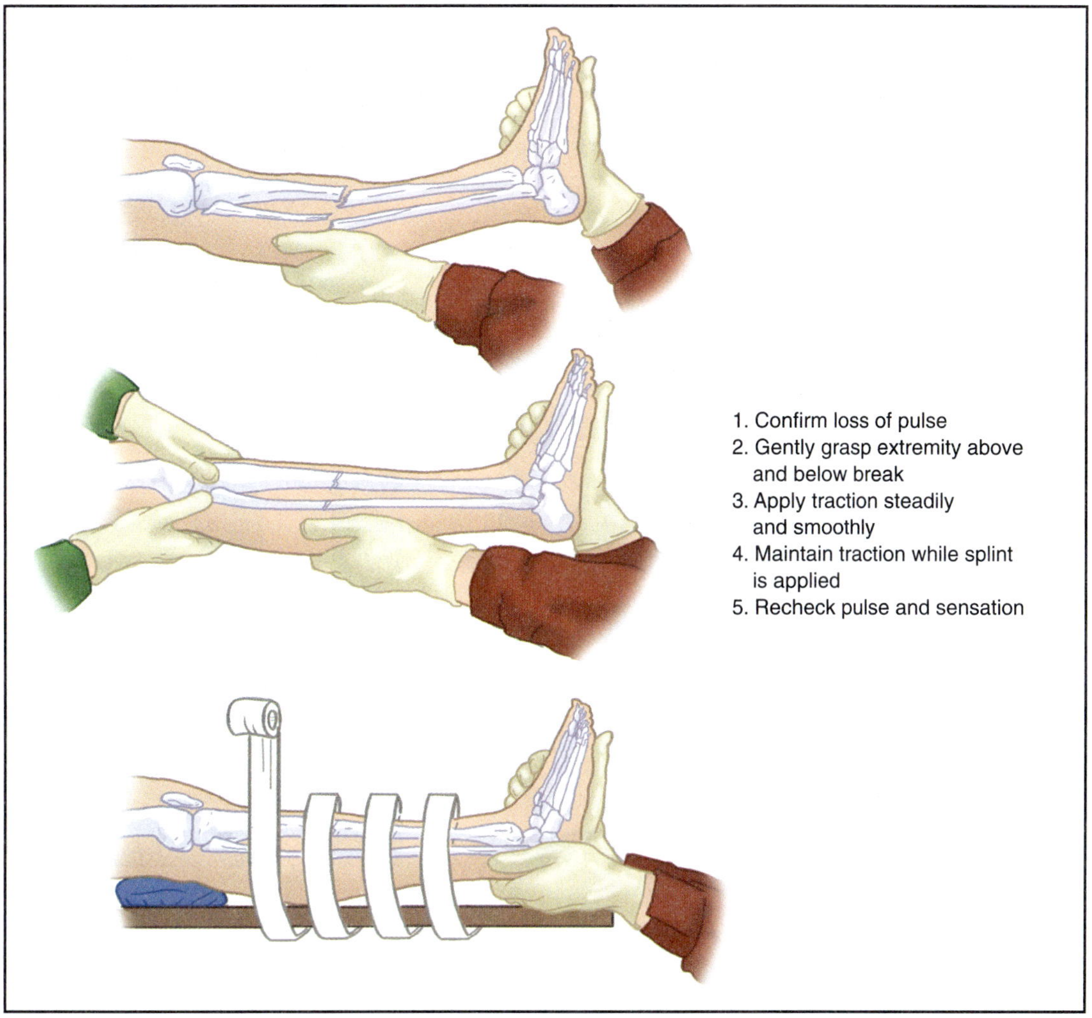

FIGURE 14-7 Straightening angulated fractures to restore pulses.

Types of Splints

For examples of splinting extremities, please see Figure 14-8.

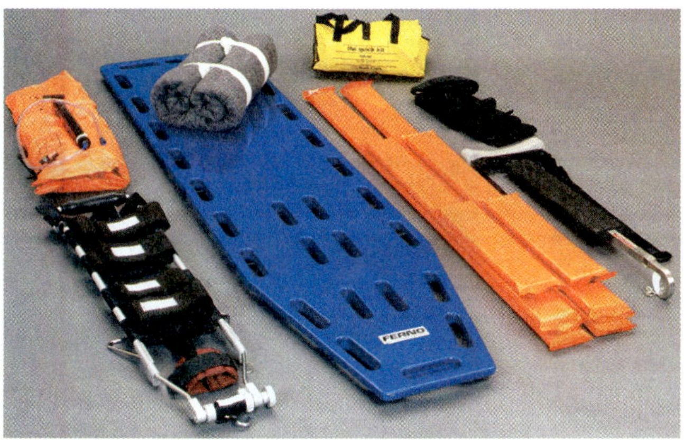

FIGURE 14-8 Examples of splints. **a.** Splinting materials.

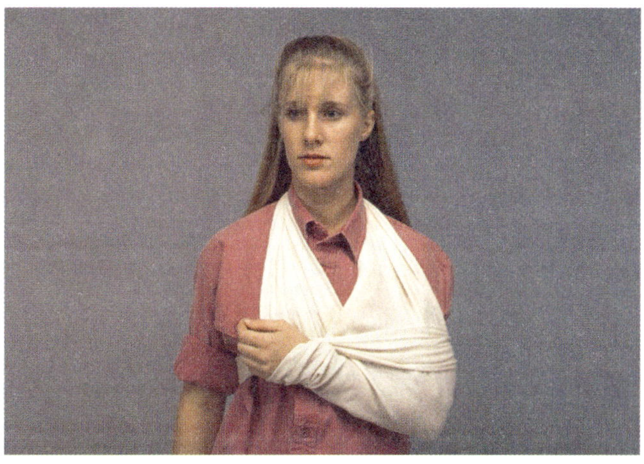

FIGURE 14-8b Sling and swathe.

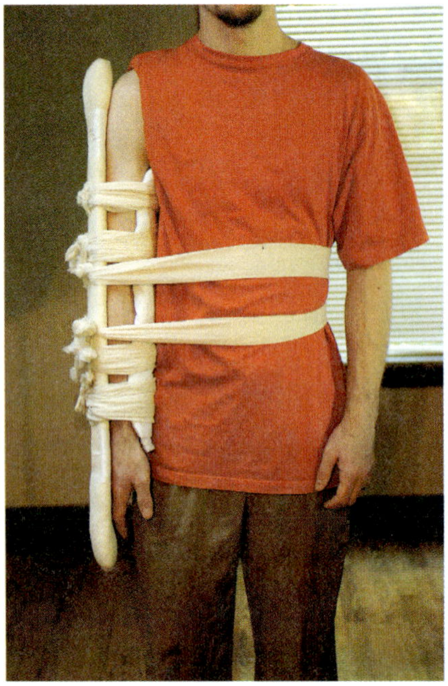

FIGURE 14-8c Rigid splint with swathes.

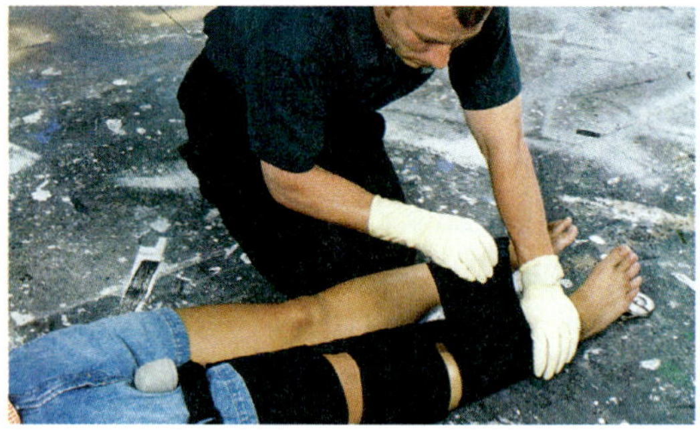

FIGURE 14-8d Traction splint.

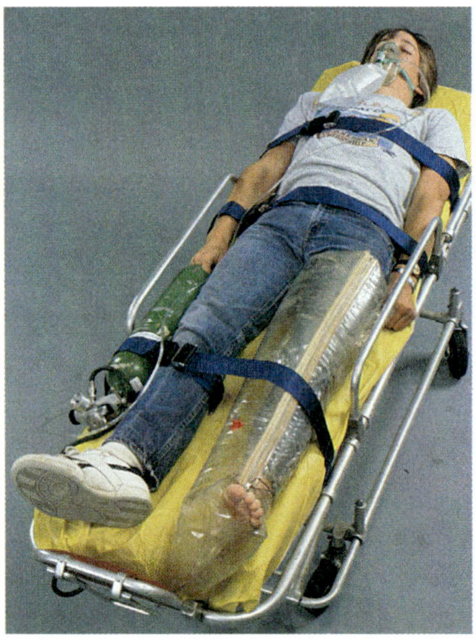

FIGURE 14-8e Air splint.

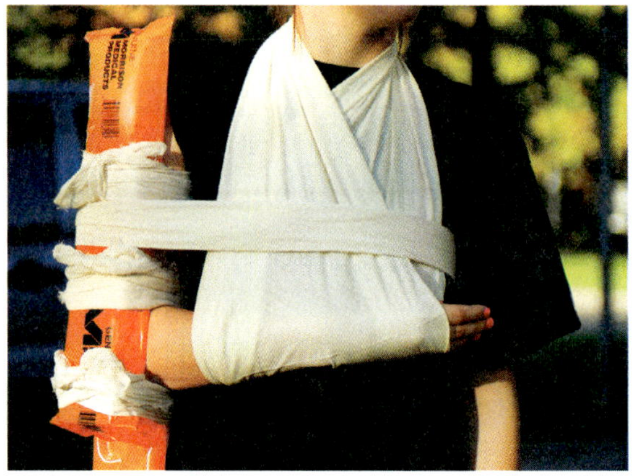

FIGURE 14-8f Fixation or rigid splint with a sling and swathe.

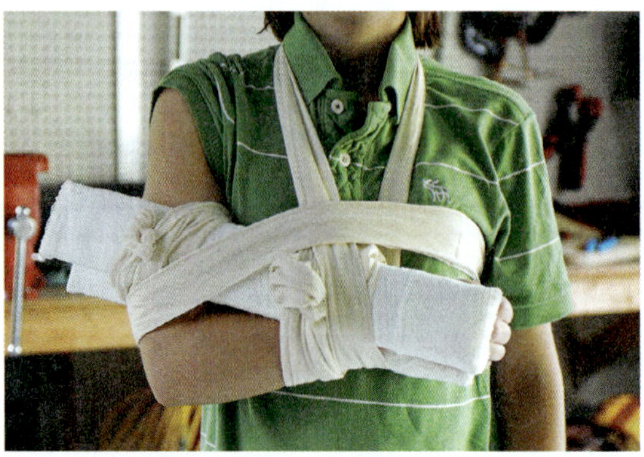

FIGURE 14-8g Injured elbow immobilized in a bent position.

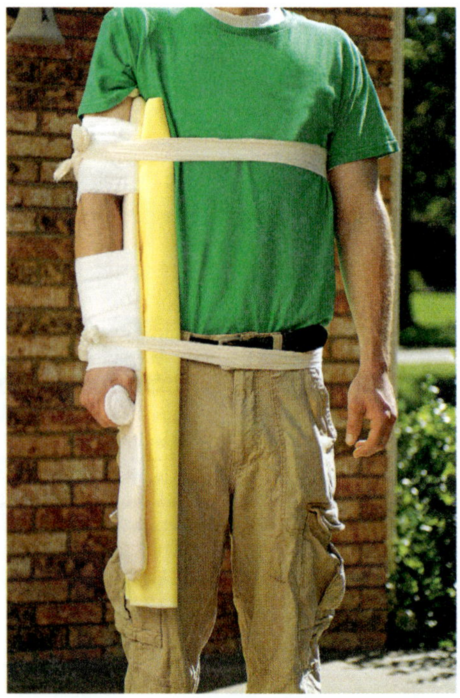

FIGURE 14-8h Injured elbow immobilized in a straight position.

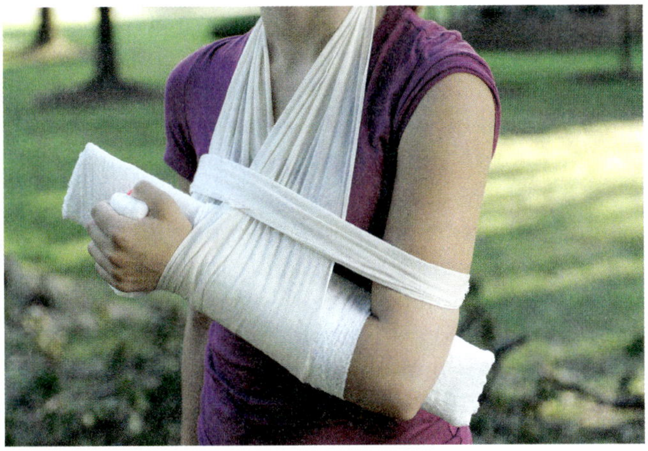

FIGURE 14-8i Immobilization of an injury to the forearm, wrist, or hand.

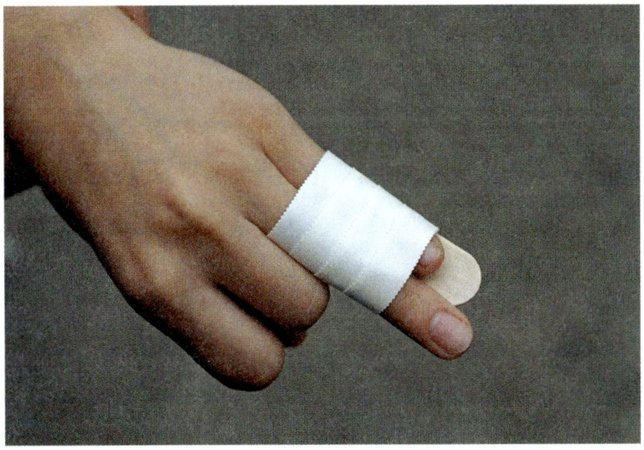

FIGURE 14-8j A tongue depressor used as a splint and then taped to an adjoining finger for stabilization.

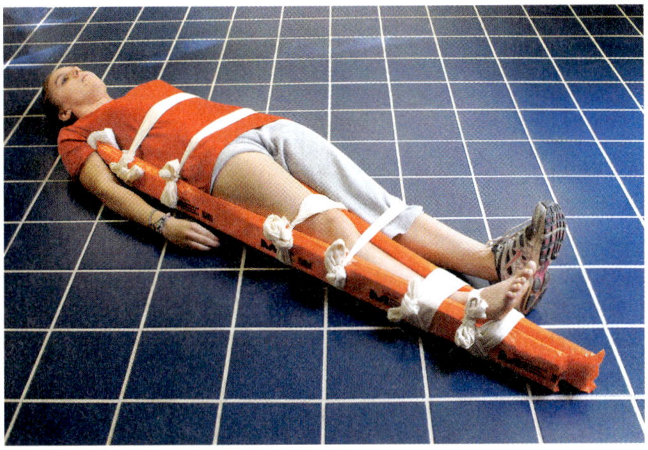

FIGURE 14-8k A high femur fracture immobilized in a fixation splint.

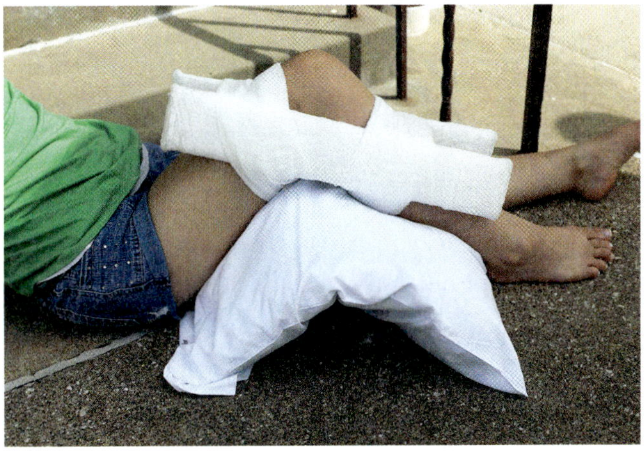

FIGURE 14-8l A splinted knee.

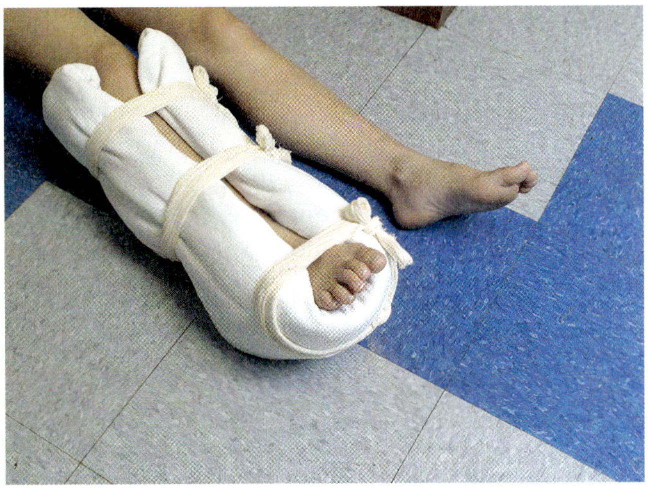

FIGURE 14-8m Blanket roll splint of the ankle and foot.

PEARLS: Spinal injuries

In major trauma, the axial skeleton is always splinted on a long backboard or appropriate scoop stretcher.

Rigid Splints. Rigid splints can be made from many different materials. They can be made of cardboard, hard plastic, metal, or wood. The type of splint that is made rigid by evacuating air from a moldable splint (vacuum splint) is also classified as a rigid splint. Rigid splints should be well padded over bony prominences and should always immobilize one joint above and one below the fracture.

Soft Splints. Soft splints include pillows, sling and swath-type splints, and air splints. Pillows make good splints for injuries to the ankle or foot, providing immobilization as well as padding to the injured area. Used with a sling and a swathe, they are useful for stabilizing a dislocated shoulder.

The sling and swathe are excellent for immobilizing injuries to the clavicle, shoulder, upper arm, elbow, and sometimes the forearm. They utilize the chest wall as a solid foundation and splint the arm against it. Some shoulder injuries cannot be brought close to the chest wall without applying significant force. In those instances, pillows are used to bridge the gap between the chest wall and the upper arm.

Air splints may be useful for fractures of the lower arm and lower leg. They provide compression, which helps to slow bleeding. Disadvantages include increasing pressure as the temperature rises or the altitude increases, inability to monitor distal pulses, and potential pain with removal. They should not be used on angulated fractures because they apply straightening pressure as they are inflated.

To apply an air splint it must be inflated by mouth or by pump (never by compressed air) until it provides good support, yet it can be dented easily with slight pressure from a fingertip. When using air splints, you must frequently check the pressure to be sure that the splint is not getting too tight or too loose (they often leak).

PEARLS: Shock

Be prepared for hemorrhagic shock when there is a pelvic or femur fracture.

Traction Splints. The traction splint is designed to stabilize fractures of the mid-femur. It holds the fracture immobile by the application of a steady pull on the ankle while applying countertraction to the ischium and the groin. This steady traction overcomes the tendency of the very strong thigh muscles to spasm. If traction is not applied, the pain worsens because the bone ends tend to impact or override. Traction also prevents free motion of the ends of the femur, which could lacerate the femoral nerve, artery, or vein.

There are many designs and types of splints available to apply traction to the lower extremity (Figure 14-9). Several of them are reviewed in Chapter 15. As with other splints, traction splints must be carefully padded and applied with care to prevent excessive pressure on the soft tissues around the pelvis.

Tourniquets

Tourniquets have returned to common use in both the military and tactical settings for uncontrollable extremity hemorrhage. They have been shown to improve survival and outcomes in these settings and are regaining acceptance in civilian use as well. Tourniquet use has been shown to be lifesaving in patients with shock due to massive blood loss from isolated extremity injuries, allowing for circulatory resuscitation. However, because tourniquets are designed to compress tissue and blood vessels to limit ongoing blood loss, they have significant consequences, and their use should be time limited, ideally to two hours or less. Complications can increase significantly after this time period, and ability to salvage the injured limb decreases.

Recommended indications for tourniquet use include significant extremity bleeding together with other ITLS Primary Survey issues (such as need for airway or breathing intervention, or shock), hostile environment, mass-casualty

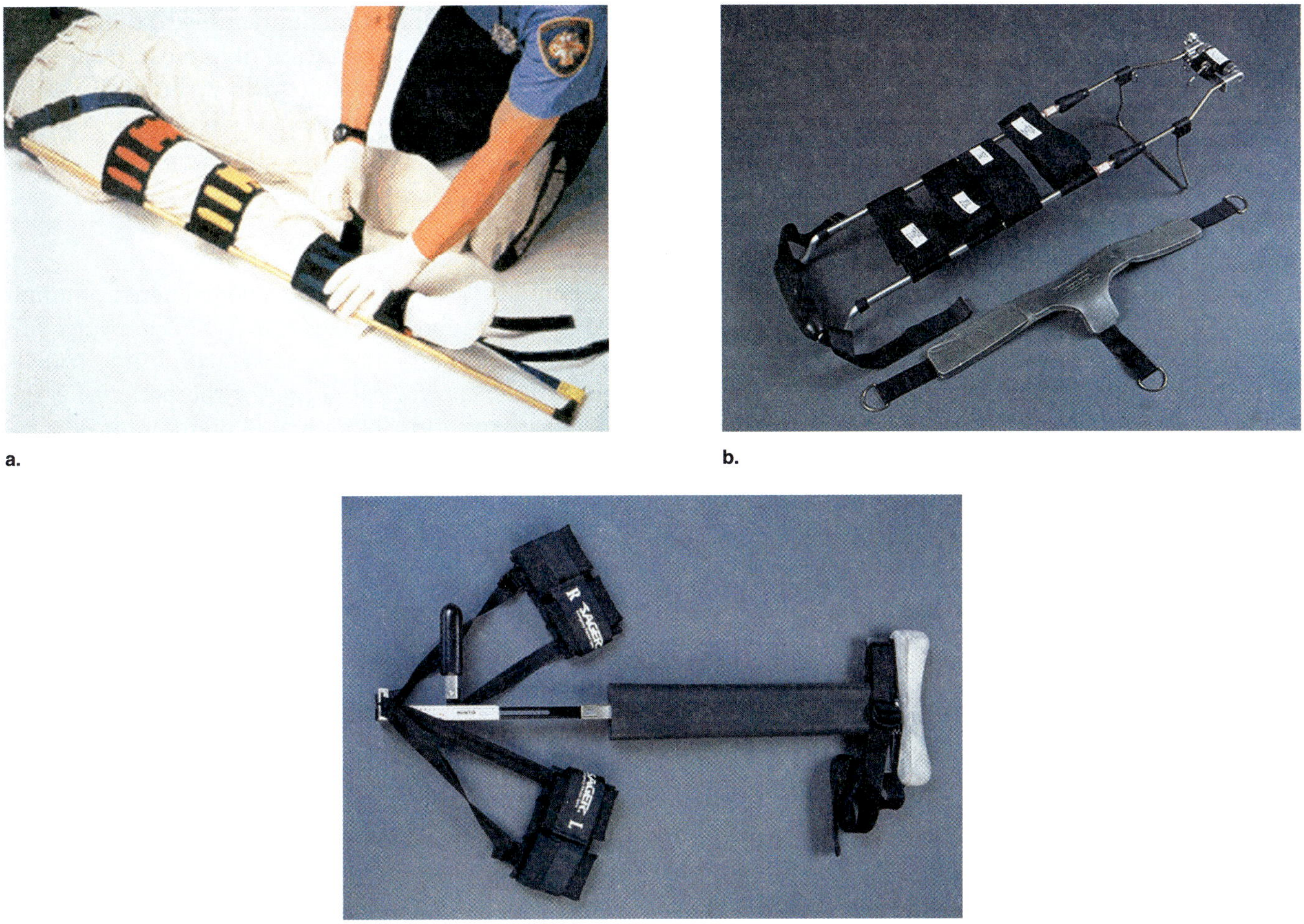

a. b. c.

FIGURE 14-9 (a) Kendrick traction device. *(Courtesy of Eduardo Romero Hicks, MD)* (b) Hare traction splint. (c) Sager traction splint.

event, or inability to manage bleeding with pressure dressings. In general, you should not remove a tourniquet you have placed for the indications noted.

You should follow the specific guidelines for the commercial tourniquet you are using. One of the most important factors is to ensure that all care providers are aware that a tourniquet has been applied to the patient. One method is to write "TK" and the time of application on the patient's forehead. Never cover a tourniquet. Commercial tourniquets offer advantages over improvised tourniquets, including rounded edges and a wider profile, which better distributes the pressure and limits damage to the tissues. Once you have placed a tourniquet, you should expedite transport to the trauma center.

Hemostatic Agents

For bleeding that is uncontrollable with direct pressure or the use of tourniquets, hemostatic agents have demonstrated the ability to reduce or stop bleeding through the promotion of clot formation. The form of the hemostatic agent (dressing, powder, packets, etc.) will depend on the specific product used. Regardless, direct application and pressure to the source of the bleeding vessel, not just the area of the wound, is required to maximize effectiveness.

Direct pressure should be maintained for a minimum of 2 minutes or until bleeding is controlled. Following cessation of bleeding, the application of a pressure dressing or gauze to the wound is recommended. To maximize effectiveness, it is recommended that prior to utilization of hemostatic agents, EMS personnel should become familiar with and follow the application instructions for each type of product used in practice.

Management of Specific Injuries

Spinal Injuries

Spinal injuries are covered in Chapter 11, but are briefly included here to remind you that if there is any chance of spinal injury, proper spinal motion restriction (SMR) must be used to prevent permanent disability or even death from a spinal-cord injury. In the most urgent cases, careful packaging of the patient on the long backboard may provide adequate splinting for a number of different extremity injuries. Remember that certain mechanisms of injury, such as a fall from a height in which the patient lands on both feet, may cause lumbar spine fracture because forces are transmitted from the heels through the legs and pelvis, all the way up to the spine.

Pelvis Injuries

It is practical to include injuries to the pelvis with extremities because they are frequently associated. Pelvic injuries are usually caused by motor-vehicle collisions or by severe trauma such as falls from heights. They are identified by instability or pain identified when gentle pressure is placed on the iliac crests, hips, and pubis during the ITLS Primary Survey. There is always the potential for serious hemorrhage in pelvic fractures, so shock should be expected, and the patient must be rapidly transported (load and go).

Internal bleeding from unstable pelvic fractures can be decreased by circumferential stabilization of the pelvis. Slings made from sheets have been used in the past for stabilization, but there are now several commercially available devices, which provide more consistent stabilization (Figure 14-10). Pelvic stabilization is most beneficial in an **open-book pelvic fracture** (Figure 14-2b) and decreases the need for blood transfusion.

Any patient with a pelvic injury should have SMR. The vacuum backboard is especially useful in these patients because it is much more comfortable than the

open-book pelvic fracture a severe pelvic fracture in which the symphysis is torn apart and the anterior pelvis is "opened" like a book. This is frequently associated with disruption of both sacro-iliac joints.

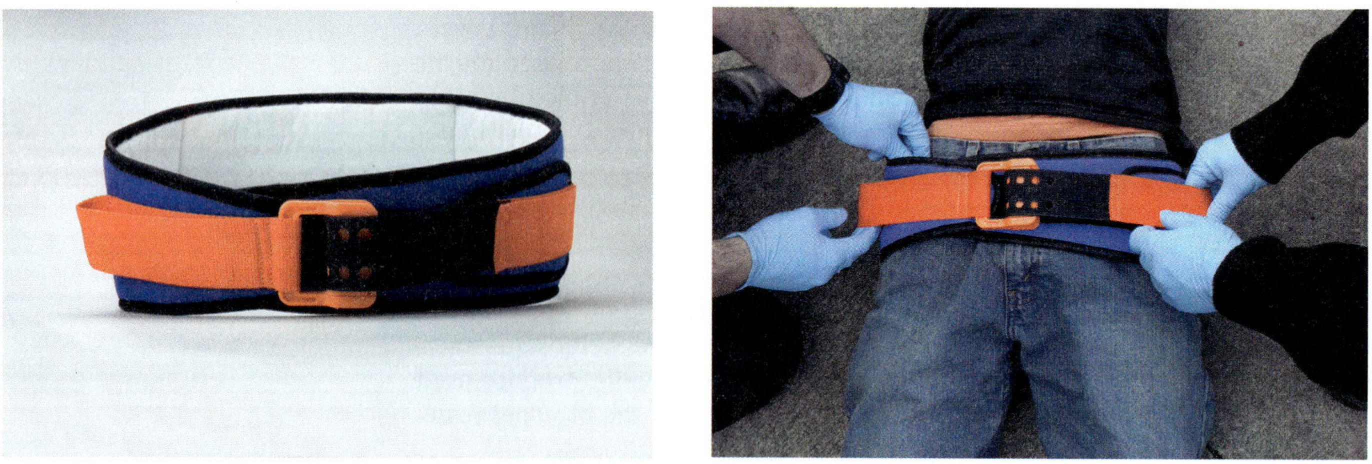

a. b.

FIGURE 14-10 (a) Commercial pelvic sling device. (b) Pelvic sling applied. *(Photos courtesy of Sam Splint)* hard backboard. Log-rolling a patient with an unstable pelvic fracture can aggravate the injury. Adequate assistance and tools such as the scoop stretcher, are potentially needed to move the patients to the backboard with limited pain and motion of the fractured pelvis. As mentioned in Chapter 2, some of the new, more rigid scoop stretchers provide SMR equal to a backboard (Figure 14-11).

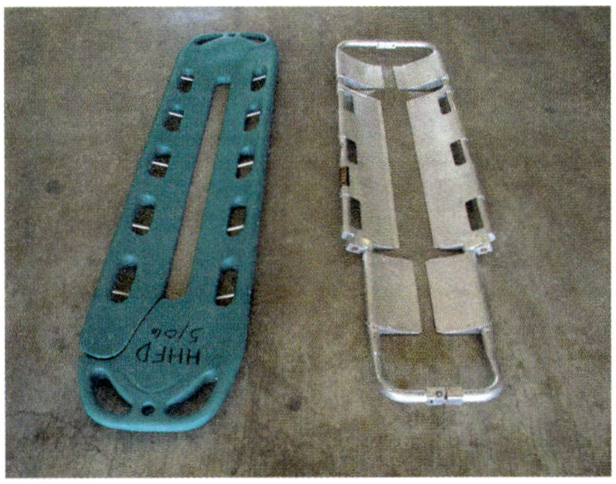

FIGURE 14-11 The scoop stretcher has been found to provide spinal stabilization equal to a backboard. *(Courtesy of Leon Charpentier, EMT-P; and Ferno Washington, Inc.)*

Femur Injuries

Femur fractures may have open wounds associated with them, and if so, they must be presumed to be open fractures. There is a lot of muscle tissue surrounding the femur, and when spasm develops after a femur fracture, it can cause the bone ends to override, causing more muscle damage, bleeding, potential nerve damage, and significant pain. Because of this, traction splints are usually used to stabilize mid-shaft femur fractures and limit additional injury and pain. As mentioned earlier, the large size of the thigh muscle can hide one to two liters of blood loss with each femur fracture. Bilateral femur fractures can be associated with a loss of up to 50% of the circulating blood volume.

Hip Injuries

Hip fractures are most often in the narrow "neck" of the femur, where strong ligaments may occasionally allow this type of fracture to bear weight. The ligaments are very strong, and there is very little movement of the bone ends in the most frequent type of hip fracture. You must consider hip fractures in any elderly person who has fallen and has pain in the knee, hip, or pelvic region. A geriatric patient who has fallen and cannot bear weight should be assumed to have a pelvic or hip fracture. The affected leg will often (but not always) be externally rotated and shortened. In the geriatric patient, fracture pain may be well tolerated and sometimes even ignored or denied. In general, the tissues in the elderly patient are more delicate, and less force is required to disrupt a given structure. Remember that isolated knee pain may well be coming from damage to the hip. Do not use a traction splint for a hip fracture.

The hip may be dislocated either posteriorly or anteriorly. Posterior hip dislocations are most common and can result when the knee is struck by the dashboard, forcing the relatively loose, relaxed hip out of the posterior side of its cup in the pelvis (Figure 14-12). Thus, any patient in a severe automobile crash with a knee injury must have the hip examined very carefully. Posterior hip dislocation is an orthopedic emergency and requires reduction as soon as possible to prevent sciatic nerve injury or necrosis of the femoral head due to interrupted blood supply.

The posteriorly dislocated hip usually is flexed, and the patient will not be able to tolerate having the leg straightened. The leg will almost invariably be rotated toward the midline. A posterior hip dislocation should be supported in the most comfortable position by the use of pillows and by splinting to the uninjured leg (Figure 14-13).

Anterior hip dislocations are rare because of the complex mechanism required to produce this injury. The patient with an anterior hip dislocation will present with external rotation of the affected leg much like a fractured hip, except you may not be able to bring the leg forward in line with the body. It may be very difficult to place this person in the supine position on a backboard or on the stretcher in the ambulance. Whereas the posterior hip

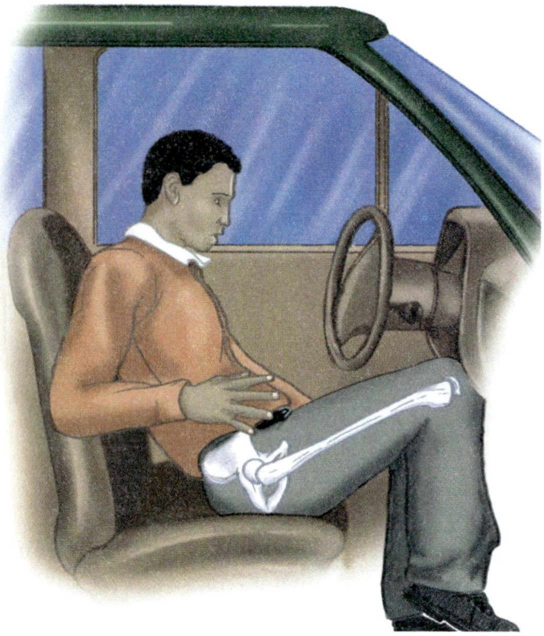

FIGURE 14-12 Mechanism of posterior dislocation of the hip, "down and under."

dislocation puts pressure on the sciatic nerve, the anterior hip dislocation puts pressure on the femoral artery and vein. If the vein has collapsed, a clot can form distally, producing a large pulmonary embolus as soon as the hip is reduced.

Knee Injuries

Fractures or dislocations of the knee (Figure 14-14) are quite serious because the blood vessels and nerves that cross the knee joint are often injured if the joint is in an abnormal position. There is no way to know whether a fracture exists in an abnormally positioned knee and, in either case, the decision must be based on the circulation and neurological function distally in the foot.

A significant number of knee dislocations have associated artery and nerve injury. It is important to restore the circulation below the knee as quickly as

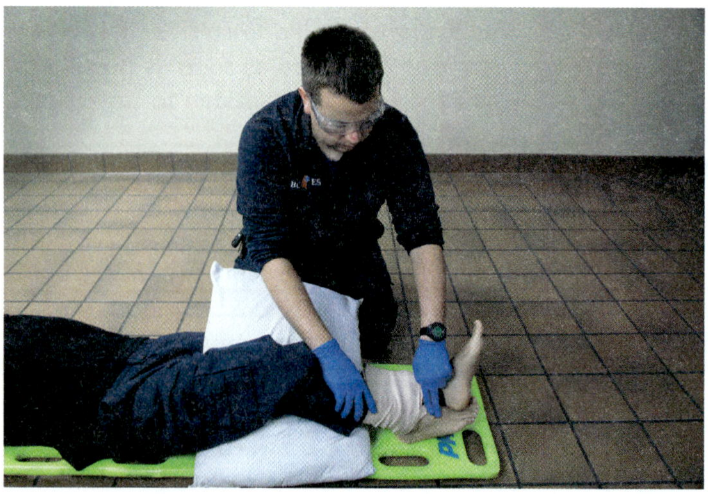

FIGURE 14-13 Splinting posterior dislocation of the hip. *(Courtesy of Louis B. Mallory, MBA, REMT-P)*

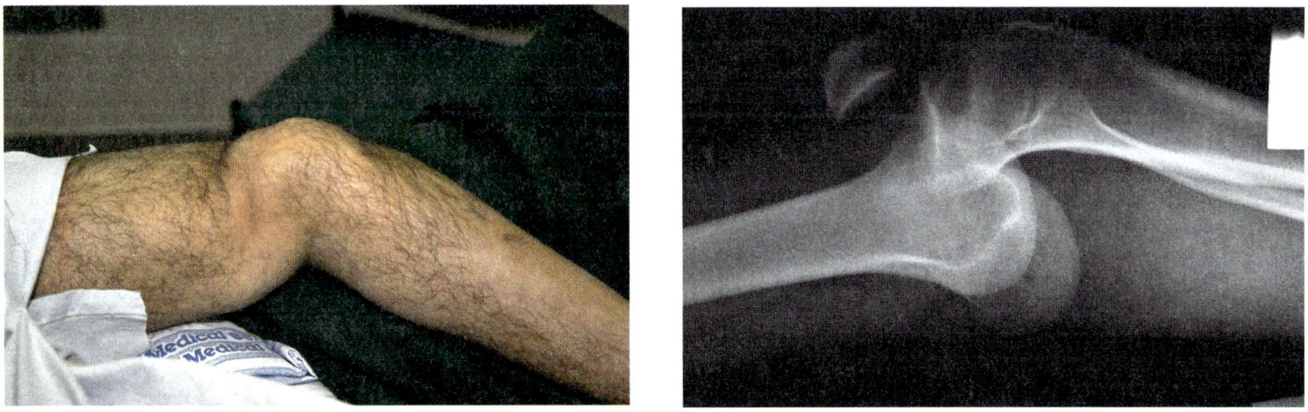

a. b.

FIGURE 14-14 Knee dislocation. (a) Presentation of a knee dislocation. (b) X-ray of the dislocation. *(Photos ©Edward T. Dickinson, MD)*

possible and to transport the patient rapidly to definitive care to avoid devastating complications like amputation. Because of this, prompt reduction of knee dislocation is very important. If there is loss of pulse or sensation, apply gentle traction by hand. Traction must be applied along the long axis of the leg. If there is resistance to straightening the knee, splint it in the most comfortable position and transport the patient rapidly. Knee dislocation is a true orthopedic emergency.

Do not confuse knee joint dislocation with patellar dislocation. The patella can dislocate to the side, and the affected leg will be held slightly flexed at the knee. You can easily see that the patella is out of place. Although painful, this is not a serious injury and should simply be splinted with a pillow under the knee and taken to the emergency department. Straightening the leg usually reduces the patella dislocation, and often the patient will spontaneously reduce this injury prior to your arrival.

Tibia and Fibula Injuries

Fractures of the lower leg are often open. Over time, swelling and internal hemorrhage can cause compartment syndrome. It is rarely possible for patients to bear weight on fractures of the tibia, but fractures of the distal fibula can be mistaken for sprains. Fractures of the lower leg and ankle may be splinted with a rigid splint, an air splint, or a pillow. As with other fractures, it is important to dress any wound, pad any bone ends under a splint, and manage the patient's pain. A dislocation of the ankle may require a gentle attempt at reduction if there is loss of circulation in the foot and you have a very long transport.

Clavicle Injuries

The clavicle is the most frequently fractured bone in the body, with injury most common in the middle third of the bone. Clavicular injuries rarely cause major complications (Figure 14-15), though rarely, there may be associated injuries to the subclavian blood vessels or to the nerves of the arm. You should carefully assess a patient with a clavicle fracture for other, more significant, chest wall injuries. This injury is best immobilized with a sling and swathe.

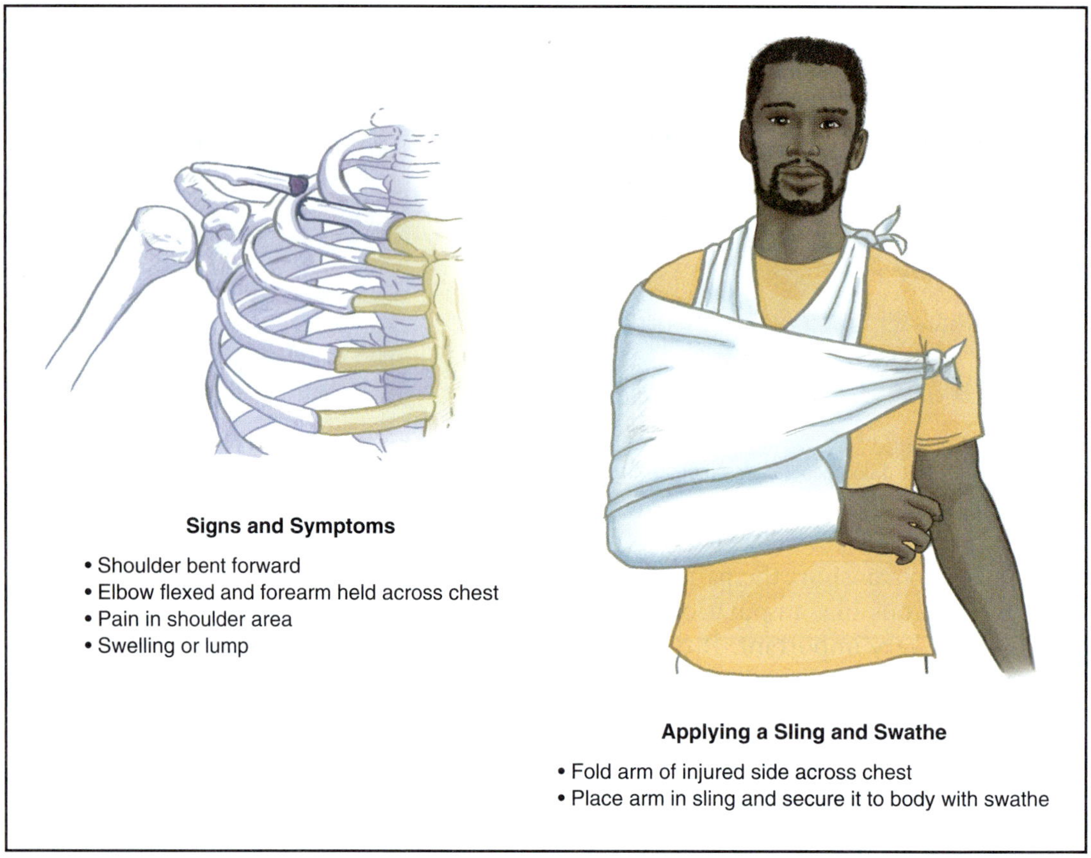

FIGURE 14-15 Fractured clavicle.

Shoulder Injuries

Most shoulder injuries are not life threatening, but because of the force required, they may be associated with severe injuries of the chest or neck. Many shoulder injuries are dislocations or separations of joint spaces and may show up as a defect at the upper outer portion of the shoulder. The upper humerus is fractured with some degree of frequency, however. The radial nerve travels quite closely around the humerus and may be injured in humeral fractures. Injury to the radial nerve results in an inability of the patient to lift the hand (wrist drop).

Dislocated shoulders are very painful and quite often require a pillow between the arm and body to hold the upper arm in the most comfortable position. Shoulders that are held in abnormal positions should never be forced into a more anatomic alignment (Figure 14-16). Scapular fractures may refer injury to the shoulder joint itself. Because considerable force is required to fracture the scapula, anyone who may have this injury should be carefully evaluated for other chest injuries such as rib fractures and pulmonary contusion.

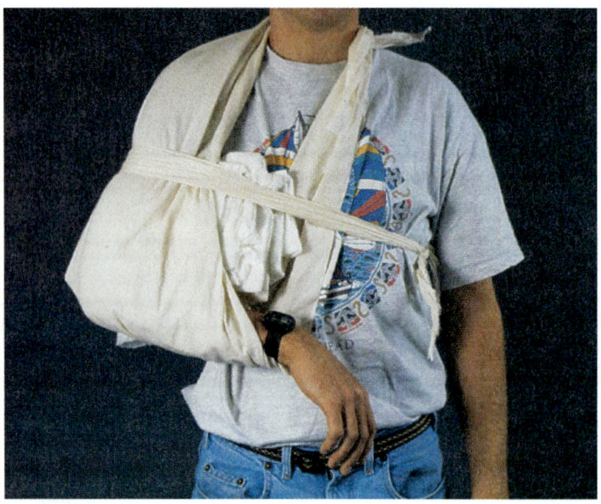

FIGURE 1 4-16 Dislocated shoulder.

Elbow Injuries

It may be difficult to see the difference between a fracture and a dislocation. Both can be serious because of the danger of damage to the vessels and nerves that run across the flexor surface of the elbow. The most common mechanism of injury is a fall onto an outstretched arm. Elbow injuries should always be

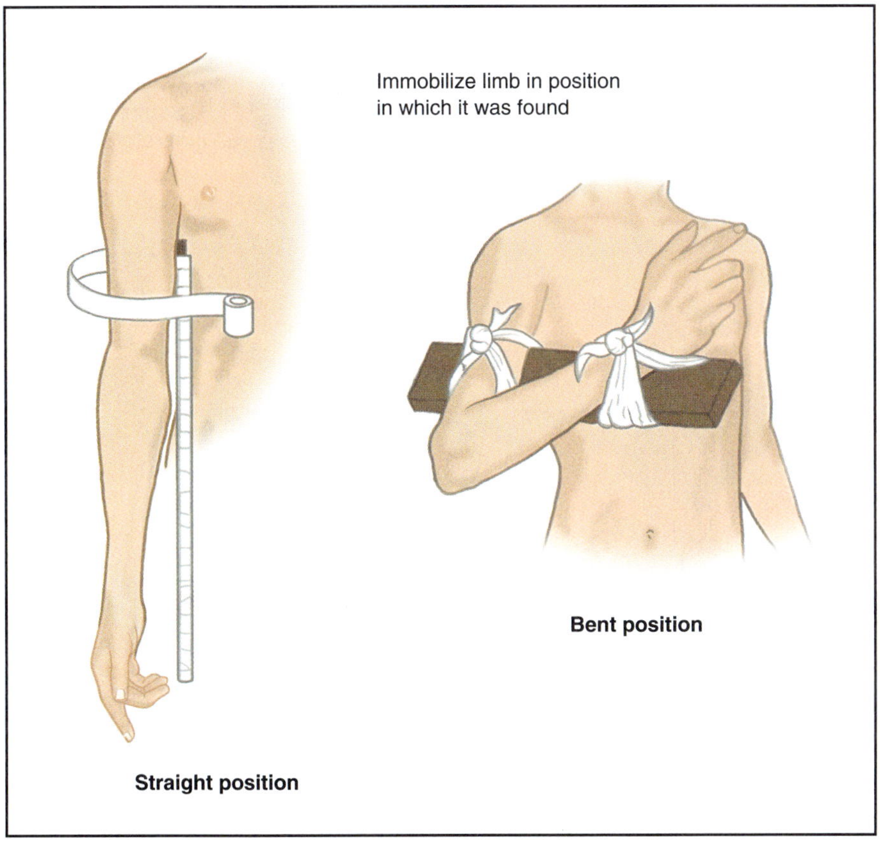

FIGURE 14-17 Fractures or dislocations of the elbow.

splinted in the most comfortable position and the distal function clearly evaluated (Figure 14-17). Never attempt to straighten or apply traction to an elbow injury due to the complexity of the anatomy.

Forearm and Wrist Injuries

Fractures to the forearm and wrist are very common (Figure 14-18). Like elbow injuries, a common mechanism is a fall onto an outstretched arm. Usually, such a

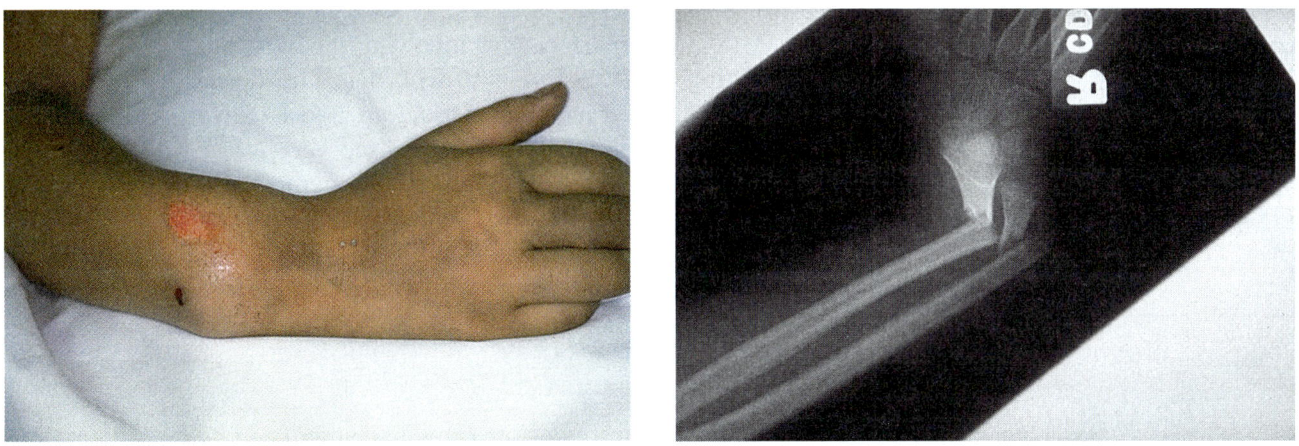

a. b.

FIGURE 14-18 Presentation of a forearm fracture. (a) A fracture will often present with deformity. (b) An x-ray of the fracture.

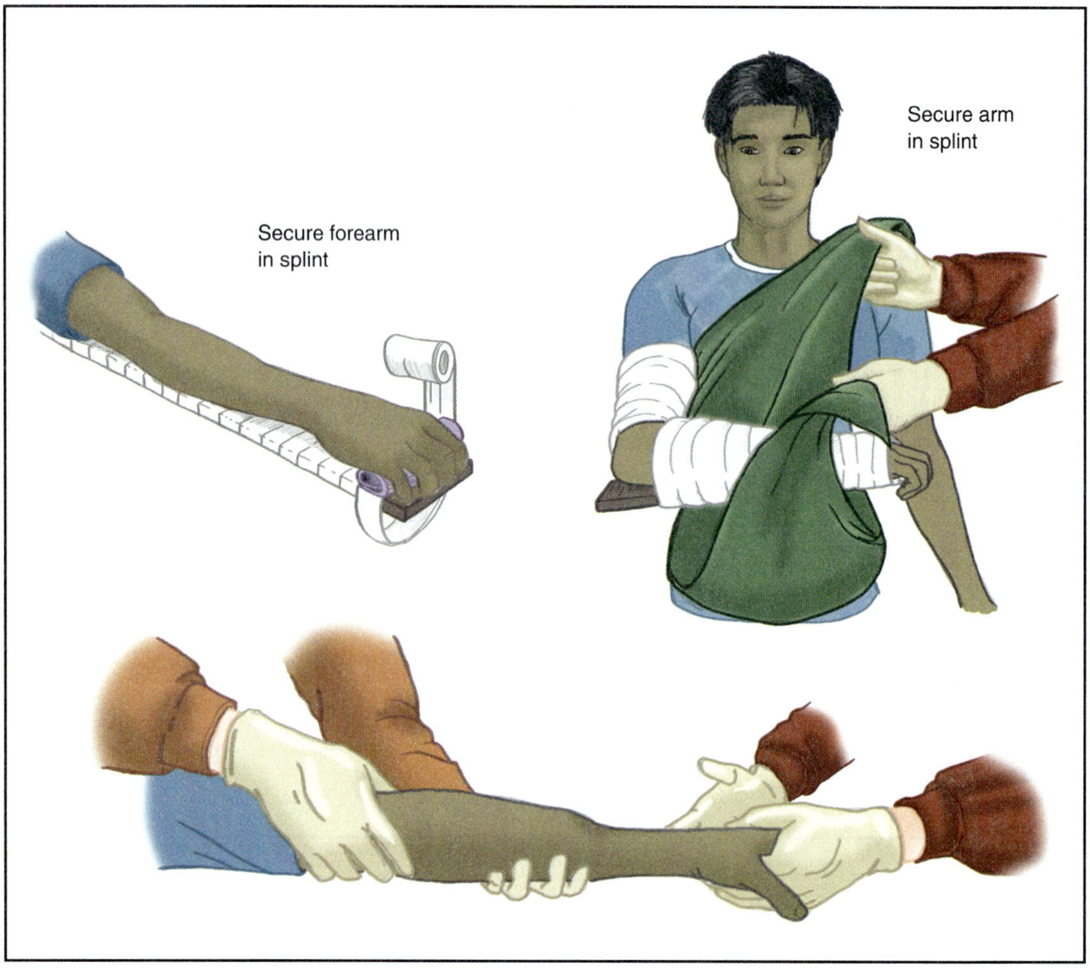

FIGURE 14-19 Fractures of the forearm and wrist.

fracture is best immobilized with a rigid splint or an air splint (Figure 14-19). If a rigid splint is used, a roll of gauze in the hand will hold the arm in the most comfortable position of function. Forearm fractures also put the patient at risk for compartment syndrome.

Hand or Foot Injuries

Many industrial accidents involving the hand or the foot produce multiple open fractures and avulsions. The injuries are often gruesome in appearance but are seldom associated with life-threatening bleeding. A pillow may be used very effectively to support them (Figure 14-20). An alternative method of dressing the hand is to insert a roll of gauze in the palm, then arrange the fingers and thumb in their position of function (Figure 14-21a). The entire hand is then wrapped as though it were a ball inside a very large and bulky dressing (Figure 14-21b).

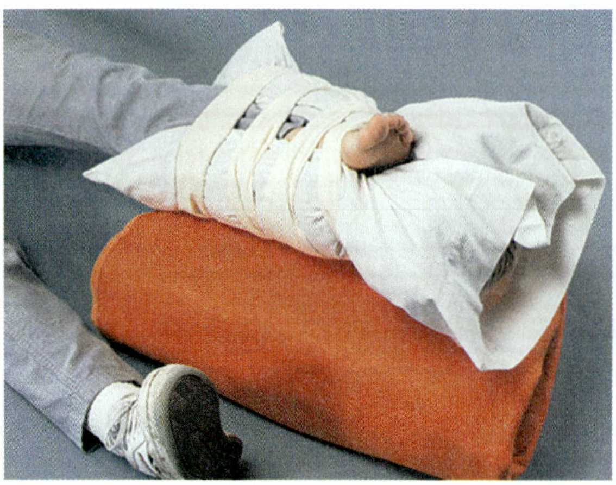

FIGURE 14-20 Pillow splinting an injured foot.

Crush Injuries

Performing frequent ongoing assessments and close monitoring of vital signs is required with patients who have experienced a crush injury. To effectively address the toxins released and

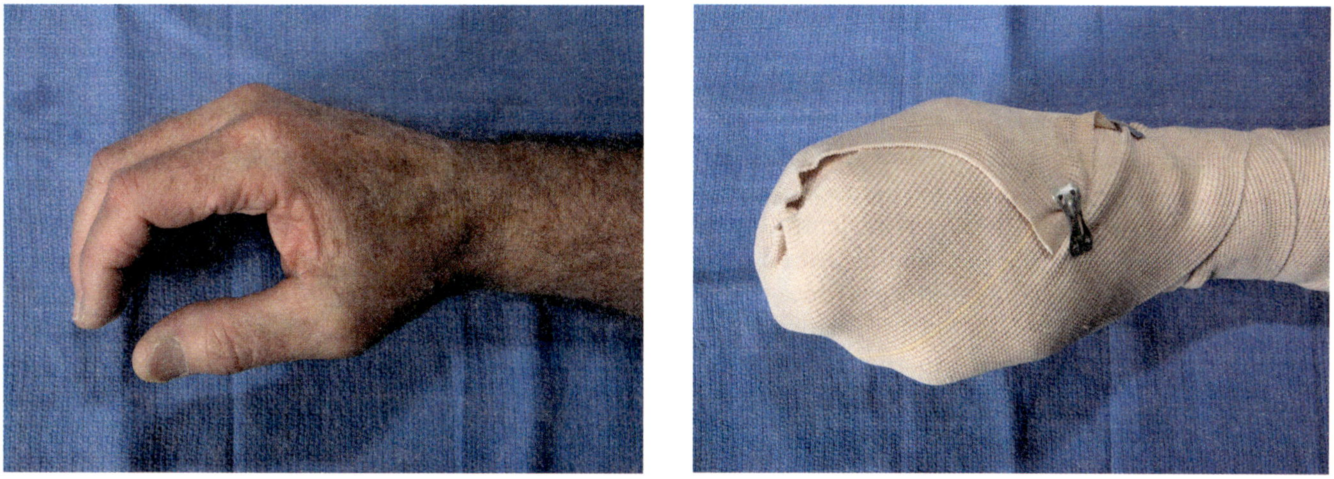

a.

b.

FIGURE 14-21 (a) Hand in position of function. (b) Hand dressing. *(Photos courtesy of Stanley Cooper, EMT-P)*

reduce the risk of crush syndrome, alkalizing the blood is necessary. This is accomplished through delivery of large volumes of intravenous fluids and potential utilization of alkalizing agents such as sodium bicarbonate and osmotic diuretics such as mannitol. The addition of sodium bicarbonate to a bag of normal saline solution versus bolus administration is preferred.

Initial administration of sodium bicarbonate should be at 1 mEq/kg followed by an infusion of 0.25 mEq/kg/hr. If administration of fluids or medications prior to releasing the entrapped body area is not possible, consider application of a tourniquet proximal to the injury site on the extremity. Although application of the tourniquet will reduce systemic toxin release, crush syndrome will continue to develop. Early contact with medical direction or the receiving trauma facility is recommended for all patients who have experienced a crush injury.

CASE PRESENTATION (continued)

An ALS ambulance has been dispatched to a nearby national park where a hiker was injured when a large rock fell on his leg. On arrival, they are met by other hikers who advise that the patient is unable to walk and is located about 15 minutes away in the wilderness. When the team arrives at the patient's location, they find him lying on the ground, holding his left leg. The scene is safe. He is the only patient.

As the ambulance crew approaches, their general impression is good. Initial assessment reveals a patient who is awake, cooperative, and in obvious pain. He says he slipped and fell while trying to climb to the top of a rock outcropping. A fairly large rock was dislodged, and it fell onto his left lower leg. He has a strong, slightly elevated radial pulse. Because of the patient's fall, the team leader performs a rapid trauma survey, which reveals that there is no deformity of the neck and the neck veins are flat. The chest has no apparent injuries, and breath sounds are present and equal. Heart sounds are easily heard. The abdomen is soft, and the patient does not have pain when the abdomen is palpated. The pelvis is stable, but the patient has a significant deformity of his lower left leg and foot.

The patient advises that he was injured about an hour ago and had to wait until some other hikers walked by with a cell phone, and they called for help. Because no life-threatening injuries were identified in the rapid trauma survey, the team leader continues with a focused exam of the patient's left leg. He begins by exposing the leg while Rescuer 2 obtains vital signs and completes the SAMPLE history.

They cut the patient's pant leg to above the knee, and stabilize the significant distal lower leg deformity, while carefully removing the patient's shoe and sock so they can assess PMS. After exposure, it is clear there is a likely fracture—dislocation of the distal lower leg and ankle, and although there are no open wounds noted, there is bruising and swelling of the calf. The patient has intact movement of his toes with significant pain, but pulses are difficult to find, and capillary refill is delayed, though sensation remains intact. The foot and knee appear uninjured.

The team is concerned about the lack of circulation distal to the fracture, and the significant time that has already passed. Before extricating the patient from the woods, the leader elects to try gentle traction to the leg in an effort to restore distal circulation. Prior to the attempt, Rescuer 2 initiates intravenous access and the patient is given morphine for pain.

Following traction, they are successful in restoring the dorsalis pedis pulse and improved capillary refill. The ankle is now aligned more normally, and it is splinted with plenty of padding over the bony prominences. The patient is extricated from the woods.

On reassessment in the ambulance prior to transport, the patient complains of significantly increasing pain, and the onset of tingling in his toes. Because of the closed lower extremity fracture and the prolonged prehospital time, the team is concerned that the patient may be developing compartment syndrome. The leader elevates the leg above the patient's heart to limit additional swelling and administers an additional dose of IV morphine for pain.

By the time they arrive at the hospital, the patient is nearly two hours postinjury, and his pain continues to be severe despite the team's efforts, although pulses and movement remain intact. On x-ray the patient is found to have a closed fracture of the distal tibia and fibula and a now reduced ankle dislocation. Evaluation of his compartments reveals increased pressure, and the patient is emergently taken for fasciotomy and repair of his orthopedic injury. After a prolonged course, the patient has recovered the ability to walk with a cane. ■

Summary

Although usually not life threatening, extremity injuries can be disabling. These injuries may be more dramatic than more serious internal injuries, but do not let them distract you from following the usual steps of the ITLS Primary Survey. The exception is that pelvic and femur fractures can be associated with life-threatening internal bleeding, so patients with these injuries are in the load-and-go category.

Proper splinting is important to protect the injured extremity from further injury. Dislocations of elbows, hips, and knees require careful splinting and rapid reduction to prevent severe disability. They are frequently load-and-go situations, not because they are life threatening, but because they are limb threatening. A high index of suspicion and early intervention for crush injuries are paramount to reducing the harmful effects of crush syndrome.

Bibliography

1. Abarbanell, N. R. 2001. Prehospital midthigh trauma and traction splint use: Recommendations for treatment protocols. *American Journal of Emergency Medicine.* 19(2): 137–140.
2. American College of Surgeons Committee on Trauma. 2004. *Advanced trauma life support.* Chicago: American College of Surgeons, 205–30.
3. Brown, D. M., J. Worley. 2007. Experience with chitosan dressings in a civilian EMS system. *Journal of Emergency Medicine*, Elsevier, Inc. In Press, Corrected Proof, Available online 19 November 2007.
4. Bledsoe, B. E., R. S. Porter, R. A. Cherry. 2009. *Paramedic care; principles and practice*, 3rd ed., pp. 884–886. Upper Saddle River, NJ: Pearson Education.
5. Bledsoe, B., D. Barnes. 2004. Traction splint. An EMS relic? *JEMS* 29(8): 64–69.
6. Brodie, S., T. J. Hodgetts, J. Ollerton, J. McLeod, P. Lambert, P. Mahoney. 2007. Tourniquet use in combat trauma: UK military experience. *J R Army Med Corps* 153: 310–313.
7. Cross, D. A., J. Baskerville. 2001. Comparison of perceived pain with different immobilization techniques. *Prehospital Emergency Care* 5(3): 270–274.
8. Dayan, L., Zinmann, C., Stahl, S., Norman, D. (2008). Complications associated with prolonged tourniquet application on the battlefield. *Military Medicine* 173(1): 63–66.
9. Demetriades, D., et al. 2002. Pelvic fractures: epidemiology and predictors of associated abdominal injuries and outcomes. *J Am Coll Surg* 195: 1–10.
10. Dischinger, P. C., K. Read, J. Kerns, et al. 2004. Consequences and costs of lower extremity injuries. *Annual Proceedings of the Association for the Advancement of Automotive Medicine* 48: 339–353.
11. Doyle G. S., P. P. Taillac. 2008. Tourniquets: A review of current use with proposals for expanded prehospital use. *Prehospital Emergency Care* 12: 241–256.
12. Friese, G., G. LeMay. 2005. Emergency stabilization of unstable pelvic fractures. *Emergency Medical Services* 34(5): 67–71.
13. Greaves, I., K. Porter, J. E. Smith 2003. Consensus statement on the early management of crush injury and prevention of crush syndrome. *Journal of the Royal Army Medical Corps* 149(4): 255–259.
14. Heightman, A. 2006. From the editor: Out of sight, out of mind. *JEMS* 31(7): 2006.
15. Baek, S. M., S. S. Kim. 1992. Successful digital replantation after 42 hours of warm ischemia. *J Reconstr Microsurg* 8: 455–458.

16. Krell, J. M., et al. 2006. Comparison of the Ferno scoop stretcher with the long backboard for spinal immobilization. *Prehospital Emergency Care* 10: 46–51.

17. Roberts, J. R. 2009. Prehospital immobilization: Lower extremity splinting in *Clinical procedures in emergency medicine*, Chap 46, 5th ed. Philadelphia: Saunders.

18. Walters, T. J., R. I. Mabry. 2005. Issues related to the use of tourniquets on the battlefield. *Military Medicine* 170(9): 770–775.

19. Wedmore, I., J. G. McManus, A. E. Pusateri, J. E. Holcomb. 2006. A special report on the chitosan-based hemostatic dressing: Experience in current combat operations. *Journal of Trauma* 60(3): 655–658.

Explore Resource Central

For additional review and practice tests, visit www.bradybooks.com and click on Resource Central to access book-specific resources for this text. To access Resource Central, follow directions on the Student Access Card provided with this text. If there is no card, go to www.bradybooks.com and follow the Resource Central link to Buy Access from there.

Extremity Trauma Skills

Donna Hastings, EMT-P
S. Robert Seitz, M Ed, RN, NREMT-P

(Photo courtesy of Regien Paassen, Shutterstock.com)

Extremity Trauma

Trauma alle Estremità

Traumatismo de Extremidades

Traumatisme d'extrémité

Obrażenia kończyn

Extremitäten Trauma

Ozljede ekstremiteta

إصابات الأطراف

trauma ekstremiteta

Poškodbe okončin

Végtagsérülés

OBJECTIVES

Upon successful completion of this chapter, you should be able to:

1. Explain when to use a traction splint.
2. Describe the complications of using a traction splint.
3. Apply the most common traction splints:
    a. Thomas splint
    b. Hare splint
    c. Sager splint
4. Demonstrate pelvic stabilization techniques.
5. Explain the use of and demonstrate the application of tourniquets on a mannequin model.
6. Explain the use of and demonstrate the application of hemostatic agents on a mannequin model.

Traction Splints

Traction splints are designed to immobilize fractures of the femur. They are not useful for fractures of the hip, knee, or lower leg. Applying firm traction to a fractured or dislocated knee may tear the blood vessels behind the knee. If there appears to be a pelvic fracture, you cannot use a traction splint because it may cause further damage to the pelvis. Fractures below the mid-thigh that are not angulated or severely shortened may just as well be immobilized by air splints.

Traction splints work by applying a padded device to the back of the pelvis (ischium) or to the groin. A hitching device is then applied to the ankle, and countertraction is applied until the limb is straight and well immobilized. Apply the splints to the pelvis and groin very carefully to prevent excessive pressure on the genitalia. Also use care when attaching the hitching device to the foot and ankle so as not to interfere with circulation.

To prevent any unnecessary movement, do not apply traction splints until the patient is on a long backboard. If the splint extends beyond the end of the backboard, be very careful when moving the patient and when closing the ambulance door so that you do not hit the splint and cause movement in the fracture site. You must check the circulation in the injured leg, so remove the shoe before attaching the hitching device.

In every case at least two people are needed to apply traction. One must hold steady, gentle traction on the foot and leg while the other applies the splint. When dealing with load-and-go situations, do not apply the splint until the patient is in the ambulance (unless the ambulance has not arrived).

PROCEDURE

Applying a Thomas Traction Splint (Half-Ring Splint)

The Thomas splint was used exclusively prior to the advent of modern traction devices. During World War I, its use decreased the mortality rate for battlefield femur fractures from 80% to 40%. At that time it was considered one of the greatest advancements in medical care. It is still used in some countries and in the absence of other options. To apply a Thomas traction splint, follow these steps (Figure 15-1):

1. Have your partner support the leg and maintain gentle traction while you cut away the clothing and remove the shoe and sock to check the pulse and sensation at the foot.
2. Position the splint under the injured leg. The ring goes down, and the short side goes to the inside of the leg. Slide the ring snugly up under the hip, where it will be pressed against the ischial tuberosity.
3. Attach the top ring strap.
4. Apply padding to the foot and ankle.
5. Apply the traction hitch around the foot and ankle (Figure 15-2).
6. Maintain gentle traction by hand.
7. Attach the traction hitch to the end of the splint.
8. Increase traction by Spanish windlass action, using a stick or tongue depressors.
9. Position two support straps above the knee and two below the knee. Do not place over fracture site.
10. Release manual traction and reassess circulation and sensation.
11. Support the end of the splint so that there is no pressure on the heel.

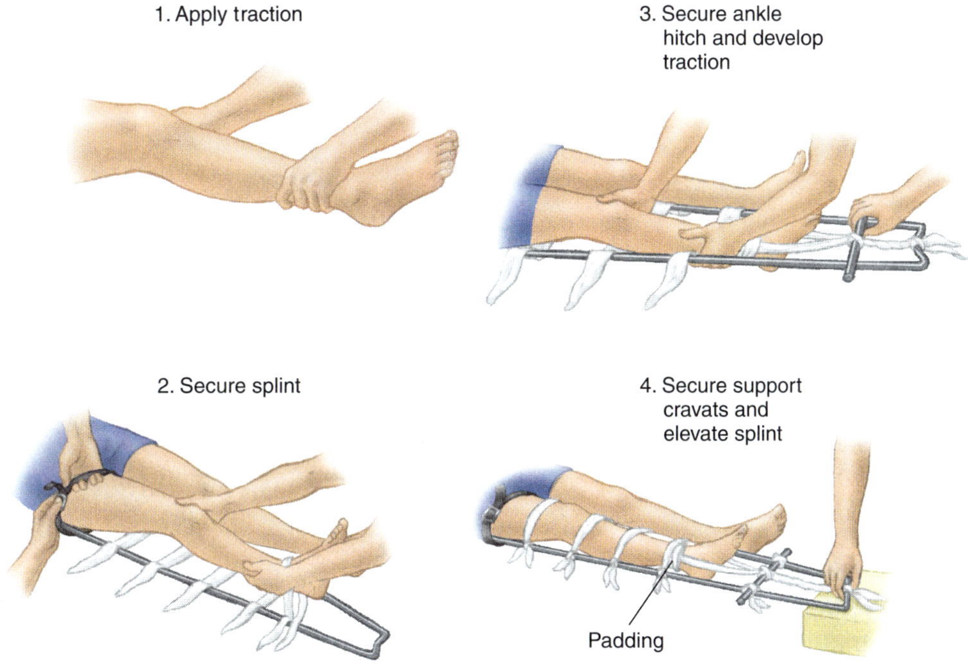

FIGURE 15-1 Applying a Thomas traction splint.

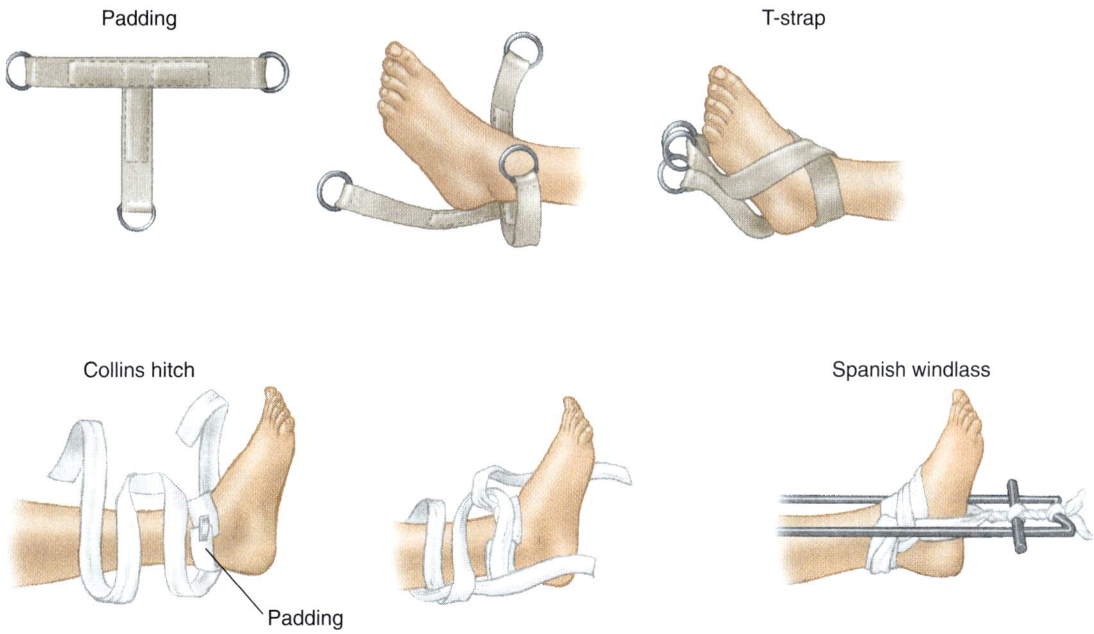

FIGURE 15-2 Applying a traction hitch to the ankle.

PROCEDURE

Applying a Hare Traction Splint

The Hare traction splint is the modern version of the Thomas splint. To apply the Hare traction splint, follow these steps (Scan 15-1):

SCAN 15-1 Applying a Hare Traction Splint

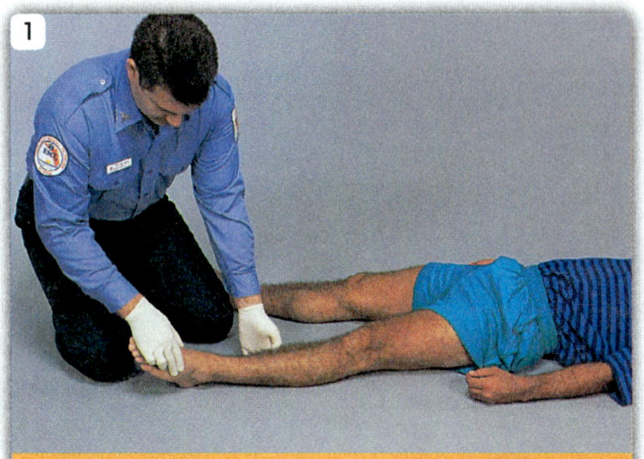

Assess distal pulses and motor and sensory function.

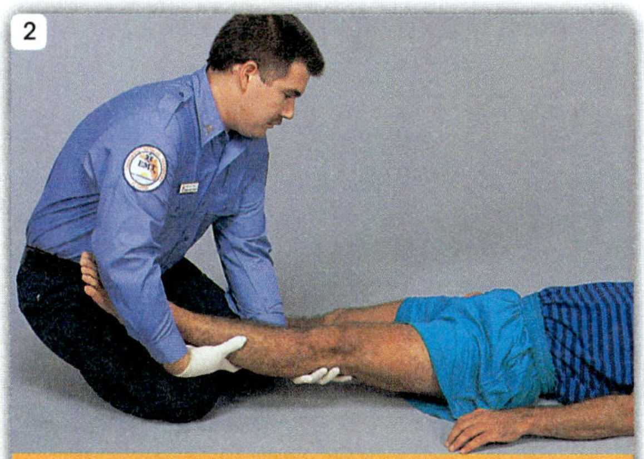

Stabilize the injured leg by applying manual traction.

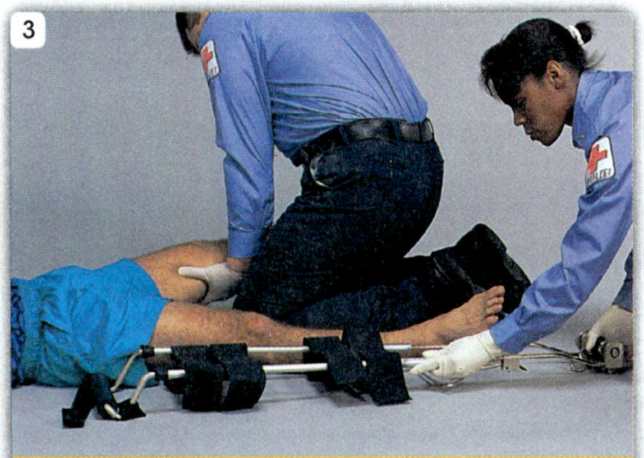

Adjust the splint for proper length.

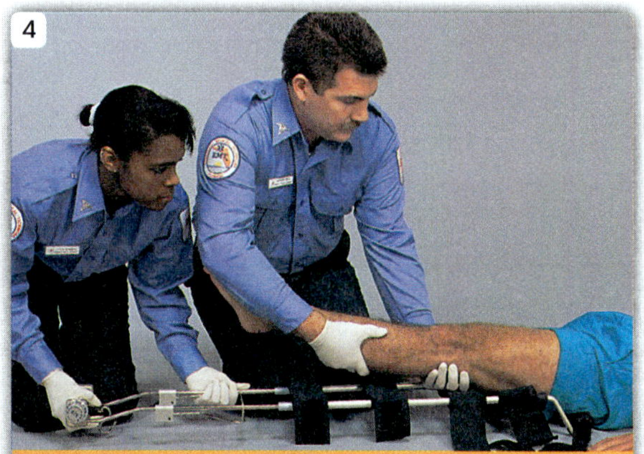

Position the splint under the injured leg until the ischial pad rests against the bony prominence of the buttocks. Once the splint is in position, raise the heel stand.

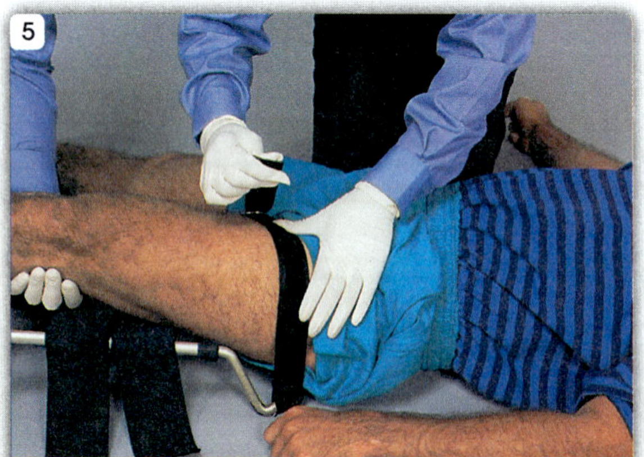

Attach the ischial strap over the groin and thigh.

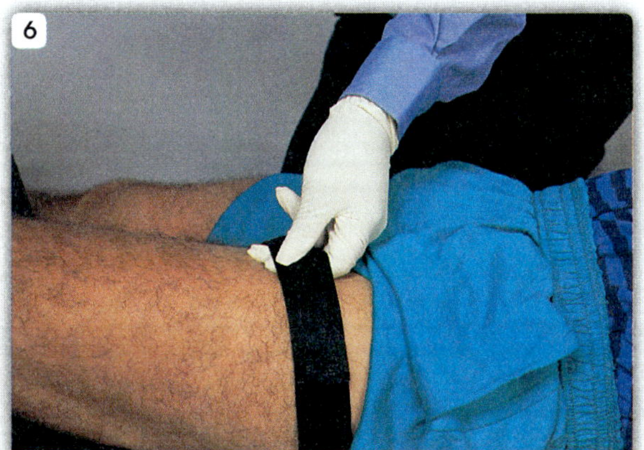

Make sure the ischial strap is snug but not tight enough to reduce distal circulation.

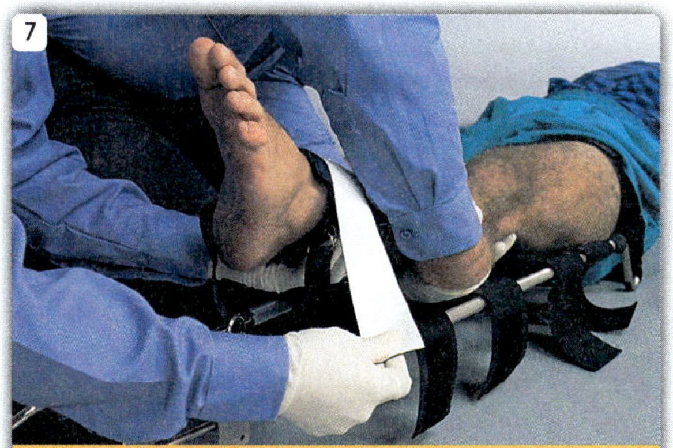

With the patient's foot in an upright position, secure the ankle hitch.

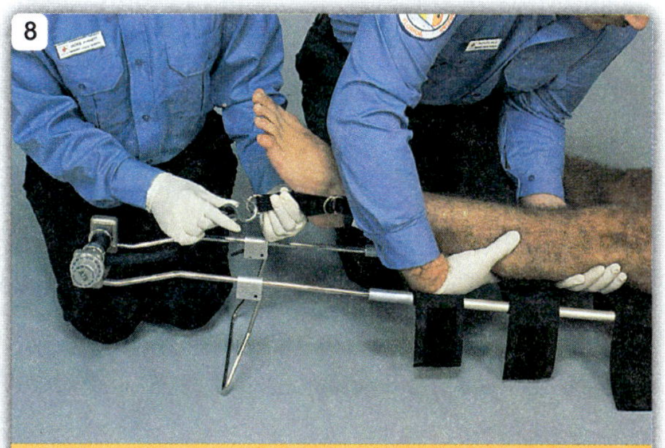

Attach the S-hook to the D-ring and apply mechanical traction. Full traction is achieved when the mechanical traction is equal to the manual traction and the pain and muscle spasms are reduced. In an unresponsive patient, adjust the traction until the injured leg is the same length as the uninjured leg.

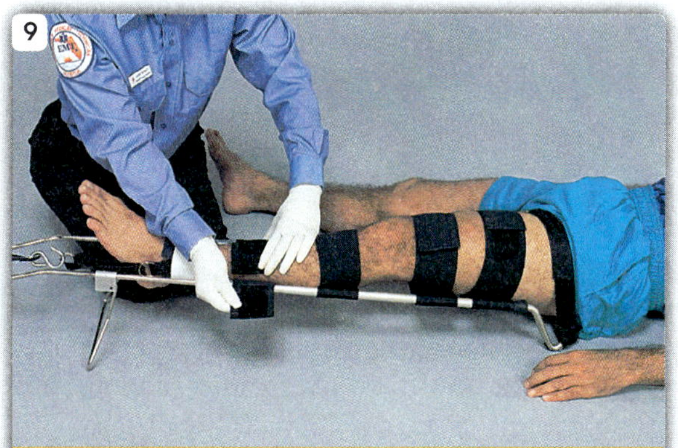

Fasten the leg support straps.

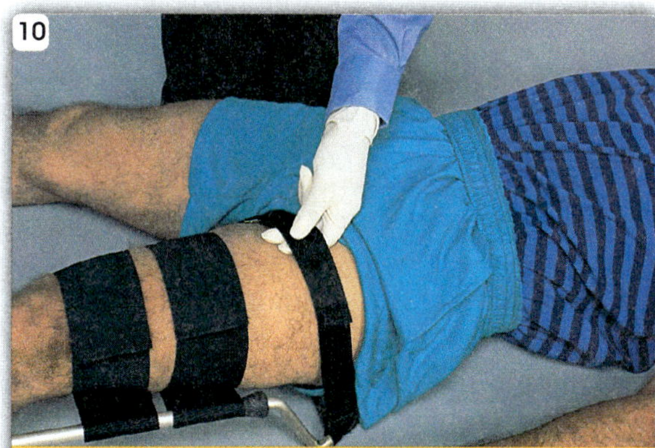

Reevaluate the ischial strap and ankle hitch to ensure that both are securely fastened.

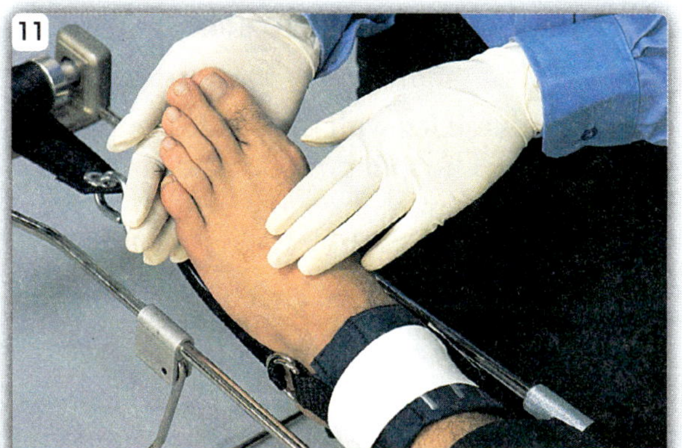

Reassess distal pulses, motor function, and sensation.

1. Position the patient on the backboard or stretcher.
2. Have your partner support the leg and maintain gentle traction, while you cut away the clothing and remove the shoe and sock to check pulse and sensation at the foot.
3. Using the uninjured leg as a guide, pull the splint out to the correct length.
4. Position the splint under the injured leg. The ring goes down, and the short side goes to the inside of the leg. Slide the ring up snugly under the hip against the ischial tuberosity.
5. Attach the ischial strap.
6. Apply the padded traction hitch to the ankle and foot.
7. Attach the traction hitch to the windlass by way of the S-hook.
8. Turn the ratchet until the correct tension is applied.
9. Reassess PMS of the leg.
10. Position and attach two support straps above the knee and two below the knee. Do not place over fracture site.
11. Release manual traction and recheck circulation and sensation.
12. To release mechanical traction (when too tight or when removing the splint), pull the ratchet knob outward and then slowly turn to loosen.

PROCEDURE

Applying a Sager Traction Splint

The Sager traction splint is different from the two splints already described in several ways. It works by providing countertraction against the pubic ramus and the ischial tuberosity medial to the shaft of the femur; thus, it does not go under the leg. The hip does not have to be slightly flexed, as with the Hare. The Sager splint is also lighter and more compact than other traction splints. You also can splint both legs with one splint if needed. The current Sager splints are significantly improved over older models and may represent the state of the art in traction splints. To apply a Sager traction splint, follow these steps (Scan 15-2):

1. Position the patient on a long backboard or stretcher.
2. Have your partner support the leg and maintain gentle traction while you cut away the clothing and remove the shoe and sock to check the pulse and sensation at the foot.
3. Using the uninjured leg as a guide, pull the splint out to the correct length.
4. Position the splint to the inside of the injured leg with the padded bar fitted snugly against the pelvis in the groin. Attach the strap to the thigh. The splint can be used on the outside of the leg, using the strap to maintain traction against the pubic ramus. Be very careful not to catch the genitals under the bar (or strap).
5. While your partner maintains gentle manual traction, attach the padded hitch to the foot and ankle.
6. Extend the splint until the correct tension is obtained.
7. Apply the elastic straps to secure the leg to the splint. Do not place over fracture site.
8. Release manual traction and recheck circulation and sensation.

SCAN 15-2 Applying a Sager Traction Splint

1
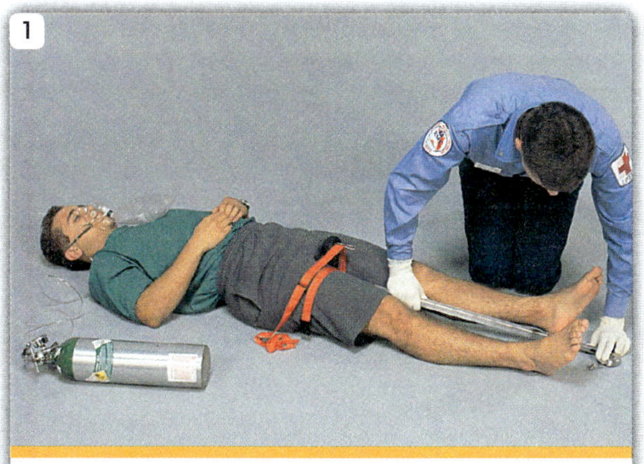

Place the splint along the medial aspect of the injured leg. Adjust it so that it extends about 4 inches beyond the heel.

2
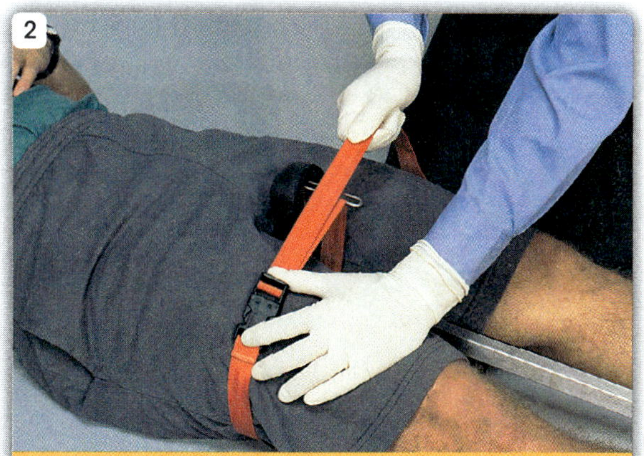

Secure the strap to the thigh.

3
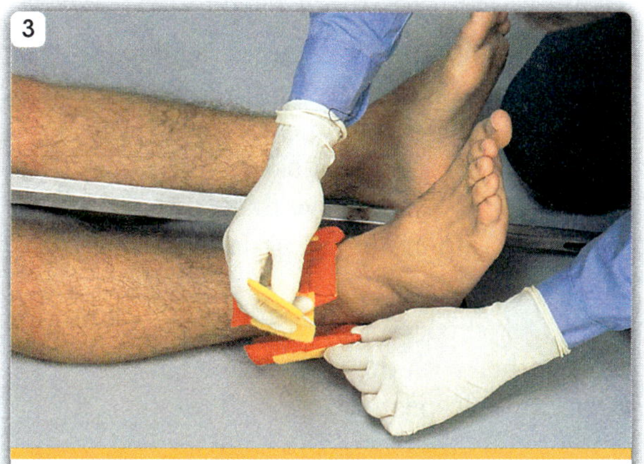

Apply the ankle hitch and attach it to the splint.

4
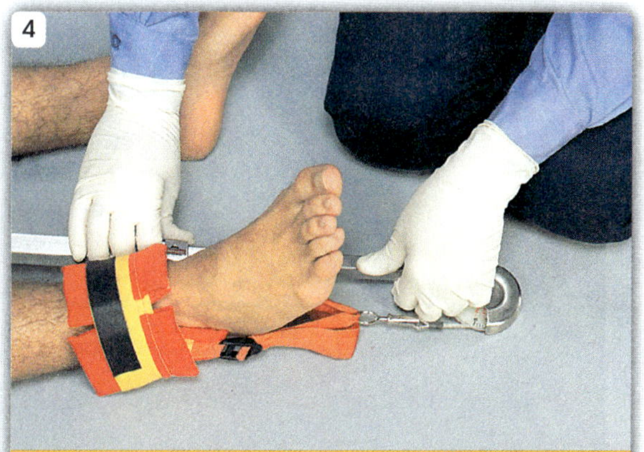

Apply traction by extending the splint. Adjust the splint to 10% of the patient's body weight.

5
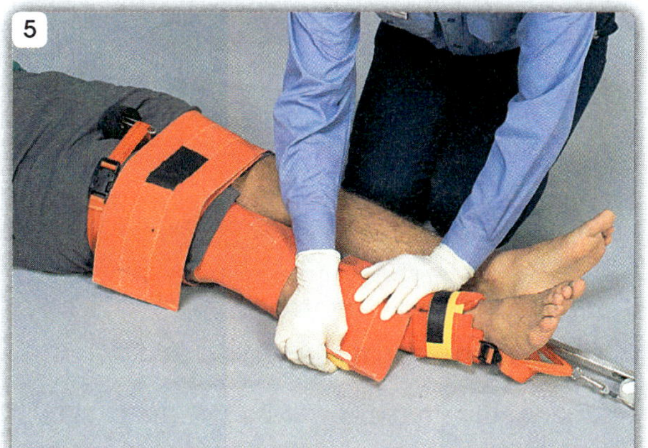

Apply the straps to secure leg to splint. Reassess distal pulse, motor function, and sensation.

Pelvic Stabilization Techniques

Pelvic fractures involve either the iliac crest or the pelvic ring. Fractures to the iliac crest indicate serious trauma. However, they are not life threatening like fractures of the pelvic ring, which have a much higher blood loss. In either case, the actual technique for stabilizing the fracture is the same and may be accomplished by either of two common approaches (described here).

PROCEDURE

Stabilizing the Pelvis with a Sheet or Blanket

1. Place a sheet or blanket horizontally on the lower half of the backboard prior to moving the patient.

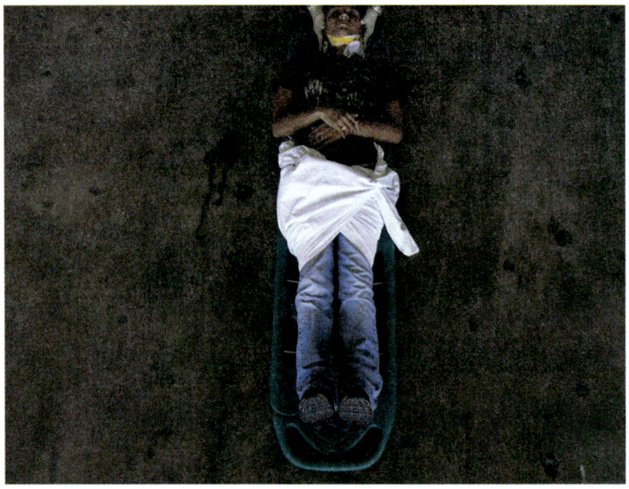

FIGURE 15-3 Manual stabilization of unstable pelvic fracture using a sheet. *(Courtesy of Leon Charpentier, EMT-P)*

2. Use a scoop stretcher, if available, to move the patient onto the backboard. If a scoop stretcher is not available, the patient will need to be log-rolled as gently and quickly as possible. If you have one of the newer, more stable scoop stretchers, you can use it instead of a backboard, but you will have to slide the sheet or blanket up under the patient after he is on the stretcher.
3. Tie two diagonal corners of the sheet or blanket together with the knot formed at the hip on one side. Repeat the tie with the remaining two corners and the knot formed on the opposite hip. In each case, gently and smoothly increase the tension until firm support is provided for the pelvis (Figure 15-3).

PROCEDURE

Stabilizing the Pelvis with a Commercial Device

1. Open the device and place it horizontally on the lower half of the backboard prior to moving the patient.
2. Use a scoop stretcher, if available, to move the patient onto the backboard. If a scoop stretcher is not available, the patient will need to be log-rolled as gently and quickly as possible. If you have one of the newer more stable scoop stretchers, you can use it instead of a backboard, but you will have to slide the device up under the patient after he is on the stretcher.

3. Tighten the device as the manufacturer recommends. Gently and smoothly increase the tension until firm support is provided for the pelvis (Figure 15-4).

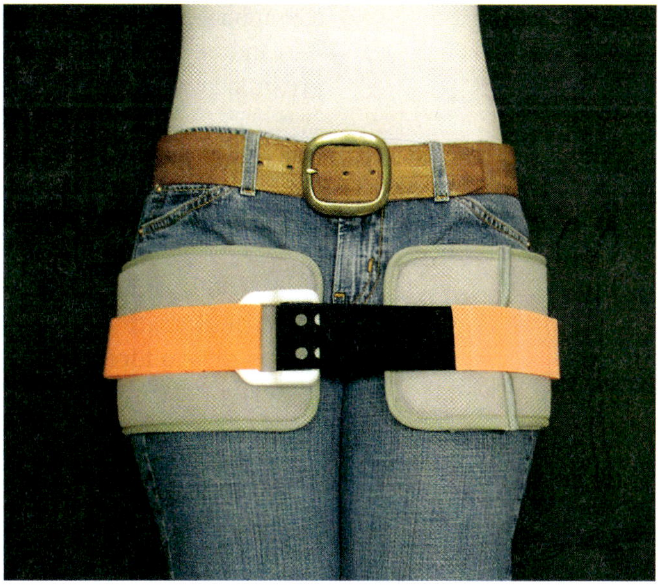

FIGURE 15-4 Stabilization of an unstable pelvic fracture using a commercial device. *(Courtesy of Sam Medical Products)*

Bleeding

The immediate control of massive bleeding from external injuries is vital to the survival and recovery of the trauma patient. Although varying definitions exist to define massive bleeding (Adams & Schwab, 1988; Carr, 2004), it may be identified by bleeding that cannot be controlled by the conventional method of direct pressure.

Direct pressure is widely accepted as a standard of practice for the control of all levels of injury severity. However, scientific research that quantifies the applicability and efficacy of this instrument has been very limited. Studies evaluating the effectiveness of tourniquets and hemostatic agents quantify bleeding in the context of a control within the design of the studies (Jackson et al., 1997; Wedmore et al., 2006). In the past, basic and advanced-level provider education presented various methodologies to control external bleeding, including direct pressure, elevation of an extremity in conjunction with direct pressure, packing with fingertips, or sterile gauze and direct pressure over pressure points (Bledsoe, Porter, & Cherry, 2009; Campbell, 2008; McSwain, Frame, & Salomone, 2005).

Currently, if direct pressure is unsuccessful, the recommendation is to immediately apply a tourniquet if the bleeding is in an area where one may be applied. If a tourniquet cannot be applied, a hemostatic agent should be used. All methods of controlling hemorrhage serve to restrict blood flow and augment the body's response to blood loss—vascular constriction, platelet aggregation, and coagulation.

Application of Tourniquets

Injuries to extremities, such as avulsions, amputations, and lacerations, with associated bleeding that is not quickly controlled by direct pressure, meet the criteria for the application of a tourniquet (Kragh et al., 2008; Lee, 2007; Alam et al., 2005). Tourniquets provide circumferential compression to the vascular structures just proximal to the wound, inhibiting distal blood flow.

Commercial Devices

A general description of the guidelines for the ideal tourniquet includes effectiveness of arterial occlusion, ease of use, lightweight, compact, and rugged (King et al., 2006). The issue of expense is applicable to EMS, and thus the addition of cost consideration is appropriate to this list. Key elements of the tourniquet design must address the width of the occluding strap/pneumatic band and ability to overcome soft tissue (Walters & Mabry, 2005). The combination of appropriate mechanical assistance and width designs of two inches or greater appears to provide adequate soft-tissue compression and stop bleeding at lower pressures, decreasing tissue damage and discomfort at the tourniquet site.

Multiple types of tourniquet devices are now commercially available. Although ITLS does not endorse any specific brand or model, studies have shown several to be more effective than others (Walters et al., 2005; Wenke et al., 2005; King et al., 2006).

The Combat Application Tourniquet® (CAT) is manufactured by Composite Resources and designed with a self-adherent Velcro band, friction adaptor buckle, and a windlass rod and clip (Figure 15-5). The self-adherent Velcro band is reportedly made from a nonstretch material long enough for application on large and obese extremities. The surface area width is sufficient for distributing the application of pressure circumferentially around the extremity.

Application of the CAT is accomplished by feeding the Velcro band around an extremity and inserting the free-running end through the buckle. Insertion into the buckle locks the band in place on the extremity. Turning the windlass rod creates circumferential tightening and is locked into place with the clip and secured with a small strap after bleeding has been controlled. A location on the top of the windlass strap is available to note the time of application. The manufacturer accentuates an independent internal band and clip that permits one-handed or self-application.

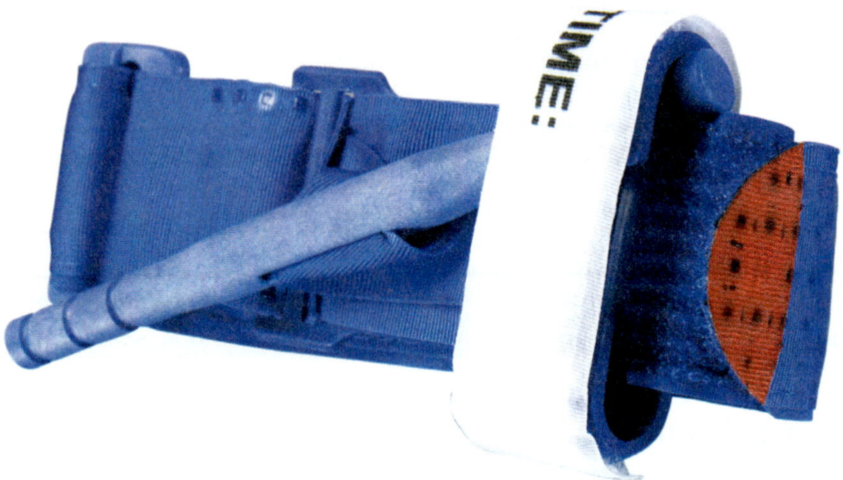

FIGURE 15-5 Combat Application Tourniquet® (CAT). *(© 2010 North American Rescue, LLC)*

The Emergency and Military Tourniquet® (EMT) by Delfi Medical (Figure 15-6) is a pneumatic-based device with an inflatable bladder and a hand bulb inflator permanently attached to the bladder by way of a flexible hose. A twist-type air release valve is included between the hand bulb inflator and the bladder to allow deflation of the bladder. The clamp secures a portion of the bladder around the limb and seals the bladder across its width, such that the portion of the bladder surrounding the limb inflates, and the remaining portion of the bladder does not inflate. The EMT is available in one size and able to encircle a 3- to 34-inch circumference around an extremity. A blood pressure cuff may be used in exactly the same way.

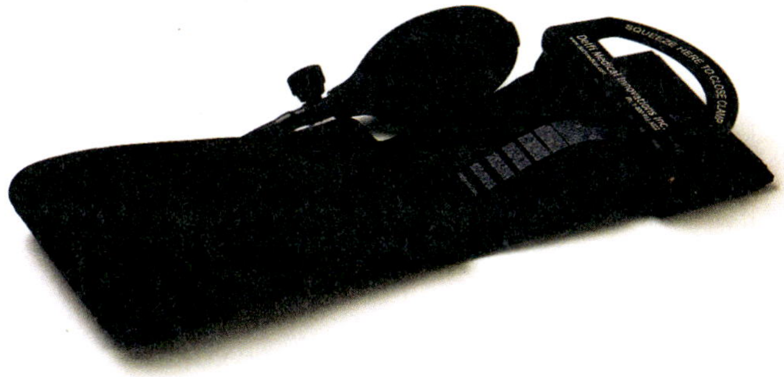

FIGURE 15-6 The Emergency and Military Tourniquet® (EMT). *(Courtesy of Delphi Medical Innovations, Inc.)*

Both the CAT and EMT advocate use of minimal pressure to control bleeding, and provide discussion of procedures for increasing and decreasing the pressure exerted by the device.

Tourniquet Application

Regardless of the device used, the following procedure may be employed for hemorrhage that is unable to be controlled with conventional methods of direct pressure and is anatomically appropriate to tourniquet application:

1. Identify massive extremity bleeding caused by avulsions, amputations, and lacerations.
2. Attempt direct pressure to control bleeding. If you are unable to control bleeding quickly, proceed immediately to application of tourniquet.
3. Position tourniquet just proximal to the source of bleeding, avoiding application over any joints on the extremity.
4. Secure the tourniquet in place and apply circumferential pressure by a method recommended by the tourniquet manufacturer.
5. Tighten the tourniquet until bleeding stops.
6. Secure the tourniquet in place.
7. Note the time of application.
8. Do not cover the tourniquet.
9. Frequently reassess for bleeding. Increase tourniquet pressure as needed.
10. Contact receiving facility and notify them of the application of a tourniquet.

The use of a tourniquet is not a benign procedure. Application of a tourniquet may cause extreme pain and discomfort at and distal to the site of application. When appropriate, the use of analgesic medications to decrease pain should be considered. Complications such as inappropriate positioning and device malfunction can occur. In addition, necrosis to the muscle at and distal to the application, compartment syndrome, and nerve palsy are all possible (Kragh et al., 2008). Unless extreme circumstances exist where delivery to definitive care is delayed, the removal of a tourniquet or reperfusion of an extremity following tourniquet application should include appropriate communications with medical direction.

Use of Hemostatic Agents

Injuries where the control of massive bleeding is not successful with direct pressure and the use of a tourniquet, or where the application of a tourniquet is not possible, such as the neck, axilla, or groin, the use of a hemostatic agent in combination with direct pressure is warranted as an additional resource to control bleeding. Laboratory studies and field trials conducted by the U.S. military and limited research completed by EMS agencies indicates hemostatic agents have benefit when used in conjunction with existing methods of bleeding control (Brown Daya, & Worley, 2007; King 2004). Within the context of education for the use of hemostatic agents, a study by Brown et al. (2007) indicated a 21% failure rate when used by EMS personnel. This outcome identifies the need to define appropriate application based on the severity of the injury in conjunction with initial and continuing educational methodologies for the use of hemostatic agents.

Hemostatic Agent Types

This is a technology that is rapidly changing, and there are many competing hemostatic products. Various chitosan, mineral, and non-mineral-based hemostatic agents are currently available to EMS personnel. Product names such as Celox™, QuikClot Combat Gauze®, HemCon®, and TraumaDex™ promote clotting (with different degrees of effectiveness) through various mechanisms of action (Acheson et al., 2005; Alam, 2003; Kheirabadi et al., 2008; King, 2004; Lawton et al., 2010; Pusateri et al., 2006; Ward et al, 2007). Most hemostatic agents are available in powder, granular, or bandage form. The U.S. military is currently using QuikClot Combat Gauze.

Common to each currently approved hemostatic agent regardless of application form is the requirement to make direct contact with the primary source of bleeding and exert external compression directly to the source of bleeding. Clotting time based on blood vessel type, size, and level of exsanguination presenting may vary, with 2 minutes of direct pressure required to facilitate cessation of bleeding (Alam, 2003; Kheirabadi, 2008). These agents are not to be used for internal bleeding.

Hemostatic Agent Application

The following procedure may be used for hemorrhage that cannot be controlled with conventional methods of direct pressure, when the injury is anatomically inappropriate for the application of a tourniquet, or when bleeding does not stop following direct pressure and tourniquet application.

PROCEDURE

Applying a Hemostatic Agent

1. Identify massive bleeding caused by avulsions, amputations, or lacerations.
2. Attempt direct pressure to control bleeding. If you are unable to facilitate rapid cessation of bleeding, proceed immediately to application of tourniquet for anatomically appropriate locations.
3. If bleeding is not controlled, apply hemostatic agent directly to the source of the bleeding.
4. With fingertip pressure and a 4 × 4 or trauma dressing, compress the wound and hemostatic agent for at least two minutes. Failure to apply direct pressure to the source of the bleeding may delay or prevent cessation of bleeding.

5. Leaving the 4 × 4 or trauma dressing in place, evaluate for cessation of bleeding. If bleeding has stopped, dress the wound as appropriate.
6. If bleeding continues, remove the 4 × 4 or trauma dressing and reapply the hemostatic agent and 4 × 4 or trauma dressing. Confirm direct pressure is being placed on the source of bleeding.

Complications include ineffectiveness of the hemostatic agent, continued bleeding (recognized and unrecognized), and tissue damage secondary to the type of hemostatic agent used. Any bleeding that cannot be controlled must be considered life threatening. Do not delay transportation for reapplication of tourniquets or hemostatic agents. Immediately package and transport the patient upon completion of the rapid survey and continue interventions en route to definitive care.

Bibliography

1. Acheson, E. M., B. S. Kheirabadi, R. M. Deguzman, E. J. Dick, J. B. Holcomb. 2005. Comparison of hemorrhage control agents applied to lethal extremity arterial hemorrhages in swine. *Journal of Trauma—Inury, Infection and Critical Care* 865–875.
2. Adams, D. B., C. W. Schwab. 1988. Twenty-one-year experience with land mine injuries. *J Trauma* 28(1 Suppl): S159–62.
3. Alam H. 2003. Comparative analysis of hemostatic agents in a swine model of lethal groin injury. *Journal of Trauma* 1077–1082.
4. Alam, H. B., D. Burris, J. A. DaCorta, P. Rhee. 2005. Hemorrhage control in the battlefield: Role of new hemostatic agents. *Military Medicine* 170(1): 63–69.
5. Bledsoe, B., R. Porter, R. Cherry. 2009. *Paramedic care principles and practices. 3rd ed.* Upper Saddle River, NJ: Pearson.
6. Brown, M., M. Daya, J.Worley. 2007. Experience with chitosan dressings in a civilian EMS system. *Journal of Emergency Medicine*. Elsevier, Inc. In Press, Corrected Proof, Available online 19 November 2007.
7. Campbell, J. E. 2008. *International trauma life support for prehospital care providers. 6th ed.* Upper Saddle River, NJ: Pearson Prentice Hall.
8. Carr, M. E., Jr. 2004. Monitoring of hemostasis in combat trauma patients. *Military Medicine* 169(12 Suppl): 11–15.
9. Jackson, M. R., S. A. Friedman, A. J. Carter, B. S. Vladislav. 1997. Hemostatic efficacy of a fibrin sealant based on topical agent in a femoral artery injury model: A randomized, blinded, placebo-controlled study. *Journal of Vascular Surgery* 26(2): 274–280.
10. Kheirabadi, B. S., E. M. Acheson, R. M. Deguzman, J. L. Sondeen, K. L. Ryan, A. P. Delgado, et al. 2005. Efficacy of two advanced dressings in an aortic hemorrhage model in swine. *Journal of Trauma* 25–35.
11. King, K. 2004. Hemostatic dressings for the first responder: a review. *Military Medicine* 169(9): 716–720.
12. King, R. B., D. Filips, S. Blitz, S. Logsetty. 2006. Evaluation of possible tourniquet systems for use in the Canadian forces. *J Trauma* 60(5): 1061–1071.

13. Kragh, J. F., Jr., T. J. Walters, D. G. Baer, C. J. Fox, C. E. Wade, J. Salinas, J. B. Holcomb. 2008. Practical use of emergency tourniquets to stop bleeding in major limb trauma. *Journal of Trauma* 64(2): Sup.S38–50.

14. Lawton, G., J. Granville-Chapman, & P. J. Parker. 2010. Novel heamostatic dressings. *JR Army Med Corps* 155(4): 309–314.

15. Lee, C., K. M. Porter, T. J. Hodgetts. 2007. Tourniquet use in the civilian prehospital setting. *Emerg Med J* 24(8): 584–587.

16. McSwain, N. E., S. Frame, J. P. Salomone. 2005, *Prehospital trauma life support: Military edition Rev. 5th ed.* St. Louis, MO: Elsevier.

17. Naimer, S. A., M. Tanami, A. Malichi, D. Moryosef. 2006. Control of traumatic wound bleeding by compression with a compact elastic adhesive dressing. *Military Medicine* 171(7): 644–647.

18. Pusateri, A. E., J. B. Holcomb, B. S. Kheirabadi, H. B. Alam, C. E. Wade, K. L. Ryan. 2006. Making sense of the preclinical literature on advanced hemostatic products. *Journal of Trauma* 674–682.

19. Walters, T. J., M. C. Mabry. 2005. Issues related to the use of tourniquets on the battlefield. *Military Medicine* 170(9): 770–775.

20. Walters, T. J., J. C. Wernke, D. S. Kauvar, J. G. McManus, J. B. Holcomb, D. G. Baer. 2005. Effectiveness of self-applied tourniquets in human volunteers. *Prehospital Emergency Care* 9(4): 416–422.

21. Ward, K. R., M. H. Tiba, W. H. Holbert, C. R. Blocher, G. T. Draucker, E. K. Proffitt, et al. 2007. Comparison of a new hemostatic agent to current combat hemostatic agents in a swine model of lethal extremity arterial hemorrhage. *Journal of Trauma* 276–284.

22. Wedmore, I., J. G. McManus, A. E. Pusateri, J. E. Holcomb. 2006. A special report on the chitosan-based hemostatic dressing: Experience in current combat operations. Lippincott Williams & Wilkins, 60(3): 655–658.

23. Wenke, J. C., T. J. Walters, D. J. Greydanus, A. E. Pusateri, V. A. Convertino. 2005. Physiological evaluation of the U.S. army one-handed tourniquet. *Military Medicine* 170(9): 776–781.

Explore Resource Central

For additional review and practice tests, visit www.bradybooks.com and click on Resource Central to access book-specific resources for this text. To access Resource Central, follow directions on the Student Access Card provided with this text. If there is no card, go to www.bradybooks.com and follow the Resource Central link to Buy Access from there.

Burns

Roy L. Alson, PhD, MD, FACEP

16

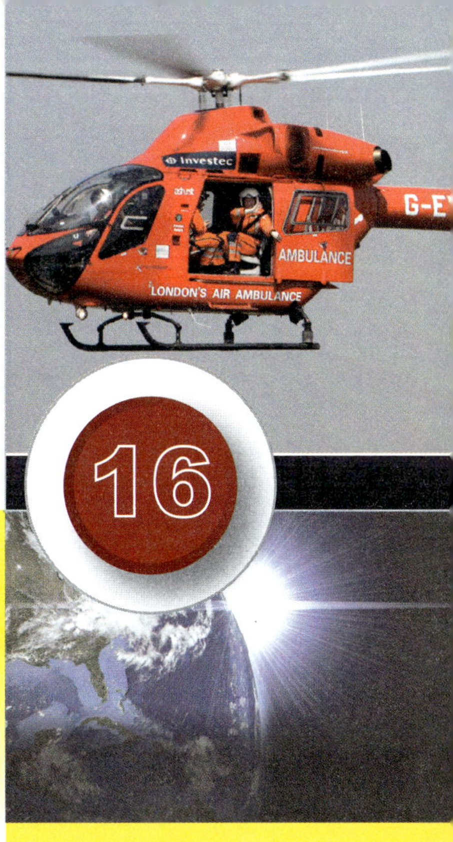

(Photo courtesy of Paul Drabot, Shutterstock.com)

Burns Ustioni Quemaduras Brûlures

Oparzenia Verbrennungen Opekline الحروق

opekotine Opekline Égés

OBJECTIVES

Upon successful completion of this chapter, you should be able to:

1. Identify the basic anatomy of the skin including
   a. Epidermal and dermal layers
   b. Structures found within
2. List the basic functions of the skin.
3. Describe types of burns as a function of burn depth.
4. Estimate depth of burn based on skin appearance.
5. Estimate extent of burn using the rule of nines.
6. Identify complications and describe the management of:
   a. Thermal burns
   b. Chemical burns
   c. Electrical burns
7. List situations and physical signs that:
   a. Indicate heat-inhalation injury
   b. Suggest carbon monoxide poisoning
8. Discuss how carbon monoxide causes hypoxia.
9. Describe the treatment for carbon monoxide poisoning.
10. Identify which patients may require transport to a burn center.

KEY TERMS

burn depth, *p. 288*
carbon monoxide poisoning, *p. 295*
chemical injury, *p. 298*
electrical injury, *p. 300*
heat-inhalation injury, *p. 295*
lightning injury, *p. 302*
Parkland formula, *p. 304*
rhabdomyolysis, *p. 302*
radiation injury, *p. 303*
rule of nines, *p. 289*
smoke-inhalation injury, *p. 297*
thermal injury, *p. 297*

Chapter Overview

According to the American Burn Association, there are over 1 million burn injuries per year in the United States, resulting in more than 4,500 deaths. Many who survive their burns are left severely disabled and/or disfigured. Although the number of those killed or injured has decreased in the last 30 years, particularly with the use of smoke detectors and the improvements in burn care, burn injury is still a major problem for our society. Applying the basic principles taught here can help decrease death, disability, and disfigurement from burn injuries. Because the rescue of burn patients can be extremely dangerous, following the rules of scene safety is extremely important. Multiple agents (Table 16-1) can cause burn injuries, but in general, pathologic damage to the skin is similar no matter what the cause. Specific differences among the types of burns will be discussed in later sections.

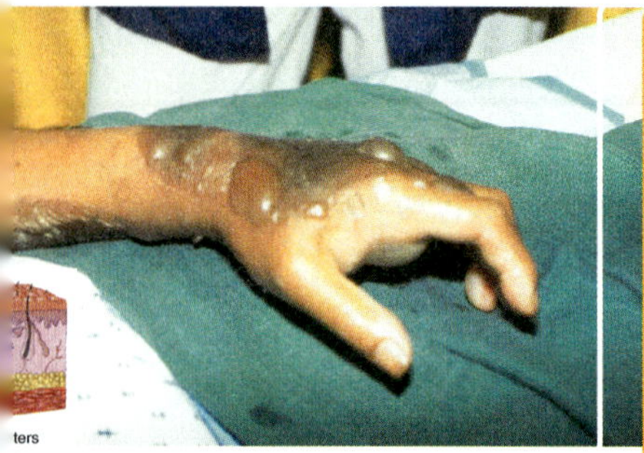

(Courtesy of Roy Alson, MD)

CASE PRESENTATION

It is a hot day in July, and an ALS ambulance has been called to the scene of a suicide attempt. They are told that a young woman has tried to kill herself by pouring gasoline in her car and then sitting in the auto and lighting the gasoline. She had driven into the woods to do this. She changed her mind as soon as the gasoline ignited. She was alone and did not have a phone, so had to hike a mile to get help. What injuries should they expect with a mechanism of this type? Are heat-inhalation injuries possible? Would she be likely to have lower respiratory system burns? Keep these questions in mind as you read the chapter. Then, at the end of the chapter, find out how the rescuers completed this call. ■

Anatomy and Pathophysiology

The Skin

The largest organ of the body, the skin, is made up of two layers. The outer layer, which we can see on the surface, is called the *epidermis*. It serves as a barrier between the environment and our body. Underneath the thin epidermis is a thick layer of collagen connective tissue called the *dermis*. This layer contains the important sensory nerves and also the support structures such as the hair follicles, sweat glands, and oil glands (Figure 16-1).

Table 16-1 Types of Burn injuries

- Thermal: flame, scald, steam
- Electrical
- Chemical
- Radiation

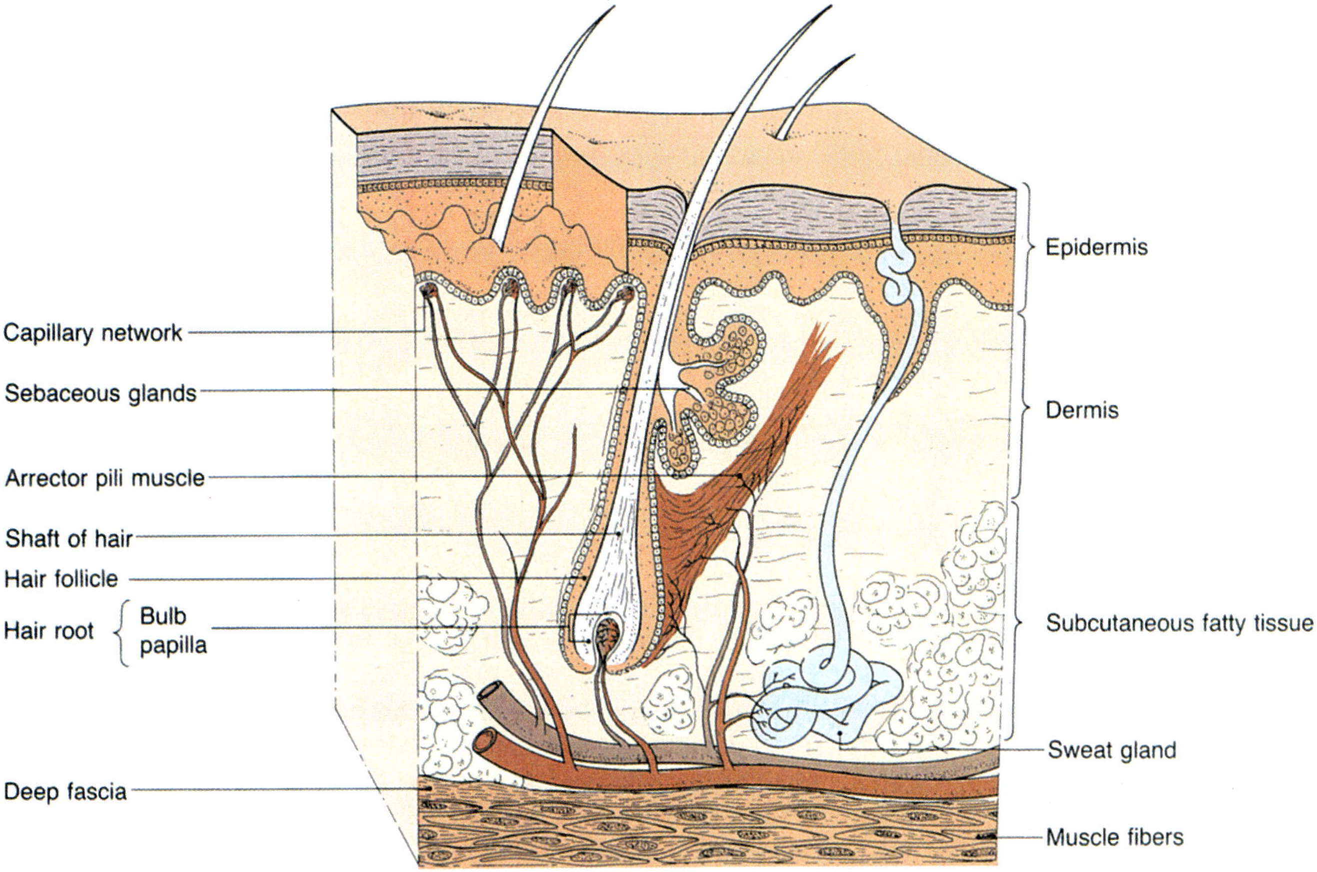

FIGURE 16-1 The skin.

The skin has many important functions, which include acting as a mechanical and protective barrier between the body and the outside world, sealing fluids inside, and preventing bacteria and other microorganisms from readily entering the body.

The skin is also a vital sensory organ that provides input to the brain on general and specific environmental data and serves a primary role in temperature regulation. Damage to the skin renders it unable to carry out these functions and puts the body at risk for serious problems.

Burn damage to the skin occurs when heat or caustic chemicals come in contact with the skin and damage its chemical and cellular components. In addition to actual tissue injury, the body's inflammatory response to the skin damage may result in additional injury or increase the severity of a burn. The portions of the skin that are necrosed by the thermal insult are referred to as the *zone of coagulation* and have suffered irreversible injury. Surrounding this area is a *zone of stasis*; blood flow is compromised and tissues will die if blood flow is not restored. This condition is seen in the deeper areas of partial-thickness burns and is helped by good burn care and fluid resuscitation. Surrounding the zone of stasis is the *zone of hyperemia*, where there is increased blood flow to the tissues as a result of the actions of inflammatory mediators released by damaged skin.

Classifying Burns by Depth

Burns are characterized, based on the depth of tissue damage and skin response, as superficial (first degree), partial thickness (second degree), or full thickness

Table 16-2 Characteristics of Various Depths of Burns

	Superficial (First Degree)	Partial Thickness (Second Degree)	Full Thickness (Third Degree)
Cause	Sun or minor flash	Hot liquids, flashes, or flame	Chemicals, electricity, flame, hot metals
Skin color	Red	Mottled red	Pearly white and/or charred, translucent and parchmentlike
Skin surface	Dry with no blisters	Blisters with weeping	Dry with thrombosed blood vessels
Sensation	Painful	Painful	Anesthetic with peripheral pain
Healing	3–6 days	2–4 weeks, depending on depth	Requires skin grafting

(third degree). Superficial burns result in minor tissue damage to the outer epidermal layer only, but do cause an intense and painful inflammatory response. The most common injury of this type is "sunburn." Although no medical treatment is usually required, various medications can be prescribed that significantly speed healing and reduce the painful inflammatory response.

Partial-thickness burns cause damage through the epidermis and into a variable depth of the dermis. These injuries will heal (usually without scarring) because the cells lining the deeper portions of the hair follicles, and sweat glands will multiply and grow new skin for healing. Antibiotic creams or various specialized types of dressings are routinely used to treat these burns, and therefore, appropriate medical evaluation and care should be provided for patients with these injuries. Emergency care of partial-thickness burns involves cooling the burn and covering it with a clean dry dressing.

burn depth a classification of severity of burns by how deep the skin is burned. In order of worsening injury: superficial burns (first degree), partial-thickness burns (second degree), and full-thickness burns (third degree).

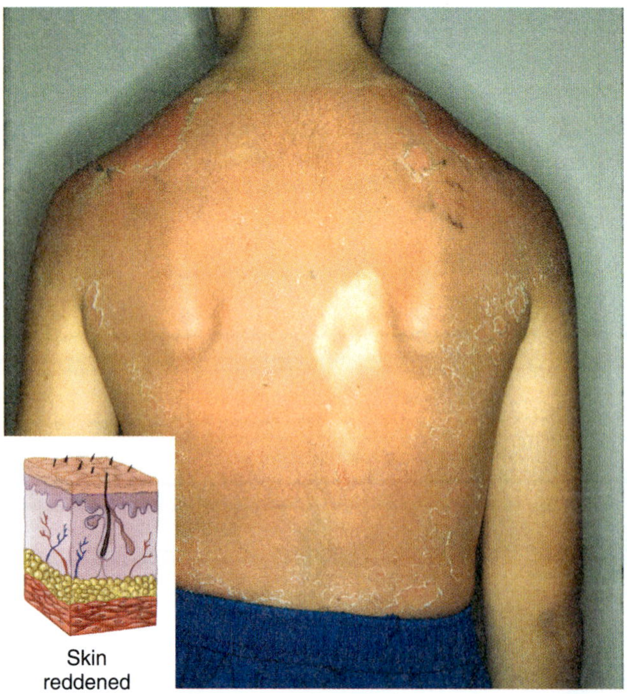

FIGURE 16-2 Superficial (first-degree) burn.

Full-thickness burns cause damage to all layers of the epidermis and dermis. No more skin cell layers are left, so healing by regrowth of epidermal cells is impossible. All full-thickness burns leave scars that later may contract and limit motion of the extremity (or restrict movement of the chest wall). Deeper full-thickness burns usually result in skin protein becoming denatured and hard, forming a firm, leatherlike covering that is referred to as *eschar*. Characteristics of these burns are listed in Table 16-2, and the depth levels and examples are shown in Figures 16-2, 16-3, and 16-4.

Determining the Severity of Burns

The body's normal inflammatory response to the burn injury can result in progressive tissue damage for a day or two following burn injury, which may well result in an increase in **burn depth**. Any condition that either reduces circulation (shock) to this damaged tissue or by itself causes further tissue damage will lead to burn progression with increasing burn depth. Because of this process of burn progression, it is not essential to determine exactly the burn

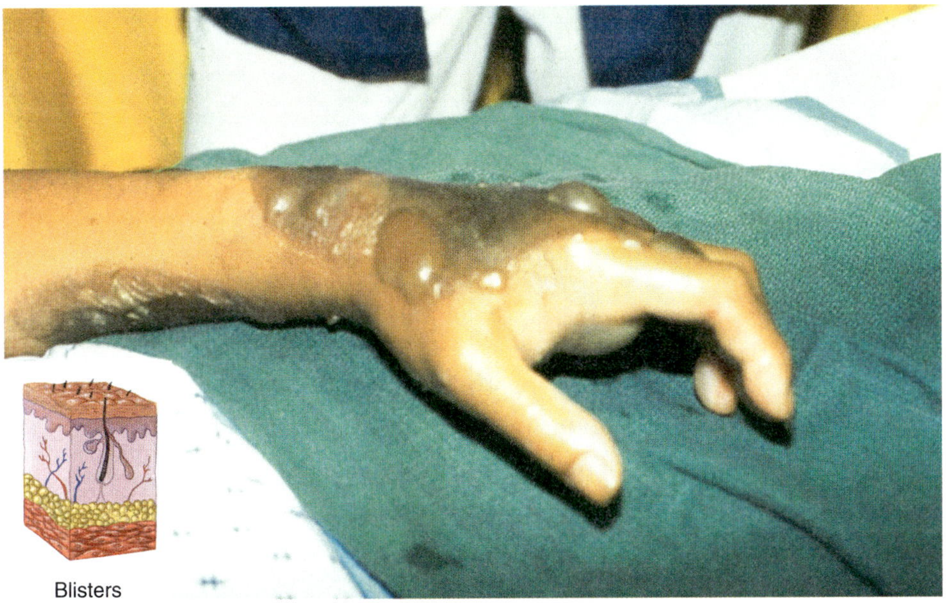

FIGURE 16-3 Partial-thickness (second-degree) burn. *(Courtesy of Roy Alson, MD)*

depth in the field. You should, however, be able to clearly discern between superficial and deep burns. Because transport to a burn center depends on both depth and extent of the burn, you also should be able to estimate the amount of body surface involved in the burn.

The burn size is best estimated in the field using the **rule of nines** (Figure 16-5). The body is divided into areas that are either 9% or 18% of the total body surface, and by roughly drawing in the burned areas, the extent can be estimated. Only partial-thickness and full-thickness burns are used for this calculation. In small children there are some differences in body size proportions, and a Lund and

rule of nines a method of estimating the body surface area burned by a division of the body into regions, each of which represents approximately 9% of the total surface area, plus 1% for the genital area.

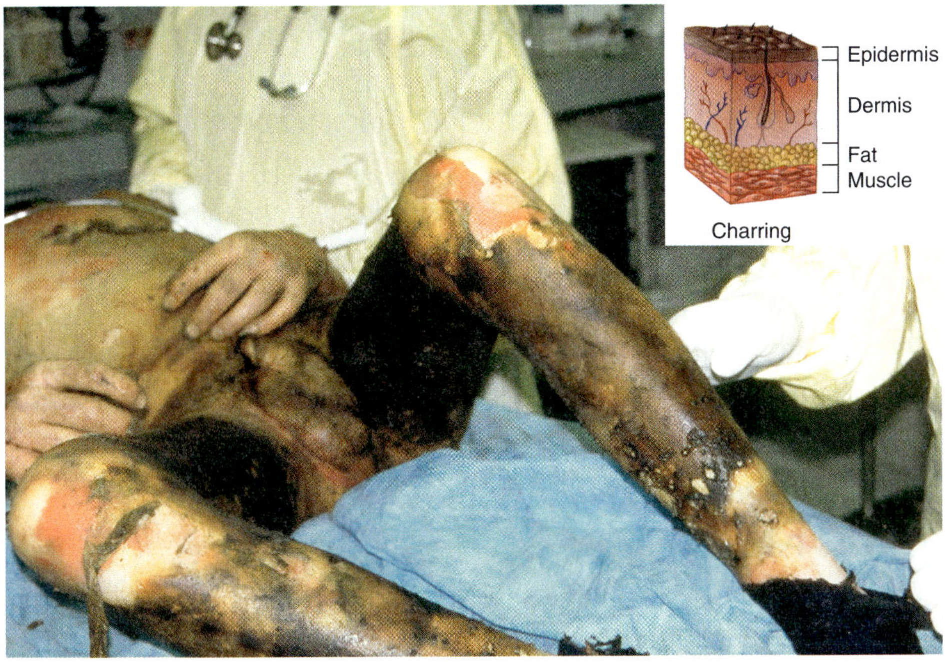

FIGURE 16-4 Full-thickness (third-degree) burn. *(Courtesy of Roy Alson, MD)*

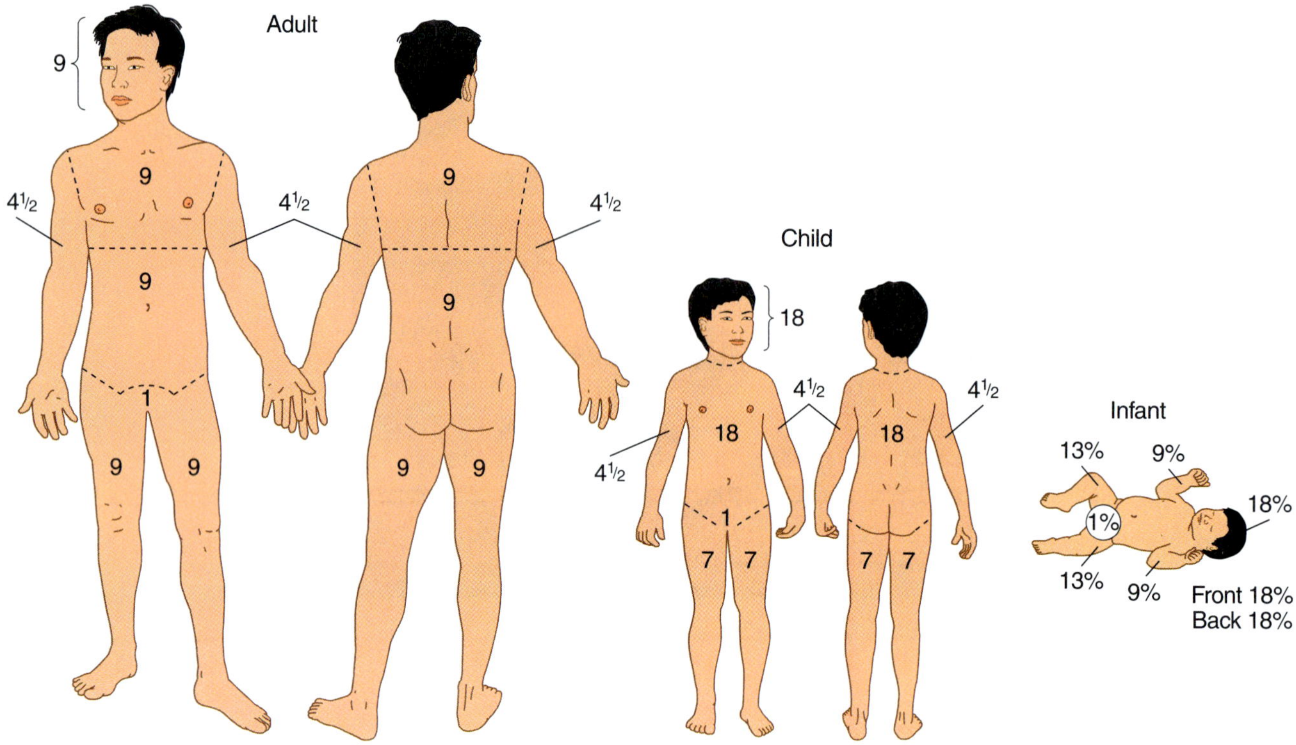

FIGURE 16-5 The rule of nines.

Browder chart is helpful (Table 16-3). For smaller or irregular burns, the size can be estimated using the palmar surface (including the fingers) of the patient's hand, which is about 1% of the total body surface area. Even small burns can be serious if they involve certain parts of the body that affect function or appearance (Figure 16-6).

Initial care that is directed specifically toward the burn should concentrate on limiting any progression of the burn depth and extent.

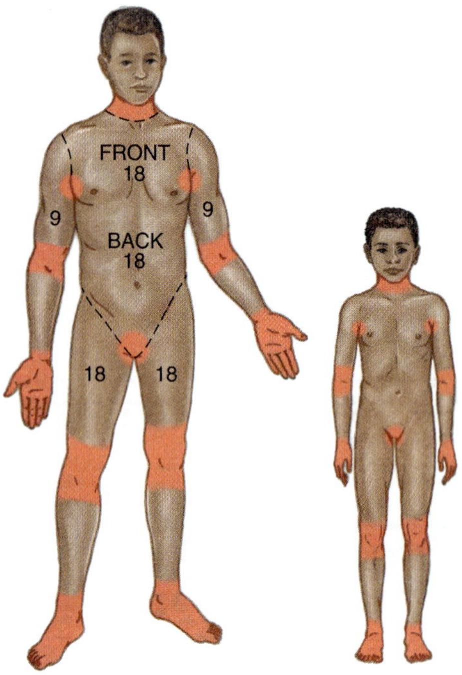

FIGURE 16-6 Areas in which small burns are more serious: Second- or third-degree burns in these areas (shaded portions) should be treated in the hospital.

Patient Assessment and Management

Evaluation of the burn patient is often complicated by the dramatic nature of the injuries. You can easily be overwhelmed by the extent of the injury. You must remember that even patients with major burns rarely expire in the initial postburn period from the burn injury. Death in the immediate postburn period is a consequence of associated trauma or conditions such as airway compromise or smoke inhalation. A careful, systematic approach to patient evaluation will allow you to identify and manage critical life-threatening problems and to improve patient outcome.

The ITLS Primary and Secondary Surveys should follow the standard format described in Chapter 2.

ITLS Primary Survey

Scene Size-up

The steps for assessing a major burn patient are the same as for any other major trauma patient. Begin by performing a scene size-up as outlined in

Table 16-3 Lund and Browder Chart

	Age (Years)					%	%	%
Area	**0–1**	**1–4**	**5–9**	**10–15**	**Adults**	**2°**	**3°**	**Total**
Head	19	17	13	10	7			
Neck	2	2	2	2	2			
Ant. Trunk	13	17	13	13	13			
Post. Trunk	13	13	13	13	13			
R. Buttock	2 ½	2 ½	2 ½	2 ½	2 ½			
L. Buttock	2 ½	2 ½	2 ½	2 ½	2 ½			
Genitalia	1	1	1	1	1			
R.U. Arm	4	4	4	4	4			
L.U. Arm	4	4	4	4	4			
R.L. Arm	3	3	3	3	3			
L.L. Arm	3	3	3	3	3			
R. Hand	2 ½	2 ½	2 ½	2 ½	2 ½			
L. Hand	2 ½	2 ½	2 ½	2 ½	2 ½			
R. Thigh	5 ½	6 ½	8 ½	8 ½	9 ½			
L. Thigh	5 ½	6 ½	8 ½	8 ½	9 ½			
R. Leg	5	5	5 ½	6	7			
L. Leg	5	5	5 ½	6	7			
R. Foot	3 ½	3 ½	3 ½	3 ½	3 ½			
L. Foot	3 ½	3 ½	3 ½	3 ½	3 ½			
					Total			

Weight ______

Height ______

Chapter 1, with an emphasis on your own safety. After the size-up is completed, your next priority is to remove the patient to a safe area away from the source of the burn.

There are specific and significant dangers in removing the burn source in all types of burn injuries. As a structure fire progresses, there is a point at which flashover occurs. Flashover is the sudden explosion into flame of everything in the room, with the temperature rising instantaneously to over 2,000°C. There is often little warning before this happens; thus removal of patients from burning buildings takes priority over all other treatment. Remember also that fire consumes oxygen and produces large quantities of toxic products and smoke. Thus, personnel making entry to carry out rescue should wear breathing apparatus or risk becoming victims themselves. Extrication of the patient from the burn source is usually the responsibility of fire department personnel rather than EMS personnel. Your responsibility should begin when the patient is delivered to you in a safe place.

Chemicals are not always easy to detect, either on patients or on objects in the environment. Rescuers have suffered severe chemical burns because of the failure to note sources of toxic and caustic chemicals and use appropriate personal protective equipment. Special training in hazardous materials management is recommended for all rescuers.

PEARLS: Assessment

Treat burn patients as trauma patients: ITLS Primary Survey, critical interventions, transport decision, ITLS Secondary Survey, and ITLS Ongoing Exam.

PEARLS: Safety

- Maintain appropriate safety when removing patients from the source of a burn injury.
- Remember that dealing with hazardous materials requires proper training and equipment. You must use appropriate personal protective equipment.

Electricity is exceptionally dangerous, and handling of high-voltage wires is extremely hazardous. Specialized training, knowledge, and equipment are required to appropriately deal with these situations, and you should not attempt to remove wires unless specifically trained and equipped to do so. Even objects commonly felt to be safe, such as wooden sticks, manila rope, and firefighter's gloves, may not be protective and may result in electrocution. If at all possible, the source of electricity should be turned off before any attempt at rescue is made.

Initial Assessment

Burn patients differ from other trauma patients in that the burning process must be halted immediately on removal of the patient from the source of the burn. This is best done with a quick irrigation of the burn with room-temperature tap water. Any source of clean water can be used, but do not use cold water. Irrigate for only a minute or two so that the patient does not become hypothermic. This can be done by another rescuer while the team leader begins the Primary Survey.

PEARLS: Airway Compromise

Early deaths from burns are not due to burn injury but to airway compromise. Perform frequent exams of the airway and be prepared to secure it with an endotracheal tube.

People do not actually die rapidly from burn injuries. Early burn deaths are usually the result of airway compromise, smoke inhalation, or associated trauma. Death from shock due to fluid loss from the burn will not be seen for many hours (or days), and sepsis usually takes days to develop. Burn victims may sustain multiple trauma from falls or other mechanisms. Hemorrhagic shock will develop rapidly compared to burn shock, so that management of the patient's blunt or penetrating trauma using ITLS guidelines is very important. Even though the burn is highly visible and makes an intense impression at the scene, other than stopping the burn process, care of the burn itself has a lower priority than airway management. You should perform an initial assessment as soon as the burn victim is in a safe area.

Begin by assessing level of consciousness, while securing the cervical spine if indicated. Assess the airway; if the patient is hoarse or exhibits stridor, protecting the airway is an immediate concern. Assessment of breathing, circulation, and control of major hemorrhage is then carried out.

Rapid Trauma Survey

Based on the findings from the scene size-up and the initial assessment, a rapid trauma survey or focused exam is then performed, a baseline set of vital signs is obtained, and if possible, a SAMPLE history is obtained. At this point a determination is made on the need for immediate transport and critical interventions. Critical problems in the burn patient that require immediate intervention include airway compromise, altered level of consciousness, or the presence of major injuries in addition to the burn. Clues from the mechanism of injury that point to critical problems include a history of being confined in a closed space with the fire or smoke, electrical burns, chemical exposure, falls from a height, or other major blunt force trauma. Oxygen at 12 to 15 L/minute by nonrebreather mask (or endotracheal tube if indicated) should be initiated as soon as possible for all major burn patients.

PEARLS: Inhalation Injury

- Any type of burn can have some degree of inhalation injury.
- Remember that a history of smoke exposure in a closed space is the best predictor of smoke inhalation or other airway injury!

The rapid trauma survey of the burn patient is directed toward identification of causes of breathing and circulatory compromise. Besides clues from the mechanism of injury, other findings that should alert the responder to potential airway problems are the presence of facial and scalp burns, sooty sputum, and singed nasal hair and eyebrows. Examine the oral cavity and look for soot, swelling, or erythema (redness). Ask the patient to speak. A hoarse voice, stridor, or persistent cough suggests involvement of deeper airway structures and is an indication for aggressive airway management. Auscultate the chest. Wheezing or rales should alert you to the presence of lower airway injury from inhalation. Examine burned areas and check for distal pulses. Based on the initial assessment and the mechanism of injury, a search for associate injuries should be the focus of the rapid trauma survey.

In your assessment of the burn patient, note and record the type of burn mechanism and the particular circumstances such as entrapment, explosion, mechanisms for other possible injuries, smoke exposure, chemical/electrical details, and so forth. An appropriate past medical history should also be documented in writing. If the patient is unable to speak, ask other witnesses and/or fire personnel about the circumstances of the injury.

ITLS Secondary Survey

Perform a standard ITLS Secondary Survey on stable patients. This survey should include an evaluation of the burn, estimating the depth based on appearance, and also estimating the burn size. Those findings are important in determining the level of medical care that is appropriate for the burn victim.

Patient Management

Once the immediate life-threats have been addressed, you should attend to the burn wound itself. As mentioned earlier, try to limit burn wound progression as much as possible. Rapid cooling early in the course of a surface burn injury can help limit this progression. Following removal from the source of the burn, the skin and clothing are still hot, and this heat continues to injure the tissues, causing an increase in burn depth and seriousness of the injury. Cooling halts this process and, if done appropriately, is beneficial. Cooling should be done with tap water or any source of clean room-temperature water, but this should be undertaken for no more than a minute or two. Cooling for longer periods of time can induce hypothermia and subsequent shock.

> **PEARLS:** Cooling
>
> Early after the burn event, properly cool the surface thermal injury with room temperature water, but do not cause hypothermia.

Following the brief period of cooling, manage the burn by covering the patient with clean, dry sheets and blankets to keep the patient warm and to prevent hypothermia. It is not necessary to have sterile sheets. Usually, nothing other than a clean sheet should be put on the burn but antimicrobial sheets (Acticoat or Silverlon) can be used if you have transport times of an hour or more. The patient should be covered even when the environment is not cold because damaged skin loses temperature regulation capacity. Patients should never be transported on wet sheets, wet towels, or wet clothing, and ice is absolutely contraindicated. Ice will worsen the injury because it causes vasoconstriction and thus reduces the blood supply to already damaged tissue. Cooling the burn wound improperly can cause hypothermia and additional tissue damage and could be worse than not cooling the burn at all. Initial management of chemical and electrical burn injuries will be described later in this chapter in the sections on those injuries.

During the evaluation of the extent of the burn injury, you should remove the patient's loose clothing and jewelry. Cut around burned clothing that is adherent, but do not try to pull the clothing off of the skin. Intravenous (IV) line insertion is rarely needed on scene during initial care unless delay in transport to a hospital is unavoidable. It takes hours for burn shock to develop; therefore, the only reason to initiate IV therapy is if other factors indicate a need for fluid volume or medication administration. Attempting to start IV therapy on scene in major burn patients is often difficult and routinely delays initial transport and

> **PEARLS:** Fluid Resuscitation
>
> Initiation of fluid resuscitation on scene is not as important as management of other potential life threats. Most burn injuries do not require fluids in the prehospital phase unless there is a long transport time.

Table 16-4 Injuries That Benefit from Care at a Burn Center

- Partial-thickness burns greater than 10% total body surface area (TBSA)
- Burns that involve the face, hands, feet, genitalia, perineum, or major joints
- Third-degree burns in any age group
- Electrical burns, including lightning injury
- Chemical burns
- Inhalation injury
- Burn injury in patients with preexisting medical disorders that could complicate management, prolong recovery, or affect mortality
- Any patients with burns and concomitant trauma (such as fractures) in which the burn injury poses the greatest risk of morbidity or mortality. In such cases, if the trauma poses the greater immediate risk, the patient may be initially stabilized in a trauma center before being transferred to a burn unit. Physician judgment will be necessary in such situations and should be in concert with the regional medical control plan and triage protocols.
- Burned children in hospitals without qualified personnel or equipment for the care of children
- Burn injury in patients who will require special social, emotional, or long-term rehabilitative intervention

Source: American College of Surgeons, Committee on Trauma. 2006. *Guidelines for the operations of burn units; Resources for optimal care of the injured patient.*

arrival at the hospital. IV or intraosseous (IO) access may be established during transport.

Pain medication administration in the multiple-trauma patient has been controversial. A risk of masking associated trauma and also both central nervous system and cardiovascular depression are associated with the use of pain medication. In the major burn patient, with or without coexisting trauma and especially with long transport times, administration of analgesics in appropriate dosages will improve patient comfort. Therefore, prior to administration of pain medication, consultation with medical direction is recommended.

All burn injuries should be evaluated at the hospital. There are now available specialized forms of therapy that offer specific advantages to the treatment of superficial, partial-thickness, and full-thickness burns. Partial-thickness burns can become infected and progress to full-thickness burns because of poor care. The sooner specialized burn therapy can be initiated, the more rapid and satisfactory the results will be.

Table 16-4 lists conditions that would benefit from care at a burn center. Based on available local resources and protocols, it may be appropriate to bypass a local facility and transport these patients directly to the burn center.

Special Problems in Burn Management

The following sections review management of specific types of burns, based on the injury mechanism. Be aware that more than one type of burn can be present in a patient. For example, a high-voltage electrical burn injury may also produce flame burns due to ignition of the patient's clothing.

Circumferential Burns

Full-thickness burns result in the formation of an eschar that is tough and unyielding. If the full-thickness burn is circumferential to an extremity, as the burn edema develops in the extremity, the eschar can act like a tourniquet and result in loss of circulation to that extremity. Thus all extremity burns should undergo regular pulse checks. Though not a prehospital procedure, consideration should be given to the performance of an escharotomy at the hospital prior to transfer to a burn center. If the chest is the site of the circumferential burn, the eschar may limit chest excursion during respiration and lead to hypoxia. Intubation and escharotomy can prevent hypoventilation in this situation.

Flash Burns

Flash burns are virtually always superficial or partial-thickness burns. A flash burn occurs when there is some type of explosion, but no sustained fire. The single heat wave traveling out from the explosions results in such short patient/heat contact that full-thickness burns almost never occur. Only areas directly exposed to the true heat wave will be injured. Typically, face and hands are involved. An example of this type of burn is seen when someone pours gasoline on a charcoal fire to get it to heat up faster. In situations of possible flash explosion risk, you should *always* wear proper protective clothing and avoid entry into explosive environments. Other injuries (fractures, internal injuries, blast chest injuries, and so on) may occur as a result of explosion.

Inhalation Injuries

Inhalation injuries account for more than half of the 4,500 plus burn-related deaths in the United States each year. Inhalation injuries are classified as carbon monoxide poisoning, **heat-inhalation injury**, or smoke (toxic) inhalation injury. Most frequently, inhalation injuries occur when a patient is injured in a confined space or is trapped; however, even victims of fires in open spaces may have inhalation injuries. Flash explosions (no fire) practically never cause inhalation injuries.

heat-inhalation injury thermal burns of the upper airway caused by inhaling flame or hot gasses. The lower airways are usually not affected because of efficient cooling by moist mucous membranes.

Carbon Monoxide Poisoning. **Carbon monoxide poisoning** and asphyxiation are by far the most common causes of early death associated with burn injury. When any material burns, oxygen in the air is consumed, and the fire environment should be considered to be an oxygen-deprived environment. Carbon monoxide is a by-product of combustion and is one of the numerous chemicals in common smoke. It is present in high concentrations in auto exhaust fumes and fumes from some types of home space heaters. Because it is colorless, odorless, and tasteless, its presence is virtually impossible to detect without special instruments.

carbon monoxide poisoning a type of inhalation injury (hypoxia) from inhalation of the colorless, odorless, and tasteless gas, carbon monoxide. Carbon monoxide binds to the hemoglobin molecule and prevents oxygenation of the cells of the body.

Carbon monoxide binds to hemoglobin (257 times stronger than oxygen), resulting in the hemoglobin being unable to transport oxygen. Patients quickly become hypoxic even in the presence of low concentrations of carbon monoxide. An alteration in level of consciousness is the predominant sign of this hypoxia (Table 16-5). A cherry-red skin color or cyanosis is rarely present as a result of carbon monoxide poisoning and, therefore, cannot be used in the assessment of patients for carbon monoxide poisoning.

Pulse oximetry will remain normal to high in the presence of carbon monoxide and cannot be used to assess patients for carbon monoxide poisoning. Some newer model pulse oximeters (Figure 16-7) can specifically measure carboxyhemoglobin levels and, if available, should be used on all those who have the possibility of exposure to carbon monoxide. Death usually occurs because of either cerebral or myocardial ischemia or myocardial infarction due to progressive cardiac hypoxia.

Table 16-5 Symptoms Associated with Increasing Levels of Carboxyhemoglobin Binding

Carboxyhemoglobin Level	Symptoms
20%	Headache common, throbbing in nature; shortness of breath on exertion
30%	Headache present; altered central nervous system function with disturbed judgment; irritability, dizziness, decreased vision
40% to 50%	Marked central nervous system alteration with confusion, collapse; also fainting with exertion
60% to 70%	Convulsions; unconsciousness; apnea with prolonged exposure
80%	Rapidly fatal

Treat patients suspected of having carbon monoxide poisoning with high-flow oxygen by mask. If such a patient loses consciousness, begin advanced life support with intubation and ventilation using 100% oxygen. If a patient is simply removed from the source of the carbon monoxide and allowed to breathe fresh air, it takes up to 7 hours to reduce the carbon monoxide/hemoglobin complex to a safe level. Having the patient breathe 100% oxygen decreases this time to about 90 to 120 minutes, and use of hyperbaric oxygen (100% oxygen at 2.5 atmospheres) will decrease this time to about 30 minutes (Figure 16-8).

All suspected cases of carbon monoxide poisoning or toxic inhalation should be transported to an appropriate hospital. The decision to transport the patient to a hyperbaric chamber should be made by medical direction.

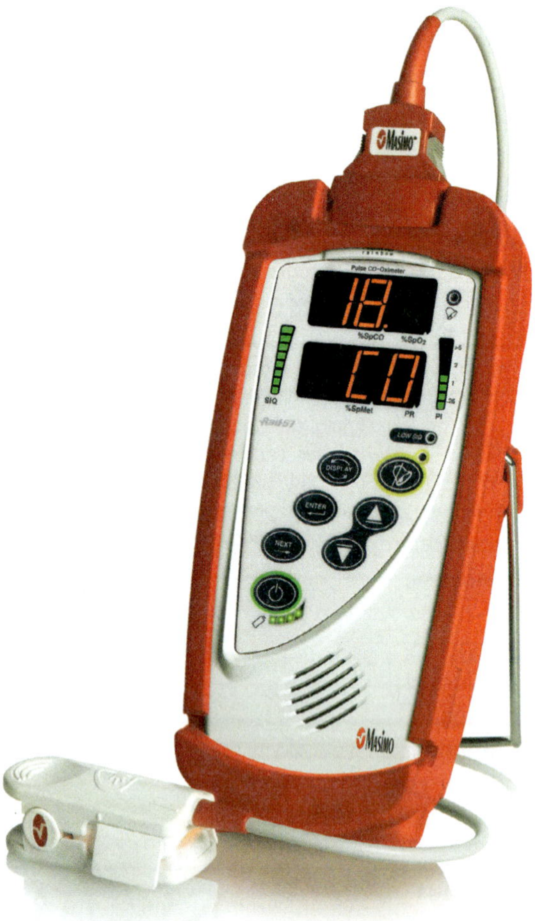

FIGURE 16-7 Example of a carbon monoxide monitor. *(Images of the Masimo Rad-57 Pulse CO-Oximeter are ©2011 Masimo Corporation. All rights reserved. Masimo, Rad-57, Pulse CO-Oximeter, and SpCO are trademarks or registered trademarks of Masimo Corporation)*

Cyanide and Smoke Inhalation. In the modern world, many items in homes and businesses are made of plastics. When combusted, many of them give off toxic gases, which can cause significant pulmonary injury. Among the toxic components in smoke is hydrogen cyanide. It is highly toxic and causes cellular hypoxia by preventing the cell from using oxygen to generate energy to function. Studies of smoke inhalation victims have shown elevated levels of cyanide in some cases.

Opinions regarding empirical treatment of smoke inhalation victims for cyanide poisoning still vary. Several studies suggest that patients who do not respond rapidly to treatment for hypoxia and carbon monoxide poisoning should be treated for cyanide exposure. The current recommended agent for such treatment is IV hydroxocobalamin, which combines with cyanide to form nontoxic cyanocobalamin (vitamin B_{12}). Hydroxocobalamin is easier and safer to use in the prehospital setting than the previous Lilly or Pasadena cyanide kits. This is an area of burn management that is continuing to evolve as more research is conducted.

Heat-Inhalation Injuries. Heat-inhalation injuries are confined to the upper airway because breathing in flame and hot gases does not result in heat transport down to the lung tissue itself. The water vapor in the air in the tracheal-bronchial tree effectively absorbs this heat. Steam inhalation is the exception to this rule, because steam is superheated water vapor. A second exception to this rule is if the patient has inhaled a flammable gas that then ignites and causes **thermal injury** to the level of the alveoli (example: a painter in a closed space where the paint fumes are ignited by a spark).

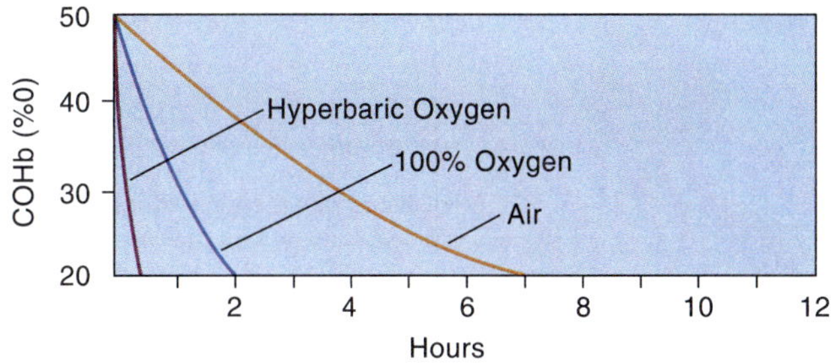

FIGURE 16-8 Decay curve for disappearance of carboxyhemoglobin from 50% lethal level to 20% acceptable level in air, 1 atm. O_2 (100% oxygen) and 2.5 atm. O_2 (hyperbaric oxygen—100% at 2.5 atmospheres).

As a result of the heat injury, tissue swelling occurs just as it does with surface burns. The vocal cords themselves do not swell because they are dense fibrous bands of connective tissue. However, the loose mucosa in the supraglottic area (the hypopharynx) is where the swelling occurs, and it can easily progress to complete airway obstruction and death (Figure 16-9). There is usually some time between the injury and the development of airway edema, so loss of airway due to direct thermal injury is rare in the initial prehospital phase. Be aware that once the swelling begins, the airway can obstruct rapidly. Development of a hoarse voice or stridor is an indication for immediate protection of the airway by endotracheal intubation. Aggressive fluid resuscitation can hasten this swelling. During secondary transport to a burn center, the risk of airway swelling can become significant and can cause airway obstruction as volume-resuscitation IV fluids are being administered. For this reason, if there is any potential for airway burns, the patient should be sedated and intubated before a transfer. It is much easier to electively intubate a patient in the emergency department than do a crash intubation in the back of an ambulance.

thermal injury injury to the skin caused by heat from flame, hot liquids, hot gases, or hot solids.

smoke-inhalation injury injury to the lungs or other body organs from inhalation of toxic gases found in smoke.

Figure 16-10 lists signs that should alert you to the danger of your patient having upper airway burns. Swollen lips indicate the presence of thermal injury at the airway entrance, and hoarseness (indicating altered air flow through the larynx area) is a warning of early airway swelling. Stridor (high-pitched inspiratory breathing and/or a seal-bark cough) indicates severe airway swelling with pending airway obstruction and represents an immediate emergency. The only appropriate treatment is airway stabilization, preferably via nasotracheal intubation or by paralysis and drug-assisted intubation (DAI). This procedure may be far more difficult than under other routine circumstances because of significant anatomic alterations due to swelling.

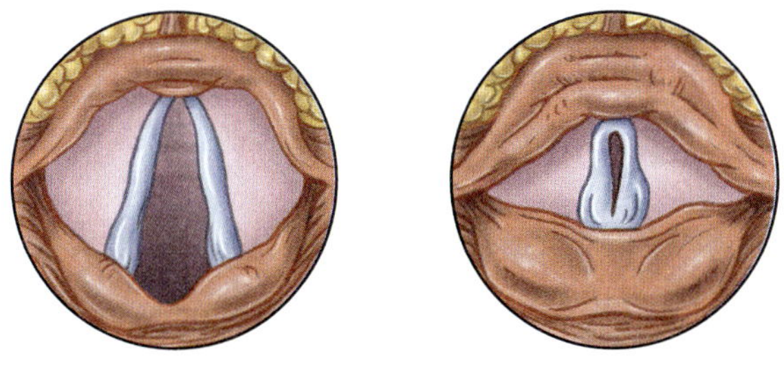

FIGURE 16-9 Heat inhalation can cause complete airway obstruction by swelling of the hypopharynx: left side—normal anatomy; right side—swelling proximal to cords.

In addition, because of irritation of inflamed damaged tissue, lethal laryngospasm may occur when the endotracheal tube first touches the laryngeal area. Therefore, this procedure is best undertaken in a hospital emergency department and should be done in the field only when absolutely necessary following communication and orders from medical direction. You should be prepared to perform a surgical airway in these patients if you are unable to intubate.

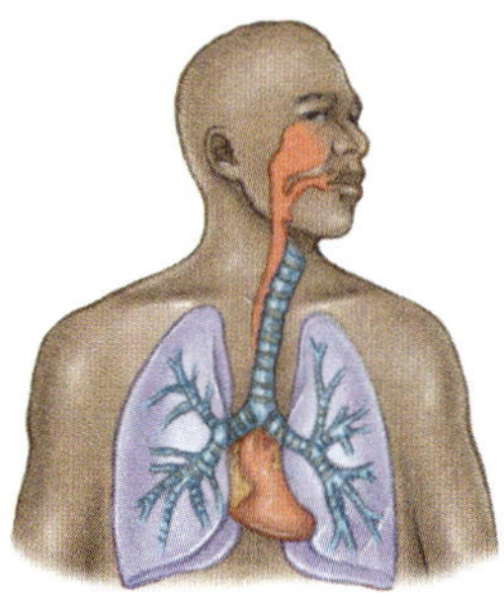

- Burns of the face
- Singed eyebrows or nasal hair
- Burns in the mouth
- Carbonaceous (sooty) sputum
- History of being confined in a closed space while being burned
- Exposure to steam

FIGURE 16-10 Danger signs of upper airway burns.

Smoke Inhalation Injuries.

Smoke-inhalation injury (Figure 16-11) is the result of inhaled toxic chemicals that cause

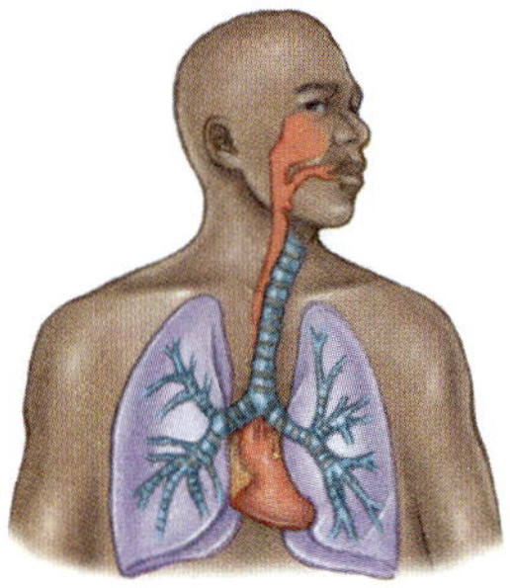

- Victims exposed to smoke in an enclosed place
- Victims who were unconscious while exposed to smoke or fire
- Victims with a cough after being exposed to smoke or fire
- Victims short of breath after being exposed to smoke or fire
- Victims with chest pain after being exposed to smoke or fire

FIGURE 16-11 Patients in whom you should suspect smoke inhalation.

structural damage to lung cells. Smoke may contain hundreds of toxic chemicals that damage the delicate alveolar cells. Smoke from plastic and synthetic products is the most damaging. Tissue destruction in the bronchi and alveoli may take hours to days. However, because the toxic products in the smoke are very irritating, they can precipitate bronchospasm or coronary artery spasm in susceptible individuals. Treat bronchospasm with inhaled beta agonists (albuterol) and oxygen.

Chemical Burns

PEARLS: Chemical Burns

Chemical injuries, in general, require prolonged and copious irrigation.

Thousands of different types of chemicals can cause burn injuries. Chemicals may not only injure the skin, but they also can be absorbed into the body and cause internal organ failure (especially liver and kidney damage). Volatile forms of chemicals may be inhaled and cause lung tissue damage with subsequent severe life-threatening respiratory failure. The effects of the chemical agents on the other organ systems, such as the lung or liver, may not be immediately apparent after exposure.

chemical injury injury to the skin or other body organs from exposure to caustic or toxic chemicals.

A **chemical injury** frequently is deceiving in that initial skin changes may be minimal even when the injury is severe. This could lead to secondary contamination of rescuers. Minimal burns on the patient may not be obvious. As a result, you can get the chemicals on your own skin unless appropriate precautions are taken.

Factors that lead to tissue damage include chemical concentration, amount, manner, and duration of skin contact, and the mechanism of action of the chemical agent. The pathological process causing the tissue damage continues until the chemical is either consumed in the damage process, detoxified by the body, or physically removed. Attempts at inactivation with specific neutralizing chemicals are dangerous because the process of neutralization may generate other chemical reactions (heat) that may worsen the injury. Therefore, you should aim treatment at chemical removal by following these four steps.

PROCEDURE

Removing the Source of Chemical Burns

1. Wear appropriate protective gloves, eyewear, and respiratory protection if needed. In some situations you will need to wear a chemical protective suit as well.
2. Remove all the patient's clothing. Place in plastic bags to limit further contact.
3. Flush chemicals off the body by irrigating copiously with any source of available clean water or other irrigant. If dry chemicals are on the skin, they should first be thoroughly brushed off before performing copious irrigation. Remember: *The solution to pollution is dilution.*
4. Remove any retained agent adhering to the skin by any appropriate physical means such as wiping or gentle scraping. Follow this with further irrigation (Figures 16-12 and 16-13).

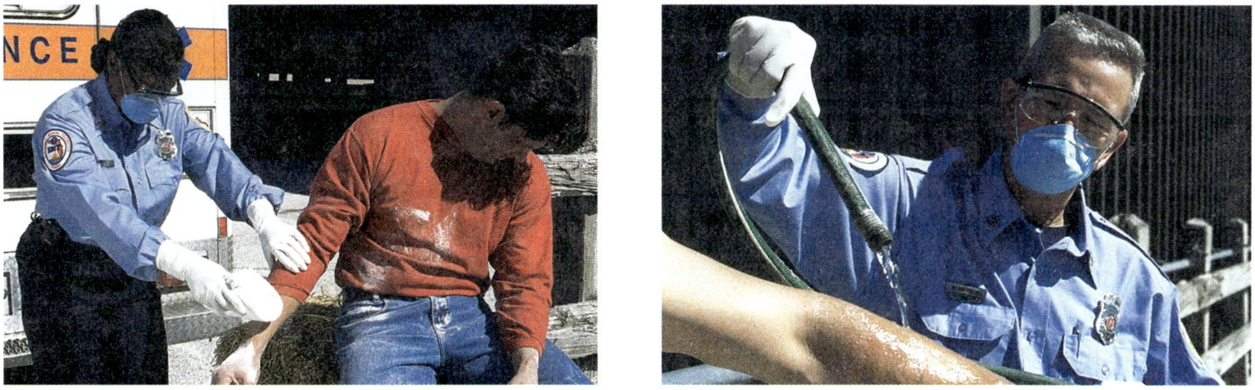

a. b.

FIGURE 16-12 For a chemical burn, (a) brush away dry powders, and then (b) flood the area with water. *(Photos courtesy of Michal Heron)*

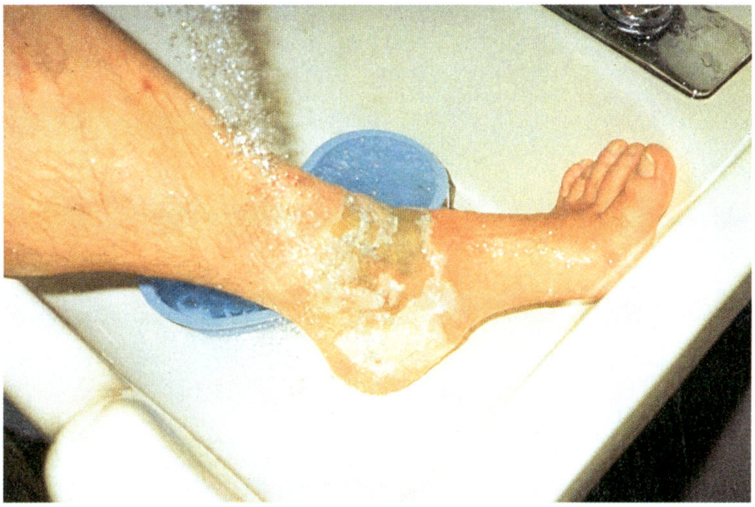

FIGURE 16-13 Acid burn of the ankle being irrigated. *(Courtesy of Roy Alson, MD)*

Ideally, all contaminated patients should be decontaminated prior to transport to limit skin damage and prevent contamination of the ambulance or hospital. Remember, removing the patient from the dangerous environment or removing the dangerous environment from the patient is your *first* priority for patient care. Critical interventions including airway management can be initiated prior to and during the decontamination process. If the patient has not been fully decontaminated prior to transport, notify the receiving hospital as soon as possible, so that they can be prepared to manage the patient.

Irrigation of caustic chemicals in the eye is exceptionally important because irreversible damage will occur in a very short period of time (less than the transport time to get to the hospital). Irrigation of injured eyes may be difficult because of the pain associated with eye opening. However, you must begin irrigation to prevent severe and permanent damage to the corneas (Figure 16-14). Check for contact lenses or foreign bodies and, if present, remove them early during irrigation. A nasal cannula hooked to an IV bag of normal saline and placed over the bridge of the nose makes an excellent bilateral eyewash system during transport.

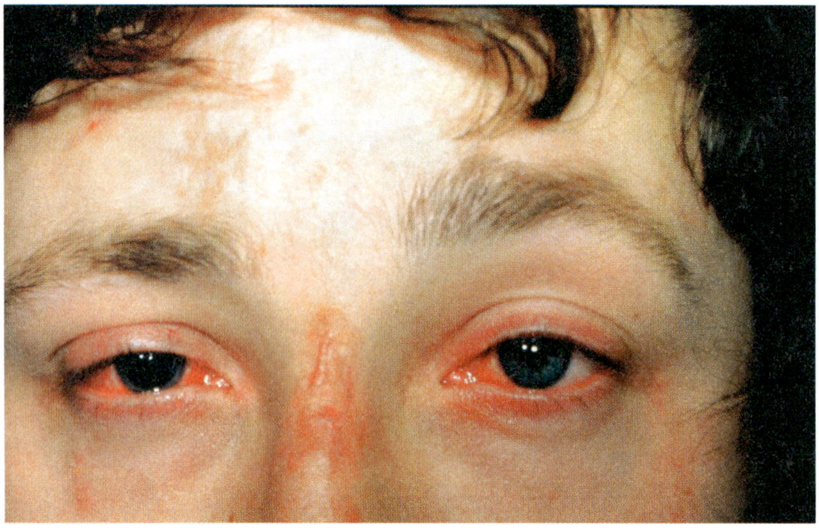

a.

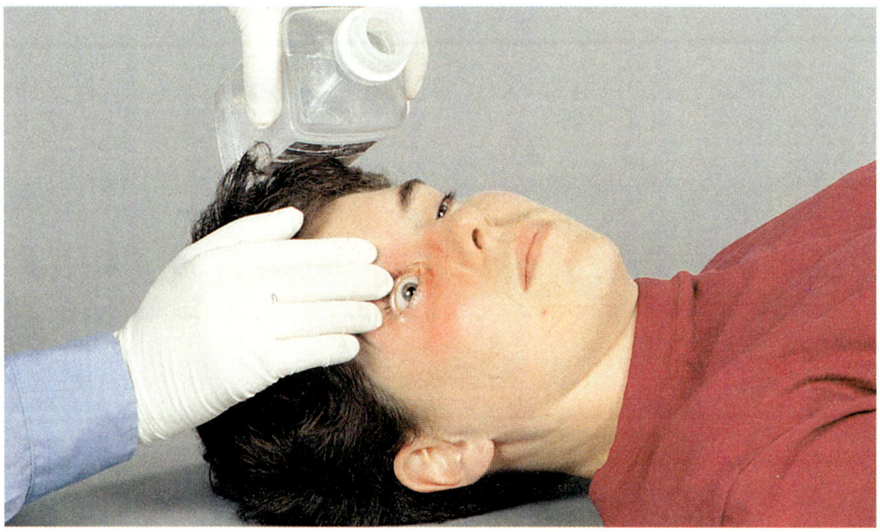

b.

FIGURE 16-14 (a) Chemical burns to the eyes; (b) emergency care of chemical burns to the eye.

PEARLS: Electrical Burns

Immediately check the cardiac status of victims of electrical injury.

electrical injury injury from the passage of electrical current through the body. The injuries can be from heat generated in tissue from electrical current passing through the body, cardiac dysrhythmias from current passing through the heart, and thermal burns from ignition of clothing.

Electrical Burns

In cases of electrical burns, damage is caused by electricity entering the body and traveling through the tissues. Injury results from the effects of the electricity on the function of the body organs and from the heat generated by the passage of the current. Extremities are at risk for more significant tissue damage, versus the torso, because their small size results in higher local current density (Figure 16-15). The factors that determine severity of **electrical injury** include the following:

- Type and amount of current (alternating versus direct current and also the voltage)
- Path of the current through the body
- Duration of contact with the current source

The most serious and immediate injury that results from electrical contact is cardiac arrhythmia. Any patient who receives an electric current injury, regardless of how stable he looks, should have a careful immediate evaluation of his

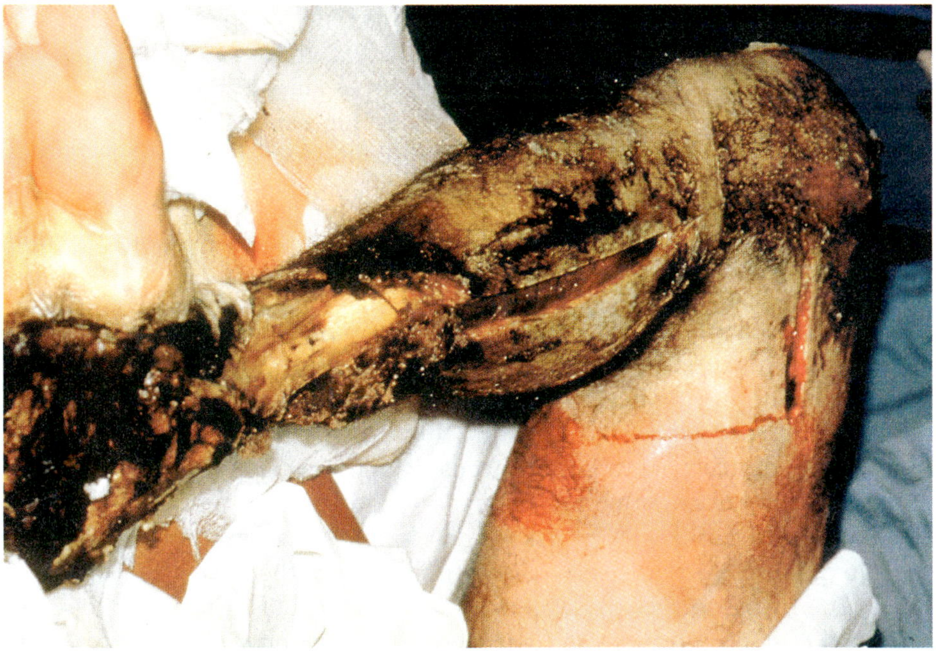

FIGURE 16-15 Electrical burn of the lower leg and foot. *(Courtesy of Roy Alson, MD)*

cardiac status and continuous monitoring of cardiac activity. The most common life-threatening arrhythmias are premature ventricular contractions, ventricular tachycardia, and ventricular fibrillation. Aggressive cardiac life support in accordance with AHA/ILCOR guidelines for the management of these arrhythmias should be undertaken because these patients are often younger and have normal healthy hearts. Most of the victims do not have preexisting cardiovascular disease, and their heart muscle tissue is usually not damaged as a result of the electricity. With good CPR, the chances for resuscitation are excellent. Even under circumstances of prolonged CPR, resuscitation is often possible. Once those efforts at managing cardiac status are complete, provide field care as previously described for thermal burns.

Electrical injuries cause skin burns at the entrance and exit sites because of high temperatures generated by the electric arc (2,500°C) at the skin surface. Additional surface flame burns may result if the patient's clothing is ignited. Fractures and dislocations may be present due to the violent muscle contractions that electrical injuries cause. Often victims are involved in construction and may sustain fractures or other injuries due to falls after an electric shock. Internal injuries usually involve muscle damage, nerve damage, and possible intravascular blood coagulation due to electrical current passage. Internal chest or abdominal organ damage due to electrical current is exceedingly rare.

At the scene of an electrical injury, your first priority is scene safety. Determine if the patient is still in contact with the electrical current. If so, you must remove the patient from contact without becoming a victim yourself (Figure 16-16). Handling high-voltage electrical wires is extremely hazardous. Special training and special equipment are needed to deal with downed wires; never attempt to move

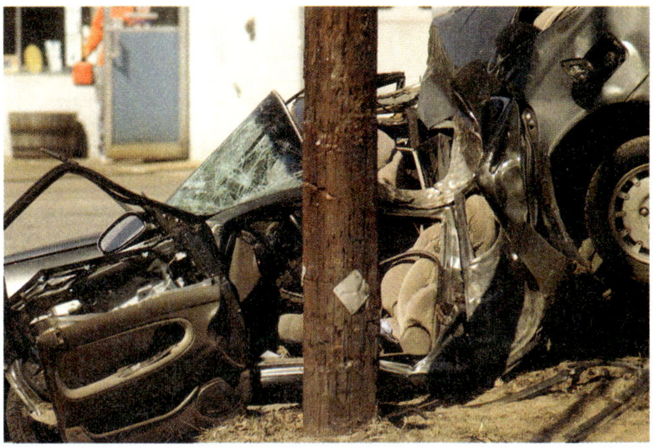

FIGURE 16-16 Removal of high-voltage electrical wires. Do not try to remove wires with safety equipment (or sticks) unless specially trained. Turn off the electricity at the source or call the power company to remove the wires. *(©Mark C. Ide)*

wires with makeshift equipment. Tree limbs, pieces of wood, and even manila rope may conduct high-voltage electricity. Even firefighter gloves and boots do not offer adequate protection in this situation. If possible, leave the handling of downed wires to power company personnel or develop a special training program with your local power company to learn how to use the special equipment designed to handle high-voltage lines. If power company personnel are turning off the electricity, be sure they test it to be sure it is off before you approach the scene.

In the field setting, it is impossible to tell the total extent of the damage in electrical burns because much of the burn injury is deep within the muscle. Therefore, all electrical burn patients should be transported for hospital evaluation. Due to the potential for arrhythmia development, routine IV access should be initiated in the ambulance, along with continuous cardiac monitoring. IV fluid resuscitation should be started during transport in this situation. Because of extensive tissue destruction, the fluid needs during interfacility transport of an electrical burn patient are often higher than for patients with thermal burns.

rhabdomyolysis disintegration (lysis) or dissolution of muscle. This releases large amounts of myoglobin into the blood, which can precipitate in the kidneys, causing renal failure.

Electrical burn patients are at risk for developing **rhabdomyolysis**, which is the breakdown of muscle with the release of myoglobin into the circulation and renal failure, as the myoglobin crystals block the kidney tubules. In those cases, the rule of nines is not applicable, and adequate fluid resuscitation is indicated by maintaining a urine output of 0.5 to 1 cc/kg body weight per hour. This level of urine flow also helps to reduce the risk of renal failure from rhabdomyolysis.

Lightning Injuries

lightning injury injury by the multiple effects of very short duration, very high voltage direct current on the body. The most serious effect is cardiac and respiratory arrest.

Lightning kills more persons in North America each year than any other weather-related phenomenon. A **lightning injury** is very different from other electrical injuries in that lightning produces extremely high voltages (> 10,000,000 volts) and currents (> 2,000 amps), but has a very short duration (< 100 msec) of contact.

Lightning produces a "flashover" phenomenon, in which the current flows around the outside of the victim's body. Consequently, the internal damage from current flow seen with generated electricity is not seen in a lightning strike. Most of the effects from a lightning strike are the result of the massive DC (direct current) shock that is received. Classic lightning strike burns produce a fernlike or splatter pattern across the skin (Figure 16-17).

The victim does not need to be struck directly to sustain an injury. Lightning can strike an adjacent object or nearby ground and still produce an injury to a victim. Often the victim's skin is wet, from either sweat or rain. This water, when heated by the lightning current, is quickly vaporized to steam, producing superficial and partial-thickness burns, and may literally explode the clothing off the victim. Because these burns are superficial, aggressive fluid resuscitation is not required.

The most serious effect of a lightning strike is cardiorespiratory arrest, with the massive current acting like a defibrillator to briefly stop the heart. Cardiac activity often spontaneously resumes within minutes. However, the respiratory drive centers of the brain are depressed by the current discharge and take longer to recover and resume the normal respiratory drive. Consequently, the victim remains in respiratory arrest, which is followed by a second cardiac arrest from hypoxia.

The essential component of the management of the lightning strike victim is restoration of cardiorespiratory function, while protecting the cervical spine. Follow standard guidelines for CPR and Advanced Cardiac Life Support (ACLS). Because lightning strikes can occur at sporting events and other outdoor gatherings, strikes often become multi-casualty events. It must be stressed that in a multi-casualty lightning strike, the conventional triage approach of a pulseless or

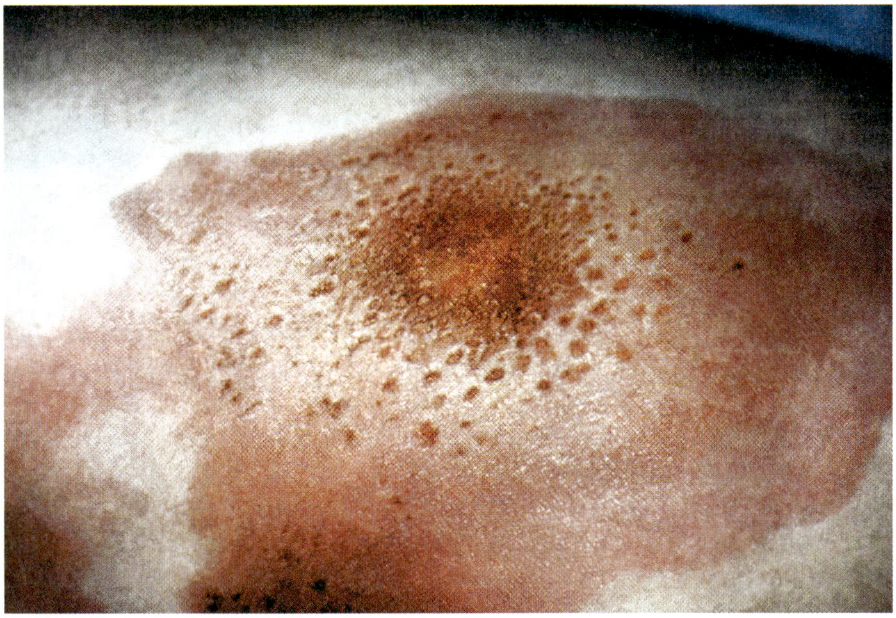

FIGURE 16-17 Flashover pattern of burns on the skin of a victim of a lightning strike.

nonbreathing patient equaling a dead patient should not be followed. If a patient is awake or breathing after a lightning strike, he will most likely survive without further intervention. Resuscitative efforts should concentrate on those victims who are in respiratory or cardiac arrest because prompt CPR and advanced cardiac life support increase the chance that these victims will survive.

Long-term problems have been seen in lightning strike patients, such as the development of cataracts, or neurological and/or psychological difficulties. Perforation of the eardrum is quite common, and rarely long bone or scapular fractures, as seen in the victims of generated high-voltage electrical injuries, may be seen. Those fractures are managed as described in Chapter 14.

There are over 200 reported deaths in North America each year due to lightning strikes. This represents only 30% of lightning strike victims; thus, it is possible that you will have to care for such a victim. These events often involve multiple victims, with varying degrees of severity. Prompt CPR greatly improves the chances of survival. When confronted with a naked (or partially unclothed) unconscious or confused patient, with perforated eardrums and a fernlike or splatter burn pattern on his body, think lightning strike.

Radiation Burns

Ionizing radiation damages cells by breaking molecular bonds. Skin burns from radiation look exactly like thermal burns and cannot be differentiated by their appearance alone. However, radiation burns develop slowly over days and so generally do not present as an emergency. Because of the damage to the skin cells, **radiation injury** heals very slowly. The burns can cause fluid loss just as thermal burns do and are even more prone to infection. Patients with radiation burns are not radioactive unless they are contaminated with radioactive material. If there is any danger that they might be contaminated, you should call for the hazardous materials team to scan them for radiation and perform decontamination if needed. Noncontaminated radiation-burn patients are treated the same as any burn patient. Decontamination of patients contaminated by radioactive material is beyond the scope of this course.

radiation injury injury to the skin and tissues from the effect of ionizing radiation. The injury is caused by the radiation breaking molecular bonds within the cell and cannot be differentiated from thermal burns by appearance alone.

Circumferential Burns

As mentioned earlier in patient management, circumferential full-thickness burns may lead to neurovascular compromise. Although this is rarely a problem on the fire scene, this may become significant during an interfacility transfer. Full-thickness burns that are circumferential around an extremity can act as a tourniquet as edema progresses. Early on, the patient may complain of loss of sensation and tingling and eventually develop ischemic pain with loss of pulses. Circumferential full-thickness burns on the extremities will require an escharotomy by the physician, especially if long transport times are involved. Circumferential burns of the chest can interfere with chest expansion and thus compromise respirations. Again, escharotomy in this setting can improve ventilatory status.

Be sure to alert the receiving facility if you are transporting a patient with full-thickness circumferential burns.

Secondary Transport

PEARLS: Secondary Transport

- Plan all secondary transports to burn centers and effectively continue resuscitation during such transports.
- Do not begin a secondary transport of a patient with a possible airway burn without the patient being intubated before transport.

Major burns often do not occur in locations where immediate transport to a burn center is possible. As a result, transport from a primary hospital to a burn center is commonly necessary. After the initial stabilization, prompt transfer to a burn center can improve patient outcome. During this transport, it is important for the ambulance crew to continue resuscitation initiated at the referring facility.

Prior to secondary transport, the transferring physician should have completed the following:

- Stabilization of respiratory and hemodynamic function, which may include intubation and IV access for fluid administration
- Assessment and management of associated injuries
- Review of appropriate lab data (specifically, blood gas analysis)
- Insertion of nasogastric tube in patients having burns covering more than 20% of the body surface area
- Placement of a Foley (urinary) catheter to allow measurement of urine output, which can assist in determining the adequacy of ongoing fluid resuscitation
- Assessment of peripheral circulation and appropriate wound management
- Proper arrangements with the receiving hospital and physician

You should specifically discuss the transport with either the referring or the receiving physician to determine what special functions may need monitoring and to determine the appropriate range for fluid administration because burns often require extremely large hourly IV rates for appropriate cardiovascular support. Initial resuscitative fluid needs in a burn patient are calculated using the **Parkland formula**:

Parkland formula a formula to calculate initial fluid resuscitation of the burn patient. The formula is: fluid needs for first 24 hours equal 4 cc of Ringer's lactate or normal saline multiplied times the % of burn area multiplied times the body weight in kilograms.

4 cc × % burn area × body weight (kg) = amount of Ringer's lactate or normal saline needed in the first 24 hours

Half of this fluid is given in the first 8 hours and the remainder over the next 16 hours. If large amounts of fluids are to be given, Ringer's lactate is preferred. Normal saline in large amounts can cause hyperchloremic acidosis.

Burn patients will need appropriate IV analgesics during transport.

It is important for you to maintain careful records indicating patient condition and treatment during transport. You should also make an in-depth report to the receiving facility.

Pediatric Burns

Children represent nearly one-half of all patients who seek treatment for burns. Because of their thinner skin, they are at greater risk for severe injury following a burn. Postburn problems, such as hypothermia, are more likely to occur in children because of their larger surface area to body mass ratio. Because of differences in anatomy, the rule of nines must be modified, because in small children the head represents a larger portion of the body surface. The Lund and Browder chart is better for estimating burn size in children (Table 16-3). The patient's palmar surface (1%) rule applies to children as well as adults.

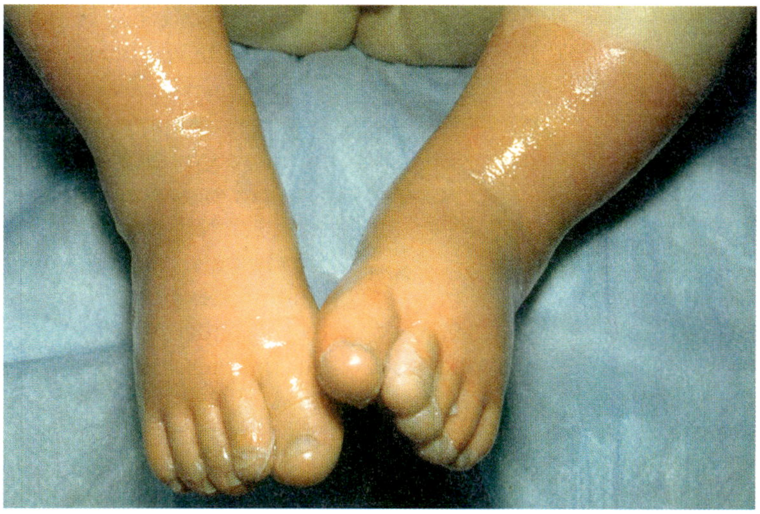

FIGURE 16-18 Scald burns on a child. This is a typical pattern of child abuse burns. *(Courtesy of Roy Alson, MD)*

Sadly, burns in children may be the result of intentional abuse, and in fact, 20% of all abuse cases in the United States involve burns. You should be alert for signs of abuse. They include burns that match shapes of objects such as curling irons, irons, or cigarette burns. Also suspicious for abuse are multiple stories of how the injury occurred or stories of the burn being caused by activities by the child that are inconsistent with the child's development. Burns to the genitalia, perineum, or in a stocking or glove distribution (Figure 16-18) should raise suspicion. If there is a suspicion of abuse, this must be reported to child protective services or law enforcement. Follow your local laws and protocols.

Fire and EMS personnel can help reduce burns in children through community education. Programs to teach parents about limiting the temperature on household water heaters to 120°F and programs to teach children about fire safety can make a significant impact on the incidence of pediatric burns in your community. You should be aware that the elderly may also be victims of abuse by burns. (See Chapter 18.)

CASE PRESENTATION (continued)

It is a hot day in July, and an ALS ambulance has been called to the scene of a suicide attempt. They are told that a young woman has tried to kill herself by pouring gasoline in her car and then sitting in the auto and lighting the gasoline. She had driven into the woods to do this. She changed her mind as soon as the gasoline ignited. She was alone and did not have a phone, so had to hike a mile to get help.

They arrive at the farmhouse to which the young woman has come for help. She is the only victim, and the scene is safe. She is dressed in a short-sleeved shirt and loose slacks. Her clothes are slightly singed but have not been on fire. She is alert and ambulatory and denies any injury other than the flash of the fireball when she ignited the gasoline. She states she poured gasoline in the floor of her car, sat in the seat, and flicked a lighter. There was a flash and immediate pain, and she scrambled out of the auto. It took her about 25 minutes to hike to the house, where the family called 911 and gave her cold compresses to put on her face and arms. The response time of the ambulance has been another 20 minutes, so close to an hour has passed since the initial burn.

The initial assessment reveals normal speaking voice and respiration, strong radial pulse that is slightly fast. A focused exam reveals singing of her hair and eyebrows and nasal hairs. Her exposed skin (face, arms) and the skin of her lower legs under her slacks are all erythematous with a few blisters. There is erythema in her nose, mouth, and pharynx.

She walks to the ambulance and is strapped to the cot. At this time the team leader notes that her voice is becoming husky, and she complains of feeling short of breath. An ITLS Ongoing Exam reveals bilateral wheezes but the pulse oximeter reading is 95% on 15 L of oxygen by nonrebreather mask. The team is worried about lower and upper airway burns and possibly losing the airway, but they don't have DAI capability, and she has an active gag reflex and won't let them insert a nasotracheal tube because it is so painful with the burns in her nose. They give her an albuterol nebulizer treatment and take her to the closest hospital, where they are able to perform DAI and insert a small endotracheal tube using a fiberoptic scope. Her oxygen saturation continues to fall, and she is admitted to the ICU, where she develops adult respiratory distress syndrome (ARDS) and has a protracted course. However, because of her youth and general good health, she survives. Her lower respiratory burns were caused by her inhaling the volatile gasoline fumes before igniting the gasoline, and when the gasoline ignited, it flashed all the way to her alveoli. ■

Summary

The mechanisms of burn injuries are potentially deadly for both you and your patient. Remember scene safety! All burns are serious and should be evaluated at the hospital. Do not forget the basics: Half of all burn deaths are from inhalation injuries. Aggressive airway management may be needed. Stop the burning process with a quick irrigation of the burn with room-temperature water. A clean sheet is all you need to put on the burn other than a blanket to prevent hypothermia. In the opposite of load and go, patients with chemical burns must be decontaminated immediately or the burn damage will continue to progress during transport. Electrical burns and lightning injury are commonly associated with cardiac arrest, but rapid evaluation and management are usually lifesaving. High-voltage electricity is extremely dangerous; get trained personnel to turn off the current before approaching the patient. Do not begin secondary transfer of a burn patient until the patient has been properly stabilized and the airway protected.

Bibliography

1. American Burn Association. 2003. Inhalation injury: Diagnosis. *Journal of the American College of Surgeons* 196(2): 307–312.

2. Borron, S. W., F. J. Baud, P. Barriot, M. Imbert, C. Bismuth. 2007. Prospective study of hydroxocobalamin for acute cyanide poisoning in smoke inhalation. *Ann Emerg Med.* 49(6): 794–801, 801.
3. Committee on Trauma, American College of Surgeons. 2009. Injuries due to burns and cold. *Advanced Trauma Life Support*. 8th ed Chicago: American College of Surgeons.
4. Danks, R. R. 2003. Burn management: A comprehensive review of the epidemiology and treatment of burn victims. *JEMS* 28(5): 118–141.
5. Fortin, J. L., J. P. Giocanti, M. Ruttimann, J. J. Kowalski. 2006. Prehospital administration of hydroxocobalamin for smoke inhalation-associated cyanide poisoning: Eight years of experience in the Paris Fire Brigade. *Clinical Toxicology* 44(Suppl 1): 37–44.
6. Goodis J., E. Schraga. 2009. Thermal burns. *Emedicine: On-line Emergency Medicine Text*. WebMD, www.emedicine.com.
7. Miller, K. 2003. Acute inhalation injury. *Emergency Medical Clinics of North America* 21(2): 533–557.
8. Miller, S. March 2009. Optimizing outcome in the adult and pediatric burn patient. *Trauma Reports* 10, # 2.
9. Shehan, H., R. Papini. 2004. Initial management of a major burn: Overview. *British Medical Journal* 328: 1555–1557.

Explore Resource Central

For additional review and practice tests, visit www.bradybooks.com and click on Resource Central to access book-specific resources for this text. To access Resource Central, follow directions on the Student Access Card provided with this text. If there is no card, go to www.bradybooks.com and follow the Resource Central link to Buy Access from there.

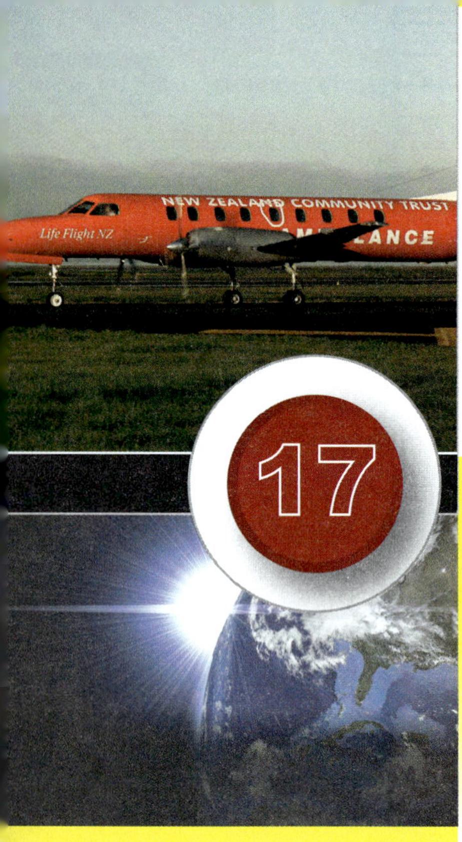

(Photo courtesy of Robert Cumming, Shutterstock.com)

Pediatric Trauma

Patrick J. Maloney, MD
Ann Marie Dietrich, MD, FACEP, FAAP
Leslie Mihalov, MD, FAAP

Trauma in Children

Traumi Pediatrici

Traumatismo en Niños

Traumatisme dans les Enfants

Urazy u dzieci

Trauma beim Kind

Ozljede u djece

إصابات الأطفال

trauma dece

Poškodbe otrok

Gyermekkori trauma

KEY TERMS

child abuse, *p. 311*
child restraint seat, *p. 327*
consent, *p. 311*
fluid resuscitation, *p. 324*
length-based tape, *p. 311*

OBJECTIVES

Upon successful completion of this chapter, you should be able to:

1. Describe effective techniques for gaining the confidence of children and their parents.
2. Predict pediatric injuries based on common mechanisms of injury.
3. Describe the ITLS Primary and Secondary Surveys in the pediatric patient.
4. Demonstrate understanding of the need for immediate transport in potentially life-threatening circumstances, regardless of the availability of immediate parental consent.
5. Differentiate the equipment needs of pediatric patients from those of adults.
6. Describe the various ways to perform spinal motion restriction (SMR) on a child and how this differs for an adult.
7. Discuss the need for involvement of EMS personnel in prevention programs for parents and children.

Note: Because of increasing demand for further training in management of the injured child, ITLS has developed a one-day course (Pediatric ITLS) that covers this subject in detail. You may get more information about this course by calling ITLS International at 888-495-4875 (outside the United States call 630-495-6442).

Chapter Overview

The goal of prehospital care is to minimize further injury, ensure patient safety, and treat life-threatening conditions. When applying those principles to the pediatric population, you must remember that children are not just little adults. They differ from adults in that they have unique patterns of injuries, frequently have different responses to those injuries, require special equipment for assessment and treatment, and can be challenging to assess and communicate with. Doctors as well as EMTs are frequently less confident treating children because of those differences and the fact that we treat them less frequently. Therefore, we do not develop as much expertise as we would like. Those of us with children of our own are further hampered by the intense emotions we feel when treating a seriously injured child. For all those reasons you should study this chapter carefully. This chapter offers a review of the ITLS Primary Survey, stresses the differences between children and adults, and describes how to manage critical injuries.

CASE PRESENTATION

An ALS ambulance has been dispatched for a 2-year-old child who was run over by a four-wheeler all-terrain vehicle. They are told that the child is unconscious. What sort of injuries should they expect from this mechanism? How does evaluation and treatment of a 2-year-old differ from an adult? Keep these questions in mind as you read the chapter. Then, at the end of the chapter, find out how the rescuers completed the call. ■

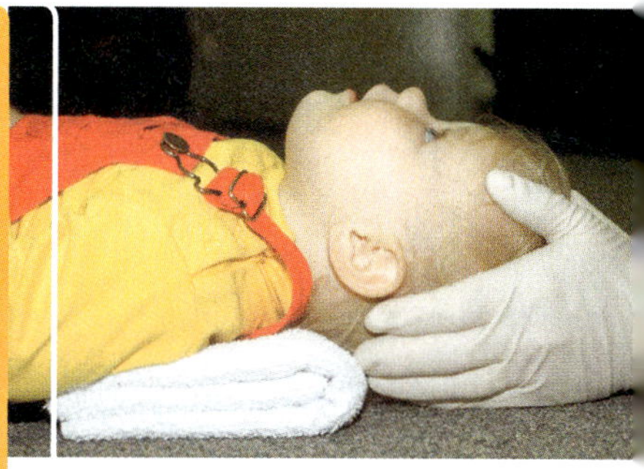

(Courtesy of Bob Page, NREMT-P)

Communication with the Child and Family

Children are part of a family unit, which is the one constant factor in their lives, so family-centered care for an injured child is ideal. (Remember that the caregiver of a child will not always be a parent, but for simplicity the generic term *parent* is used in this chapter when referring to the guardian of a child.) Following an injury to their child, parents should be involved as much as possible in his or her care. Parents who receive careful instructions and guidance may be helpful to the emergency provider. Explain to them what you are doing and why you are doing it, and then use their trust relationship with the child to enhance your history gathering, physical examination, and care of the patient. Inclusion and respect of the family will improve the performance of all aspects of the stabilization of an injured child.

The best way to get parent confidence is to demonstrate your competence and compassion in managing the child. Parents are more likely to be cooperative if they see that you are confident, organized, and using equipment that is designed for children. Show the parents you know how important they are by involving them in the care of their child. Whenever possible, keep parents in physical and verbal contact with the child. They can perform simple tasks such as holding a pressure dressing or holding the child's hand. Parents can explain to the child what is going on or sing their favorite songs.

When evaluating an injured child, remember to speak and act in a way that is understandable and calming to the child and parents. This will not only help console the scared and hurt child, but it also will help you accurately assess the child's condition. A child who can be consoled and interacts normally with a parent likely has a normal mental status. In contrast, a child who cannot be consoled or cannot interact in the usual way may have a head injury, may be in shock, may be hypoxic, or may be in severe pain. Because they are familiar with a child's baseline mental status, the parents are your best resource for detecting subtle changes in the child's behavior. They will notice when the child is "not acting right" before you will. Record and report your observations just as you would report changes in level of consciousness of an adult.

A child younger than 9 months old likes to hear "cooing" sounds, the jingle and sight of keys, and often feels more comfortable when swaddled. For the child under 2 years of age, the flashlight is a good distraction. Use appropriate language for the developmental level of the child. Children younger than 1 year of age know many "ah" sounds, like "mama" and "papa." Try to use them. Older children, especially 2-year-olds, are typically negative and often difficult to distract or comfort. Expect all questions to be answered by "no." Therefore, tell the child and the parents what you are going to do and do it. For example, "We are going to hold your head still. Mom, this is important in case he has hurt his neck." Speak simply, slowly, and clearly. Be gentle and firm. The toddler and young child can benefit from a toy or doll being with them. Ask the parent to get one favorite belonging, if easily available, for the ride to the hospital. It will make the trip to and through the hospital easier.

Do not get caught in the trap of asking the child if he wants to take a trip in the ambulance or to be placed in a cervical collar. The child will answer "no" most of the time. Tell the child what you are doing with a smile on your face. Show it does not hurt, perhaps by doing it to a parent or yourself. Size is intimidating. When approaching a child, try to make yourself small by getting on the child's level. In the care of a child, it is appropriate that EMTs spend much field time on their knees.

Whenever possible, provide the child and family members with options. It will help relieve anxiety and encourage cooperation. Frightened children, especially around the ages of 2 to 4 years, may bite, spit, or hit. They are acting out of fear. Stay calm, recognize that the behavior is normal, reassure the child, and use firm, not painful, physical control of the patient as needed. Parents and children do not understand packaging, which makes them more likely to resist it. Most parents will understand if you explain that even though the chances are low that there is anything seriously wrong with the spine, the stakes are high if there is. Make a game of packaging with the child. If the parent still refuses to let you package the child, write it down on your run report and get the parent to sign it.

Whenever possible, allow parents to accompany their child in the vehicle. It is very frightening for a child and family to be separated, especially if the injuries are potentially severe. Give the parents specific instructions and position them to provide comfort and support to their child without interfering with the care that must be given. Make sure that any family member who accompanies the child in the ambulance is properly restrained with a seat belt.

Before you leave the scene with the child, be sure to ask the parent about other children. Sometimes they are so concerned about one that they forget other small children who may be in a high-risk situation, such as alone in the house.

Parental Consent

Many jurisdictions have **consent** laws that exist to protect children. Although consent to treat is necessary for children who are stable and desirable in children who are injured, any critically injured child should *not* have care delayed while attempting to obtain consent. Prehospital care providers have to assess the situation quickly and decide whether delaying emergency care to obtain parental consent could possibly harm the child. In a situation in which a child needs emergency care (such as a child in a bicycle/motor-vehicle collision and no parent present), you must treat that child immediately. When in doubt, always err on the side of treating and transporting any seriously injured child, regardless of the ability to obtain appropriate consent. Remember to document why you are transporting without permission, and always notify medical direction of this action.

If the parents or legal guardians do not want you to transport or treat, try to persuade them. If you cannot, document your actions on the written report and ask them to sign it. If the child has a critical injury and the parents refuse transport, notify law enforcement and the appropriate social authorities immediately and try to continue care of the child until they arrive. If you suspect **child abuse**, notify authorities at the appropriate time. You should not confront the possible abuser but act in the best interests of the child.

PEARLS: Abuse

You are the only one to see the scene of the injury. Be alert to signs of child abuse.

consent the granting of permission to treat a child. It is usually given by the parents or legal guardian but is not required in an emergency situation if neither are present.

child abuse physical or emotional violence or neglect toward a person from infancy until age 15.

Assessment and Care

Pediatric Equipment

Table 17-1 contains a list of suggested pediatric equipment for the prehospital provider. A more detailed list can be downloaded from the American Academy of Pediatrics website. Keep pediatric equipment separate from your adult equipment. It would be ideal to keep equipment for each sized child in separate compartments. However, lack of storage space and high expense makes multiple containers and duplicate equipment impractical. Using a **length-based tape** has become an essential component for determining the appropriate equipment and medication doses for a child.

The length-based tape helps you measure the length of a child, estimate the child's weight, appropriately choose correctly sized equipment, and administer precalculated doses of fluid and medications (Figures 17-1 and 17-2). The device allows you to focus on the patient instead of remembering the correct equipment size and drug dose. The length-based tape estimates weight and equipment size better than medical professionals. Although there is some controversy regarding the accuracy of length-based medication dosages because of the increased incidence of childhood obesity, standard length-based resuscitation systems continue to be recommended as safe, rapid, and accurate tools.

PEARLS: Equipment

Children require special equipment. Without this equipment, you cannot provide the pediatric patient with adequate care.

length-based tape a method of estimating the appropriate size equipment and doses of medications for children. The method is based on the fact that a child's weight is proportional to his length.

Table 17-1 Prehospital Pediatric Equipment and Supplies

BLS Equipment and Supplies

Essential	Desirable
• Oropharyngeal airways: infant, child, and adult sizes (sizes 00–5) with tongue blades for insertion • Self-inflating resuscitation bag, child and adult sizes • Masks for bag-mask device: neonatal, infant, child, and adult sizes • Oxygen masks; infant, child and adult sizes • Nonrebreathing mask: pediatric and adult sizes • Stethoscope • Pediatric femur traction splint • Pediatric backboard with head immobilizer • Pediatric cervical collars (rigid) • Blood pressure cuff, infant and child • Portable suction unit with a regulator • Suction catheter: tonsil-tip and 6F–14F • Extremity splints: pediatric size • Bulb syringe • Obstetric pack • Thermal blanket • Water-soluble lubricant	• Infant car seat • Nasopharyngeal airways: sizes 18F–34F, or 4.5–8.5 mm • Glasgow Coma Score reference • Small stuffed toy • Finger-stick blood glucose device • Pulse oximeter

ALS Equipment and Supplies

ALS units should carry everything on the BLS list, plus the following items:

Essential	Desirable
• Transport monitor • Defibrillator with adult and pediatric paddles • Monitoring electrodes: pediatric sizes • Endotracheal tubes, uncuffed sizes 2.5–6 mm; cuffed sizes 6–8 mm • Endotracheal tube stylets: pediatric and adult sizes • Infant and child laryngoscope straight blades sizes 0–3 and curved blades sizes 2–4 • Nasogastric tubes, sizes 8F–16F • KID (immobilization device) • Magill forceps: pediatric and adult • IO needles, sizes 16, 18, 20 • Butterfly cannulae, 23 and 25 gauge • Over-the-needle catheters, 16–24 gauge • Pediatric armboards • Broselow tape • Nebulizer	• Disposable CO_2 detection device • End-tidal CO_2 monitors • Blood glucose analysis system

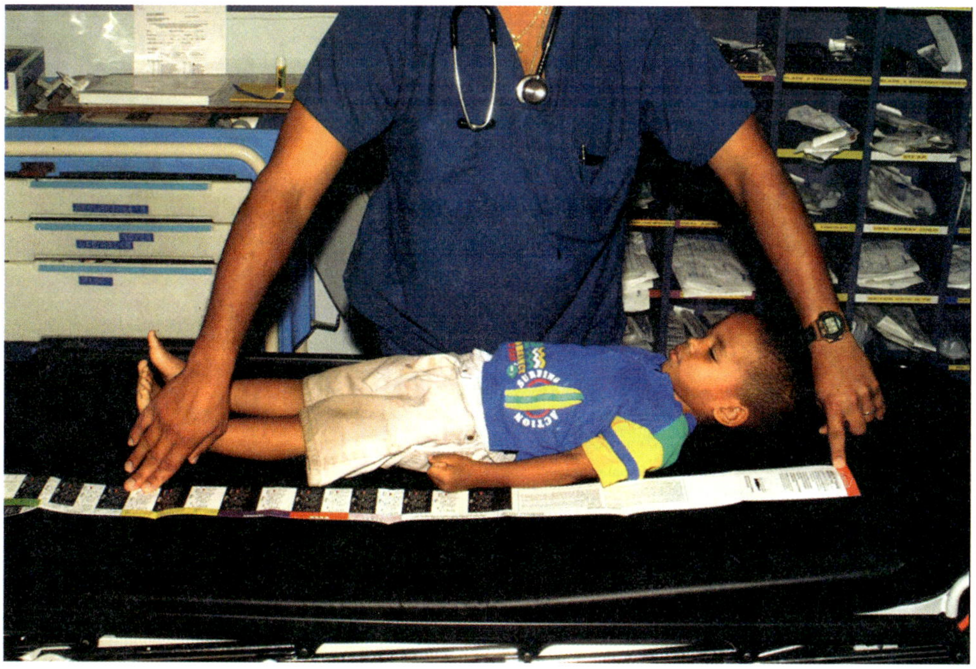

FIGURE 17-1 Use of length-based tape. *(Courtesy of James Broselow, MD)*

Common Mechanisms of Injury

Children are most commonly injured from falls, motor-vehicle collisions, auto-pedestrian crashes, burns, airway obstruction from a foreign body, submersion injuries (drownings), and child abuse. Children who fall usually land on their heads because the head is the largest and heaviest part of a small child's body. Fortunately, when children fall from a height of less than three feet, they rarely sustain serious head injuries. The use of motorcycles and dirt bikes, especially if a helmet is not worn, often results in serious injury. Motor-vehicle collisions,

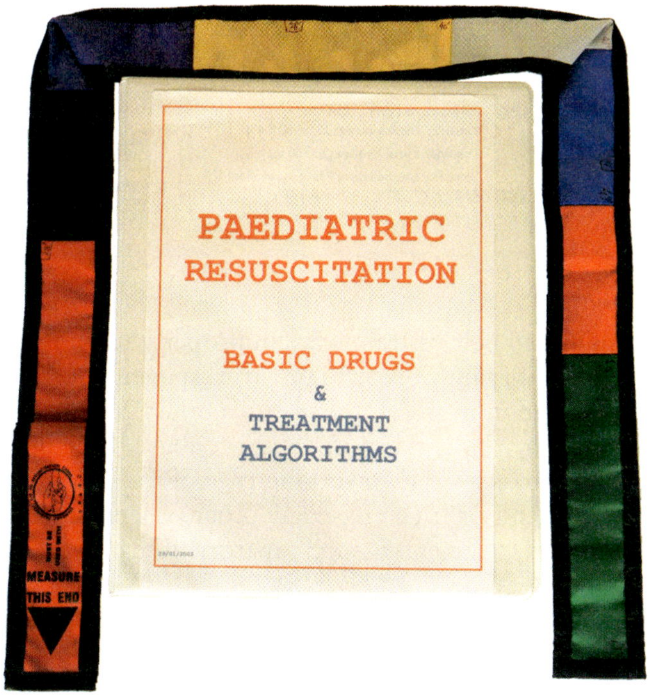

a.

FIGURE 17-2 Standard Pediatric Aid to Resuscitation Card system has color-coded tape and a booklet of precalculated doses of fluids, medications, and equipment (a). Examples of information included is shown in (b) and (c) on the next page. *(Photos courtesy of Kyee Han, MD)*

FIGURE 17-2 *(Continued)*

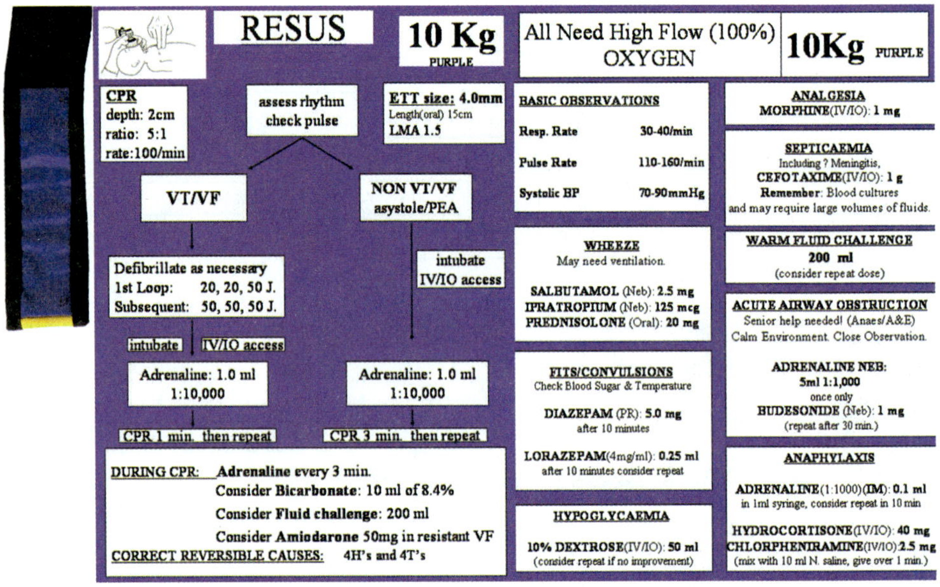

b.

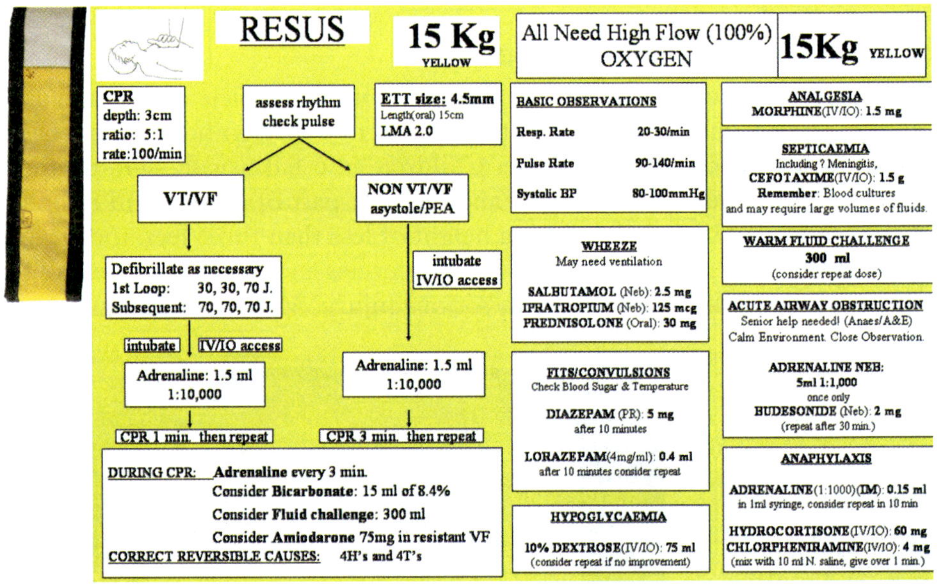

c.

especially if lap belt restraints are improperly used, may result in seat-belt syndrome and injury may occur to the liver, spleen, intestines, and/or lumbar spine.

Any situation in which the victim's injury pattern is not consistent with the mechanism may be child abuse. Suspect abuse if the history does not match the injury, if there is a delay in seeking care, if the story frequently changes during your assessment, or if you have any other concerns. Remember to report any of these findings to the emergency department team.

General Assessment

When arriving at the scene of an accident or injury, it is very important to quickly assess the situation and the injured child. After ensuring your own safety, your next step is to develop a general impression of the injured child,

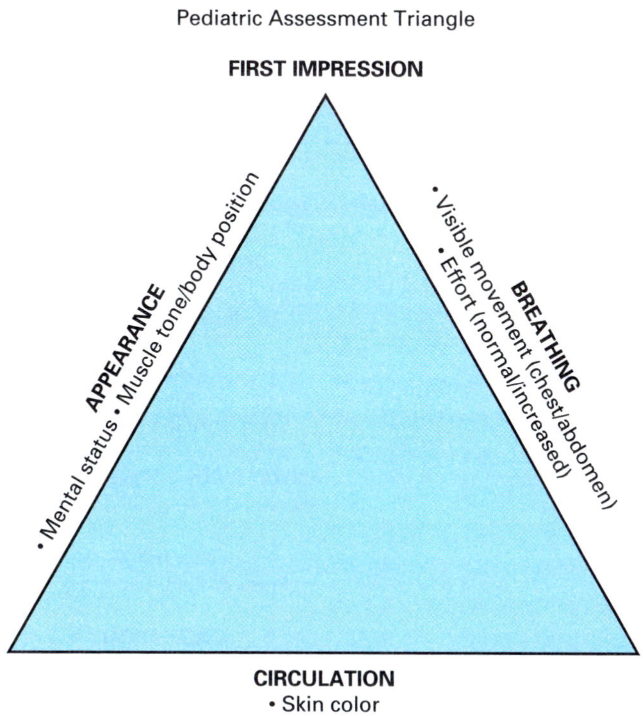

FIGURE 17-3 Pediatric Assessment Triangle. *(Copyright American Academy of Pediatrics. Used with permission.)*

usually from across the room or scene. Before ever touching an injured child, try to decide whether he or she appears to be severely injured or in distress. Make a mental note of the child's initial level of consciousness, work of breathing, and overall circulation as you begin your survey. Although a preschool child may appear to be sleeping rather than unconscious from an injury, remember that most children will not sleep through the arrival of emergency vehicles. Following a traumatic event, a decreased level of consciousness may suggest hypoxia, shock, head trauma, or seizure. One tool to help you develop this overall impression of the severity of the child's condition is the Pediatric Assessment Triangle, an objective tool developed by the American Academy of Pediatrics (Figure 17-3). It will help you efficiently prioritize your care.

Assessment of the Airway

As you begin your assessment, stabilize the neck in a neutral position with your hands. Do not take time to apply a cervical collar until you have finished the ITLS Primary Survey (Figure 17-4). Inspecting the airway is easier in the child than in the adult. It is true that the child's tongue is large, the tissue is soft, and the airway obstructs easily, but other characteristics make it easier to manage the child's airway. For example, neonates are obligatory nose breathers, so clearing the nose with a bulb syringe can be lifesaving. To use the bulb syringe, collapse the bulb end of the syringe, put the point end in the nose of the child, and release the bulb. Remove the syringe from the nose, squeeze the bulb to empty the mucus, blood, or vomit, and repeat. The bulb syringe can be used to remove secretions from the posterior pharynx of infants as well.

Look for signs of airway obstruction in the child, including apnea, stridor, and "gurgling" respirations. If identified, perform a jaw-thrust maneuver without moving the neck. That will help lift the relatively large tongue out of the way of the

FIGURE 17-4 Steps in the assessment and management of the trauma patient are the same for both children and adults.

ITLS PRIMARY SURVEY

SCENE SIZE-UP

Standard Precautions

Hazards, Number of Patients, Need for additional resources, **Mechanism of Injury**

INITIAL ASSESSMENT

GENERAL IMPRESSION

Age, Sex, Weight, General Appearance, Position, Purposeful Movement, Obvious Injuries, Skin Color

Life-threatening Bleeding

LOC

A-V-P-U

Chief Complaint/Symptoms

AIRWAY (WITH C-SPINE CONTROL)

Snoring, Gurgling, Stridor; Silence

BREATHING

Present? Rate, Depth, Effort

CIRCULATION

Radial/Carotid Present? Rate, Rhythm, Quality

Skin Color, Temperature, Moisture; Capillary Refill

Has bleeding been controlled?

RAPID TRAUMA SURVEY

HEAD and NECK

Wounds?

Neck Vein distention? Tracheal Deviation?

CHEST

Asymmetry (Paradoxical Motion?), Contusions, Penetrations, Tenderness, Instability, Crepitation

Breath Sounds

Present? Equal? (If unequal: percussion)

Heart Tones

ABDOMEN

Contusions, Penetration/Evisceration; Tenderness, Rigidity, Distension

PELVIS

Tenderness, Instability, Crepitation

LOWER/UPPER EXTREMITIES

Obvious Swelling, Deformity

Motor and Sensory

POSTERIOR

Obvious wounds, Tenderness, Deformity

If radial pulse present:

VITAL SIGNS

Measured Pulse, Breathing, Blood Pressure

If altered mental status: Brief Neurological exam

PUPILS

Size? Reactive? **Equal?**

GLASGOW COMA SCALE

Eyes, Voice, Motor

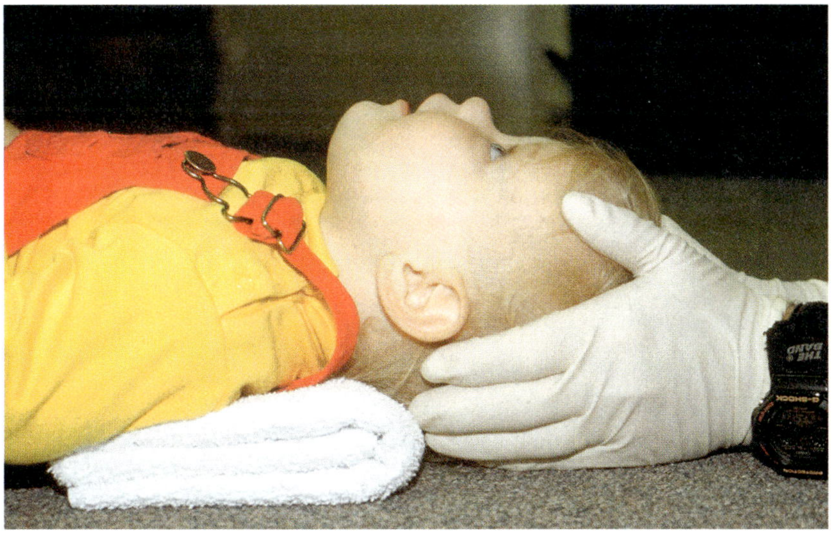

FIGURE 17-5 Most children require padding under their back and shoulders to keep the C-spine in a neutral position. *(Courtesy of Bob Page, NREMT-P)*

airway. Suctioning oral secretions and any vomit from the posterior pharynx also can help. Inserting an oropharyngeal airway may help keep the obstructed airway patent. (See Chapter 5.) If a tooth is loose, be sure to remove it from the mouth so that the child does not choke on it. Also, remember that in small children, the occiput is so big that it will often flex the neck and occlude the airway when the child is lying flat. It is often necessary to place a pad underneath the torso to keep the neck in a neutral position. (See Figure 17-5 and Chapter 11.) Hyperextension of the neck also may cause airway occlusion.

Assessment of Breathing

Assess the child for breathing difficulty. Count the child's rate of breathing. Most children breathe fast when they are having trouble, and then, when they can no longer compensate, they have periods of apnea or a very slow respiratory rate. Note whether the child is "working" to breathe, demonstrated by retractions, flaring, or grunting. Look at the chest rise, listen for air going in and out, and feel the air coming out of the nose. If there is no movement, reposition the jaw to remove any anatomical obstruction. If you still do not sense any air exchange, you must breathe for the child. If you have any doubt that the child is adequately breathing on his or her own, immediately assist the child's breathing.

Artificial Ventilation

The most important skill that you must master is artificial ventilation with a bag-mask resuscitation device. Remember, if you can artificially oxygenate and ventilate a child, you can keep that child alive!

It is crucial that your bag-mask device has a good seal around the face. If the face mask does not fit well, try a different size face mask or try turning the mask upside down for a better seal. Pay attention to your hand placement as well (Figure 17-6). Large adult hands can easily obstruct the airway or injure the child's eyes. Give each breath slowly over 1 second. Try to use the lowest pressure necessary to see good chest rise with each breath. If the chest is rising, air is getting into the lungs. If you do not see good chest rise, too little air is entering the lungs. Check air entry on both sides of the chest with your stethoscope. If the

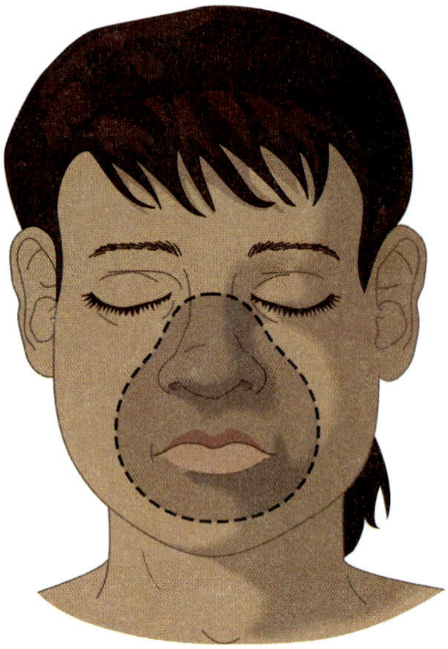

a.

FIGURE 17-6a The mask should fit on the nose and the cleft above the chin.

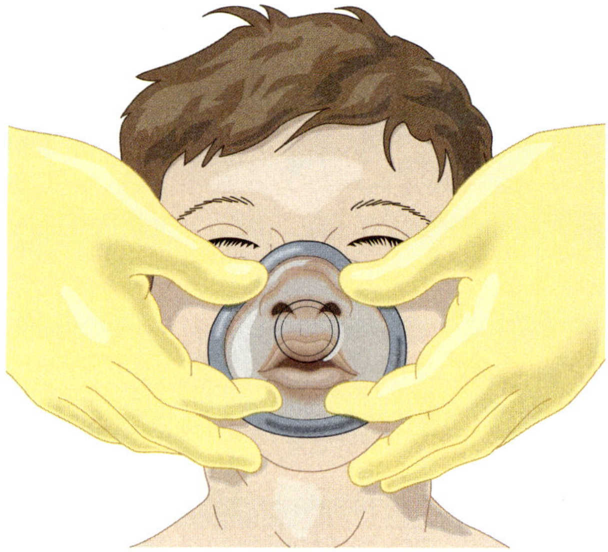

b.

FIGURE 17-6b Two-handed face mask seal.

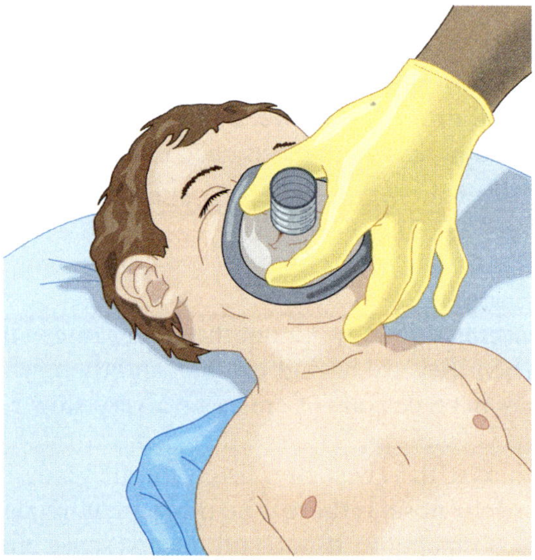

c.

FIGURE 17-6c One-handed face mask seal.

child is not getting good chest rise with each breath, make sure that air entry is not obstructed, and if still unsuccessful, you may need to provide more pressure with each rescue breath. Be careful not to provide too much pressure because that may cause a pneumothorax or overinflate the stomach and cause vomiting. Remember that most pediatric resuscitation bags have a pop-off valve. In the prehospital setting, it is usually best to ensure that this valve is turned off.

When providing artificial ventilation, typical rates are 20 per minute for a child less than 1 year of age, 15 per minute for greater than 1 year of age, and 10 per minute for an adolescent. Studies have found that rescuers tend to hyperventilate even when consciously trying not to. Always make sure that your bag is connected to oxygen and that it is flowing (usually 10–15 L/minute). Gentle cricoid pressure (Sellick maneuver; see Chapter 4) is useful and recommended in a child. However, beware that excessive cricoid pressure can easily obstruct a child's airway.

Endotracheal Intubation. If bag-mask ventilation of the child is effective, then intubation is an elective procedure. Studies have not shown that prehospital intubation improves the outcome of children. *It is usually better not to intubate the child in the field if you can ventilate successfully with a bag-mask.* Rapid and safe transportation to a trauma center, where definitive care is readily available, is one of the most important prognostic factors in trauma patients. Therefore, any unnecessary time spent at the scene should be avoided.

Intubation is extremely difficult to perform even in an emergency department, so if you must intubate in the field, be prepared! While you prepare your equipment, your partner should preoxygenate (not hyperventilate) the child with five to seven breaths with high-flow oxygen at the normal rate for the age of the child or apply a nonrebreather mask, if the child is breathing on his or her own adequately. The oral route should be used on all children. There are several ways to choose the right size for the endotracheal tube. The simplest is to refer to your length-based tape system. Other techniques include choosing a tube that is about the same diameter as the tip of the child's little finger or using the following equation:

$$4 + \frac{\text{age in years}}{4} = \text{size of tube (mm)}$$

In small children the smallest part of the airway is just below the cords. As a result, traditional practice is to use an uncuffed tube in children less than 8 years old. However, many experts now recommend using cuffed endotracheal tubes in all patients. If you decide to use a cuffed tube, choose a tube that is 0.5 mm smaller except for 3.0 mm tubes. In general, you should not inflate the cuff, however, unless directed to do so by your medical control because a cuff that is inflated too much may damage the child's airway.

There is a significant risk of neck movement with any tracheal intubation, so have someone stabilize the neck with his hands during intubation. Using a straight blade, enter the mouth on the right and gently sweep the tongue to the left; place the blade in the vallecula, and lift. Compared to adults, the small child's larynx is closer to the mouth as well as more anterior (higher up). If you cannot see the cords because of the relatively large and floppy epiglottis, advance the laryngoscope blade to the epiglottis and lift again. The cords should be easily seen. The laryngeal mask (LMA) and the King LT airways are available in pediatric sizes and can be used as rescue airways. They should not be used for airway burns or airway swelling from allergic reactions because they are supraglottic and so do not keep the glottis open.

It is recommended that pulse oximetry is used during every intubation. Pulse oximetry is a good tool for knowing when you need to stop your intubation attempt and oxygenate the patient again prior to another attempt (usually when the SpO_2 drops below about 90%). Other ways to make sure that you remember to ventilate include holding your breath when no one is breathing for the child. As soon as you get an urge to breathe, but after no more than 15 seconds, stop trying to intubate, bag the child to reoxygenate, and try again in a few minutes. An alternative effective method is to have the team member who is stabilizing the neck count aloud to 15 slowly.

PEARLS: Endotracheal Intubation

The endotracheal tube in a child may become dislodged easily, especially during movement of the child. Frequent reassessment is very important. Constant expired CO_2 monitoring (capnography) is very helpful.

Confirm the endotracheal tube is in the correct place by following the confirmation protocol. (See Chapter 5.) Although a disposable, qualitative end-tidal carbon dioxide detection device can be used to confirm that it is correctly positioned within the airway, capnography is the best way to both confirm the tube is in place and continually monitor its position. Be sure to secure the tube in place. Apply benzoin to the cheek and lip. Firmly tape (or tie with linen tape or plastic oxygen tubing) the tube to the corner of the mouth. Alternatively, a commercial endotracheal tube holder may be used, if available. Beware that simple flexion of the neck can push the tube into the right mainstem bronchus, and extension of the neck can pull the tube out of the trachea. Fortunately, the rigid cervical collar is an easy and practical adjunct to limit any unnecessary head and neck movement. Therefore, in trauma patients, applying a rigid cervical collar not only protects the patient's cervical spine from potential further injury but also helps reduce the likelihood of endotracheal tube movement and malpositioning.

Supplemental Oxygen. As you package a child, you often have to improvise. Tape and straps can restrict the child's chest movement, so assess ventilation frequently en route. Any child with a significant injury should receive supplemental oxygen (as close to 100% oxygen as possible), even if there seems to be no difficulty breathing. Injury, fear, and crying all increase oxygen demands on tissues. Children with any type of injury are likely to vomit, so be prepared. Remember to give ventilation instructions to your teammate before moving to assessment of circulation.

Assessment of Circulation

In a child, the brachial and femoral pulses are usually easy to feel, whereas the carotid pulse is not. Because tachycardia also occurs with fear and anxiety, the child should then be assessed for signs of poor perfusion, weak peripheral pulses compared to central pulses, cool distant extremities, and delayed capillary refill. A weak rapid pulse with a rate over 130 is usually a sign of shock in children of all ages except neonates (Table 17-2). An easy peripheral pulse to check in a child is the dorsalis pedis pulse.

Prolonged capillary refill, cool extremities, and skin mottling may indicate decreased tissue perfusion. Capillary refill may be used along with other methods to assess the circulation, but do not depend on it alone to diagnose shock because it is prolonged by anything that causes vasoconstriction, such as cold environment or fear. To test capillary refill, compress the nail bed, the entire foot, or the skin over the sternum for 2 seconds and release to see how quickly the blood returns. Skin color should return to the precompressed state within 2 seconds. If it does not, the child has vasoconstriction, which can be a sign of shock.

PEARLS: Shock

Because of strong compensatory mechanisms, children can look surprisingly good in early shock. When they deteriorate, they often "crash." If you have a long transport time and the mechanism of injury or the assessment suggests the possibility of hemorrhagic shock, be prepared. When you give fluid resuscitation to a child, give 20 mL/kg in each bolus, then reassess. Make sure the total amount of fluid you give is reported to the hospital.

Table 17-2 Ranges for Vital Signs

Age	Weight (kg)	Respiration (per minute)	Pulse (per minute)	Systolic Blood Pressure (mm Hg)
Newborn	3–4	30–50	120–160	> 60
6 mo–1 yr	8–10	30–40	120–140	70–80
2–4 yr	12–16	20–30	100–110	80–95
5–8 yr	18–26	14–20	90–100	90–100
8–12 yr	26–50	12–20	80–100	100–110
> 12 yr	> 50	12–16	80–100	100–120

Control of Bleeding. Obvious bleeding sources must be controlled to maintain circulation. Remember, the child's blood volume is about 80–90 mL/kg, so a 10-kg child has less than 1 liter of blood. Three or four lacerations can cause a 200-mL blood loss, which is about 20% of the child's total volume. Therefore, pay closer attention to blood loss in a child than you do in an adult. Remember that bleeding may not be immediately evident if the child is fully clothed or lying on an absorbent surface such as carpet or grass. Be sure to examine the child from head to toe for any bleeding. Posterior scalp lacerations are especially notorious for causing unnoticed bleeding. Use pressure firm enough to control arterial bleeding if necessary. If you ask the parent or a bystander to help hold pressure, monitor them to be sure they are applying enough pressure to stop the bleeding.

One mistake parents as well as emergency medical personnel commonly make is using a large bulky dressing, towel, or piece of clothing to attempt to stop bleeding. Unfortunately, the bulky dressings often do not provide enough direct pressure to stop the bleeding. Instead, they simply absorb large amounts of blood and disguise potentially serious bleeding. Your gloved hand and fingers in combination with a 4×4 sterile gauze pad is usually your best tool for applying constant firm pressure to the site of bleeding. Once the bleeding is under control, you may attempt to apply a more secure dressing. Be sure to recheck the dressing and wound often to ensure that the bleeding has not recurred.

Hemostatic agents also can be used to control hemorrhage in children. Although tourniquets are not routinely recommended, in life-threatening bleeding that cannot be controlled by other means, the lifesaving benefits of a tourniquet outweigh the small potential risk of further limb injury and loss. (See Chapter 14.)

Rapid Trauma Survey or Focused Exam

Perform a rapid head-to-toe exam (rapid trauma survey) on children who have been injured by a generalized mechanism or when you do not know the mechanism of injury. Children who have a focused (isolated) injury or an insignificant injury may have a focused exam of the injured part only. Children with insignificant mechanisms of injury may not require an ITLS Secondary Survey.

Rapid Trauma Survey. The rapid trauma survey is a quick examination of the head, neck, chest, abdomen, pelvis, and extremities. Also perform a brief neurological exam if there is altered level of consciousness. Look for life-threatening injuries. By this time, the child should be adequately exposed to assess all the injuries. Parents may be able to assist with this because most children are taught not to allow strangers to disrobe them. *You cannot assess what you cannot see!*

Rapidly check the head and neck for signs of injury, such as bruises, abrasions, lacerations, and puncture wounds. Also look for distended neck veins and tracheal deviation. What appears to be minor trauma to the neck can be life threatening because any bleeding or swelling within the neck can compress and obstruct the child's airway very quickly.

Look at, listen to, and feel the chest. Look for deformities, contusions, abrasions, perforations, burns, tenderness, lacerations, and swelling (DCAP-BTLS). Listen to breath sounds on each side and note any abnormalities. Feel for tenderness, instability, or crepitus (TIC). If not already done, have one of your partners stabilize flail segments, seal open wounds, or decompress a tension pneumothorax.

Gently palpate the abdomen and note any contusions, abrasions, penetrations, or distention. If there is no complaint of pain in the pelvic area, gently palpate the pelvis noting any TIC. Quickly evaluate the extremities for obvious injury.

As soon as you finish the rapid trauma survey, transfer the child to a spinal motion restriction device. Remember to log-roll the child the same way you would an adult (Chapter 12). This is the time to check the child's back carefully for any injuries. If an appropriate size cervical collar is available, place it on the child and secure the child's body and then the head to the SMR device. It may be difficult to prevent all movement of the cervical spine, especially in the young child.

Critical Trauma Situation

If you have found a critical trauma situation, the child needs rapid transport. Once you have the child packaged, you should leave the scene as quickly as possible. Remember to use a pad under the torso to align the neck in a neutral position. Appropriately sized rigid cervical collars are useful, especially in children over 1 year of age, and can help remind the patient and providers not to move the head. Do not depend on the cervical collar alone. Restrict motion of the head with tape and a head motion-restriction device. There are very few procedures that should be done in the field. Minutes count, especially in children. On-scene times of less than 5 minutes are desirable.

Administer 100% oxygen to all potentially seriously injured pediatric patients. There is strong evidence to support the policy that bag-mask ventilation of the critical child is preferable to placing an endotracheal tube if the transport time to an appropriate emergency department is short. When considering transportation options, providers should be aware of local and regional resources and policies. This includes deciding on the appropriate destination for a particular patient (the nearest emergency department versus a regional pediatric trauma center) as well as choosing the best transportation mode (BLS versus ALS versus air ambulance). As a general rule, any child with life-threatening injuries or hemodynamic instability should be transported to the nearest facility with the capabilities to stabilize the patient further. See Table 17-3 for a partial list of mechanisms of injury that are criteria for transport to an emergency department that is approved for pediatrics or a pediatric trauma center.

Table 17-3 Suggested Criteria for Transfer to an Emergency Department Approved for Pediatrics or a Pediatric Trauma Center

Criteria
• Obstructed airway
• Need for an airway intervention
• Respiratory distress
• Shock
• Altered mental status
• Dilated pupil
• Glasgow Coma Scale score < 13
• Pediatric Trauma Score < 8
• Mechanism of injury (less reliable indicators) associated with severe injuries:
• Fall from a height of 10 feet or more
• Motor-vehicle collision with fatalities
• Ejection from an automobile in an MVC
• In an MVC, significant intrusion into the passenger compartment
• Hit by a car as a pedestrian or bicyclist
• Fractures in more than one extremity
• Significant injury to more than one organ system

If the child needs a procedure, you must decide whether it is worth the time. You should consider how long it will take to perform, how urgent the procedure is, how difficult it will be at the scene versus in the back of the ambulance or at the hospital, and how much it will delay reaching definitive care. If you have a 3-minute procedure (an IV) and a 30-minute transport, the intravenous (IV) line probably should be started. If you are awaiting the arrival of a helicopter, you also may attempt the procedure, but be sure to have the child packaged and ready when transportation arrives. Your lifesaving procedures can be performed in an ambulance while en route to the hospital. Call ahead so that the emergency department can have the necessary equipment and personnel ready. Perform the ITLS Ongoing Exams and ITLS Secondary Survey en route if there is time.

If, after completing the ITLS Primary Survey, you find no critical trauma situation, place the child on a backboard and do a methodical ITLS Secondary Survey.

ITLS Secondary Survey

As in adults, record accurate vital signs, take a SAMPLE history, and perform a complete head-to-toe exam, including a more detailed neurological exam. During your neurological exam make a notation of the child's behavior and response to the environment (alert and reaching for mom) and calculate the Glasgow Coma Scale (GCS) score or Pediatric GCS score (Table 17-4). Finish bandaging and splinting, and transport the child while continuously monitoring. Notify medical direction.

Table 17-4 Glasgow Coma Scale

		> 1 year	< 1 year	
Eyes Opening	4	Spontaneously	Spontaneously	
	3	To verbal command	To shout	
	2	To pain	To pain	
	1	No response	No response	
		> 1 year	**< 1 year**	
Best Motor Response	6	Obeys		
	5	Localizes pain	Localizes pain	
	4	Flexion—withdrawal	Flexion—normal	
	3	Flexion—abnormal (decorticate rigidity)	Flexion—abnormal (decorticate rigidity)	
	2	Extension (decerebrate rigidity)	Extension (decerebrate rigidity)	
	1	No response	No response	
		> 5 years	**2–5 years**	**0–23 months**
Best Verbal Response	5	Oriented and converses	Appropriate words and phrases	Smiles, coos, cries appropriately
	4	Disoriented and converses	Inappropriate words	Cries
	3	Inappropriate words	Cries and/or screams	Inappropriate crying and/or screaming
	2	Incomprehensible sounds	Grunts	Grunts
	1	No response	No response	No response

Potentially Life-Threatening Injuries

Hemorrhagic Shock

The most common sites of severe internal bleeding in children are the chest, abdomen, pelvis, and long bones (femur fractures). Although intracranial blood loss rarely causes hemorrhagic shock, this may infrequently occur in the very young infant. Of course, external bleeding from wounds is also an important source of blood loss. Early shock (often referred to as compensated shock) is far more difficult to diagnose in a child than an adult because of a child's ability to maintain a normal blood pressure despite life-threatening bleeding. Persistent tachycardia is the most reliable early indicator of shock in a child.

Individual variances and environmental factors may make some of the signs of shock normal for a particular child. Tachycardia may occur because of fear or fever. Mottling may be normal in an infant younger than 6 months of age, but it also may be a sign of poor circulation, so note it.

Extremities may be cold because of cold exposure or poor perfusion. Capillary refill may be prolonged in a child who is cold. In general, a child should be carefully evaluated and assumed to have signs of shock if there is persistent tachycardia or signs of poor peripheral perfusion (prolonged capillary refill or cool extremities).

Low blood pressure is a late sign of shock (also called *decompensated shock*). Do not be falsely reassured by a normal blood pressure. A child may still have a serious injury and be compensating to maintain a normal blood pressure. The rule of thumb for cuff size is to use the largest one that will fit snugly on the patient's upper arm. If there is too much noise, you can perform a blood pressure by palpation. Find the radial pulse, pump up the blood pressure cuff until you no longer feel the pulse, and allow air to leak slowly while observing the dial on the blood pressure cuff. Record the pressure at which you first feel the pulse and label it "p," for palpation. This will be a systolic blood pressure only and will be slightly lower than a blood pressure that can be auscultated. As a general estimate, the lower limit of normal (95th percentile) for systolic blood pressure is approximately 70 mm Hg in infants and (70 + 2 [age in years]) mm Hg in children 1 year and older. (Remember that these are not *normal* parameters, but rather low values that should prompt you to be very concerned.) A systolic blood pressure below those values should be treated as decompensated shock, which means the child has lost a very significant amount of blood.

It is useful to routinely measure blood pressures in all children to enhance your comfort and skill with this procedure so you are able to obtain a blood pressure quickly and efficiently in a frightened or significantly injured child. With repeated practice in healthy children you will be more prepared for the difficult situations.

Fluid Resuscitation

fluid resuscitation the replacement of intravascular volume in a hypovolemic child by infusing a crystalloid solution.

If shock is present (compensated with a normal blood pressure or decompensated with a low blood pressure), the child requires **fluid resuscitation**. You should establish vascular access quickly and give a fluid bolus. The initial bolus should be 20 mL/kg of normal saline given as rapidly as possible. If there is no response, another 20 mL/kg may be given. When considering a peripheral IV, try to insert the largest practical catheter available to give the fluid bolus quickly. If the child is in shock it may be difficult to see or feel a peripheral vein. If you cannot start an IV in two attempts or 90 seconds, you will need to insert an intraosseous (IO)

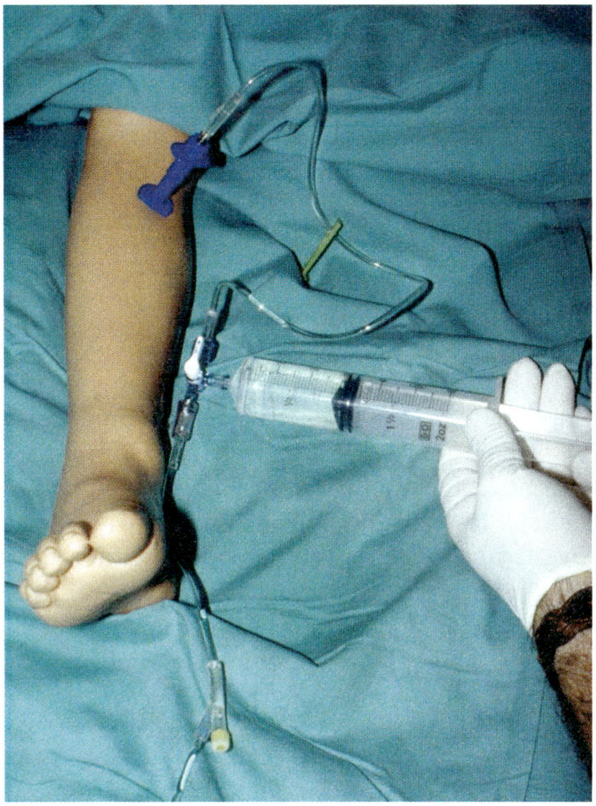

FIGURE 17-7 An IO needle in a child's proximal tibia being used for venous access. *(Courtesy of Bob Page, NREMT-P)*

needle. (See Figure 17-7 and Chapter 9 for technique.) There is *no* scientific data available at this time to suggest that any child in hemorrhagic shock should not be given IV fluids. Remember that cardiac output equals stroke volume times heart rate. Children cannot increase their stoke volume, so when hypovolemic and less blood is returning to the heart, they can only maintain perfusion by vasoconstriction and increasing their heart rate. Sometimes children in severe shock develop bradycardia, and this can cause a severe and frequently fatal decrease in perfusion. Treat hypovolemia early.

Head Injury

Head injuries are the most common cause of death in pediatric patients. The head is the primary focus of injury because the child's head is proportionately larger than the adult's. Fortunately, children with head injury often fare much better than adults with the same degree of injury. The goal of managing head injuries is twofold. First, it is important to quickly recognize all life-threatening intracranial emergencies such as an epidural hematoma. In the prehospital setting, this means transporting all children with potentially serious head injuries to an emergency department equipped to provide definitive care. Second, although some of the injury to the brain occurs from the initial impact, further injury to the brain results from preventable causes (secondary brain injury) such as hypoxia and shock. To minimize those risks, you should prioritize three simple principles:

1. *Give oxygen.* Head injury increases brain cell metabolic rate and decreases blood flow in at least part of the brain. So all pediatric patients with a head injury should receive 100% oxygen and similar to adults, should not be hyperventilated unless they have evidence of the cerebral herniation syndrome. (See Chapter 10.) Remember to monitor ventilation with capnography, if available.

2. *Keep blood pressure normal.* Blood must get to the brain to carry oxygen. It is therefore critical to recognize early signs of shock (tachycardia and poor perfusion) and aggressively correct hypovolemia. Remember, a systolic blood pressure less than 80 mm Hg in the preschool child and less than 90 mm Hg in older children should be considered hypotension and has been shown to be a predictor of poor outcome.
3. *Be prepared to prevent aspiration.* Head-injury patients frequently vomit. The Sellick maneuver should be used during bag-mask ventilation and any intubation attempts. Suction should be readily assessable for any child with a head injury.

Changing level of consciousness is the best indicator of head trauma. A child entering the emergency department with a GCS of 10 that has come down from 13, will be approached very differently from the child who has a GCS score of 10 that has come up from 7. Assessments using vague words like *semiconscious* are not helpful. Instead, note specific points such as whether the child is alert and interactive, asking for parent/crying, reaching for the parent, or reacting to pain or voice.

Assessment of pupils is as important in the child with altered level of consciousness as in the adult. Note also whether the eyes are moving both left and right or whether they remain in one position. Do not move the head to determine this!

Overall, it may be difficult at the scene to assess the extent of a child's head injury. Priorities should be focused on prevention of secondary brain injury and rapid transport to a trauma center equipped to provide definitive care.

Chest Injury

Children with chest injuries generally give visible signs of respiratory distress, such as tachypnea, grunting, nasal flaring, and retractions. Any injured child with any respiratory distress would benefit from supplemental oxygen. Be aware that children's normal respiratory rates are higher than those of adults (Table 17-2). A child breathing faster than 40, or an infant faster than 60, usually has respiratory distress.

Other signs of respiratory distress include flaring (the nose moves like a rabbit), and retractions, which are the caving in of the suprasternal, intercostal, or subcostal areas with inspiration. Grunting is usually abnormal and indicates significant respiratory distress or a severe intra-abdominal injury and indicates a need for ventilatory assistance. Observe the child's breathing pattern as well. Shallow breathing, apnea spells (10–20 seconds of no breathing), or agonal respirations are all signs of respiratory failure and mandate ventilatory assistance.

Children with blunt chest injury are at risk for pneumothorax. Because the chest is small, a difference in breath sounds from side to side may be more subtle than in the adult. You may not be able to tell a difference, even by listening carefully. It is also difficult to diagnose tension pneumothorax in young children, who usually have short, fat necks that mask both neck vein distention and tracheal deviation. If a tension pneumothorax develops, the trachea should eventually shift away from the side of the pneumothorax, although this is a very late finding. Needle thoracostomy can be lifesaving. (See Chapter 7.)

Children in the preadolescent age group have highly elastic chest walls. Rib fractures, flail chest, pericardial tamponade, and aortic rupture are, therefore, seldom seen in this group. However, pulmonary contusion is common. If a child does have rib fractures or a flail chest, he has sustained a significant force to his chest and should be assumed to have serious internal injuries.

Abdominal Injury

The second leading cause of traumatic death in pediatric centers is blunt abdominal trauma resulting in solid organ injury and bleeding. Common mechanisms include motor-vehicle collisions, bicycle crashes, sports-related injuries, and child abuse. In children, the liver and spleen are relatively large and both protrude below the ribs, exposing these organs to blunt trauma.

Abdominal injuries are difficult to diagnose in the field and are frequently missed because the presentation may be subtle. Children may have a difficult time communicating that they have abdominal pain, or the history may be limited secondary to the age of the child or other injuries the child has sustained. Any injured child who complains of abdominal pain should be assumed to have an intra-abdominal injury. The physical exam also may be challenging because of fear, pain, and the age of the child. A child may have a severe abdominal injury with minimal signs of trauma. Findings on examination that suggest significant abdominal injury include tenderness, bruising, and signs of shock. Seat-belt marks and bicycle handlebar marks are also worrisome.

Your assessment should be quick. If a child with blunt trauma is in shock with no obvious source of bleeding, your decision should be to load and go. Remember, however, that normal vital signs (heart rate and systolic blood pressure) do not rule out serious intra-abdominal injury.

Lifesaving interventions should be made en route to the hospital. If you have a short (5- to 10-minute) transport time to a trauma center, it is not necessary to attempt an IV line. If the child is critical and the transport time is long, you should make no more than two attempts at IV lines before going to an IO needle. Any child who has been crying or suffered an abdominal injury may develop gastric distention and a tendency to vomit, so be prepared.

Spinal Injury

Although children have short necks, big heads, and loose ligaments, cervical-spine injuries are uncommon before adolescence. When they do occur, children younger than 9 years of age usually have upper cervical-spine injuries in contrast to older children and adults, who usually have lower cervical-spine injuries. There is no proven protocol for "clearing" the spine of a child in the field. A cervical collar is not necessary if the head is properly restricted in a padded device. Again, try to make a game of packaging the child. You can promise you will give him a ride in the ambulance as a reward after you get him all wrapped up and ready. Have a parent or other familiar person assist, if possible. Be sure your packaging does not restrict chest movement. As mentioned before, children up to about 8 years of age will need a pad under the torso to keep the neck in a neutral position.

Child Restraint Seats

A child in a motor-vehicle collision while properly restrained in a **child restraint seat** is much less likely to have a serious injury than an unrestrained passenger. If in a car seat, usually the child can be transported without being removed from the device. Assess the child as you would other trauma patients. If no injury is found and the seat's integrity appears to be intact, place padding around the child's head, and tape the head directly to the car seat (Scan 17-1). This method of transportation should be used only after a complete assessment that has revealed *no* injury to the child. Be aware of your local protocols regarding this. If the child has evidence of any serious injuries, then remove the child

child restraint seat a piece of safety equipment in which a child sits and that is designed to protect a child in case of a motor-vehicle collision. It must fit the child, and the child must be properly strapped into the seat for it to be effective.

SCAN 17-1 Stabilizing an Apparently Uninjured Child in a Car Seat

1

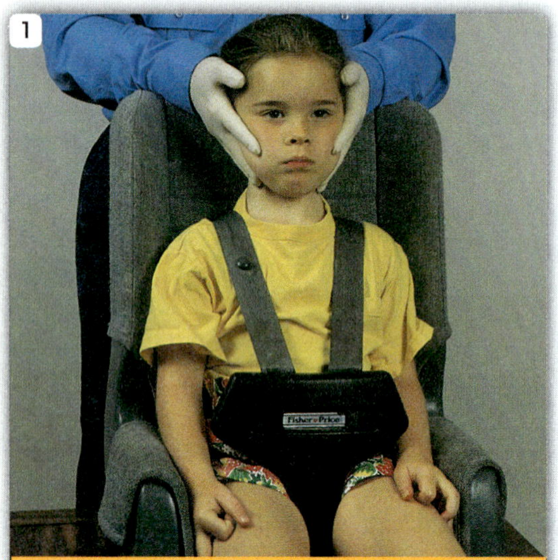

One EMT stabilizes the car seat in an upright position and applies and maintains manual in-line stabilization throughout the SMR process.

2

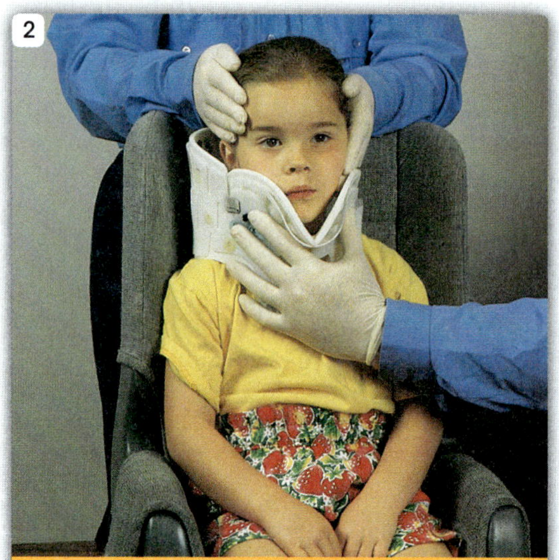

A second EMT applies an appropriately sized cervical collar. If one is not available, improvise using a rolled hand towel.

3

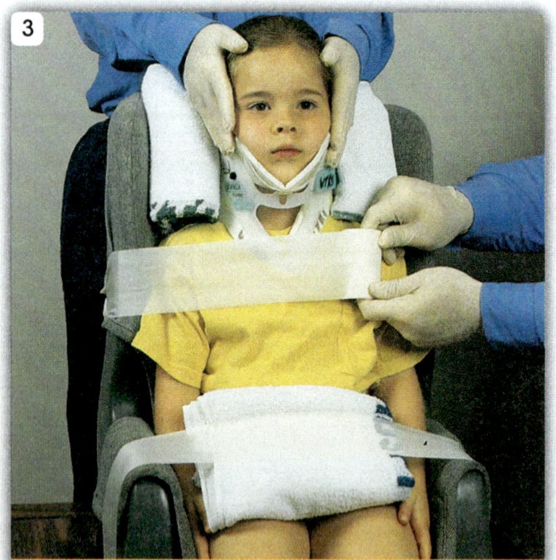

The second EMT places a small blanket or towel on the child's lap, then uses straps or wide tape to secure the chest and pelvic areas to the seat.

4

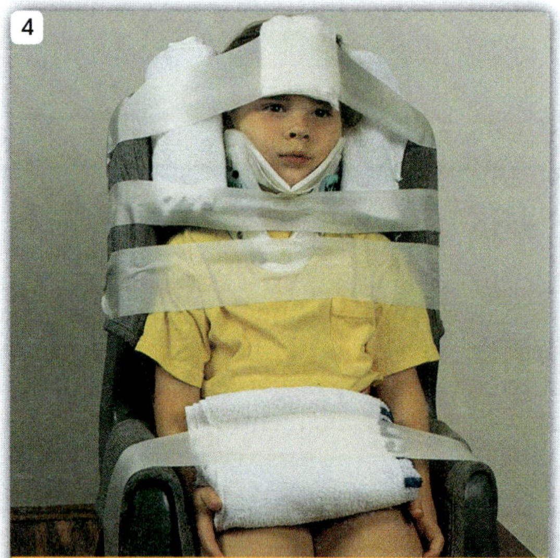

The second EMT places towel rolls on both sides of the child's head to fill the voids between the head and seat. He tapes the head into place, taping across the forehead and the collar, but avoiding taping over the chin, which would put pressure on the neck. The patient and seat can be carried to the ambulance and strapped to the stretcher, with the stretcher head raised.

from the car seat and package. Some cars have built-in infant restraint seats. Those seats cannot be removed, so the child who is restrained in one of them will have to be extricated and placed on a pediatric spinal motion-restriction device.

CASE PRESENTATION (continued)

An ALS ambulance has been dispatched for a 2-year-old child who was run over by a four-wheeler all-terrain vehicle. They are told that the child is unconscious. When they arrive at a house in the country, they are told the father has brought the child into the house from where he was injured in the backyard. The distraught father says, "I was with Freddy in the back yard while his older brother was riding the four-wheeler. I was distracted by a call on my cell phone and Freddy ran to his brother who didn't see him in time to stop. He ran over him."

They see a 2-year-old child lying on the couch. There is no obvious external bleeding. The general appearance is not good because the child is not moving. The child does not respond to the team leader when she speaks to him. While rescuer 2 stabilizes the neck, she immediately checks the airway and finds it open but respiration is slow and shallow. The pulse is normal and strong at the wrist.

She asks rescuer 3 to assist respiration with the bag-mask. She immediately cuts off his shirt and shorts and begins the rapid trauma survey. The child has an obvious hematoma of the left temporal area, with bruising of the face. The neck has no obvious deformities. The neck veins are flat and trachea is in the midline. There are some abrasions of the left chest but no instability and breath sounds are present and equal. There are also abrasions of the left abdomen and the child moans and localizes with his hands when she palpates the left upper abdomen. The pelvis feels stable and the extremities appear normal.

The leader places a clean sheet on the backboard and they carefully logroll Freddy onto it and move him to the ambulance. The team leader tells the family that they are going to the trauma center and the mother can ride with them but the rest of the family will have to follow in their automobile. In the ambulance the leader notes that the left pupil is slightly larger than the right but responds to light. Rescuer 2 takes vital signs: blood pressure 100/70, respiration 16 per minute when not ventilating, and pulse 100 per minute. The leader calculates the GCS as 9 (eyes, 2; motor, 5; and verbal, 2) and then starts a large-bore IV at a keep-vein-open rate. She also attaches the cardiac monitor (sinus rhythm) and pulse oximeter (95 on 100% oxygen).

The leader notifies medical direction that they have an unconscious 2-year-old child who was run over by an ATV. He has blunt head trauma, abrasions to the left chest and abdomen, and probably a ruptured spleen. The ITLS Ongoing Exam does not change during the brief transport to the trauma center, where the child is found to have a small cerebral contusion that required no surgery and a subcapsular hematoma of the spleen that resolved with observation. The father sold the ATV. ■

Summary

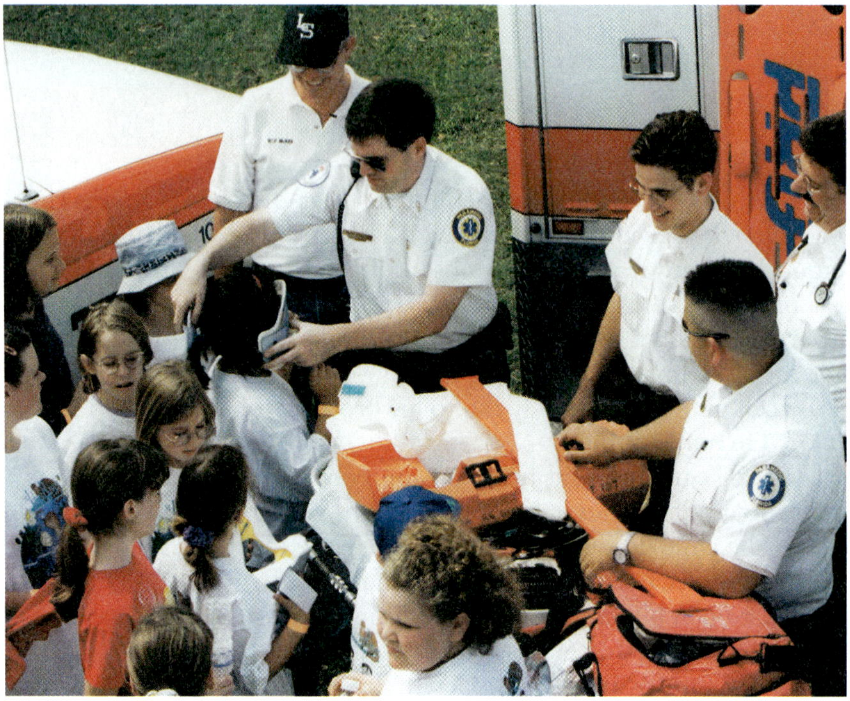

FIGURE 17-8 It is important to organize or participate in programs that educate children about injury prevention and health care. *(© Craig Jackson/In the Dark Photography)*

To provide good trauma care for children, you must have the proper equipment, know how to interact with frightened parents, know the normal vital signs for various ages (or have them posted in your trauma box), and be familiar with the injuries that are more common in children. Fortunately, the assessment sequence is the same for children as for adults. If you perform your assessment well, you will obtain the information needed to make the right decisions in management. Focusing on assessment and management of the child's airway (with cervical-spine control), breathing, and circulation will result in the best possible outcome.

Although assessment and management of the injured child are lifesaving skills, all responders involved in the care of the seriously injured child should be concerned also about prevention. Car seats, bicycle helmets, seat belts, all-terrain vehicle injuries, water safety, scald burn injuries, firearm safety, and fire drills are within our area of concern. We should donate our time to teaching safety (Figure 17-8), and we should speak out for laws (infant seat restraints, seat belts, drunk driving) that save lives.

Bibliography

1. Bliss, D., M. Silen. 2002. Pediatric thoracic trauma. *Crit Care Med* 20: S409– 415.
2. Dietrich, A., S. Shaner, J. Campbell. 2009. *Pediatric International trauma life support*. 3rd ed. Oakbrook Terrace, IL: International Trauma Life Support.

3. DiRusso, S. M., et al. 2005. Intubation of pediatric trauma patients in the field: Prediction of negative outcome despite risk stratification. *Journal of Trauma* 59(July): 84–91.

4. Fleicher, G. R., S. Ludwig, M. Henretig (eds.). 2005. *Textbook of pediatric emergency medicine.* 5th edition. Philadelphia: Lippincott Williams & Wilkins.

5. Gausche, M., R. J. Lewis, et al. 2000. Effect of out-of-hospital pediatric endotracheal intubation on survival and neurological outcome: A controlled clinical trial. *JAMA* 283(6): 783.

6. Holmes, J. F., P. E. Sokolove, W. E. Brant, M. J. Palchak, C. W. Vance, J. T. Owings, et al. 2002. Identification of children with intra-abdominal injuries after blunt trauma. *Ann Emerg Med* 39(5): 500–509.

7. Holmes, J. F., P. E. Sokolove, W. E. Brant, et al. 2002. A clinical decision rule for identifying children with thoracic injuries after blunt torso trauma. *Ann Emerg Med* 39: 492–499.

8. Kokoska, E. R., M. S. Keller, M. C. Rallo, et al. 2001. Characteristics of pediatric cervical-spine injuries. *J Pediatr Surg* 36: 100–105.

9. Kuppermann, N., et al. 2009. Identification of children at very low risk of clinically-important brain injuries after head trauma: A prospective cohort study. *Lancet* 374(9696): 1160–1170.

10. Marx, J. A., R. S. Hockberger, R. M. Walls. 2010. *Rosen's emergency medicine.* 7th ed. Philadelphia: Mosby/Elsevier.

11. Viccellio, P., H. Simon, B. D. Pressman, et al. 2001. A prospective multicenter study of cervical-spine injury in children. *Pediatrics* 108: E20.

12. Vitale, M. G., J. M. Goss, H. Matsumoto, et al. 2006. Epidemiology of pediatric spinal cord injury in the United States. *J Pediatr Orthop* 26: 745–749.

13. Walls, R. M., M. F. Murphy (eds.). 2008. *Manual of emergency airway management.* 3rd ed. Philadelphia: Lippincott Williams & Wilkins.

Explore Resource Central

For additional review and practice tests, visit www.bradybooks.com and click on Resource Central to access book-specific resources for this text. To access Resource Central, follow directions on the Student Access Card provided with this text. If there is no card, go to www.bradybooks.com and follow the Resource Central link to Buy Access from there.

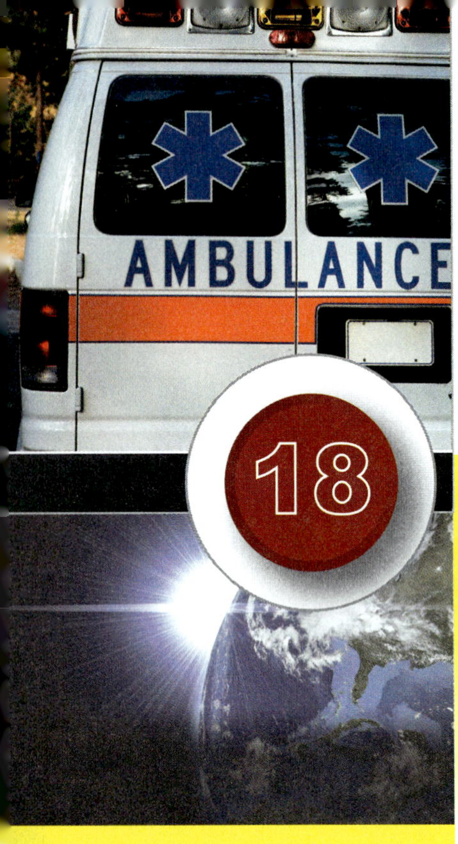

(Photo courtesy of Jupiterimages, Photos.com/Thinkstock.com)

Geriatric Trauma

Leah J. Heimbach, JD, RN, EMT-P
Jere F. Baldwin, MD, FACEP, FAAFP

Trauma in the Elderly

Traumi dell'anziano

Traumatismo en el Adulto Mayor

Traumatisme dans les Personnes âgées

Urazy u osób w podeszłym wieku

Trauma im Alter

Ozljede u osoba starije životne dobi

إصابات الكبار

trauma starih osoba

Poškodbe pri starostnikih

Időskori trauma

KEY TERMS

altered mental status, *p. 338*
compensate, *p. 335*
chronic disease, *p. 337*
kyphotic deformity, *p. 335*
osteoporosis, *p. 335*
pathophysiology of aging, *p. 334*

OBJECTIVES

Upon successful completion of this chapter, you should be able to:

1. Describe the changes that occur with aging, and explain how they can affect your assessment of the geriatric trauma patient.
2. Describe the assessment of the geriatric trauma patient.
3. Describe the management of the geriatric trauma patient.

Chapter Overview

Citizens over the age of 65 comprise over 12% of the U.S. population, but that number is expected to double in the next 25 to 30 years. The age group 85 and older is the fastest-growing segment of the U.S. population. The geriatric population already comprises a significant number of patients being transported by ambulance. In the United States, over 30% of all patients transported by ambulance are over the age of 65.

"Elderly" is often understood as being 65 years or older because retirement benefits are usually initiated at about this point in life. However, chronological age is not the most reliable definition of "elderly." It is more appropriate to consider the biological processes that change with time, such as fewer number of neurons, decreased functioning of the kidneys, and decreased elasticity of the skin and tissues.

As a group, geriatric patients tend to respond to injury less favorably than younger adults. Geriatric patients who are injured are more likely to experience fatal outcomes, even if the injury is of a relatively low severity. According to the U.S. National Safety Council, falls, thermal injury, and motor-vehicle collisions have been identified as common causes of traumatic death in the geriatric population. This is an even greater concern given that, as a whole, the elderly population continues to assume more active lifestyles, making them more prone to injury.

Falls account for the majority of injuries in the geriatric population, the most common pathology being fractures of the hip, femur, and wrist and head injuries. Motor-vehicle collisions account for approximately 25% of geriatric deaths, although the elderly drive fewer miles. The geriatric population has a higher incidence of collision than other age groups, second only to those under the age of 25. Eight percent of deaths are attributable to thermal injuries, which include inhalation, contact with a heat source resulting in scalding and flame burns, and electrical injury.

Little has been written on the response of the geriatric patient to trauma. In addition, existing literature is retrospective in nature and offers little explanation for the more adverse outcomes experienced by the elderly. By gaining an understanding of the normal physiological changes involved in the aging process, you will be prepared to provide optimum care to the geriatric trauma victim.

This chapter addresses aging processes, highlights illnesses to which the geriatric patient is susceptible, and shows how those processes and illnesses make it difficult to predict the physiological response to trauma in the geriatric patient.

CASE PRESENTATION

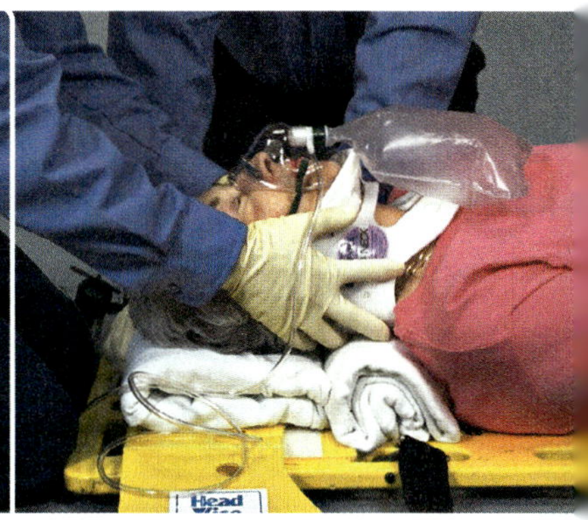

An ALS ambulance has been dispatched to a report of an elderly male who has fallen down stairs. The dispatcher advises the patient's wife is on the phone with them and says her husband is conscious but has a large bump on his head. Upon arrival, crew's scene size-up reveals the scene is safe, and they observe an elderly male, approximately 80 years old who is at the bottom of a 10-step stairway. The patient appears conscious with purposeful movement of the extremities, and a large hematoma is noted on the left temporal area. The wife states her husband is not acting his normal alert and spirited self. What type of assessment would you perform? Is this patient at higher risk of having additional injuries than someone younger? Is this a load-and-go situation? Should this patient be managed without SMR? Keep these questions in mind as you read the chapter. Then, at the end of the chapter, find out how the rescuers completed this call. ■

Pathophysiology of Aging

pathophysiology of aging the process of aging that consists of the gradual decline in the normal function of many body systems, which may in part be responsible for greater risk of injury in the elderly population.

The **pathophysiology of aging** is a gradual process whereby changes in bodily functions may occur. The changes are in part responsible for the greater risk of injury in the geriatric population.

The Aging Body

Airway

Changes in airway structures of the geriatric patient may include tooth decay, gum disease, and use of a dental prosthesis. Caps, bridges, dentures, and fillings all present potential airway obstructions in the geriatric trauma patient.

Respiratory System

Changes in the respiratory system begin to appear in the early adult years and increase markedly after the age of 60. Circulation to the pulmonary system decreases 30%, reducing the amount of carbon dioxide and oxygen exchanged at the alveolar level. There is a decrease in chest wall movement and in the flexibility of the muscles of the chest wall. The changes cause a decreased inhalation time, resulting in rapid breathing. There is a decrease in vital capacity (the amount of air exchanged per breath) because of an increased residual volume (volume of air in the lungs after deep exhalation). Overall breathing capacity and maximal work rate may decrease. If there is a history of cigarette smoking, or a history of working in an area with pollutants, the changes in breathing are even more significant.

Cardiovascular System

Circulation is reduced due to changes in the heart and the blood vessels. Cardiac output and stroke volume may decrease, and the conduction system may degenerate. The ability of the valves of the heart to operate efficiently may decline. Those changes may predispose the patient to congestive heart failure and pulmonary edema. Arteriosclerosis occurs with increasing frequency in the course of the aging process, resulting in an increased peripheral vascular resistance (and perhaps systolic hypertension). There may be a normally higher blood pressure in the elderly. Thus, a significant change in tissue perfusion may occur in a patient when the normal blood pressure of 160 drops to 120 as a result of trauma.

Neurological and Sensory Function

Several changes occur in the brain with age. The brain shrinks, and the outermost meningeal layer, the dura mater, remains tightly adherent to the skull. This creates a space or an increased distance between the brain and the skull. Instead of protecting the brain during impact, this space allows an increased incidence of subdural hematoma following trauma. There is also a hardening, narrowing, and loss of elasticity of some arteries in the brain. A deceleration injury may cause blood vessel rupture and potential bleeding inside the skull.

There is decreased blood flow to the brain. The patient may experience a slowing of sensory responses such as pain perception and decreases in hearing, eyesight, or in other sensory perceptions. Many older patients may have a higher pain tolerance from living with conditions such as arthritis or from being on analgesic medications chronically. This can result in their failure to identify areas in which they have been injured. Other signs of decreased cerebral circulation due to the aging process may include confusion, irritability, forgetfulness, altered sleep patterns, and mental dysfunctions such as loss of memory and regressive behavior. There may be a decrease in the ability, or even an absence of the ability, to **compensate** for shock.

compensate the body's natural ability to adapt to a range of conditions. In the elderly patient there may be a decrease in the ability, or even an absence of the ability, to compensate for shock or other conditions.

Thermoregulation

Mechanisms to maintain normal body temperature may not function properly. The geriatric patient may not be able to respond to an infection with a fever, or the patient may not be able to maintain a normal temperature in the face of injury. The geriatric patient with a broken hip who has been lying on the floor in a room where the temperature is 64°F can experience hypothermia.

Renal System

A decrease in the number of functioning nephrons in the kidneys of the geriatric patient can result in a decrease in filtration and a reduced ability to excrete urine and drugs.

Musculoskeletal System

The geriatric patient may exhibit signs of changes in posture. There may be a decrease in total height due to the narrowing of the vertebral discs, slight flexion of the knees and hips, and decreased muscle strength. This may result in a **kyphotic deformity** of the spine, resulting in an "S" curvature of the spine often seen in the stooped elderly. The geriatric patient also may have advanced **osteoporosis**—a thinning of the bones resulting in a decrease in bone density. This renders the bones more susceptible to fractures.

There is frequently diminished subcutaneous tissue that decreases protection from falls and blunt trauma. This lack of subcutaneous tissue can decrease the person's ability to respond to temperature changes. Finally, there may be a weakening in the strength of the muscle and bone from the decrease in physical activity. This also will render the geriatric patient more susceptible to fractures with only a slight fall.

kyphotic deformity a condition caused by narrowing of the vertebral discs and gradual collapse of the osteoporotic thoracic vertebral bodies often seen in the elderly who present in a stooped posture with an "S" shape to the spine.

osteoporosis a condition frequently seen in the elderly in which there is gradual loss of calcium from the bones with decrease in bone mass and density making the bones more easily fractured.

Gastrointestinal System

Saliva production, esophageal motility, and gastric secretion may decrease. This may result in decreased ability to absorb nutrients. Constipation and fecal impactions are common. The liver may be enlarged because of disease processes or may be failing due to disease or malnutrition. This may result in a decreased ability to metabolize medications.

Immune System

As the aging process continues, the geriatric patient may be less able to fight off infection. The patient in a poor nutritional state will be more susceptible to infection from open wounds, IV access sites, and lung and kidney infections. The geriatric trauma patient who is not otherwise severely injured may die from sepsis from an impaired immune system.

Other Changes

The total body water and total number of body cells may be decreased, and there is an increase in the proportion of the body weight as fat. There may be a loss in the capacity of the systems to adjust to illness or injury.

Medications

Many geriatric patients take several medications that can interfere with the ability to compensate after sustaining trauma. Anticoagulants may increase bleeding time. Antihypertensives and peripheral vasodilators can interfere with the body's ability to constrict blood vessels in response to hypovolemia. Beta-blockers can inhibit the heart's ability to increase the rate of contraction even in hypovolemic shock.

A number of the aging processes contribute to the increased risk of injury to the geriatric patient. The changes that may increase susceptibility to injury include the following:

- Slower reflexes
- Failing eyesight
- Hearing loss
- Arthritis
- Fragile skin and blood vessels
- Fragile bones

Causative factors related to the aging process have been linked with specific injuries such as tripping over furniture and falling down stairs. Further investigation reveals that those falls are often related as much to a decrease in the function of special senses, such as loss in peripheral vision, as they are to syncope, postural instability, transient impairment of cerebrovascular perfusion, alcohol ingestion, or medication usage. Alterations in perception and delayed response to stressors may contribute to injury in the geriatric patient. When treating the geriatric trauma patient, remember that the priorities are the same as for all trauma patients. However, you must give consideration to three important issues:

- General organ systems may not function as effectively as those in the younger adult, especially the cardiovascular, pulmonary, and renal systems.
- The geriatric patient may have a chronic illness that may complicate the effectiveness of trauma care.
- Bones may fracture more easily with less force. Fractures of major bones such as hips or femurs can be life threatening even with proper care.

Assessment and Management

Geriatric patient assessment, as any assessment, must take into account priorities, interventions, and life-threatening conditions. However, you must be acutely aware that geriatric patients can die from less-severe injuries than younger patients. In addition, it is often difficult to separate the effects of the aging process or of a chronic illness from the consequences of the injury. The chief complaint may seem trivial because the patient may not report truly important symptoms. You must search for important signs or symptoms. In the geriatric patient, it is not uncommon for the patient to suffer from more than one illness or injury at the same time. Remember that the elderly patient may not have the same response to pain, hypoxia, or hypovolemia as a young person. Do not underestimate the severity of the patient's condition.

You may have difficulty communicating with the patient. This could result from the patient's diminished senses, hearing or sight impairment, or depression. The geriatric patient nonetheless should not be approached in a condescending manner. Do not allow others to take over the reporting of events from the patient who is able and willing to communicate reliable information. Unfortunately, the patient may minimize or even deny symptoms out of fear of becoming dependent, bedridden, institutionalized, or even of losing a sense of self-sufficiency. It is important that you explain any actions, including removing any clothing, before initiating the physical assessment.

There are other considerations in assessing the geriatric trauma patient. Peripheral pulses may be difficult to evaluate. Older patients often wear many layers of clothing, which can impede physical assessment. You also must distinguish between signs and symptoms of a **chronic disease** and an acute problem; for instance:

chronic disease a long-lasting or recurrent illness that may be underlying the acute problem that prompted need for emergency care. Signs and symptoms between the chronic disease and trauma may need to be distinguished.

- The geriatric patient may have nonpathologic rales.
- The loss of skin elasticity and the presence of mouth breathing may not necessarily represent dehydration.
- Dependent edema may be secondary to venous insufficiency with varicose veins or inactivity rather than congestive heart failure.

Pay attention to deviation from expected ranges in vital signs and other physical assessment findings in the geriatric patient. An injury that is isolated and uncomplicated in the young adult may be debilitating in the older adult. This may be due to the patient's overall condition, lowered defenses, or inability to keep the effects of an injury localized.

When obtaining the past medical history, it is important to note what medications the patient may be taking. Medications may not only account for an abnormal pulse, but also may mask normal circulatory responses that would indicate deterioration in the circulatory system. The result can be a rapid decompensation without warning. Knowledge of the medications that the patient is taking can alert you to the fact that the patient's condition may be more unstable than that presented by current signs and symptoms. Antihypertensives, anticoagulants, beta-blockers, sedatives, and hypoglycemic agents may profoundly influence the response of the geriatric patient to traumatic injury.

ITLS Primary Survey

Scene Size-up

Size up the scene to decide if it is safe, to determine the number of patients, and to identify the mechanism of injury. After the ITLS Primary Survey, it may be helpful to obtain further information and to verify the patient's history from reliable family members or neighbors. This is best done in an area where the patient is unable to overhear the conversation; otherwise it may suggest that the geriatric patient is less than a competent adult. Observe the surrounding area for indications that the patient is able to provide his own care; for signs of alcohol abuse or ingestion of multiple medications; and for signs of violence, abuse, or neglect. Unfortunately, abuse and neglect of the elderly are common. When your assessment of the patient and surroundings is suspicious for abuse or neglect, do not fail to notify the proper authorities. Be sure to gather the patient's medications and bring them to the hospital.

PEARLS: Altered Mental Status

Elderly patients with **altered mental status** should always be checked for hypoglycemia, shock, and head trauma, rather than assuming that they are senile.

altered mental status a diminished level of awareness or consciousness. It has more significance in the elderly trauma patient as a benchmark for other health-care providers who will assess the patient.

Initial Assessment

As with any trauma patient, you must evaluate and provide an adequate airway and maintain spinal motion restriction (SMR) while assessing the initial level of consciousness. It has more significance with elderly patients than with younger patients, because subsequent health-care providers may attribute a decreased level of consciousness to a preexisting condition rather than to the trauma. This is more likely to occur if you have not clearly indicated that the patient was clear, lucid, and cooperative at the scene.

If patients respond appropriately to initial verbal statements, they have an open airway and are conscious. If they do not respond, gently open the airway with a modified jaw-thrust maneuver while maintaining the neck in a neutral position. This position may be difficult to determine with certainty because of arthritis and kyphosis of the spine. It is important to recognize this and not to forcibly place the occiput flat on the backboard or ground. You should add padding to the backboard to maintain the patient's usual spinal position. The vacuum backboard is very helpful here.

The airway is likely to be partially obstructed. Clear the airway, being alert to possible teeth fragments due to decay and gum disease and dental devices such as caps, bridges, dentures, and fillings. Look, listen, and feel for movement of air. Ensure that the rate and volume of air exchange is adequate. The geriatric patient with unresolved airway difficulty or a decreased level of consciousness should be transported immediately. In such a case, frequently monitor the respiratory effort and level of consciousness (remember to check blood glucose). Consider in-line endotracheal intubation.

Place your face over the patient's mouth to look at the chest rise, to listen to the quality of the breath sounds from the mouth, and to feel the patient's breath against your ear. If the breathing is so fast that there is inadequate air exchange (more than 20 breaths per minute), or if it is too slow (fewer than 10 breaths per minute), or if the volume of air being exchanged is inadequate, provide assisted ventilation with 100% supplemental oxygen. Capnography is an effective way to objectively monitor the patient's ventilation.

Check the rate and quality of the pulse at the wrist (check at the neck if there is no pulse at the wrist). Evaluate skin color and condition. Scan the patient for bleeding, and control any bleeding with pressure.

Rapid Trauma Survey or Focused Exam

The choice between the rapid trauma survey and the focused exam depends on the mechanism of injury and/or the results of the initial assessment. If there is a dangerous generalized mechanism of injury (auto crash or fall from a height, for instance) or if the patient is unconscious, you should perform a rapid trauma survey. If there is a dangerous focused mechanism of injury suggesting an isolated injury (such as a bullet wound of thigh or a stab wound to the chest), you may perform the focused exam, which is limited to the area of injury. If there is no significant mechanism of injury, and the initial assessment was normal (the patient is alert with no history of loss of consciousness, breathing normally, and a radial pulse less than 120, not complaining of dyspnea or chest, abdominal, or pelvic pain), you may move directly to the focused exam based on the patient's chief complaint.

To perform a rapid trauma survey, examine the head, neck, chest, abdomen, pelvis, and extremities. That is, briefly assess the head and neck for injuries and to see if the neck veins are flat or distended and if the trachea is midline. You may apply a rigid extrication collar at this time. Then look, feel, and listen to the chest. Look for both asymmetrical and paradoxical movement. Note if the ribs rise with respiration or if there is only diaphragmatic breathing. Look for signs of blunt trauma or open wounds. Feel for tenderness, instability, or crepitation (TIC). Listen to see if breath sounds are present and equal bilaterally.

Make appropriate interventions for chest injuries. Remember that chest injuries are more likely to cause serious problems in older people with poor pulmonary reserve. Be especially alert to problems in patients with chronic lung disease. Those patients usually have borderline hypoxia even when they are not injured. Briefly notice heart sounds so you will have a baseline for changes such as development of muffled heart sounds. Rapidly expose and look at the abdomen (distention, contusions, penetrating wounds), and gently palpate the abdomen for tenderness, guarding, and rigidity. Check the pelvis and extremities for wounds, deformity, and tenderness, instability, crepitation (TIC). Note whether the patient can move fingers and toes before transferring to a backboard.

PEARLS: Chronic Illnesses

Chronic illnesses such as congestive heart failure and COPD should be taken into account as you make judgments about interventions needed to care for the elderly trauma patient.

Critical Transport Decisions

A few procedures may be initiated on scene, but do not delay transport. Examples of critical interventions that may be initiated at the scene are the following:

- Provide airway management.
- Assist ventilation.
- Begin CPR.
- Control major bleeding.
- Seal sucking chest wounds.
- Stabilize flail chest.
- Decompress a tension pneumothorax.
- Stabilize impaled objects.

Consider whether or not the time delay in initiating those procedures outweighs the risks of delaying transportation. The chance of survival decreases with a corresponding increase in the length of scene time. The same indications for immediate transport apply for the elderly as for younger patients. (See Chapter 2.) Remember that you may not have as dramatic a response to injury in the elderly, so you should ensure early transport. If one of the critical conditions is present, immediately transfer the patient to a long backboard (vacuum backboard is recommended) with appropriate padding, apply oxygen, load the patient into the ambulance, and transport rapidly to the nearest appropriate trauma facility.

PEARLS: SMR

- When performing SMR on an elderly patient, take into consideration the fact that she might remain on a hard backboard for extended periods of time. You should use some extra padding, such as a folded blanket, for the entire body. The vacuum backboard is far superior to a hard backboard for use with the elderly patient.
- Extra padding also may be required under the head and shoulders to maintain the cervical spine in its normal alignment.

Packaging and Transport

Package or prepare the elderly patient for transport as quickly and gently as possible. Take extra care when performing SMR on the geriatric trauma patient. This includes padding void areas that may be exaggerated due to the aging process. The elderly patient with kyphosis will require padding under the shoulders and head to maintain the neck in its usual alignment (Figures 18-1). Do not force the neck into a neutral position if it is painful to do so, or if the neck is obviously fused in a forward position. Remember to treat

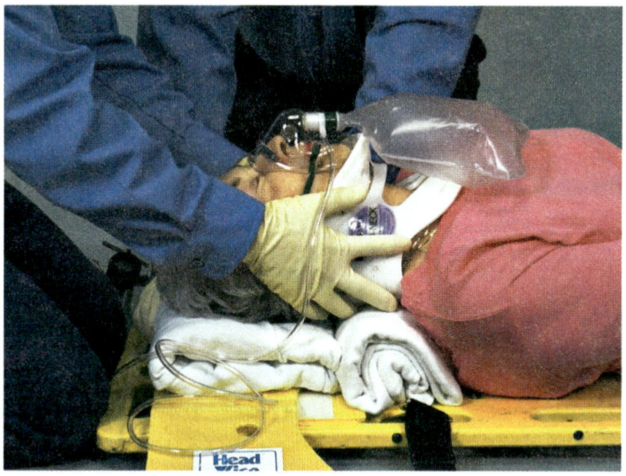

FIGURE 18-1 Elderly patients with kyphosis require padding under the head and shoulders to maintain the spine in its usual alignment.

and transport the geriatric trauma patient, as you do all trauma patients, gently and quickly.

ITLS Secondary Survey and Ongoing Exams

Perform an ITLS Secondary Survey on scene if the patient is stable. If there is any question about the patient's condition, you should transport and perform the ITLS Secondary Survey en route. Perform frequent ITLS Ongoing Exams. If IV therapy is to be started, it should be done en route to the hospital. If you start large-bore IV lines en route, monitor the patient's response to IV fluid infusion very closely. Volume infusion may precipitate congestive heart failure in patients with underlying cardiovascular disease. Frequently assess the patient's pulmonary status, including lung sounds and cardiac rhythm. All elderly patients should have cardiac monitoring, pulse oximetry, and capnography, if available.

CASE PRESENTATION (continued)

An ALS ambulance has been dispatched to a report of an elderly man who has fallen down a 10-step stairway. Upon arrival, the scene size-up reveals the scene is safe, and the responders observe an elderly man, who appears conscious with purposeful movement of the extremities and a large hematoma on the left temporal area. The wife states her husband is not acting his normal alert and spirited self.

The team leader begins the initial assessment by introducing the team, while one of the team members manually stabilizes the patient's cervical spine. Another team member applies nonrebreather oxygen. The initial assessment reveals the patient has nonlabored respirations at a normal rate, and the peripheral pulses are present, strong, and regular. The rapid trauma survey reveals the hematoma of the left temporal area, flat neck veins, breath sounds that are clear and equal, a normal chest exam, a soft and nontender abdomen, and normal pelvis and femurs, and the brief scan of the lower and upper extremities is normal. Glasgow Coma Scale (GCS) score is 14 (E4, M6, V4). Pupils are equal and reactive.

Full SMR precautions are taken because of the mechanism of injury. The patient is loaded into the ambulance, and his wife rides along in the passenger seat. Baseline vitals are respiratory rate 20, pulse rate 76, and blood pressure 130/70. Additional history is obtained from the wife: the patient has a history of hypertension and is taking a beta-blocker. He also takes warfarin.

During transport the patient's GCS decreases to 9 (E2, M4, V3), respiratory rate to 10, and pulse rate to 60. Blood pressure increases to 140/90. The left pupil is larger than the right, but is equally reactive. The team leader decides to assist ventilations while monitoring end-tidal CO_2. The receiving hospital was notified of the changes in the patient.

Upon arrival at the hospital, the patient is briefly evaluated in the emergency department and then a CAT scan is performed, where an epidural hematoma is identified. Because of the patient's history of normal mental status before the injury, it is decided that surgery is warranted. A burr hole is placed to relieve the epidural hematoma, and the patient leaves the hospital with a normal mental status a week later. ■

Summary

You will be called on to treat and transport an increasing number of geriatric trauma patients. Although the mechanisms of injury may be different from those of younger adults, the prioritized evaluation and treatment is the same. As a general rule, elderly patients have more serious injuries and more complications than younger patients. Some suggest that age greater than 60 years is sufficient reason to take an injured patient to a level 1 trauma center. The physiological processes of aging and frequent concurrent illnesses make evaluation and treatment more difficult. You must be aware of the differences to provide optimal care to the patient.

Bibliography

1. Bergeron, E., et al. 2003. Elderly trauma patients with rib fractures are at greater risk of death and pneumonia. *Journal of Trauma* 54(3): 478–485.
2. Bledsoe, B. E., R. S. Porter, R. A. Cherry. 2009. *Paramedic care: Principles & practice.* 3rd ed., Book 5, Chapter 3, pp. 146–214, Upper Saddle River, NJ: Pearson Education.
3. Diku, M., K. Newton. 1998. Geriatric trauma. *Emergency Medicine Clinics of North America* 16(1): 257–274.
4. Jacobs, D. G. 2003. Special considerations in geriatric injury. *Current Opinions in Critical Care* 9(6): 535–539.
5. Patel, V. I., H. Thadepalli, P. Patel, A. Mandal. 2004. Thoracoabdominal injuries in the elderly: 25 years of experience. *Journal of the National Medical Association* 96(12): 1553–1557.
6. Pudelek, B. 2002. Geriatric trauma: Special needs for a special population. *AACN Clinical Issues* 13(1): 61–72.
7. Stevenson, J. 2004. When the trauma patient is elderly. *J Perianesthesia Nursing* 19(6): 392–400.
8. Centers for Disease Control and Prevention. http://www/cdc.gov/fieldtriage/index.html. http://www.cdc.gov/HomeandRecreationalSafety/Falls/adultfalls.html.

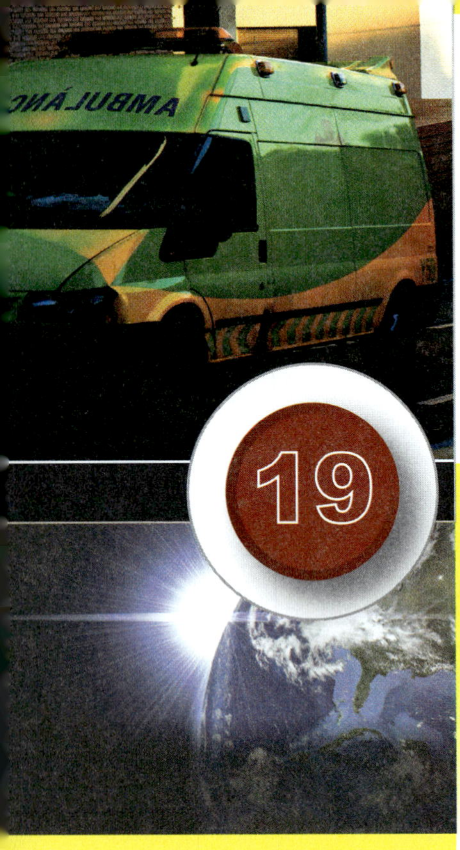

(Photo courtesy of Jupiterimages, Photos.com/Thinkstock.com)

Trauma in Pregnancy

Walter J. Bradley, MD, MBA, FACEP

Trauma in Pregnancy il trauma nel pregancy

Trauma en el embarazo | Traumatisme de la grossesse

Urazy psychiczne w ciąży | Trauma in Schwangerschaft

traume u trudnoći | صدمة في الحمل | traume u trudnoći

travme v nosečnosti | trauma a terhesség alatt

KEY TERMS

abruptio placenta, *p. 349*
domestic violence, *p. 349*
physiological changes, *p. 344*
supine hypotension syndrome, *p. 347*

OBJECTIVES

Upon successful completion of this chapter, you should be able to:

1. Understand the dual goals in managing the pregnant trauma patient.
2. Describe the physiological changes associated with pregnancy.
3. Understand the pregnant trauma patient's response to hypovolemia.
4. Describe the types of injuries most commonly associated with the pregnant trauma patient.
5. Describe the initial assessment and management of the pregnant trauma patient.
6. Discuss trauma prevention in pregnancy.

Chapter Overview

When the crossroads of pregnancy and trauma meet, there are unique challenges. The vulnerability of the pregnant trauma patient and potential injuries to the unborn child serve as reminders of the dual roles of providing care to both mother and fetus. In addition, the pregnant patient is often at risk for a higher incidence of accidental trauma. The increase in fainting spells, hyperventilation, and excess fatigue that are commonly associated with early pregnancy, as well as the physiological changes that affect balance and coordination, add to risks.

Trauma is a leading cause of morbidity and mortality in pregnancy. Although maternal mortality due to other causes such as infection, hemorrhage, hypertension, and thromboembolism, has declined over the years, the number of maternal deaths due to penetrating trauma, suicide, homicide, and motor-vehicle collisions has risen steadily. Approximately 6% to 7% of all pregnant women experience some degree of trauma. Significant trauma occurs in approximately 1 in 12 patients who are injured. Injuries requiring ICU admission occur in three to four pregnancies per 100 deliveries. Motor-vehicle collisions account for 65% to 70% of trauma in pregnant patients. Falls, abuse, and domestic violence, penetrating injuries, and burns follow. Because minor injuries rarely present problems for EMS providers, the following discussion focuses on the more severe traumatic injuries to the pregnant patient.

CASE PRESENTATION

An ALS ambulance is on the scene of a single-car motor-vehicle collision. The driver of the car swerved to avoid hitting a dog and hit a tree at an approximate speed of 30 miles per hour. The patient was restrained, and the airbag deployed from the steering wheel. The scene is safe, and law enforcement is interviewing the driver, who is ambulatory. EMS is asked to evaluate the driver because she is concerned about her unborn baby. She is eight months pregnant. She denies loss of consciousness and head, neck, or back pain. Her only complaint is a tender abdomen. Upon inspection there is a superficial abrasion running horizontally across her abdomen. What is likely to have caused this abrasion? Should this patient be transported and evaluated at the emergency department or the birthing center at the hospital? Might the incident induce premature labor? If she goes into labor, is the fetus old enough to be viable? Could this patient be managed without spinal motion restriction (SMR)? If SMR is indicated for a pregnant patient, are there special precautions to consider? Keep these questions in mind as you read the chapter. Then, at the end of the chapter, find out how the rescuers completed this call. ■

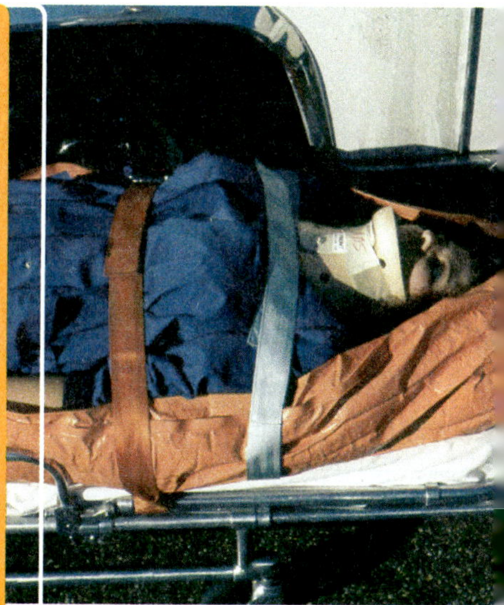

Pregnancy

Fetal Development

The effect of trauma on pregnancy depends on the gestational age of the fetus, the type and severity of the trauma, and the extent of disruption of normal uterine and fetal physiology. The fetus is formed during the first three months of

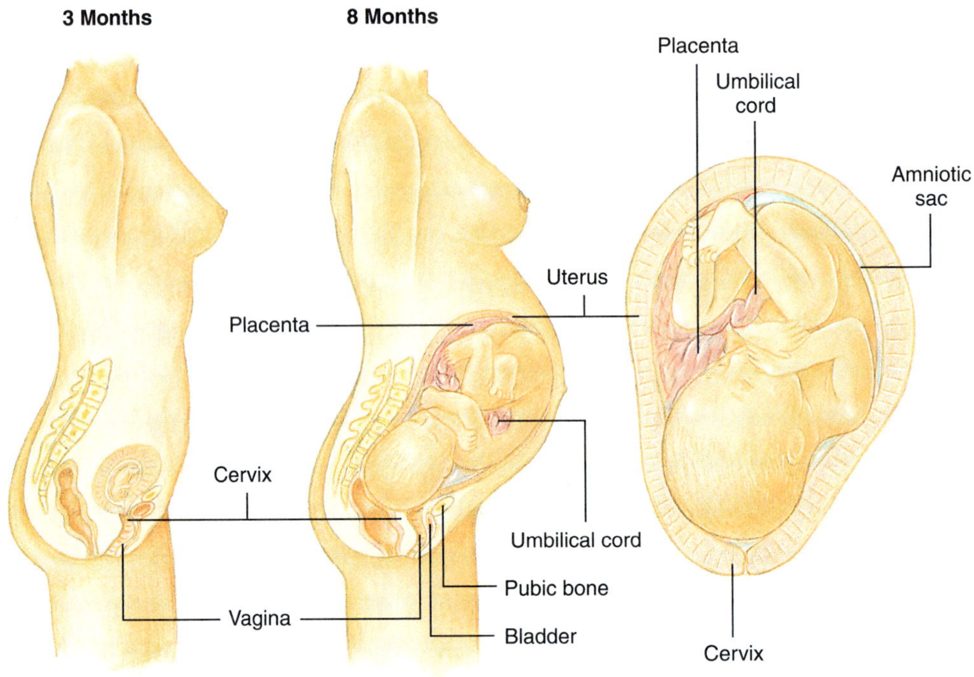

FIGURE 19-1 Anatomy of pregnancy: uterus at three months and at eight months gestation.

pregnancy. After the third month of gestation, the fully formed fetus and uterus grow rapidly, reaching the umbilicus by the fifth month and the epigastrium by the seventh month (Figure 19-1 and Table 19-1). The fetus is considered viable at 24 weeks.

Physiological Changes During Pregnancy

physiological changes the normal changes that occur to the body of a woman as she progresses through her pregnancy. These affect blood volume, vital signs, and even response to hypovolemia.

During pregnancy, dramatic **physiological changes** occur. The changes that are unique to the pregnant state affect and sometimes alter the physiological response by both the mother and fetus. Changes include blood volume (increases), cardiac output (increases), and blood pressure (decreases; Figure 19-2). The respiratory system also has significant changes due to an enlarging uterus that will elevate the diaphragm and decrease the overall volume of the thoracic cavity. That leads

Table 19-1 Assessment of a Pregnancy

	First Trimester (1–12 weeks)	Second Trimester (13–24 weeks)	Third Trimester (25–40 weeks)
Viability	Fetus not viable	Potential viability	Fetus viable
Vaginal bleeding	Potential for miscarriage	Potential miscarriage	Potential preterm birth
Fetal heart tones	Not obtainable	120–170 beats per minute	120–160 beats per minute
Height of fundus above symphysis pubis	Difficult to measure	Halfway to umbilicus equals 16 weeks; to the umbilicus equals 20 weeks	1 cm equals 1 week until 37 weeks, then uterus height decreases as the baby settles into the pelvis

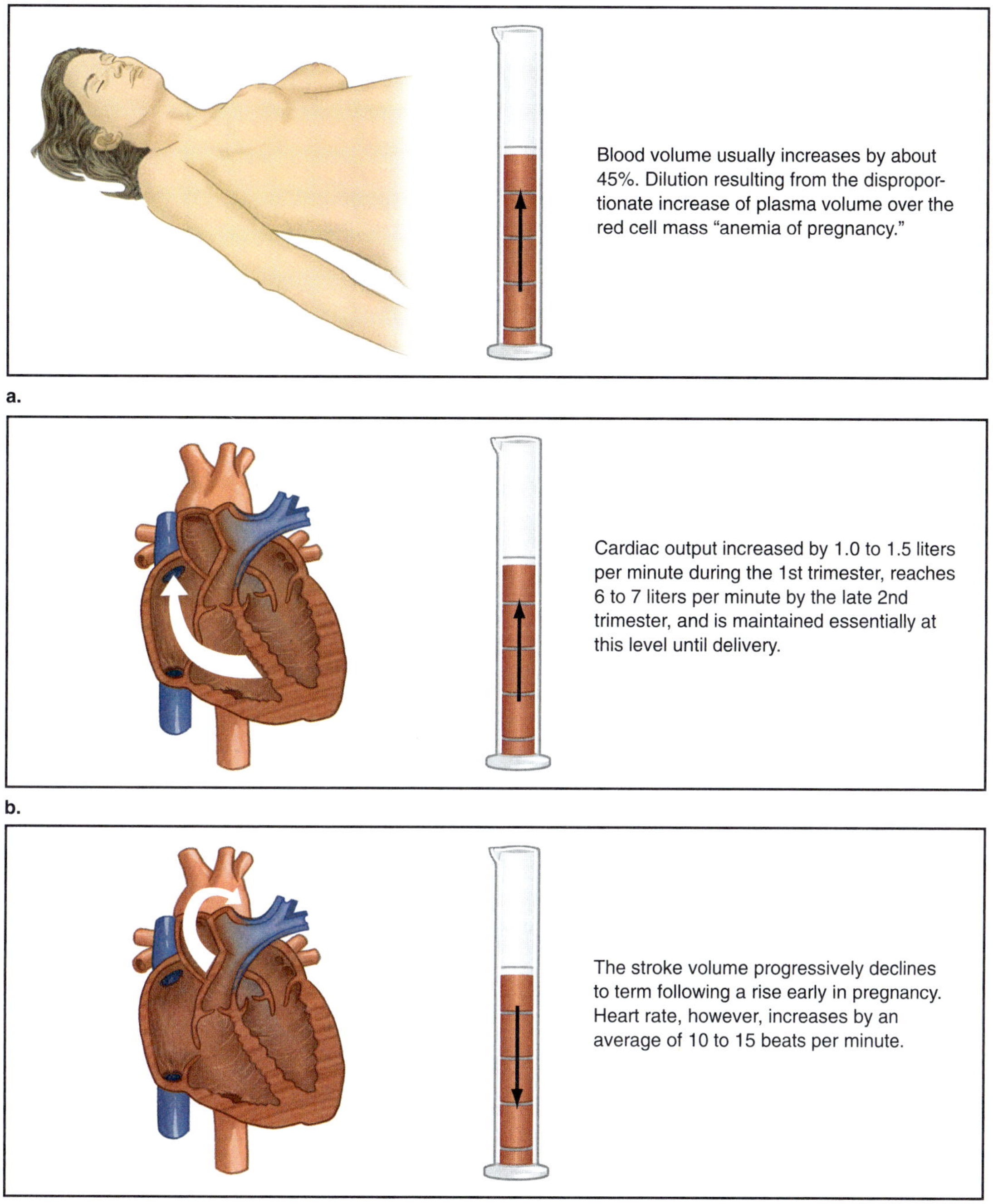

FIGURE 19-2 Physiological changes during pregnancy.

to a relative alkalosis and predisposes the patient to hyperventilation. There is, in addition, an increase in both red blood cells and plasma. With the increase of plasma greater than red blood cells, the patient will appear to be anemic (physiological anemia of pregnancy). However, many pregnant patients have poor nutritional intake during pregnancy and because the fetus draws iron stores, may develop an absolute anemia. Gastric motility is also decreased; thus, always assume the stomach of a pregnant patient is full. Always guard against vomiting and aspiration. Table 19-2 illustrates changes during pregnancy.

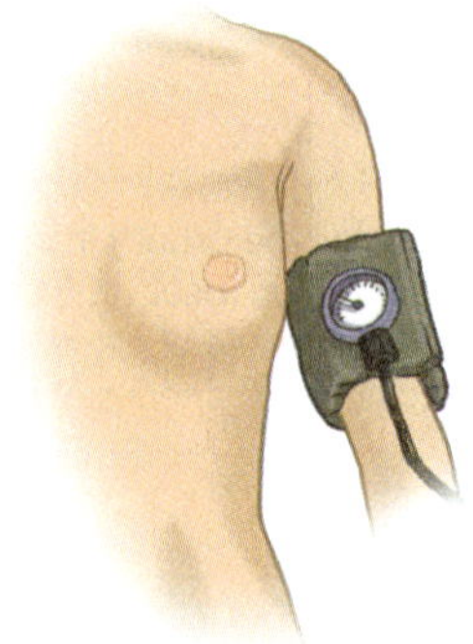

The mean level of blood pressure is characteristically 10 to 15 mm HG lower during pregnancy, the decline usually apparent by the end of the 1st trimester. Widened pulse pressure results from a proportionately greater reduction in the diastolic component.

d.

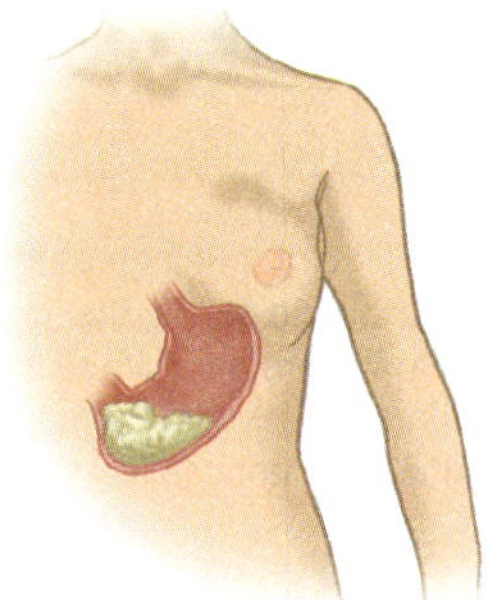

Peristalsis is slowed; thus, the stomach may still contain food hours after a meal. Be alert to the danger of vomiting and aspiration.

e.

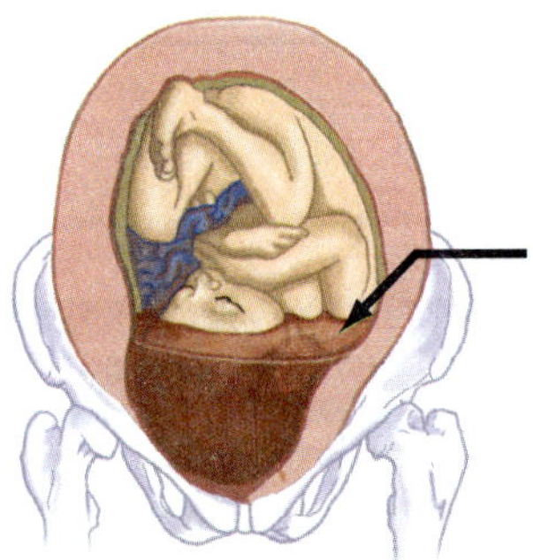

Injury to the uterus or pelvis may cause massive hemorrhage.

f.

FIGURE 19-2 *(Continued)*

Table 19-2 Physiological Changes During Pregnancy

Parameter Monitored	Normal Female	Change
Blood volume	4,000 mL	Increased 40% to 50%
Heart rate	70	Increased 10% to 15%
Blood pressure	110/70	Decreased 5 to 15 mm Hg
Cardiac output	4 to 5 Lpm	Increased 20% to 30%
Hematocrit/hemoglobin	13/40	Decreased
PCO_2	38	Decreased
Gastric motility	Normal	Decreased

Responses to Hypovolemia

Acute blood loss results in a decrease in circulating blood volume. The cardiac output decreases as the venous return falls. This hypovolemia causes the arterial blood pressure to fall, resulting in an inhibition of vagal tone and the release of catecholamines. The effect of this response is to produce vasoconstriction and tachycardia. This vasoconstriction profoundly affects the uterus. Uterine vasoconstriction leads to reduction in uterine blood flow by 20% to 30%. Because of her increased blood volume, the pregnant patient may lose up to 1,500 cc of blood before any detectable change is noted in her blood pressure. The fetus reacts to this hypoperfusion by a drop in the arterial blood pressure and a decrease in heart rate. The fetus then begins to suffer from reduced oxygen concentration in the maternal circulation. Therefore, it is important to give 100% oxygen to the mother to provide sufficient oxygen to the fetus, who suffers from both oxygen starvation and inadequate blood supply. A shock state in the mother is associated with an 80% fetal mortality rate.

PEARLS: Hypovolemia

- Do not mistake normal vital signs in pregnant patients as signs of shock. The pregnant patient has a normal resting pulse that is 10 to 15 beats faster than usual, and the blood pressure is 10 to 15 mm Hg lower than usual. However, it is also important to realize that a blood loss of 30% to 35% can occur in these patients before there is a significant change in blood pressure. Therefore, be especially alert to all signs of shock, and monitor the vital signs with frequent ITLS Ongoing Exams.
- Cardiac arrest in the pregnant patient is treated the same as for other victims. Defibrillation settings and drug dosages are the same. For hypovolemic arrest, the volume of required fluid increases, and four liters of normal saline should be given as fast as possible during transport.

Assessment and Management

Special Considerations

Major goals in caring for the pregnant trauma patient are evaluation and stabilization. The ITLS Primary Survey is the same for the pregnant patient as for other patients. (See Chapter 2.) All prehospital interventions are directed toward optimizing both fetal and maternal outcome. If the patient is pregnant, there are two patients being treated. Optimal care for the fetus is appropriate treatment of the mother. Oxygen administration (100% by nonrebreather mask or by endotracheal intubation) should be rapid. Promptly obtain venous access and begin administration of IV fluids. Monitoring of this patient should be immediate and constant because the anatomic and physiological changes of pregnancy make the trauma assessment more difficult.

supine hypotension syndrome the drop in blood pressure seen when a woman who is greater than 20 weeks pregnant is in the supine position. The hypotension is caused by the weight of the pregnant uterus pressing on the inferior vena cava and decreasing the return of blood to the heart by up to 30%.

Acute hypotension in the pregnant patient due to decreased venous return requires special mention. This **supine hypotension syndrome** usually occurs when the patient is in a supine position with a 20-week (uterus up to umbilicus) or larger uterus (Figure 19-3). This can lead to maternal hypotension, syncope, and fetal bradycardia. Left uterine displacement increases cardiac output by 30% and restores circulation. Uterine displacement must be maintained at all times during resuscitation, transport, and perioperatively for nonobstetrical surgery. Therefore, the transport of all pregnant trauma patients, if no contraindication exists, should be by one of the following methods to alleviate vena cava compression:

- Tilt or rotate the backboard 15 to 30 degrees to the patient's left.
- Elevate the right hip 4 to 6 inches with a towel and manually displace the uterus to the left.

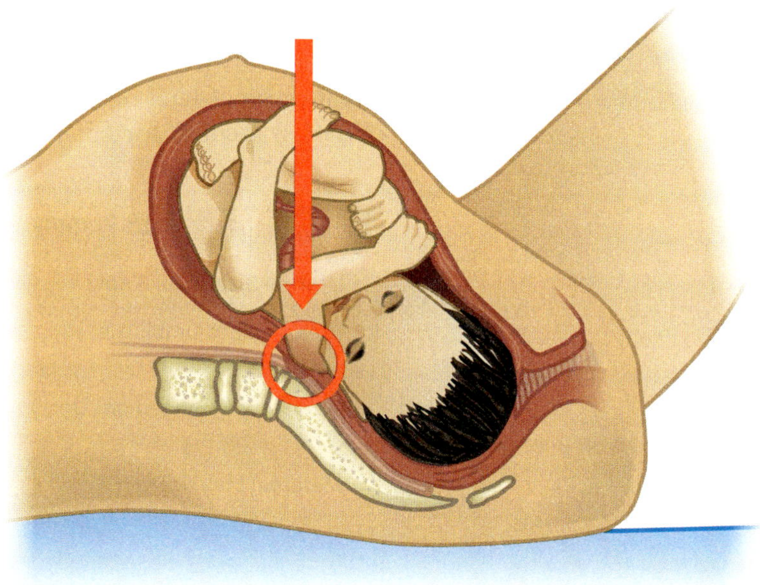

FIGURE 19-3 Venous return to the maternal heart may be decreased up to 30% because of vena cava compression by the fetus. Transport the patient.

PEARLS: Treatment

- You are treating two patients. However, the mortality of the fetus is related to the treatment provided to the mother. The goal of prehospital intervention is to maximize the chances of maternal survival, which will provide the fetus with the best chance for survival.
- If the mother dies, continue CPR and notify the hospital to be prepared for immediate cesarean section. Have them bring a sonogram machine to the emergency department for immediate evaluation of the fetus.
- Hypoxemia of the fetus may go unnoticed in the injured pregnant patient. Treatment should include high-flow oxygen.

PEARLS: Transport

Transport must include appropriate spinal motion restriction (SMR), extremity splints, and prevention of vena cava compression.

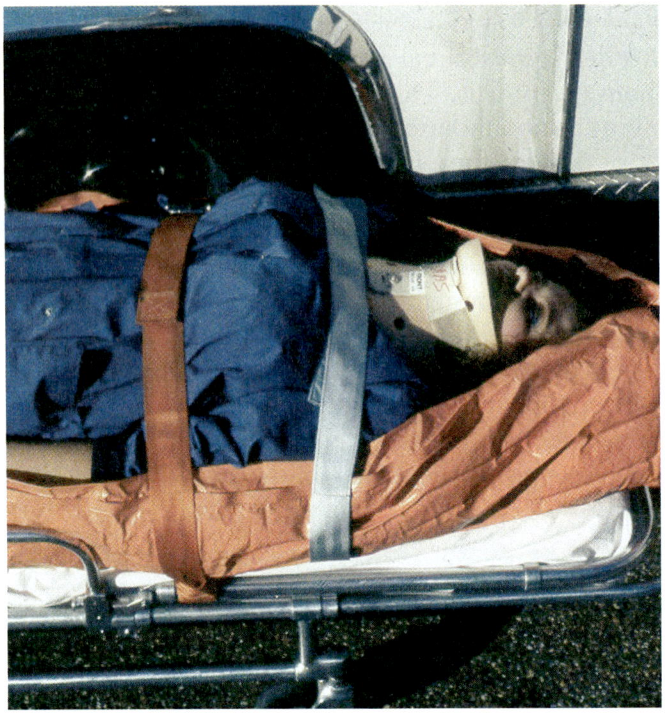

FIGURE 19-4 The pregnant patient is better stabilized and more comfortable in a vacuum backboard than a hard backboard.

You must be very careful when strapping a third-trimester pregnant patient onto a long backboard. Many patients (and backboards) will roll right over onto the ambulance floor if the tilted backboard is not secured to the stretcher. The vacuum backboard (Figure 19-4) is more comfortable and makes it easier to maintain SMR of the pregnant patient. Table 19-3 illustrates evaluation of uterine size and its effect on management of the pregnant patient.

Types of Trauma

Motor-Vehicle Collisions

Though relatively minor abdominal trauma can cause fetal death, the most common cause of fetal death in trauma is maternal death. Motor-vehicle collisions (MVCs) account for 65% to 75% of pregnancy-related trauma. Fetal distress,

Table 19-3 ITLS Primary Survey Brief Evaluation of Uterine Size

Uterine Size < 20 Weeks	Uterine Size > 20 Weeks
Uterus Not to Umbilicus	Uterus to Umbilicus or Higher
↓	↓
Pregnancy Management Unchanged	Lateral Displacement of Uterus
↓	↓
Maternal Stabilization	Brief Confirmation of Fetal Heart Activity (if possible)
	↓
	Maternal Stabilization Secondary Fetal Stabilization

fetal death, **abruptio placenta**, uterine rupture (Figure 19-5), and preterm labor are often seen in pregnant patients who have been in MVCs. A review of the literature indicates that less than 1% of pregnant patients will sustain injury when there is only minor damage to the vehicle.

Head injury is the most common cause of death in pregnant patients involved in MVCs. This is closely followed by uncontrolled hemorrhage. Pregnant victims of MVCs have associated injuries, such as pelvic fractures, that often result in concealed hemorrhage within the retroperitoneal space. The retroperitoneal area, because of its low-pressure venous system, can accommodate the loss of four or more liters of blood into that area with few clinical signs. Seat-belt use with both a shoulder restraint and lap belt can significantly decrease patient mortality and has not shown any increase in uterine injuries.

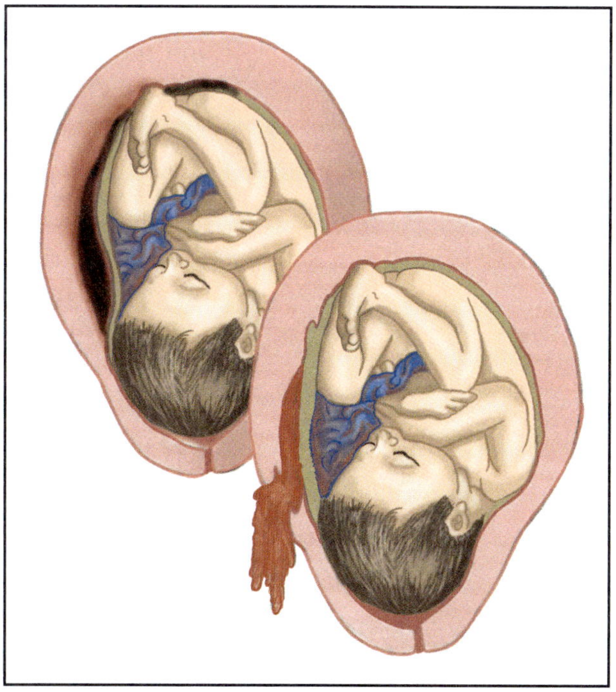

FIGURE 19-5 Blunt trauma to the uterus may cause separation of the placenta (abruptio placenta) or rupture of the uterus. Massive bleeding may occur, but there may not be visible vaginal bleeding early.

Penetrating Injuries

Gunshot wounds and stabbings are the most common injuries encountered. If the path of entry is below the fundus, the uterus will often offer protection to the mother, absorbing the force of the bullet or knife. Upper abdominal wounds will often injure the bowel due to its compression in a smaller than normal space by the uterus. Studies have shown that gunshot wounds to the pregnant abdomen carry a high mortality rate for the fetus (40% to 70%). They are lower for the mother (4% to 10%) because the large uterus usually protects vital organs. Stab wounds follow much the same pattern of outcome, with fetal mortality rates of about 40%. Definitive care will depend on several factors, involving degree of shock, associated organ injury, and time of gestation.

abruptio placenta the separation of the placenta from the wall of the uterus.

PEARLS: Abdominal Trauma

Trauma to the abdominal compartment can cause occult bleeding in either the intrauterine or retroperitoneal area. Keep in mind that gradual stretching of the abdominal wall during pregnancy, along with hormonal changes within the body, make the peritoneal surface less sensitive to irritable stimuli. Therefore, bleeding can occur intraperitoneally, and the signs of rebound, guarding, and rigidity may not be present.

Domestic Violence

A large number of pregnant women experience **domestic violence**. The frequency appears to worsen as pregnancy progresses. Through the second and third trimesters, it is estimated that 1 in 10 women experiences abuse during pregnancy. Physical abuse is more likely to be manifest with proximal and midline injuries than the distal injuries of accidental trauma. The face and neck are most common. Domestic abuse has also been associated with low birth weight. The pregnant patient who is under great stress produces hormones (high circulating adrenaline levels, and so on) that are not good for her pregnancy. The folklore that pregnant patients should be shielded from frightening or disturbing situations is probably true. Spouses and boyfriends are the perpetrators of the violence in 70% to 85% of cases.

domestic violence physical abuse in the home. Through the second and third trimester, it is estimated that 1 in 10 pregnant women experiences physical abuse.

Falls

The incidence of falls increases with the progression of pregnancy. This is in part due to an alteration in the patient's center of gravity. The incidence of significant injury is proportionate to the force of impact and the specific body part that sustains the impact. Pelvic injuries may result in abruption placenta (separation of the placenta from the uterine wall causing hemorrhage and fetal hypoxia and often death) and fetal fractures. Emergency department evaluation and monitoring is recommended for even minor abdominal trauma during pregnancy.

Burns

Of the 2.2 million patients that suffer burn injuries in the United States annually, less than 4% are pregnant. The overall mortality and morbidity resulting from thermal injuries to the pregnant patient is not markedly different from the nonpregnant patient. However, it is important to remember that the fluid requirement for the pregnant patient is greater than that of the nonpregnant woman. Fetal mortality increases when the maternal surface burn exceeds 20%.

Trauma Prevention in Pregnancy

Upon reviewing major causes of trauma in pregnancy, it is clear that specific recommendations such as proper seat belt use in motor vehicles, reporting and counseling for domestic violence, as well as education of the multiple physiological, anatomical, and emotional changes associated with pregnancy will all serve to reduce trauma in pregnancy. Some patients get very little if any prenatal care, and even less prenatal education. If the situation is not critical, you should not hesitate to educate your pregnant patients when you are called to see them.

CASE PRESENTATION (continued)

An ALS ambulance is on scene of a single-car motor-vehicle collision. The driver of the car swerved to avoid hitting a dog and hit a tree at an approximate speed of 30 miles per hour. The patient was restrained, and the airbag deployed from the steering wheel. The scene is safe, and law enforcement is interviewing the driver, who is ambulatory. EMS is asked to evaluate the driver because she is concerned about her unborn baby. She is eight months pregnant. She denies loss of consciousness and head, neck, or back pain. Her only complaint is her abdomen is tender. Upon inspection there is a superficial abrasion running horizontally across her abdomen. Because of the mechanism of injury, the team performs a rapid trauma survey that is normal with the exception of generalized tenderness of the abdomen but no rebound. The fundus of the uterus is at the xyphoid. The vital signs are normal. It appears the patient had her lap belt across her abdomen instead of her pelvis, and it could have caused uterine or intrauterine injury so the patient is placed on the ambulance stretcher in the semireclining position, with no SMR, and transported nonemergency to the hospital where her obstetrician practices. A sonogram was done in the emergency department, and no abnormality was seen, so a fetal monitor was applied, and the patient was observed overnight. She developed premature labor during the night and delivered a healthy 5-pound, 6-ounce boy. She had a normal postpartum course, and she and the baby did well. ■

Summary

Management of the pregnant trauma patient requires knowledge of the physiological changes that occur during pregnancy. Pregnant patients require rapid evaluation and also rapid interventions for stabilization, including aggressive oxygen administration and fluid resuscitation. They require special techniques in packaging and transport to prevent the vena cava compression syndrome. Because of the difficulty in early diagnosis, you should have a low threshold for load and go, if there is any danger of the development of hemorrhagic shock. Pregnant patients with serious injuries should be directly transported to a facility (trauma center) capable of managing these complex patients. Optional fetal care is dependent on care of the mother.

Bibliography

1. Chang, J., C. Berg, L. Saltzman, J. Herndon. 2005. Homicide: A leading cause of injury deaths among pregnant and postpartum women in the United States. *American Journal of Public Health* 95(3): 471–477.
2. Coker, A., M. Sanderson, B. Dong. 2004. Partner violence during pregnancy and risk of adverse pregnancy outcomes. *Paediatric and Perinatal Epidemiology* 18(4): 260–269.
3. El Kady, D., W. Gilbert, J. Anderson, et al. 2004. Trauma during pregnancy: An analysis of maternal and fetal outcomes in a large population. *American Journal of Obstetrics and Gynecology* 190(6): 1661–1668.
4. Esposito, T. J. 1994. Trauma during pregnancy. *Emergency Medicine Clinics of North America* 12: 167–199.
5. Fildes J., L. Reed, N. Jones, et al. 1992. Trauma: The leading cause of maternal death. *The Journal of Trauma* 32: 643.
6. Hill, D. A., J. J. Lense. 1996. Abdominal trauma in the pregnant patient. *American Family Physician* 53: 1269–1274.
7. Maghsoudi, H., R. Samnia, et al. 2006. Burns in pregnancy. *Burns* 32(2): 246–250.
8. Pons, P. T. 1994. Prehospital considerations in the pregnant patient. *Emergency Medical Clinics of North America* 12: 1–7.
9. Vaizey, C. J., M. J. Jacobson, F. W. Cross. 1994. Trauma in pregnancy. *British Journal of Surgery* 81: 1406–1415.
10. Weiss, H., T. Songer, A. Fabio. 2001. Fetal deaths related to maternal injury. *JAMA* 286(15): 1863–1868.

Explore Resource Central

For additional review and practice tests, visit www.bradybooks.com and click on Resource Central to access book-specific resources for this text. To access Resource Central, follow directions on the Student Access Card provided with this text. If there is no card, go to www.bradybooks.com and follow the Resource Central link to Buy Access from there.

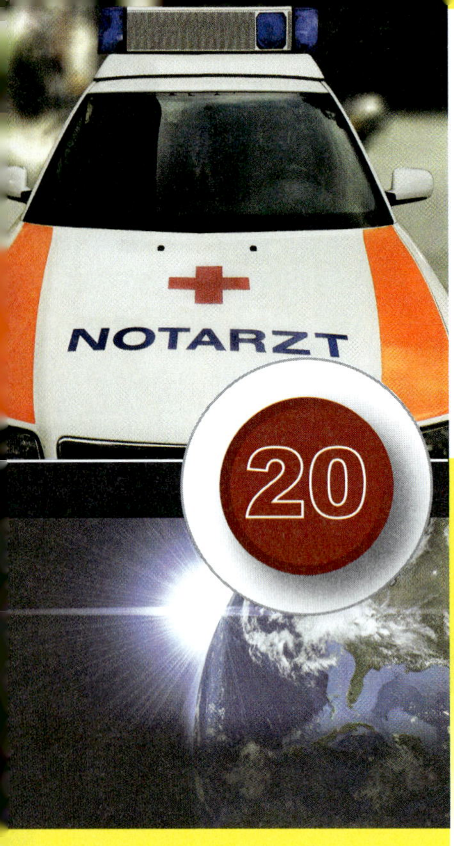

(Photo courtesy of Alexander Ivanov, Shutterstock.com)

20

The Impaired Patient

Jonathan G. Newman, MD, MMM, FACEP, EMT-P

Patients under the influence of alcohol or drugs

Paziente Intossicato da Alcool o Droghe

Pacientes Intoxicados por alcohol o drogas

Les Patients sous l'influence d'alcool ou de drogues

Pacjent pod wpływem alkoholu lub narkotyków

Patienten unter dem Einfluss von Alkohol oder Drogen

Ozljeđenici pod utjecajem alkohola ili droga

المخدر مريض تحت تأثير الكحول أو

pacijent pod uticajem alkohola ili droga

Pacienti pod vplivom alkohola ali drog

Ittas vagy kábítószer hatása alatt lévő sérült

KEY TERMS

closed-ended questions, *p. 355*
interactive style, *p. 355*
patient restraint, *p. 355*
Reeves sleeve, *p. 356*
uncooperative patient, *p. 355*

OBJECTIVES

Upon successful completion of this chapter, you should be able to:

1. List signs and symptoms of patients under the influence of alcohol and/or drugs.
2. Describe the five strategies you would use to best ensure cooperation during assessment and management of a patient under the influence of alcohol and/or drugs.
3. Describe situations in which you would restrain patients, and tell how to handle an uncooperative patient.
4. List the special considerations for assessment and management of patients in whom substance abuse is suspected.

Chapter Overview

The relationship between alcohol and trauma is well documented. For instance, it is reported that car crashes involving alcohol result in injuries to about 500,000 people a year. Studies of individuals who are substance abusers note that those persons are at greater risk to suffer an injury than the general population and that they are more likely to have repeated injuries.

Substance abuse includes individuals who have abused alcohol, drugs, or both. It has been associated with a number of traumatic events, often resulting from accidents, car crashes, suicides, homicides, and other violent crimes. Further, a study reported in the *Journal of the American College of Surgeons* found a high rate of alcohol and illicit drug use in patients who die from trauma (Demetriades et al., 2004). Therefore, it would not be surprising to find that a number of seriously injured trauma patients are under the influence of alcohol or some other substance. This group of trauma patients often presents with unique challenges that can require some special patient management techniques along with good ITLS care.

A high index of suspicion combined with the results of the physical exam, the history obtained from the patient or bystanders, and evidence at the scene can clue you into whether your patient is under the influence of alcohol or drugs. Table 20-1 includes commonly abused drugs, along with signs and symptoms of their use.

Table 20-1 Commonly Abused Drugs with Their Associated Signs and Symptoms

Drug Category	Common Names	Signs and Symptoms of Use or Abuse
Alcohol	Beer, whiskey, wine, mouthwash	Altered mental function, confusion, polyuria, slurred speech, coma, hypertension, hyperthermia
Amphetamines, methamphetamines	Bennies, ice, speed, uppers, dexies, Ecstasy, MDMA, Adderall	Excitement, hyperactivity, dilated pupils, hypertension, tachycardia, tremors, seizures, fever, paranoia, psychosis
Cocaine	Coke, crack, blow, rock	Same as amphetamines plus chest pain; lethal dysrhythmias
Hallucinogens	Acid, LSD, PCP	Hallucinations, dizziness, dilated pupils, nausea, rambling speech, psychosis, anxiety, panic
Marijuana	Grass, hash, pot, tea, weed	Euphoria, sleepiness, dilated pupils, dry mouth, increased appetite
Narcotics/Opiates	Heroin, horse, big H, Darvon, codeine, stuff, morphine, smack	Altered mental status, constricted pupils, bradycardia, hypotension, respiratory depression, hypothermia
Sedatives and psychoactive medications (The list is far too long to record a significant portion of the legitimate mediations)	GHB; barbiturates; benzodiazepines (e.g., Librium, Valium, Xanax, Ativan, Rohypnol) Antidepressants: Elavil, Prozac, Sinequan, Effexor Antipsychotics: Thorazine; Zyprexa, Abilify	Altered mental status, dilated pupils, cardiac dysrhythmias, hypotension, respiratory depression, hypothermia

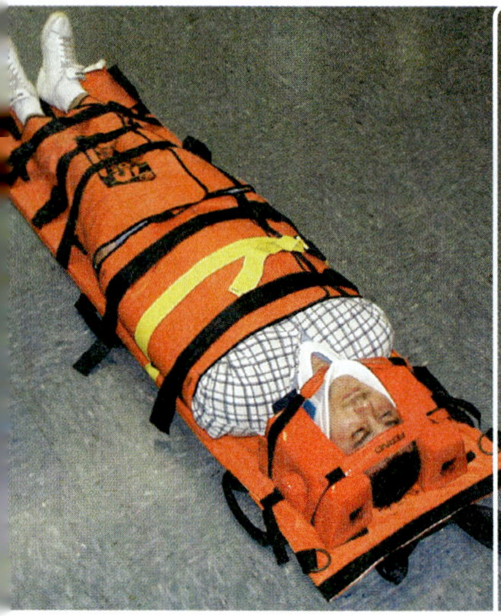

CASE PRESENTATION

A BLS team is on medical standby at a sporting event when rescuers are summoned to a report of a fan who fell off the bleachers. Their scene size-up reveals the scene is currently safe; however, it is very noisy, and there are many spectators in the bleachers watching from above. The fall was approximately 15 feet onto a grassy surface. Friends of the patient state he was drinking alcohol during the entire event, including a pregame tailgating party. The patient is unresponsive with sonorous respirations at a rate of 12 per minute, and peripheral pulses are present, strong, and regular. What type of assessment would you perform? Could some effects of alcohol intoxication mimic trauma-related signs and symptoms? Is this a load-and-go patient? Could the scene dynamics change and become unsafe? Keep these questions in mind as you read the chapter. Then, at the end of the chapter, find out how the rescuers completed this call. ■

Assessment and Management

Your ITLS Primary and Secondary Surveys should follow the ITLS guidelines that have been described in this book. (See Chapter 2.) However, there are some particular aspects to be aware of when conducting an exam on a patient for whom you suspect substance abuse. Pay particular attention to mental status, pupils, speech, and respiration, and note any needle marks you may discover. An altered mental status can be seen in every form of substance abuse. However, *remember that an altered level of consciousness is always due to a head injury, shock, or hypoglycemia until proven otherwise. Also remember that all patients have an emergency medical condition until proven otherwise.*

Pupils often are constricted in patients who have abused opiates. Dilated pupils are common in patients exposed to amphetamines, cocaine, hallucinogens, and marijuana. Patients who use barbiturates will have pupils that are constricted early on. However, if high doses have been consumed, the pupils can eventually become fixed and dilated. Speech can be slurred when patients use alcohol or sedatives, and patients who are under the influence of hallucinogens may seem to ramble when they talk. Respiration can be significantly depressed with opiates and sedatives.

The history supplied by the patient or bystanders can help to establish whether substance abuse is involved. Try to find out what was used, when it was taken, and how much was taken. *If you know the name of the drug taken, you may need to check with your local poison control center because the number of even prescription medications that are abused is in the hundreds, and many have serious toxic effects.*

However, be aware that patients often deny that they have used or abused any substance. If possible, inspect the patient's surroundings for clues that drugs or alcohol may have been used. Note any alcoholic beverage bottles, pill containers, injection equipment, smoking or snorting paraphernalia, or unusual odors.

Trauma patients under the influence of alcohol or drugs can challenge the provider not only by their traumatic injuries but also by their attitudes. The way in which you interact with patients who have abused substances can determine if the

PEARLS: Under the Influence

It is extremely difficult to differentiate between patients under the influence and those experiencing a medical and/or trauma emergency. You may have to alter your usual management techniques. Many patients will initially refuse treatment. You may have to consult local protocol, medical direction, and appropriate law enforcement personnel for assistance.

PEARLS: Attitude

The standard ITLS approach to patient care will work well, even with patients under the influence. Your attitude can help determine if your patient approach will be accepted or not. Be positive and nonjudgmental.

patient will be cooperative or uncooperative. How you speak to them can be as important as what you are doing for them. Your interaction style, if offensive, can make patients uncooperative and force you both to lose precious minutes of the Golden period. If your **interactive style** is positive and nonjudgmental, the patient is more likely to be cooperative and to allow all the appropriate medical interventions, thus decreasing on-scene time. As noted before, all the substances that are abused can cause an altered mental state. When interacting with patients, you must be prepared to deal with euphoria, psychosis, paranoia, or confusion and disorientation.

interactive style your speech and body language as you interact with a patient. A positive, nonjudgmental interactive style facilitates assessment and interventions while decreasing scene time.

Five interaction strategies that can help you gain your patient's cooperation are as follows:

- Identify yourself to the patient and orient him to the surroundings. Tell him your name and your title (for example, "EMT, Paramedic"). Ask for his name and how he would like to be addressed. Avoid using generic names like "Bub" or "Honey." With this patient population it may be necessary to orient the patient to place, date, and what is going on frequently.
- Treat the patient in a respectful manner and avoid being judgmental. Often a lack of respect can be heard in the tone of your voice or how you say things, not just in what you say. Never forget that you are there to save lives; this includes all patients. You are not a police officer (do not gather evidence), and you are not there to pass judgment on the patient's worth to society. Also take care not to destroy evidence.
- Acknowledge the patient's concerns and feelings. The patient who is scared or confused may be more comfortable with what is taking place if you recognize and address those feelings. Be gentle but firm. Explain all treatment interventions before they are performed. Be honest; backboards and extrication collars are uncomfortable and IV lines hurt.
- Let the patient know what will be required of him. For instance, he may be confused and not realize that he needs to hold still while you are trying to stabilize him on a backboard.
- Ask **closed-ended questions** when getting your history from the patient. Close-ended questions can be answered with a yes or no. The patient may only be able to concentrate for short periods of time, and he may ramble when asked open-ended questions that require a full answer. Consider getting as much of the history as you can from relatives, friends, or bystanders. This may help improve the reliability of what you discover. Get as much relevant history as you can, but do not delay transport.

closed-ended questions questions that can be answered with a "yes" or "no." This is often the best approach with patients under the influence of alcohol or drugs due to their limited ability to concentrate.

The Uncooperative Patient

A small percentage of your patients may be uncooperative. You must be firm with them. Set limits to their behavior, and let them know when their behavior is inappropriate. Consider physical **patient restraint** only if you are not able to secure enough cooperation to provide adequate care. Often a show of force may be enough to convince an **uncooperative patient** to allow medical care to be provided.

patient restraint methods of limiting the patient's motion and mobility to prevent him from becoming a danger to himself or others.

uncooperative patient a patient who behaves inappropriately and does not respond to reasonable requests and limits placed on him for his own safety and that of caregivers. Based on jurisdiction, a range of options are available for restraining patients against their will when warranted for patient safety, assessment, and care.

Plan for patient encounters. First, check with your local jurisdiction to determine what protocol you must use when restraining patients against their will. Most municipalities allow police officers to place people in custody if they are a threat to themselves or others. Severely injured trauma patients who refuse or will not cooperate with care may be considered a threat to themselves.

Once the decision has been made to restrain the patient, it must be carried out with care. Securely strapping a patient to a backboard with use of a cervical collar

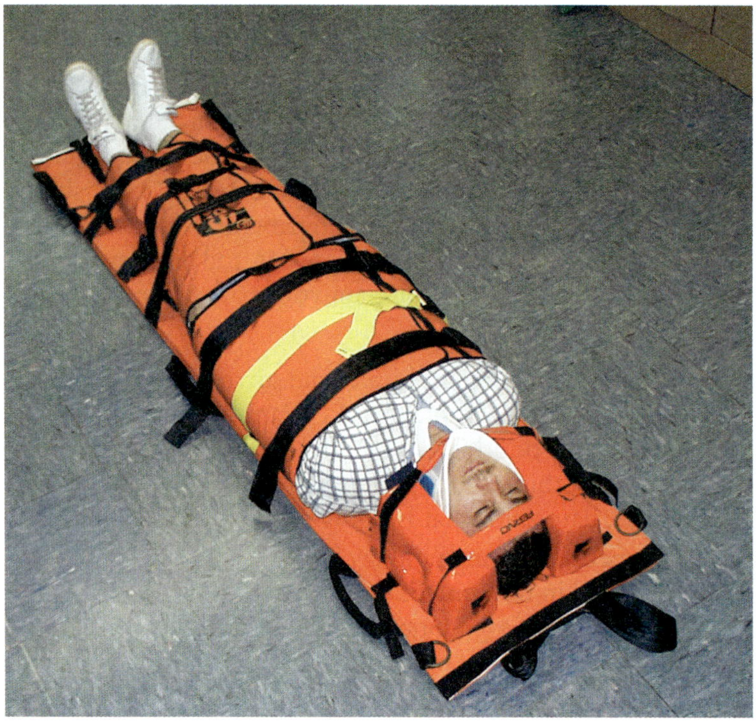

FIGURE 20-1 Reeves sleeve.

and head motion-restriction device will serve to restrain most patients. Caution must be taken not to worsen any current injuries or to inflict any new ones. There is often no good solution to this predicament. Restrained patients could struggle so hard that spinal motion restriction (SMR) is rendered ineffective. The **Reeves sleeve** is one of the few pieces of equipment that is very effective in providing both restraint and motion restriction (Figure 20-1). Crews should plan and practice procedures for restraining patients. The trauma scene is not the place to learn new skills. Reassess restrained patients often. You do not want to be the one providing care for a drug-impaired patient who dies by asphyxiation during prehospital restraint.

Reeves sleeve a dual-purpose motion-restriction device that is effective for both SMR and patient restraint.

The standard ITLS approach to patient care will work well, even with patients under the influence of alcohol or drugs. Ensure that the scene is safe, determine the number of injured, and discover the mechanism of injury. Use standard precautions. This patient population includes people who are at high risk for infection with hepatitis B, hepatitis C, and HIV. Follow the ITLS Primary and Secondary Surveys as recorded in Chapter 2. Remember to note any mental status changes that might be associated with substance abuse.

PEARLS: Management

- Check finger-stick glucose and provide ECG monitoring on every patient with altered mental status.
- In this population, hypothermia, hypotension, and respiratory depression are common and must be treated aggressively. Involve the poison control center early if the person has taken a drug with which you are not familiar.

When performing the ITLS Secondary Survey, be sure to include the specific areas that can provide clues to substance abuse. As with all trauma patients, treatment includes the consideration of oxygen, an IV line, cardiac monitoring, and O_2 saturation or expired CO_2 monitoring. Check a blood sugar in all patients with altered mental status.

Table 20-2 lists drug categories and associated specific treatments or areas to pay close attention to when substance abuse is suspected. Based on a 2009 survey of teenagers, The National Institute on Drug Abuse (NIDA) concluded that many drug use trends are declining. However, they reported that the perception of 3, 4-Methylenedioxymethamphetamine (MDMA or Ecstasy) as harmful is going down, and this might be a precursor to an increase use of this drug. The NIDA also expressed concern about the nonmedical use of the narcotics Vicodin (hydrocodone) and OxyContin (oxycodone).

Table 20-2 Drug Categories and Specific Treatments to Consider or Areas to Assess Closely

Drug Category	Specific Treatments and Areas to Assess
Alcohol	Administer IV thiamine and glucose; use $D_{50}W$ if indicated; watch for hypothermia.
Amphetamines/ Methamphetamine	Monitor for seizures and dysrhythmias; treat seizures with diazepam or lorazepam.
Cocaine	Monitor for seizures and dysrhythmia; treat rhythm disorders. Avoid beta-blockers, as these may increase myocardial ischemia.
Hallucinogens	Provide reassurance.
Marijuana	Provide reassurance.
Narcotics/Opiates	Try naloxone*, watch for hypothermia, hypotension, and respiratory depression (CO_2 monitor).
Sedatives	Try naloxone* and consider flumazenil**, watch for hypothermia, hypotension, and respiratory depression (CO_2 monitor).

*Naloxone should be titrated to the patient's respirations. Repeated doses may be indicated because the narcotic may last longer than the effects of the naloxone.

**Flumazenil use is controversial; it can precipitate seizures in patients dependent on benzodiazepines. Further, flumazenil use may cause seizures in those who have been using benzodiazepines to prevent seizures and in those patients who have overdosed on tricyclic antidepressants. Flumazenil should be given only on direct order of medical direction.

CASE PRESENTATION (continued)

A BLS team on medical standby at a sporting event are summoned to a report of a fan who fell off the bleachers. Their scene size-up reveals the scene is currently safe; however, it is very noisy, and there are many spectators in the bleachers watching from above. The patient's fall was approximately 15 feet onto a grassy surface. Friends of the patient state he was drinking alcohol during the entire event, including a pre-game tailgating party.

The patient is unresponsive with sonorous respirations at a rate of 12 per minute, and peripheral pulses are present, strong, and regular. The mechanism of a 15-foot fall with altered mental status (even if possibly due to alcohol ingestion) requires a rapid trauma survey. Rescuer 2 immediately stabilizes the patient's neck and begins oxygen by nasal cannula. The team leader does a rapid trauma survey and finds no definite injuries, but because of the combination of a significant fall and unresponsiveness, the patient is immediately spinal packaged and taken to the trauma center. Evaluation there reveals an elevated serum alcohol level as well as a nondisplaced fracture of the posterior elements of the fourth and fifth cervical vertebra.

There was no intracranial injury, and the patient woke after several hours. He required spinal stabilization surgery but survived with no spinal-cord injury. In any instance where there are multiple intoxicated bystanders (potentially unsafe scene), it is wise to load the patient and transport as soon as the ITLS Primary Survey is completed. ■

Summary

Knowing the signs and symptoms of alcohol and drug abuse will allow you to recognize the patient who may be impaired. Assessing the patient for signs and symptoms outlined in this chapter can help you confirm your suspicions. Determining that your patient has abused some substance will allow you to pay attention to specific areas for critical changes as well as provide lifesaving interventions that may be indicated for individual substances. The five interaction strategies for improving patient cooperation are very important when dealing with the patient under the influence of alcohol or drugs, but those strategies also should be used with all patients. Remember that the patient's safety is a primary concern. If you must restrain a patient for his or her safety, do so in a planned manner that is most sensitive to your patient's needs.

Bibliography

1. Bledsoe, B., R. Porter, R. Cherry. 2009. *Paramedic care: Principles and practice.* 3rd ed. Vol. 5, pp. 206–207 and 3rd ed., Vol. 3, pp. 499–507. Upper Saddle River, NJ: Prentice Hall.
2. Demetriades D., G. Gkiokas, G. C. Velmahos, et al. 2004. Alcohol and illicit drugs in traumatic deaths: Prevalence and association with type and severity of injuries. *Journal of the American College of Surgeons* 199(5): 687–692.
3. Elling, B., K. M. Elling. 2009. *AAOS paramedic: Pharmacology applications*, pp. 274–278 Sudbury, MA: Jones and Bartlett.
4. Miller, T. R., D. C. Lestina, G. S. Smith. 2001, April. Injury risk among medically identified alcohol and drug abusers. *Alcoholism, Clinical and Experimental Research* 25(1): 54–59.
5. National Institute on Drug Abuse. NIDA InfoFacts: Nationwide Trends. http://www.drugabuse.gov/infofacts/nationtrends.html.

Explore Resource Central

For additional review and practice tests, visit **www.bradybooks.com** and click on Resource Central to access book-specific resources for this text. To access Resource Central, follow directions on the Student Access Card provided with this text. If there is no card, go to www.bradybooks.com and follow the Resource Central link to Buy Access from there.

Trauma Arrest

Ray Fowler, MD, FACEP
Ahamed Idris, MD
Jeremy Brywczynski, MD

Trauma Cardiopulmonary Arrest

Arresto CardioRespiratorio Post Traumatico Paro Cardiopulmonar Traumático Arrêt Cardiorespiratoire

Zatrzymanie krążenia u chorego po urazie Herz- Kreislaufstillstand nach Trauma

Zastoj srca i disanja u traumi إصابات توقف القلب والرئة kardiorespiratorni zastoj usled traume

Kardiopulmonalni zastoj zaradi poškodbe Traumás eredetű keringés-légzésleállás

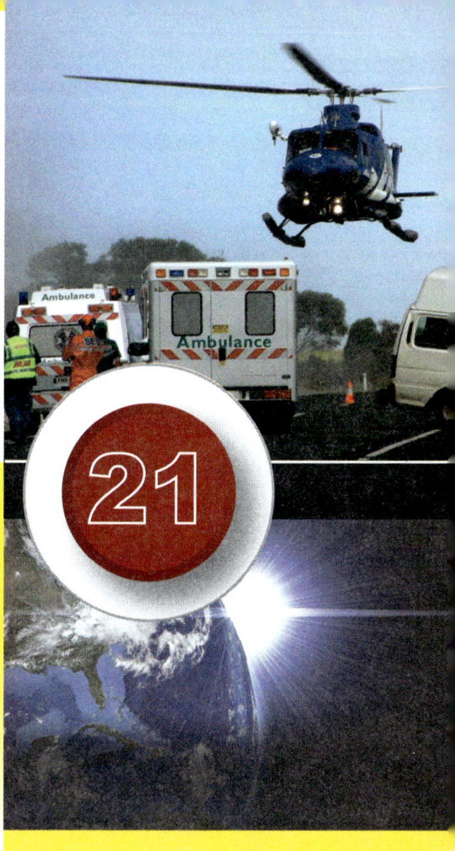

(Photo courtesy of David Hancock, Shutterstock.com)

OBJECTIVES

Upon successful completion of this chapter, you should be able to:

1. Identify treatable causes of traumatic cardiopulmonary arrest.
2. Describe the proper evaluation and management of the patient in traumatic cardiopulmonary arrest.
3. Identify patients in traumatic cardiac arrest for whom you should withhold resuscitation attempts.

KEY TERMS

foreign body airway obstruction (FBAO), *p. 365*
traumatic cardiopulmonary arrest (TCPA), *p. 360*
unsalvageable patient, *p. 360*
withholding or termination of resuscitation, *p. 360*

Chapter Overview

You will encounter trauma patients who are found either pulseless or apneic on scene or who deteriorate rapidly and develop those signs while under your care. Although CPR in pulseless arrest is considered futile, there are several causes of traumatic cardiac arrest that are correctable, and prompt recognition and intervention could be lifesaving. This chapter will discuss guidelines for when to attempt resuscitation and when it would be futile. You also will review the causes of the traumatic cardiac arrest and the best plan of action to rapidly identify the cause and match your response to that cause.

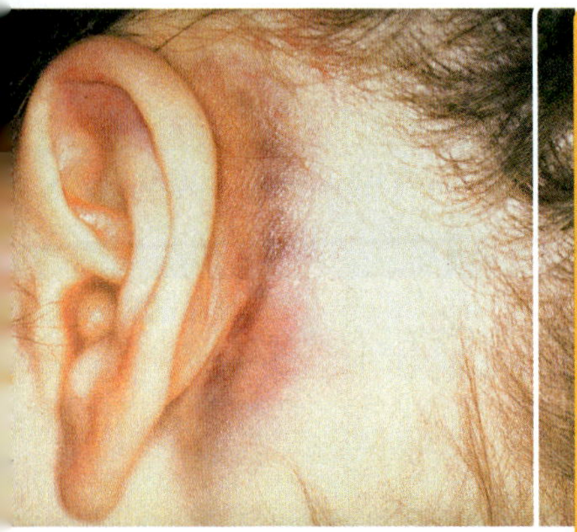

(Courtesy of David Effron, MD, FACEP)

CASE PRESENTATION

A BLS ambulance just arrives on scene of a motorcycle crash in a very rural area. The closest rural hospital is 15 miles away, and the closest level 2 trauma hospital is 45 miles away. In this EMS system, ALS is only dispatched on request of the BLS ambulance on scene. The scene size-up reveals a safe scene with one patient (approximately 20 years old) from a motorcycle that appears to have failed to negotiate a curve in the road. The motorcycle and helmetless driver left the roadway and struck a tree.

The patient is unresponsive, is not breathing, and has no pulses. There is an obvious deformity to the skull, multiple rib fractures, and deformity to the left femur. There were no witnesses to the crash, and it is difficult to determine when the crash occurred. An AED is applied, and it indicates, "No shock advised." Should CPR be initiated? Should the BLS ambulance request an ALS response? If ALS does respond, should they respond with "lights and sirens"? What are likely causes of this cardiac arrest? Keep these questions in mind as you read the chapter. Then, at the end of the chapter, find out how the rescuers completed this call. ■

traumatic cardiopulmonary arrest (TCPA) a grouping of conditions defined by the common precipitating factor of being trauma as the origin for the cardiac arrest.

unsalvageable patient one who does not have a reasonable expectation for resuscitation and survival based on defined clinical indicators and parameters. It is acceptable to withhold resuscitation under those conditions.

withholding or terminating resuscitation based on research and published guidelines, attempting to resuscitate the patient in cardiac arrest may be withheld or terminated in certain instances.

The Unsalvageable Patient

Attempting to resuscitate the patient in **traumatic cardiopulmonary arrest (TCPA)** can put you and the public in danger. Research has shown that emergency "lights and sirens" traffic can be hazardous to both prehospital providers and to the safety of the public (Saunders & Heye, 1994). Do not attempt resuscitation unless there is some chance of the patient's survival. One review of 195 trauma patients who presented unconscious, without palpable pulse or spontaneous respiration, found that patients with sinus rhythm and nondilated (< 4 mm) reactive pupils had a good chance of survival. However, in those patients with asystole, agonal rhythm, ventricular fibrillation, or ventricular tachycardia (**unsalvageable patients**), there were no survivors (Cere et al., 2003). The National Association of EMS Physicians and the American College of Surgeons Committee on Trauma have jointly developed guidelines for **withholding or termination of resuscitation** in

Table 21-1 Guidelines for Withholding or Terminating Resuscitation of Prehospital Traumatic Cardiopulmonary Arrest*

1. Resuscitation should be withheld in cases of:
   a. Blunt trauma with no breathing, pulse, or organized rhythm on ECG on EMS arrival at the scene.
   b. Penetrating trauma with no breathing, pulse, pupillary reflexes, spontaneous movement, or organized ECG activity.
   c. Any trauma with injuries obviously incompatible with life (e.g., decapitation).
   d. Any trauma with evidence of significant time lapse since pulselessness, including dependent lividity, rigor mortis, etc.
2. Cardiopulmonary arrest patients in whom the mechanism of injury does not correlate with the clinical condition, suggesting a nontraumatic cause of the arrest, should have standard resuscitation initiated.
3. Termination of resuscitation efforts should be considered (consult medical direction):
   a. With EMS-witnessed cardiopulmonary arrest and 15 minutes of unsuccessful resuscitation.
   b. When transport time to the hospital emergency department is more than 15 minutes.
4. Special consideration should be given to victims of near drowning, lightning strike, and hypothermia.

*Joint Position Statement of the National Association of EMS Physicians and the American College of Surgeons Committee on Trauma (Hopson, Hirsch, Delgado, et al., 2003)

prehospital traumatic cardiopulmonary arrest (Table 21-1). You also should be familiar with your local protocols that relate to traumatic cardiac arrest.

Advanced Cardiac Life Support (ACLS) has always been directed toward dealing with a cardiac cause for the pulseless patient. In trauma cases, however, cardiopulmonary arrest is usually not due to primary cardiac disease such as coronary atherosclerosis with acute myocardial infarction. You must direct your treatment by identifying the underlying cause of the arrest, or you will almost never be successful in resuscitation. Use the ITLS Primary Survey to determine both the cause of the arrest and to identify those patients for whom you should attempt resuscitation.

PEARLS: Cardiac Arrest

Cardiac arrest following trauma is usually not due to cardiac disease.

Airway and Breathing Problems

Hypoxemia is the most common cause of traumatic cardiopulmonary arrest. Acute airway obstruction or ineffective breathing will be clinically manifested as hypoxemia. Carbon dioxide accumulation from inadequate breathing will play a role in your being unable to resuscitate the patient. Airway problems such as those listed in Table 21-2 lead to hypoxemia by preventing the flow of oxygen to the lungs. Drugs and alcohol, often in conjunction with minor head trauma, can result in airway obstruction by the tongue as well as by respiratory depression.

Careful monitoring of the intoxicated patient may prevent respiratory or cardiac arrest. The same is true of the patient who is unconscious from a head injury. The lax muscles in the pharynx allow the tongue to fall back and obstruct the airway. Obtaining and maintaining an open airway by the modified jaw-thrust maneuver along with an oro- or nasopharyngeal airway is paramount for patients with no gag reflex. You may use a blind insertion

Table 21-2 Causes of Prehospital Traumatic Cardiopulmonary Arrest

1. Airway Problems
   a. Foreign body
   b. Tongue prolapse
   c. Swelling
   d. Tracheal damage
   e. Hemorrhage into the airway
   f. Misplaced advanced airway
2. Breathing Problems
   a. Tension pneumothorax
   b. Open pneumothorax (sucking chest wound)
   c. Flail chest
   d. Diaphragmatic injury
   e. High spinal-cord injury
   f. Carbon monoxide inhalation
   g. Smoke inhalation
   h. Aspiration
   i. Near-drowning
   j. Central nervous system depression from drugs/alcohol
   k. Apnea secondary to electric shock or lightning strike
3. Circulatory Problems
   a. Hemorrhagic shock (empty heart syndrome) from any cause, including traumatic aortic dissection and other vascular injuries
   b. Tension pneumothorax
   c. Pericardial tamponade
   d. Myocardial contusion
   e. Acute myocardial infarction
   f. Cardiac arrest secondary to electric shock

supraglottic airway device (King Airway, LMA, and others) if tolerated by the patient. The role of endotracheal intubation (ETI) in the major trauma patient is an area of wide debate and study. Theoretically, management of the airway should be simpler with ETI, but studies have questioned its benefit and any role in improving survival. In any case, the provider should use all efforts available to prevent aspiration, including having an effective suction device readily available.

Patients with TCPA caused by airway obstruction may respond to advanced life support if the anoxic period was not prolonged.

Patients with hypoxia secondary to a breathing problem have an adequate airway, but they are unable to oxygenate their blood because they cannot get oxygen and blood together at the alveolar-capillary membrane of the lungs. This could be from one or more of the following:

- Inability to ventilate, as in a tension pneumothorax, open pneumothorax, flail chest, pulmonary contusion, or high spinal-cord (C-3 or above) injury.
- Lung tissue filled with fluid, as in the patient with aspiration of blood or vomitus or adult respiratory distress syndrome (ARDS, also known as *non-cardiogenic pulmonary edema*). Near-drowning patients have hypoxemia early from lack of oxygen, and later their lungs develop ARDS.
- Lungs filled with gas (smoke inhalation) that does not contain the appropriate amount of oxygen but instead contains harmful gases such as carbon monoxide or cyanide. In addition, the hot vapor can result in pulmonary edema, further preventing oxygenation by increasing the

distance (by alveolar capillary membrane swelling) between the red blood cells and oxygen.

- Hypoventilation caused by head injury, lightning strike, and/or drugs and alcohol.

Patients with breathing problems should have aggressive appropriate airway management and assisted ventilation with high-flow oxygen. Many of these patients will respond quickly if they have not been anoxic for too long. It is important for you to remember that the patient in shock is very sensitive to positive pressure (also known as "assisted") ventilation. Positive pressure ventilation will diminish venous return to the heart. This lowers cardiac output and hence blood pressure, worsening the shock state. This will be covered in more detail later in this chapter.

Circulatory Problems

The causes of TCPA due to circulatory failure are found in Table 21-2.

Hypovolemic shock (hypovolemic shock is due to blood loss) is the most common circulatory cause of the TCPA. Blood loss may be external, internal, or both, and it may be classified as controlled or uncontrolled. Massive internal bleeding causing cardiac arrest is usually fatal, displaying any of the cardiac arrest ECG rhythms on the monitor.

> **PEARLS:** ACLS Protocols
>
> Do not rely on Advanced Cardiac Life Support (ACLS) protocols alone. Protocols should be modified to provide adequate volume replacement and chest decompression when indicated.

Massive external bleeding causing TCPA often can be controlled in such conditions as amputations, and tourniquets may be lifesaving in such cases. Prompt intravenous (IV) fluid replacement—especially with blood and blood products—presents an opportunity for salvage of the patient.

Massive internal bleeding producing cardiac arrest is due to a transected blood vessel, injury to an internal organ (e.g., liver and spleen), or both. TCPA in these patients is usually fatal. Arrival at a trauma center with some cardiac electrical activity presents slight hope for successful resuscitation with prompt care by the trauma team.

Traumatic tension pneumothorax reduces venous return due to increased intrathoracic pressure in the affected pleural space, accompanied by pressure against the mediastinum late in its course. Decreased venous return reduces cardiac output, and shock occurs. Jugular venous distention, tachycardia, and cyanosis occur, appearing similar to pericardial tamponade, and the patient's trachea may deviate away from the affected side with increasing pressure against the mediastinum late in the course of the condition.

It is vital to diagnose tension pneumothorax if it is present during TCPA. This is one potentially correctable cause of TCPA, and needle decompression of the pleural space on the affected side may be lifesaving.

Traumatic pericardial tamponade (another form of "mechanical" or obstructive shock) producing TCPA is quickly fatal. This condition is usually encountered in a patient with penetrating trauma to the chest wall. The heart is squeezed by blood and clots in the pericardial sac and cannot fill with blood during each beat. The pressure within the pericardial sac is transmitted to the chambers of the heart, preventing them from filling. That reduces venous return to the heart, and cardiac arrest and shock occur. Because of poor lung perfusion, cyanosis usually develops.

These patients often show "Beck's triad," which is a "quiet heart" (muffled heart tones because the heart is nearly empty), evidence of blood not getting into the heart (jugular venous distention), and hypotension (due to low cardiac output) in the setting of equal bilateral breath sounds (unless a lung injury is also present).

Peripheral pulses diminish as hypotension worsens, and indeed, cardiac output may be so low that you cannot feel a pulse. Tachycardia is usually present on the monitor until cardiac arrest is imminent. The peripheral pulses may decrease or disappear with inspiration (termed *pulsus paradoxus*), which is an exaggeration of the slight (less than 10 mm Hg) decrease in systolic blood pressure that occurs during normal inspiration.

Importantly, the multiple trauma victim may have massive hemorrhage in addition to cardiac tamponade (or tension pneumothorax), reducing the distention of neck veins and making the tamponade (or tension pneumothorax) harder to detect.

Patients with pericardial tamponade may appear to be in pulseless electrical activity (PEA) and commonly will not respond to ACLS protocols.

Acute myocardial infarction and myocardial contusion can produce inadequate blood flow (circulation) by either one or a combination of three mechanisms. Those mechanisms are dysrhythmias, acute pump failure, and pericardial tamponade. The patient with a myocardial contusion has usually been in a deceleration accident. There may be a chest wall or sternal contusion.

Ventricular fibrillation (VF) triggered by a blow to the anterior chest wall during cardiac repolarization is most commonly seen in teenage boys who are engaged in sporting activities or from compression of the chest against a steering wheel. This condition is known as *commotio cordis*. Prompt recognition that the VF may have been caused by a blow to the chest is critical, and rapid defibrillation is often lifesaving.

TCPA from an electrical shock usually presents as ventricular fibrillation. It may respond to ACLS protocols if you are able to initiate resuscitation early enough following TCPA. The cardiac arrest is frequently due to the prolonged apnea that may follow electrocution or lightning strike. The victim of an electrical shock has suffered severe muscle spasm and may well have been thrown down or fallen a great distance. Thus the same systematic approach to the patient is required to identify all associated injuries and to give the patient the best chance for a good outcome. However, it should be remembered that patients in TCPA after electrical or lightning injury have a higher rate of survival than arrest from other causes, and full resuscitation should always be attempted when they are encountered (Fontanarosa, 1993). Be sure the patient is no longer in contact with the electricity source. Do not become a victim yourself!

In summary, patients with cardiopulmonary arrest related to inadequate circulation have either of the following:

- Inadequate return of blood to the heart because of
  - Increased pressure in the chest causing decreased venous return to the heart, as in tension pneumothorax or pericardial tamponade
  - Hemorrhagic shock with inadequate circulating blood volume because of blood loss
- Inadequate pumping of the heart because of
  - Rhythm disturbances as in myocardial contusion, acute myocardial infarction, commotio cordis, or electrical shock
  - Acute heart failure with pulmonary edema, as in large myocardial contusion or acute myocardial infarction

Approach to Trauma Patients in Cardiac Arrest

TCPA patients are a special group. Many are young and do not have preexisting cardiac conditions or coronary disease. Ensuring a complete scene size-up is important because many cases involve criminal activity (stabbings, shootings), so carefully record (after the run) your observations of the scene. Some of these patients may be resuscitated if you arrive soon enough and you pay attention to the differences from the usual medical cardiac arrest.

The extremely poor resuscitation rate for TCPA patients is probably due to the fact that many of them have been hypoxic for a prolonged period of time before the arrest occurred. Prolonged hypoxia causes such severe acidosis that the patient may not respond to attempted resuscitation. One study concluded that of 138 patients requiring prehospital CPR at the scene or during transport because of the absence of blood pressure, pulse, and respirations, none of the patients survived, whether the victim of blunt or penetrating trauma (Rosemurgy, 1993). In addition, there has been no survival benefit noted in traumatic cardiac arrest patients transported by ground or air EMS services (DiBartolomeo, 2005).

Patients who suffer TCPA from isolated head injury usually do not survive. However, they should be aggressively resuscitated because the extent of injury cannot always be determined in the field, and therefore, you cannot predict the outcome for the individual patient. (They are also potential organ donors.) With suspected head injured patients, it is important to avoid hyperventilation because it decreases oxygen supply to the already injured brain tissue (Warner et al., 2007). Patients who are found in asystole after massive blunt trauma are dead, and their resuscitation may be terminated in the field.

Children are a special case. Although some reports show the same dismal results for resuscitation of children in cardiac arrest in the field as for adults, one review of over 700 cases of children who received CPR in the field found that 25% survived to discharge (Perron et al., 1997). This may be in part because sometimes the pulse is difficult to find in a child. In any case, you should be especially aggressive in attempting to resuscitate children with no palpable pulse. Limit pulse check to 10 seconds. If no pulse has been found after 10 seconds, begin CPR.

PEARLS: Pregnant Patients

Cardiac arrest in the pregnant patient is treated the same as in other patients. Defibrillation settings and drug dosages are exactly the same. For hypovolemic arrest, the volume of fluid needed increases, and 4 liters of normal saline should be given as fast as possible during transport.

PEARLS: Children in Cardiac Arrest

Because children who are in traumatic cardiac arrest are more likely to respond to resuscitation than adults, they are treated aggressively unless obviously unsalvageable.

General Plan of Action

As you approach the patient, note obvious injuries. The patient in cardiac arrest will have no active bleeding, but if he is in a pool of blood, that is strong evidence he may have arrested from exsanguination. After determining unresponsiveness and that the victim is not breathing (or only gasping), restrict the motion of the cervical spine. Take no longer than 10 seconds to check for a pulse, and then begin chest compressions immediately. For one rescuer the ratio of chest compressions to breaths is 30:2. For two rescuers, the ratio is 15:2 compressions to breaths.

More than 90% of childhood deaths are from foreign body aspiration that occurs in children under 5 years of age, with 65% occurring in infants. The management of a **foreign body airway obstruction (FBAO**; airway is blocked and no coughing) in a victim who is responsive or unresponsive is as follows.

PEARLS: Proper Response

An adequate number of rescuers are required to handle this situation well: one to drive the ambulance, one to ventilate, one to do chest compressions, and one to diagnose and treat the cause of the arrest.

foreign body airway obstruction (FBAO) any foreign body (vomitus, blood, food, etc.) that obstructs the airway.

FBAO Responsive Patient

- *Child or adult.* Start with supradiaphragmatic abdominal thrusts.
- *Infant.* Start with five back blows followed by five chest compressions until the object is expelled.

FBAO Unresponsive Patient

If the cause of the collapse is known to be FBAO, start CPR with chest compressions. (Do not perform pulse check.) After 30 compressions, check the airway. (Do not perform blind finger sweeps.) Ventilate two times.

Open the airway with the modified jaw-thrust maneuver. You will need assistance to maintain cervical motion restriction. The patient must be on a firm flat surface because there is a chance of injuring the spine if there is an associated vertebral injury, but this is of less concern if the patient is dying of an airway obstruction. If still unsuccessful, you may attempt cricothyroidotomy or translaryngeal jet ventilation if you are trained in the procedures and if your protocols permit them.

If the airway is not obstructed, give two full breaths and then check the pulse. If no pulse is palpable, you must begin chest compressions immediately. Prepare for immediate transport, if you are not planning to terminate resuscitation. Allow two of your teammates to do the cardiopulmonary resuscitation while you get the monitor. Perform at least two minutes of continuous chest compressions, and then check the cardiac rhythm. If either ventricular fibrillation or pulseless ventricular tachycardia (VF/pVT) is present, continue compressions while charging the defibrillator. Defibrillate with the energy recommended in your treatment guidelines. Evidence suggests that higher energy settings may have some benefit. Resume compressions for 2 minutes after defibrillation before reanalyzing the rhythm.

PEARLS: Asystole

Patients found in asystole after massive blunt trauma are dead. There is no reasonable expectation of resuscitation.

If asystole or PEA is present—or if VF/pVT persists after the shock—you should evaluate the patient for the cause of the arrest, while continuing CPR. If the patient is a victim of blunt trauma, consider termination of resuscitation. If the patient has penetrating trauma, quickly check the pupils. If the pupils are dilated and nonreactive, consider termination of resuscitation. As mentioned earlier, it may be beneficial to attempt bilateral needle decompression in the second intercostal space anteriorly (or fourth intercostal space laterally) because tension pneumothorax is one reversible cause of traumatic cardiac arrest. Resuscitation efforts should not be initiated for patients with either injuries incompatible with life or for those who have evidence of prolonged time since the arrest (Table 21-1). If resuscitation attempts have already begun on these patients, it is appropriate to terminate resuscitation efforts as directed by your local medical direction.

PEARLS: ITLS Primary Survey

The pulseless trauma patient requires attention in the ITLS Primary Survey to identify treatable problems in the proper priority.

For patients with an organized rhythm on ECG, you must quickly evaluate and treat for the cause of the arrest. This should be done in the ambulance during transport, if possible. Use the ITLS Primary Survey that you follow for every trauma patient to try to determine the cause of the TCPA.

PROCEDURE

Initial Assessment and Critical Actions

1. Establish and control the airway using the appropriate airway adjunct according to your treatment guidelines. Ventilate with 100% oxygen. While the other rescuers are ventilating and performing chest compressions, you must systematically look for reversible causes of the arrest.
2. Look for breathing problems as a cause of the arrest. Answering the following questions may allow you to identify any breathing problems that may be the cause or a contributing factor:
   a. Look at the neck.
      (1) Are the neck veins flat or distended?
      (2) Is the trachea midline?
      (3) Is there evidence of soft-tissue trauma to the neck?

b. Look at the chest.
   (1) Does the chest rise symmetrically each time you ventilate?
   (2) Are there chest injuries (penetrations, bruising, flail segment)?
   (3) If there is spontaneous respiration, is there any paradoxical motion noted?
c. Feel the chest:
   (1) Is there any instability or asymmetry?
   (2) Is there any crepitation?
   (3) Is there any subcutaneous emphysema?
d. Listen to the chest:
   (1) Are breath sounds present on both sides?
   (2) Are the breath sounds equal?

If breath sounds are not equal, percuss the chest. Is the side with the absent or decreased breath sounds hyperresonant or dull? If the patient has been intubated, is the endotracheal tube inserted too far?

If there are distended neck veins, decreased breath sounds on one side of the chest, with the trachea deviated away from the side of the injury, and hyperresonance to percussion of the chest on the affected side, then the patient probably has a tension pneumothorax. An improperly positioned endotracheal tube can cause unequal breath sounds and may be harmful to the patient because only one lung is being ventilated. You should always recheck the position of the endotracheal tube before you make a diagnosis of tension pneumothorax because it is much more common to have a poorly positioned endotracheal tube than to have a tension pneumothorax. A tension pneumothorax requires needle decompression of the affected side of the chest, if you are trained in the procedure and your protocols allow for this. If required, call medical direction immediately for permission to decompress. Continue ventilation with 100% oxygen.

Do not discontinue chest compressions until either there is a palpable pulse or resuscitation is terminated. Even though you have found a cause, there may be other causes for the patient's arrest. Other breathing problems (sucking chest wound, flail chest, simple pneumothorax) will be adequately treated by airway control and ventilation with high-flow oxygen. Once you have established an airway and are applying positive pressure ventilation to the TCPA patient, you no longer have to seal sucking chest wounds or apply external stabilization to flails. Remember, though, that positive pressure ventilation can convert a simple pneumothorax to a tension pneumothorax.

Now that the patient has both adequate airway management and is being ventilated, you may concentrate on the circulatory system. As soon as IV access is obtained, rapidly give 2 liters of normal saline. Once again, do not delay at the scene. All treatment past establishing the airway should be done during transport, if the decision has been made to continue resuscitation.

PEARLS: Transport

Rapid transport to a surgical facility is necessary. Perform procedures in the ambulance during transport. Do not waste valuable time.

Hemorrhagic shock is the most common circulatory cause of traumatic cardiopulmonary arrest. If there is a large amount of blood on or around the patient, you should note the source of the bleeding because this must be controlled if you resuscitate the patient. If there is no external bleeding, the patient must be carefully examined for evidence of internal bleeding. Reexamine the neck veins. Flat neck veins in the presence of sinus tachycardia on the monitor favor the presence of hypovolemic shock. Attempt to start two large-bore IV lines while en route.

Intraosseous (IO) lines are acceptable alternatives to IV lines, though the flow rate of the IO needle may not always approach that of large-bore IV catheters. A 10 cc flush of normal saline into the IO needle after placement into the bone often improves flow rate.

Decreased breath sounds on one side with percussion dullness on the same side suggests a hemothorax of such degree that shock will be present, though dullness to percussion may also suggest a ruptured diaphragm. Obvious bleeding, distended abdomen, multiple fractures, or an unstable pelvis also suggest that hemorrhagic shock is the cause of the TCPA. Transport rapidly while rapidly infusing 2 liters of normal saline.

Penetrating wounds of the chest or upper abdomen, or contusions of the anterior chest, are associated with pericardial tamponade and/or myocardial contusion. If the neck veins are distended, the trachea is midline, and breath sounds are equal, you should suspect pericardial tamponade. Attempt to start two large-bore IV lines while proceeding with all possible haste to the emergency department.

Electrical shock creates a special situation. It usually presents as ventricular fibrillation. Severe acidosis can develop rapidly, making resuscitation more difficult. TCPA secondary to electric shock may respond readily to ACLS protocols if you arrive before the acidosis is too severe. Do not forget to restrict the motion of the spine. A victim of high-voltage electrical shock may have fallen from a power line or have been thrown several feet by the violent muscle spasm associated with the shock. Be sure the patient is no longer in contact with the electrical source. Do not become a victim!

Considerations in Traumatic Cardiac Arrest Management

Research continues into how to optimize patient evaluation and management in TCPA patients. These patients present many challenges, requiring the ITLS provider to maintain current understanding in the care of these critically ill trauma victims.

Airway Management

It is unclear what the optimal airway is for the patient in TCPA. Prolonged periods of hypoxia have been demonstrated for patients on whom ETI is attempted in the prehospital phase of care (Davis et al., 1993). Excessive manipulation of the airway during ETI has been associated with increased risk of aspiration (Wang & Yealy, 2006). A recent study has revealed no difference in survival to hospital discharge in cardiac arrest patients when comparing the use of ETI to Combitube placement in the prehospital phase of care.

What is apparent is that the airway needed in managing a TCPA patient is that which can adequately do the job. If a bag-mask is adequate, then use that. Laryngeal fracture from blunt trauma or severe vocal cord edema due to inhaling burning gases may require cricothyrotomy. "One size fits all" does *not* apply in airway management of the patient in TCPA.

Ventilation

We now know that positive pressure ventilations reduce venous return, whether via bag-mask, ETI, or supraglottic airways. You must attempt to provide adequate air exchange while avoiding overventilation. In the TCPA patient it is reasonable to begin with an assisted ventilation rate of one breath every 8 seconds with a tidal volume of 750 cc, which is about eight times per minute using roughly a one-hand squeeze on a standard bag. This should provide good chest rise and provides a minute ventilation of about 5 liters per minute. The patient should be reassessed continuously during the resuscitation to determine if this rate of assisted ventilation is appropriate, too high, or too low.

Capnography

Oxygen is supplied to cells by the lungs and vascular system. The oxygen is transported to the cells of the body, where energy substrate (such as carbohydrate) is enzymatically burned in the cells, producing energy, water, and carbon dioxide (CO_2). CO_2 is produced proportionally to the supply of O_2 to the cells by the lungs and vascular system. The CO_2 is returned to the lungs to be exhaled. CO_2 can be measured at the airway through a technique called "waveform capnography" (literally: graphing the wave of exhaled CO_2). Thus waveform capnography provides a glimpse of the actual metabolism of the body, and the normal level measured at the airway is approximately 40 mm Hg during exhalation. A low measured level of CO_2 at the airway in TCPA patients is an indication that O_2 supply to the cells is low. Rising CO_2 levels during resuscitation of TCPA patients is an indication of improving circulation.

Overventilation of the TCPA patient can reduce cardiac output. This lowers O_2 delivery to the tissues, reducing CO_2 production and measured capnography. Thus, measuring capnography at the airway is a useful guide to establishing the correct ventilation rate and tidal volume (literally: minute ventilation) in the TCPA patient, adjusting the ventilation rates downward if capnography measures under 10 mm Hg. Specific guidelines to ventilation rate and capnography measurements should come from your local medical direction.

CASE PRESENTATION (continued)

A BLS ambulance just arrived on scene of a motorcycle crash. The closest hospital is 15 miles away and the closest level 2 trauma hospital is 45 miles away. In this EMS system, ALS is only dispatched on request of the BLS ambulance on scene. The scene size-up reveals a safe scene with one patient (approximately 20 years old) from a motorcycle that failed to negotiate a curve in the road and struck a tree. The driver was helmetless. The patient is unresponsive, is not breathing, and has no pulses. There is an obvious deformity to the skull, multiple rib fractures, and deformity to the left femur. There were no witnesses to the crash, and it is difficult to determine when the crash occurred. An AED is applied, and it indicates, "No shock advised."

Because the cardiac rhythm could not be determined by the AED, CPR is initiated, and an ALS unit is requested to respond. ALS arrives within 5 minutes of being summoned. The ALS team assesses the patient and finds him unresponsive, no spontaneous respirations, and no pulses (with or without CPR). The heart monitor is applied, and the ECG reveals asystole in two leads. The ALS team contacts medical direction to request stopping resuscitative efforts. Medical direction approves the request, and resuscitative efforts are stopped.

The autopsy revealed massive cerebral trauma, rib fractures, pulmonary contusion, a lacerated liver, and pelvic and left femur fractures. Cause of death was cited as accidental traumatic brain injury and exsanguination. ■

Summary

The trauma patient in cardiopulmonary arrest is usually suffering from a breathing or circulatory problem. If you are to save this patient, you must identify the cause of the arrest with the ITLS Primary Survey and then rapidly transport the patient while performing those procedures that specifically address the cause of the arrest. Although it is very rare to successfully resuscitate a patient suffering from a trauma arrest secondary to hemorrhagic shock, attention to detail will allow you the best chance to "bring one back from the dead," which is the greatest challenge and greatest satisfaction in EMS.

Bibliography

1. American Heart Association. 2010. Guidelines for Cardiopulmonary Care Resuscitation (CPR) and Emergency Cardiovascualar Care (ECC) *Science* 122 (18) Supplement 3.
2. Cera, S., G. Mostafa, R. Sing, et al. 2003. Physiologic predictors of survival in post-traumatic arrest. *The American Surgeon* 69: 140–144.
3. Davis, D. P., D. Hoyt, et al. 1993. The effect of paramedic rapid sequence intubation on outcome in patients with severe traumatic brain injury. *Journal of Trauma—Injury Infection & Critical Care* 54 (3): 444–453.
4. DiBartolomeo S., G. Sanson, G. Nardi, V. Michelutto, F. Scian. 2005. HEMS vs. ground-BLS care in traumatic cardiac arrest. *Prehosp Emerg Care* 9: 79–84.
5. Fontanarosa P. 1993. Electric shock and lightning strike. *Ann Emerg Med* 22(2): 378–387.
6. Hopson, L., E. Hirsh, J. Delgado, et al. 2003. Guidelines for withholding or termination of resuscitation in prehospital traumatic cardiopulmonary arrest: Joint position statement of the National Association of EMS Physicians and the American College of Surgeons Committee on Trauma. *Journal of the American College of Surgeons* 196: 106–112.
7. Perron, A. D., R. Sing, et al. 1997. Research forum abstracts. Predicting survival in pediatric trauma patients receiving CPR in the prehospital setting. *Annals of Emergency Medicine* 30: 381.
8. Rosemurgy A. S., P. Norris et el. 1993. Prehospital traumatic cardiac arrest: the cost of futility. *J Trauma* 35(3):468–73.
9. Saunders C. E., C. Heye. 1994. Ambulance collisions in an urban environment. *Prehosp Disaster Med* 9(2): 118–124.
10. Wang H. E., D. Yealy. 2006. How many attempts are required to accomplish out-of-hospital endotracheal intubation? *Acad Emerg Med* 13(4): 372–377.
11. Warner K. J., J. Cuschieri, M. Copass, et al. 2007. The impact of prehospital ventilation on outcome after severe traumatic brain injury. *J Trauma* 62: 1330–1338.

Explore Resource Central

For additional review and practice tests, visit www.bradybooks.com and click on Resource Central to access book-specific resources for this text. To access Resource Central, follow directions on the Student Access Card provided with this text. If there is no card, go to www.bradybooks.com and follow the Resource Central link to Buy Access from there.

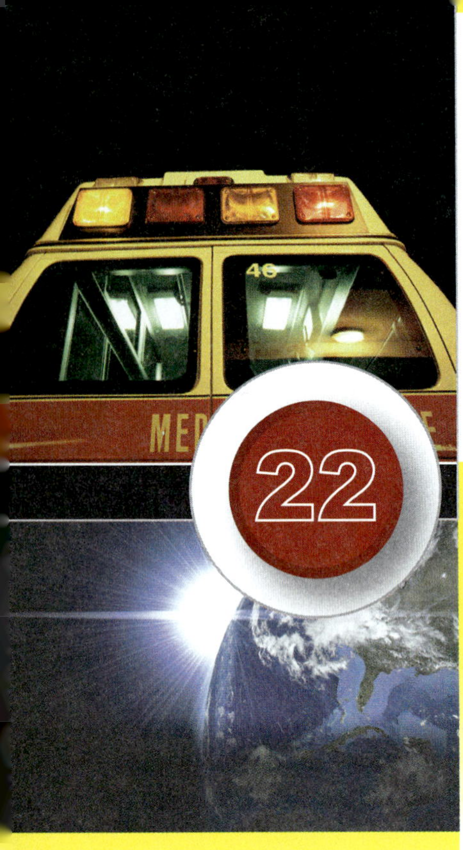

(Photo courtesy of Ryan McVay, Digital Vision, Thinkstock.com)

Standard Precautions

Katherine West, BSN, MSEd, CIC
Howard Werman, MD, FACEP
Richard N. Nelson, MD, FACEP

Standard Precautions

Precauzioni Standard

Precauciones Estándar

Précautions standard

Środki ostrożności

Eigenschutz

Standardne mjere zaštite

الاحتياطات الواجب اتباعها

standarne mere opreza

Standardni varnostni ukrepi

Általános óvintézkedés

KEY TERMS

blood and OPIM, *p.375*
hepatitis B virus (HBV), *p.374*
hepatitis C virus (HCV), *p.375*
human immunodeficiency virus (HIV), *p.376*
postexposure prophylaxis (PEP), *p.377*
standard precautions, *p.377*

OBJECTIVES

Upon successful completion of this chapter, you should be able to:

1. Discuss the three most common blood-borne viral illnesses to which EMS providers are likely to be exposed in the provision of patient care.
2. Discuss the signs and symptoms of tuberculosis, and describe protective measures to reduce possible exposure to it.
3. Describe precautions EMS providers can take to prevent exposure to blood and other potentially infectious materials (CSF, synovial fluid, amniotic fluid, pericardial fluid, pleural fluid, or any fluid with gross visible blood).
4. Identify appropriate use of personal protective equipment.
5. Describe procedures for EMS providers to follow if they are accidentally exposed.
6. Discuss multidrug-resistant organisms and prevention measures.
7. List vaccines and immunizations recommended for EMS personnel.

Chapter Overview

All occupations carry some risk. For EMS, risks have included highway hazards, fires, downed electrical wires, toxic substances, and scene security problems. The provision of patient care may pose the additional possibility of exposure to blood-borne and other diseases. Fortunately, there are precautions that can be taken to markedly reduce those risks. In addition, if personal protective equipment could not be used or failed, treatment is available to reduce the chances of acquiring those diseases following an exposure event. And of course, there are vaccines and immunizations that protect personnel from many diseases to which they may be exposed. Exposure does not mean infection. Exposure can be treated or prevented.

The spectrum of diseases to which you are potentially exposed is beyond the scope of this book. However, the three most common types of viral blood-borne infections are appropriate to discuss in conjunction with trauma management because their modes of spread are primarily by contaminated blood and other potentially infectious materials (OPIM). They are hepatitis B (HBV), hepatitis C (HBC), and HIV infection. It is a common misconception that all body fluids are potentially infectious. Body fluids that do not pose a risk for HBV, HBC, and HIV are tears, sweat, saliva, urine, stool, vomitus, nasal secretions, and sputum unless they contain visible blood contamination. This chapter offers a review of the three most common types of viral blood-borne infections plus a brief review of the bacterial disease tuberculosis and infections by multidrug-resistant organisms.

CASE PRESENTATION

An ALS tactical medical team is on scene with law enforcement's special response team (SRT). The team is preparing to enter a dwelling where there is known crack/cocaine and methamphetamine sales and usage. Just prior to entry, a NFDD (noise, flash, diversionary device) is detonated inside the dwelling. Entry is made, and the scene is secured. However, during the initial commotion one of the occupants of the dwelling tried to escape by jumping through a large glass window. The tactical medics are cleared to assess the patient who tried to escape. The nearly naked male patient is approximately 25 years old and has multiple lacerations on his face, neck, and arms. There is severe, active bleeding from the medial aspect of the patient's left upper arm. It is believed the brachial artery has been lacerated. The patient is still conscious and is physically and verbally abusive. How should the "bleeder" be managed? Is a tourniquet indicated? Are the medics, and others, at risk of being exposed to blood or other potential infectious material (OPIM)? Does the patient's lifestyle (suspected drug user) make him at high risk for having infectious diseases? What personal protective equipment (PPE) should the medics don? Keep these questions in mind as you read the chapter. Then, at the end of the chapter, find out how the rescuers completed this call . ■

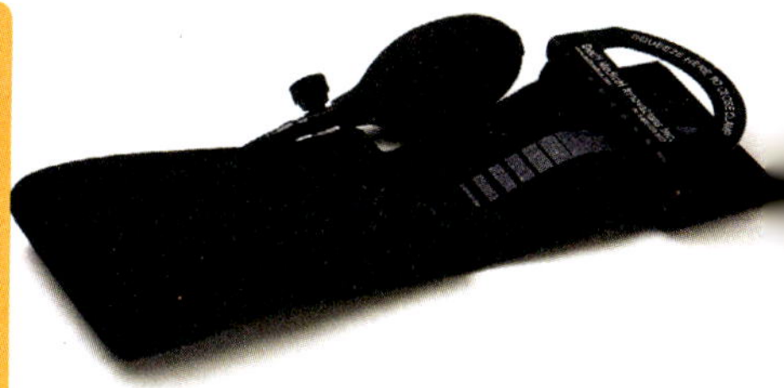

(Courtesy of Delphi Medical Innovations, Inc.)

PEARLS: An EMS Standard

All patients are potential carriers of infectious disease. That is why standard precautions are the EMS standard for practice.

Diseases of Concern

Hepatitis B

The term *viral hepatitis* is used to describe a group of viral infections involving the liver. At least five types of hepatitis virus have been described: hepatitis A, B, C, D, and E. Hepatitis A and E are spread primarily through contact with contaminated fecal material and are not blood borne. They are most prevalent in Africa. Hepatitis D is transmitted through blood and body fluid exposure to patients already infected with hepatitis B. Because of their frequent contact with blood and needles, health-care workers are considered at risk of becoming infected with the **hepatitis B virus (HBV)**. Fortunately, hepatitis B is the one form of hepatitis for which there is an effective preventive vaccine.

hepatitis B virus (HBV) an infectious virus usually spread by exposure to infected blood. It is the major cause of acute and chronic hepatitis, cirrhosis, and liver cancer. There is an effective vaccine to prevent infection.

HBV is a major cause of acute and chronic hepatitis, cirrhosis, and liver cancer. An estimated 3,000 people in the United States are infected each year. In 2009, the CDC reported that hepatitis B infection in health-care workers acquired through occupational exposure is infrequent. Because of the universal vaccination program, those numbers have decreased 90% since 1992. Following acute infection, 3% to 5% continue to be chronic carriers of the virus. These carriers are potentially infectious.

HBV is spread by contact with contaminated blood or OPIM, sexual transmission, and direct contact with a contaminated item and nonintact skin. Infection usually occurs from contaminated needlesticks or through sexual contact. The risk for acquiring HBV infection by occupational exposure is only an issue for personnel who have not been vaccinated and do not report an exposure. In those situations there is an estimated 6% to 30% risk for contracting HBV infection, if the source patient is positive for active disease. If the nonvaccinated EMS provider reports the exposure, he or she can be treated after the exposure. There is also a special treatment protocol for those who did not previously mount an antibody response to the vaccine and have an exposure.

Passage of the Needlestick Safety and Prevention Act of 2000 by the U.S. Congress requires the use of needle-safe or needleless devices (Figure 22-1). This legislation has cut the number of sharps injuries by more than half since 2003. Infection also can occur by contact of infectious bloody secretions with open skin lesions or mucosal surfaces. Routine testing of donor blood for HBV makes transmission from blood transfusions very rare.

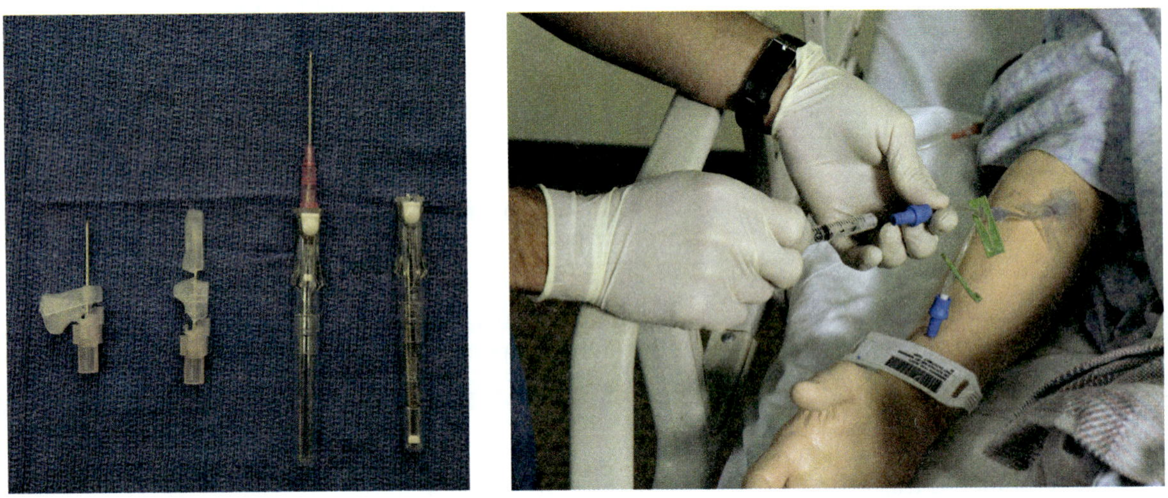

a. b.

FIGURE 22-1 (a) Safety needles and (b) needleless medication administration system. *(Photos courtesy of Stanley Cooper, EMT-P)*

Although HBV infection is uncommon in the general population, members of certain groups are considered much more likely to harbor the virus. High-risk groups are immigrants from areas where HBV is prevalent (Asia and Pacific Islands, for example), incarcerated individuals, institutionalized patients, intravenous drug users, male homosexuals, hemophiliacs, household contacts of HBV patients, and hemodialysis patients.

In the United States, the Occupational Safety and Health Administration (OSHA) mandated in 1991 that all employers of health-care workers offer HBV vaccine to any health-care worker who is at risk of occupational exposure to **blood and OPIM**. This must occur within 10 days of being hired. The vaccine offers lifelong protection. Vaccines available today are recombinant; they contain no human components. A titer (blood test) is performed 1 to 2 months after completion of the vaccine series to document response to the vaccine. If positive, no further titer testing is needed or recommended. The vaccine is safe and produces immunity in over 90% of people vaccinated.

The second form of protection is hepatitis B immunoglobulin (HBIG). This preparation contains antibodies to HBV and provides temporary, passive protection against HBV. HBIG is only 70% effective and when effective, provides protection for only 6 months. HBIG is used only when there has been a significant exposure to HBV in an unimmunized person but is given in conjunction with vaccine to offer full coverage postexposure. There are four protocols for medical follow-up for exposure to HBV based on the vaccine status of the EMS provider. Thus, it is important for the department's designated officer for infection control to have easy access to medical records 24/7 should an exposure occur.

PEARLS: Immunizations

Be prepared! Stay up to date on all your immunizations.

PEARLS: OPIM

The abbreviation "OPIM" refers to other (than blood) potentially infectious materials. Those materials include

- Cerebrospinal fluid (CSF)
- Synovial fluid
- Amniotic fluid
- Pericardial fluid
- Pleural fluid
- Any fluid with gross visible blood

blood and OPIM anything that can carry infectious disease and for which each health-care worker must take precautions to prevent exposure.

Hepatitis C

The **hepatitis C virus (HCV)** was identified in 1988–1989. This virus is thought to be responsible for the majority of what had been identified as non-A, non-B hepatitis infections. The incubation period is 6 to 7 weeks. Antibodies to the HCV have been used to identify patients with previous HCV infection. Those exposed to HCV are test-positive 4 to 6 weeks after exposure. The incidence rate for this disease is low in the United States. For 2009, there were 844 new cases reported nationwide.

hepatitis C (HCV) an infectious virus primarily spread by exposure to infected blood. It is no longer spread by blood transfusions. There is no current vaccine.

Prior to 1992, HCV was the leading cause of hepatitis resulting from blood transfusions. The virus also appears to be spread by sharing of intravenous needles, sexual contact, tattooing, and body piercing, much like HBV. Health-care workers can acquire infection through hollow-bore needlesticks with contaminated needles. The likelihood of becoming infected with HCV after a single high-risk needlestick is estimated at 1.5%. This risk is further reduced by the use of needle-safe devices.

HCV infection tends to be less severe than HBV during the initial infection. However, there appears to be a greater likelihood of becoming a chronic carrier of HCV following infection. Liver failure and cirrhosis occur in 10% to 20% of chronic HCV carriers.

There is currently no vaccine available to protect against HCV infection. Evidence suggests that there is no protective effect provided by administering immune globulin following exposure to HCV. Now, rapid HCV testing can be performed on the source patient. Rapid testing is termed *signal-to-cut-off ratio (s/co)*. Several companies make this test. It is inexpensive and takes 23 minutes to perform on source patient blood. If the source is positive, the exposed provider may be offered a follow-up test (HCV-RNA) in 4 to 6 weeks postexposure. This latter test detects the virus itself. This reduces the concern about having acquired the disease to 4 to 6 weeks instead of 6 months of follow-up. Treatment is available for people who acquire the disease. Current treatment is with peginterferon alfa-2a, a combination of long-acting interferon and another antiviral agent, ribavirin. Together, this treatment has resulted in 56% becoming clear of infection. It appears that with early treatment, chronic infection with HCV can be prevented.

Human Immunodeficiency Virus Infection

human immunodeficiency virus (HIV) a virus that weakens the immune system, predisposing a patient to a wide range of unusual infections.

HIV infection is caused by the **human immunodeficiency virus (HIV)**. Patients with HIV infection have difficulty fighting certain infections due to their compromised immune systems. This predisposes the HIV-infected patient to a variety of unusual infections not generally seen in healthy patients of similar age. They are called "opportunistic infections" and pose a risk to the patient but not to the care provider. An example is *Pneumocystis carinii* pneumonia (PCP). Most individuals have PCP in their lungs, but it does not cause illness because the immune system maintains a balance of organisms. PCP is not transmissible from an infected patient to care providers with intact immune systems.

Patients infected with HIV can present with a wide spectrum of clinical manifestations. Many patients with HIV infection are asymptomatic. An HIV-positive patient may not always present a risk. It has been documented that about 10% of Caucasians carry a mutated gene that protects them from HIV disease. They test HIV positive because they had an exposure at some time but do not have the disease and cannot transmit the disease to others. HIV patients being treated with current drugs may be free of virus circulating in their blood and, as such, pose only a minute risk. Knowing that a patient is HIV positive may not be enough information to assess risk for infection; testing the source patient's blood for viral load may be needed.

HIV appears to be transmitted in a manner similar to HBV. Although the virus has been cultured from a variety of body fluids, only blood has been implicated in the transmission of the virus in the workplace. This is because other body fluids do not carry enough virus particles to transmit the disease. Semen and vaginal secretions have been shown to transmit the virus during sexual activity only. There is no evidence to suggest that HIV is transmitted by casual contact.

Transmission to health-care workers has been documented only after accidental parenteral exposure (needlestick) or exposure of mucous membranes and open wounds to large amounts of infected blood. Measurable risk data for occupational exposure is 0.3% for needlestick injuries and 0.09% for mucous membrane exposure. There is one documented case of transmission from infected blood on nonintact skin. This case was reported in 2002 and involved a health-care worker with extensive dermatitis who did not always use gloves appropriately when caring for a patient coinfected with HIV and HCV.

HIV appears to be different from the hepatitis B virus (HBV) in two ways.

- HIV does not survive outside the body. No special cleaning agents are required.
- HIV is transmitted far less efficiently than HBV.

Several groups have been identified as having a high risk of HIV infection. They include male homosexuals or bisexuals, intravenous drug abusers, patients who have received blood transfusions or pooled-plasma products prior to 1992 (such as hemophiliacs), and heterosexual contacts of HIV-positive people. However, because of the difficulty in identifying HIV-infected patients, all contacts with blood and OPIM should be considered a potential HIV exposure. This concept (all patients are potentially infective) is why **standard precautions** are "universally" applied.

standard precautions steps each health-care worker takes to protect himself and his patient from exposure to infectious agents; includes treating each patient and himself as if they were infectious.

There is currently no available vaccine to protect against HIV infection. Antiretroviral drug regimens, though not a cure, have been shown to prolong the lives of HIV/AIDS patients. Some studies have suggested that antiretroviral agents may reduce the risk of HIV transmission in health-care workers if administered within hours following a significant exposure to HIV-infected blood and OPIM. The decision to administer such agents should be based on the nature of the exposure, the likelihood that the patient is infected with HIV, and the duration of time following exposure (Table 22-1 and Table 22-2). In general, large-gauge hollow-needle exposures are more significant than solid instruments (such as a scalpel).

If the exposure meets the CDC criteria for **postexposure prophylaxis (PEP)**, or offering drugs postexposure to the health-care worker, they can be administered within "hours but not days." Employees need to be counseled about the side effects and the unknown issues involving the use of these drugs before they are started. Baseline lab work also needs to be drawn. This can all be avoided by performing rapid HIV testing on the source patient, thus preventing a health-care provider from being placed on drugs unnecessarily while awaiting blood work on the source. Remember, all postexposure medical follow-up begins with testing the source, not the exposed employee.

postexposure prophylaxis (PEP) the administration of medications to prevent infection from the agent to which the person was exposed.

Table 22-1 Recommended HIV Postexposure Prophylaxis (PEP) for Percutaneous Injuries

Exposure Type	HIV-Positive, Class 1*	HIV-Positive, Class 2*	Source of Unknown HIV Status†	Unknown Source§	HIV-Negative
Less severe¹	Recommend basic two-drug PEP	Recommend expanded ≥ three-drug PEP	Generally, no PEP warranted; however, consider basic two-drug PEP** for source with HIV risk factors††	Generally, no PEP warranted; however, consider basic two-drug PEP** in settings in which exposure to HIV-infected persons is likely	No PEP warranted
More severe§§	Recommend expanded three-drug PEP	Recommend expanded ≥ three-drug PEP	Generally, no PEP warranted; however, consider basic two-drug PEP** for source with HIV risk factors††	Generally, no PEP warranted; however, consider basic two-drug PEP** in settings in which exposure to HIV-infected persons is likely	No PEP warranted

*HIV-positive, class 1—asymptomatic HIV infection or known low viral load (e.g., < 1,500 ribonucleic acid copies/mL). HIV-positive class 2—symptomatic HIV infection, acquired immunodeficiency syndrome, acute seroconversion, or known high viral load. If drug resistance is a concern, obtain expert consultation, initiation of PEP should not be delayed pending expert consultation. Initiation of PEP should not be delayed pending expert consultation, and because expert consultation alone cannot substitute for face-to-face counseling, resources should be available to provide immediate evaluation and follow-up care for all exposures.

†For example, deceased source person with no samples available for HIV testing

§For example, a needle from a sharps disposal container.

¹For example, solid needle or superficial injury.

**The recommendation "consider PEP" indicates that PEP is optional; a decision to initiate PEP should be based on a discussion between the exposed person and the treating clinician regarding the risks versus benefits of PEP.

††If PEP is offered and administered and the source is later determined to be HIV-negative, PEP should be discontinued.

§§For example, large-bore hollow needle, deep puncture, visible blood on device, or needle used in patient's artery or vein.

Table 22-2 Recommended HIV Postexposure Prophylaxis (PEP) for Mucous Membrane Exposures and Nonintact Skin* Exposures

Exposure Type	HIV-Positive, Class 1†	HIV-Positive, Class 2†	Source of Unknown HIV Status§	Unknown Source¶	HIV-Negative
Small volume**	Consider basic two-drug PEP††	Recommend basic two-drug PEP	Generally, no PEP warranted§§	Generally, no PEP warranted	No PEP warranted
Large volume¶¶	Recommend basic two-drug PEP	Recommend expanded ≥ three-drug PEP	Generally, no PEP warranted; however, consider basic two-drug PEP†† for source with HIV risk factors§§	Generally, no PEP warranted; however, consider basic two-drug PEP†† in settings in which exposure to HIV-infected persons is likely	No PEP warranted

*For skin exposures, follow-up is indicated only if evidence exists of compromised skin integrity (e.g., dermatitis, abrasion, or open wound)

†HIV-positive, class 1—asymptomatic HIV infection or known low viral load (e.g., < 1,500 ribonucleic acid copies/mL). HIV-positive, class 2—symptomatic HIV infection, AIDS, acute seroconversion, or known high viral load. If drug resistance is a concern, obtain expert consultation. Initiation of PEP should not be delayed pending expert consultation, and, because expert consultation alone cannot substitute for face-to-face counseling, resources should be available to provide immediate evaluation and follow-up care for all exposures.

§For example, deceased source person with no samples available for HIV testing.

¶For example, splash from inappropriately disposed blood.

**For example, a few drops.

††The recommendation "consider PEP" indicates that PEP is optional; a decision to initiate PEP should be based on a discussion between the exposed person and the treating clinician regarding the risks versus benefits of PEP.

§§If PEP is offered and administered and the source is later determined to be HIV-negative, PEP should be discontinued.

¶¶For example, a major blood splash.

Tuberculosis

PEARLS: TB

If your patient has a persistent cough plus other symptoms suggestive of TB, place a mask on the patient, not on yourself. You should wear a mask if the patient requires oxygen and cannot wear a mask.

From 1985 to 1993, the incidence of active tuberculosis increased significantly to over 25,000 cases in the United States. This was the result of an increase in cases among people infected with HIV and an increase in immigration of people from areas where tuberculosis infection is endemic (Asia, Latin America, the Caribbean, Africa). Because of better public health measures, tuberculosis has been declining in the past several years. Cases decreased by 71.4% from 1997 to 2007. In fact, the number of cases in 2007 to 2009 was the lowest ever reported in the United States. Risk factors for tuberculosis include homeless people, certain immigrant populations, patients at risk for HIV infection, and people who live in congregate settings (correction facilities, nursing homes, homeless shelters). On a global perspective, tuberculosis is still the deadliest infectious disease in Third World countries, with eight million new infections and three million deaths annually.

Tuberculosis is caused by a bacterium, *Mycobacterium tuberculosis*, which is spread from an infected person to susceptible people through the air, especially by coughing or sneezing. This is *not* a highly communicable disease. Contracting tuberculosis requires prolonged direct contact, as in a family living situation. Only persons with active infection of the lung or throat spread tuberculosis.

Clinical manifestations of the disease become apparent only when the patient's immune system fails to keep the bacteria in check. The bacteria then begins to infect the lungs and may spread to other portions of the body, particularly the kidneys, spine, or brain. Cases are termed extrapulmonary and are not communicable to the care provider. Symptoms of active tuberculosis are most prominent in the lungs and include a productive cough that lasts longer than three weeks in conjunction with two or more of the following: pain in the chest, coughing up bloody sputum, weakness or fatigue, unexplained weight loss, loss of appetite, fever, chills, night sweats, or hoarseness.

Treatment of tuberculosis includes antibiotic agents. A positive TB skin test (PPD) means the person is infected with TB (*TB infection*), but it does not necessarily indicate active disease. *TB disease* is the term for active disease. If there is a positive skin test but no indication of active TB, isoniazid (INH) or rifampin is used for a period of 6 to 9 months to eradicate the infection.

Three to four antibiotic agents are used when TB disease is confirmed. Although some strains of TB are developing resistance to many of the agents used to treat the disease, multidrug-resistant TB is still treatable and is rare (116 cases in the United States in 2007). Multidrug-resistance means that the organism has become resistant to two of the first-line antibiotics. Additional drugs are available. In 2007, extensively drug-resistant TB (XDR-TB) gained media attention. XDR-TB occurs when the organism has become resistant to two of the first-line oral antibiotics and two of the first-line injectible antibiotics. There are other drugs currently available to treat XDR-TB.

Since 1995, the U.S. Centers for Disease Control and Prevention (CDC) has recommended placing a surgical mask on any patient suspected of having TB. Thus the care provider does not need to wear a mask of any kind. Health-care workers should receive tuberculin skin testing prior to employment and periodically thereafter, depending on the TB risk assessment in their work area, to ensure that tuberculosis has not been acquired. This is in keeping with the CDC guidelines published on December 30, 2005, which OSHA is enforcing. Annual TB skin testing is *only* continued if more than three active untreated TB patients were transported by an EMS service in the previous 12 months. It should be noted that to continue annual testing in low-risk areas leads to false-positive tests. The IAFF and the NFPA 1581 Infection Control Standard defer to the CDC guidelines.

Multidrug-Resistant Organisms

Since the early 1960s the incidence rate for multidrug-resistant organisms has been increasing. The incidence began in the hospital care setting, and hospital-associated infections (HAIs) are now the leading cause of extended hospital stay and increased costs.

Methicillin-resistant *Staphylococcus aureus* (MRSA) is perhaps the most prevalent HAI, but now there is a community acquired (CA-MRSA) strain that is more common and more easily transmissible than the HA form. The new CA strain is called *USA 300* or *USA 400*. This can be transmitted by close personal contact with nonintact skin, close contact sports (wrestling/football), and poor personal hygiene. Household pets have also been identified as a source for transmission. Infection often is misdiagnosed as a "spider bite."

Referring to MRSA as methicillin resistant is a bit misleading. MRSA strains are currently resistant to several different antibiotics, including penicillin, oxacillin, and amoxicillin. HA-MRSA is often also resistant to tetracycline and erythromycin. Generally, it presents as a localized soft-tissue infection and is easily treated by incision and drainage. However, the organism can affect organs and joints. Complications of MRSA infection may include endocarditis, necrotizing fasciitis, osteomyelitis, sepsis, and death.

Prehospital care personnel are not at high risk for contracting MRSA when performing job tasks. Gloves, good handwashing, and cleaning surfaces and

PEARLS: Artificial Ventilation

Be prepared! Have appropriate barrier devices with you so you are not required to do mouth-to-mouth breathing. However, you have an obligation to perform mouth-to-mouth resuscitation if your patient needs it and you forgot your equipment.

equipment are important for protection of patients and care providers. EMS agencies also should have cleaning routines established for exercise equipment and enforce CDC work-restriction guidelines for personnel with nonintact skin that is not able to be covered with a dressing. There is *no* postexposure treatment for exposure to MRSA recommended.

Multidrug-resistant organisms will continue to be an issue until several key influencing factors are addressed. They include good handwashing practice, cleaning of vehicles and equipment, education regarding the nonuse of antibiotics when not needed, removal of antibiotics from animal foods, and altering prescription habits.

Ensuring Protection from Other Diseases of Concern

Many diseases that were once felt to be eradicated in the United States have returned. Currently there are many unvaccinated children in this country. It is important for EMS agencies to follow the CDC guidelines for vaccination and immunization of health-care workers. Current recommendations include HBV vaccine, Td booster every 10 years. However, due to the increasing rate of pertussis (whooping cough) all health-care workers are to receive one booster dose of Tdap (tetanus, diphtheria, acellular pertussis), chickenpox (varicella) vaccine, measles, mumps, rubella (MMR) if not immune, and annual flu vaccine. TB testing is performed based on the annual TB risk assessment for each EMS agency.

Precautions for Prevention of Transmission of Infectious Agents

Standard precautions refer to treating everyone (including you) as if they are infectious. Your goal is to prevent the spread of infection from you to the patient and from the patient to you. In today's environment, you must use appropriate precautions based on each and every patient's care needs. Consider the use of personal protection based on the task being performed (Table 22-3).

Table 22-3 Recommended Personal Protective Equipment for Worker Protection Against HIV and HBV Transmission in Prehospital Settings*

Task or Activity	Disposable Gloves	Gown	Mask	Protective Eyewear
Bleeding control with spurting blood	Yes	Yes	Yes	Yes
Bleeding control with minimal bleeding	Yes	No	No	No
Emergency childbirth	Yes	Yes	Yes	Yes
Blood drawing	Yes	No	No	No
Starting IV line	Yes	No	No	No
ET intubation or use of BIAD	Yes	No	No, unless splashing is likely	No, unless splashing is likely
Oral/nasal suctioning, manually cleaning airway	Yes	No	No, unless splashing is likely	No, unless splashing is likely
Handling and cleaning instruments with microbial contamination	Yes	No, unless soiling is likely	No	No
Measuring blood pressure	No	No	No	No
Measuring temperature	No	No	No	No
Giving an injection	No	No	No	No

*From CDC Guidelines for Public Safety Personnel & U.S. OSHA Guidelines

PROCEDURE

General Considerations

- Be knowledgeable about infection from hepatitis B, hepatitis C, and HIV. Understand their etiologies, signs and symptoms, routes of transmission, and epidemiology (relationships of the various factors determining the frequency and distribution of a disease).
- If you have open or weeping lesions, take special precautions to prevent exposure of those areas to blood and OPIM. Lesions should be covered with a bandage. If the lesions cannot be adequately protected, get placed on work restriction; avoid invasive procedures, other direct patient care activities, or handling of equipment used for patient care.
- Perform routine handwashing before and after all patient contact. Wash hands as soon as possible following exposure to blood or OPIM. Wash hands after glove removal. Alcohol-based foam or gel is best for in-field use. Patient-care providers should not have artificial nails or extensions (Chapman et al., 2008).
- Become immunized against the hepatitis B virus.
- Report any exposure event to your designated infection control officer (DICO).

PROCEDURE

Handling and Cleaning of Items Exposed to Blood or OPIM

- Prevent sharps injuries by using needle-safe or needleless devices. It is the law and in your best interest.
- Any disposable equipment such as masks, gowns, gloves, mouthpieces, and airways that have been contaminated by blood or OPIM should be collected in an impervious plastic bag. The plastic bags should then be disposed of according to state definitions of medical waste, in proper waste containers available in hospital emergency departments or other health-care locations. Nondisposable gowns can be laundered using simple laundry procedures. Your hospital should have linen bags or linen containers designated for contaminated gowns, etc.
- Use a low-sudsing detergent with a neutral pH to wash any surface spills on nondisposable equipment that does not usually come in contact with skin or mucous membranes. The equipment should then be wet down or soaked in a 1:100 dilution of household bleach (or 70% isopropyl alcohol). In this concentration, bleach will not cause corrosion of metal objects (U.S. Centers for Disease Control and Prevention, 1989).
- Using a low-sudsing detergent with a neutral pH, wash nondisposable medical devices that will frequently contact skin or mucous membranes. Check manufacturer's recommendations for disinfection so the warranty is not voided. If appropriate, then soak them for 30 to 40 minutes or more in 2% alkaline glutaraldehyde (e.g., Cidex) or similar solution in a well-ventilated area, rinse in sterile water, and package until reuse.

PROCEDURE

Personal Protection During Patient Exposures

(See Table 22-3.)

- Wear gloves if exposure to blood or OPIM is anticipated. Always take this precaution when performing an invasive procedure or handling any item soiled with blood or body fluids. Almost all trauma patients are risks for exposure to blood or body fluids.
- Disposable gowns, masks, and eye coverings are necessary only when extensive contact with blood or body fluids is anticipated. Those precautions are advised when airborne spread of blood or body fluids is likely (such as with endotracheal intubation, blind insertion airway device, vaginal deliveries, and major trauma).
- When treating any patient with respiratory complaints, mask the patient with a surgical mask or nonrebreather oxygen mask. It is also important to get a travel history.
- Direct mouth-to-mouth ventilation of patients during CPR is discouraged. Use disposable mouthpieces when artificial ventilation is indicated.

PROCEDURE

Reporting Accidental Exposure to Blood or OPIM

- Thoroughly wash or irrigate the exposed area immediately following an exposure to blood or contaminated body fluids. In the United States, you must contact your designated officer (mandated by federal law, March 1994, October 30, 2009). All employers of health-care workers must have a designated officer (DO). The DO will deal with the incident and the medical facility from this point.
- The DO will make the first determination regarding whether or not an exposure occurred and will notify the receiving facility of the possible exposure at the time of the incident. The DO will ask the facility to cooperate in determining the serologic status of the source. In some areas, informed consent need not be obtained to determine serologic status of the source. Know your local laws.
- Write a report of the incident as soon as possible. The minimum information that should be recorded on the report is included in Figure 22-2. The written ambulance report may be used to supplement, but not replace, the exposure report. In the United States, you will fill out a confidential exposure report form. Only the exposed employee, the DO, and the treating physician are allowed to see the form and be involved in the communication process. An exposed employee has become a patient and has a right to privacy.
- Blood tests (if any) to be done on the exposed employee depend on reports of testing of the source patient. If the results of rapid HIV testing are negative, then no further testing of the employee is needed. If the source patient is positive for HIV, then the exposed employee should undergo HIV serology determination close to the time of the incident. Repeat testing should be done at 6 weeks and 3 months. If the source patient is HCV positive, the exposed employee can be tested for HCV-RNA in 4 to 6 weeks. If the source patient is HBV positive and the exposed care provider has not already been immunized, hepatitis B vaccine should be administered. The administration of HBIG should be determined by the serologic testing of both the source (where possible) and the exposed health-care provider, as well as by the assessment of the risk of the exposure.

REPORT OF EXPOSURE TO BLOOD OR OPIM

NAME OF EMS PERSONNEL ______________________
NAME OF EMS SERVICE ______________________
SSI ______________________
ADDRESS OF EMS SERVICE ______________________
PHONE NUMBER (HOME) ______________ (WORK) ______________
DATE OF EXPOSURE ______________ TIME OF EXPOSURE ______________
NAME OF PATIENT ______________________
HOSPITAL ID NUMBER ______________________
PATIENT ADDRESS ______________________
PHONE NUMBER (WORK) ______________ (HOME) ______________
ROUTE OF EXPOSURE: ______________________

( ) Parenteral exposure (needlestick or sharp instrument)
( ) Mucous membrane
( ) Open skin
( ) Intact skin
( ) Other ______________________

TYPE OF FLUID:

( ) blood	( ) emesis	( ) saliva
( ) stool	( ) urine	( ) other ______

SOURCE OF EXPOSURE:

HIV:	( ) Yes	( ) No	( ) Unknown	
Hepatitis B:	( ) No	( ) Acute	( ) Chronic Carrier	( ) Unknown
Hepatitis C:	( ) No	( ) Acute	( ) Chronic Carrier	( ) Unknown
Tuberculosis:	( ) No	( ) Yes		

RISK FACTORS:

( ) Homosexual ( ) IV Drug Abuser
( ) Hemophilia ( ) Dialysis Patient
( ) Sexual Contact of the Above
( ) Other ______________________

HIV Test:	( ) Pos.	( ) Neg.	( ) Unknown

Date of HIV Test: ______________________

HBsAg:	( ) Pos.	( ) Neg .	( ) Unknown

Date of HBsAg Test ______________________

Description of Circumstances Surrounding the Exposure, Including Measures Taken After Exposure:
____
____
____

INSTITUTION NOTIFIED: ______________________
PHYSICIAN OR RESPONSIBLE PERSON: ______________________
DATE OF NOTIFICATION: ______________ TIME OF NOTIFICATION: ______________
NAME OF EXPOSED PERSONNEL ______________ DATE ______________
SIGNATURE ______________________

FIGURE 22-2 Sample report form.

PEARLS: Reporting an Exposure

Any possible exposure to blood or OPIM or an airborne transmissible disease should be immediately reported to your designated officer. (Know who this is and how to reach him or her 24/7.)

PEARLS: Mandatory Reporting

Reporting of exposure to HBV, HBC, HIV and other exposure to blood or OPIM is mandatory in the United States and has significantly reduced the incidence and spread of infection in health-care providers in the last 15 years.

CASE PRESENTATION (continued)

An ALS tactical medical team is on scene with law enforcement's special response team (SRT). The team is preparing to enter a dwelling where there is known crack/cocaine and methamphetamine sales and usage. Just prior to entry, a noise, flash, diversionary device (NFDD) is detonated inside the dwelling. Entry is made, and the scene is secured. However, during the initial commotion, one of the occupants of the dwelling tried to escape by jumping through a large glass window. The tactical medics are cleared to assess the patient who tried to escape. The nearly naked male patient is approximately 25 years old and has multiple lacerations on his face, neck, and arms. There is severe, active bleeding from the medial aspect of the patient's left upper arm. It is believed the brachial artery has been lacerated. The patient is still conscious and is physically and verbally abusive.

The medics and law enforcement officers don supplemental personal protective equipment (gloves, face shields, and gowns). The patient is physically restrained, and the bleeding cannot be controlled by pressure alone. A commercially made tourniquet is applied proximal to the bleeder. Bleeding is controlled with the device. The ITLS Primary Survey reveals the patient is conscious and combative, verbally abusive, and spitting. Although being manually and mechanically restrained, the patient continues to resist.

Respiratory rate is 30, pulse rate is 120, and breath sounds are clear and equal. Minor lacerations, with minimal bleeding, are noted on the chest, forearms, and upper legs. The patient is immediately transported. No useful additional information is gathered during the ITLS Secondary Survey. Due to combativeness a blood pressure is not obtained, but skin color is good, capillary refill is normal, and peripheral pulses, although rapid, are present and weak. An IV is established, with 4 mg of lorazepam and a 20 mL/kg bolus of normal saline administered. During transport the receiving hospital is notified of the incoming patient status and the suspicions of drug use and excited delirium syndrome.

The patient is admitted to the hospital, after the repair of the lacerated brachial artery, for treatment for polydrug abuse and hepatitis C virus infection. Because of the proper use of personal protective equipment, none of the EMS personnel were found to be at risk of infection . ■

Summary

Like most health-care workers, you are at risk of exposure to many contagious diseases. Because of the presence of blood and contaminated secretions in many trauma victims, you must take extra precautions to avoid exposure to the viruses that cause hepatitis B, hepatitis C, and HIV and to the bacteria that cause tuberculosis. Knowledge of the modes of exposure, as well as adherence to barrier precautions, or postexposure medical follow-up will reduce your risk of contracting any of those infections. In the United States, the recent standards released by OSHA make adherence to precautions mandatory for health-care workers at risk for exposure to contaminated blood or OPIM with the exception of not delaying care if personal protective equipment is not readily available. Taking recommended vaccine and immunizations also lowers risk for exposure to vaccine preventable diseases.

Bibliography

1. APIC Text of Infection Control and Epidemiology. 2009. Association for Professionals in Infection Control and Epidemiology, Inc.
2. Chapman, L. E., E. E. Sullivent, L. A. Grohskopf, E. M. Beltrami, J. F. Perz, K. Kretsinger, et al. 2008. Centers for Disease Control and Prevention (CDC). Recommendations for postexposure interventions to prevent infection with hepatitis B virus, hepatitis C virus, or human immunodeficiency virus, and tetanus in persons wounded during bombings and other mass-casualty events—United States, 2008: Recommendations of the Centers for Disease Control and Prevention (CDC). *MMWR Recomm Rep.* 57(RR-6): 1–21.
3. Immunization of Health-Care Workers: Recommendations for the Advisory Committee on Immunization Practices (ACIP) and the Hospital Infection Control Practices Advisory Committee (HICPAC), *MMWR*, December 26, 1997.
4. NIOSH Alert. 1997, June. Latex allergy.
5. Ryan White Comprehensive AIDS Resources Emergency Act; Emergency Response Employees; Notice, Centers for Disease Control, Department of Health and Human Services, Federal Register, March 21, 1994—Reauthorized September 30, 2009, Part G.
6. Updated U.S. Public Health Service Guidelines for the Management of Occupational Exposures to HIV, Recommendations for Postexposure Prophylaxis, Centers for Disease Control and Prevention, September 30, 2005.
7. U.S. Centers for Disease Control and Prevention. 2002, October 25. Hand hygiene guidelines.
8. U.S. Centers for Disease Control and Prevention. 2001. Updated U.S. Public Health Service guidelines for the management of occupational exposures to HBV, HCV, and HIV and recommendations for postexposure prophylaxis. *Morbidity and Mortality Weekly Report* 50(RR11): 1–42.
9. U.S. Centers for Disease Control and Prevention. 1989. Guidelines for Public Safety.
10. U.S. Congress. 2000. Needlestick Safety and Prevention Act.
11. U.S. Department of Labor. 2001, November 27. Compliance directive for occupational exposure to bloodborne pathogens (CPL 2-2.69).
12. U.S. Public Health Service. 2005, December 30. Guidelines for the prevention of transmission of *Mycobacterium tuberculosis* in health-care settings.
13. Weiner H. R. 2008. Community-associated methicillin-resistant *Staphylococcus aureus*: Diagnosis and treatment. *Compr Ther.* 34(3-4): 143–146.

Explore Resource Central

For additional review and practice tests, visit www.bradybooks.com and click on Resource Central to access book-specific resources for this text. To access Resource Central, follow directions on the Student Access Card provided with this text. If there is no card, go to www.bradybooks.com and follow the Resource Central link to Buy Access from there.

Glossary

A

abruptio placenta: the separation of the placenta from the wall of the uterus.

altered mental status: a diminished level of awareness or consciousness.

amputation: an open injury caused by the cutting or tearing away of a limb, body part, or organ.

AVPU: an abbreviated description of the patient's level of consciousness. The letters AVPU stand for alert, responds to verbal stimuli, responds to pain, unresponsive.

B

Beck's triad: the three clinical signs of cardiac tamponade (distended neck veins, muffled heart sounds, and pulsus paradoxus).

BIAD: short for blind insertion airway device, which can be inserted without having to visualize the larynx. Also called supraglottic airway devices.

blast injuries: injuries commonly produced by the mechanisms associated with an explosion (air blast, shrapnel, burns, etc.).

blood and OPIM: short way of referring to anything that can carry infectious disease and for which each health-care worker must take precautions to prevent exposure. The letters OPIM stand for other potentially infectious material.

BLS: short for basic life support.

BSA: short for body surface area; usually refers to percent of a patient's body surface area affected by a burn.

burn depth: a classification of severity of burns by how deep the skin is burned. In order of worsening injury that includes superficial burns (first degree), partial-thickness burns (second degree), and full-thickness burns (third degree).

C

capillary refill time (CRT): a test for shock performed by pressing on the palm of the hand or sides of the fingertips and noting how quickly color returns to the blanched area. The test is suspicious for shock if the blanched area remains pale for longer than 2 seconds. It has been found to be unreliable for early shock and neurogenic shock.

capnography: a noninvasive device that detects or measures the amount of carbon dioxide in the expired breath of a patient.

carbon monoxide poisoning: a type of inhalation injury (hypoxia) from inhalation of carbon monoxide, a colorless, odorless, and tasteless gas. Carbon monoxide binds to the hemoglobin molecule and prevents oxygenation of the cells of the body.

cerebral herniation syndrome: a critical syndrome in which swelling of the brain forces portions of the brain tissue down through the opening at the base of the skull, squeezing the brain stem and causing coma, dilatation of pupils, contralateral paralysis, elevated blood pressure, and bradycardia. Unless corrected, it is always fatal.

cerebral perfusion pressure (CPP): the pressure of the blood flowing through the brain. Its value is obtained by subtracting the intracranial pressure from the mean arterial blood pressure. It must be maintained above 60 mm Hg to perfuse the brain.

chemical injury: an injury to the skin or other body organs from exposure to caustic or toxic chemicals.

child abuse: the physical or emotional violence or neglect toward a person from infancy until age 15.

child restraint seat: a piece of safety equipment in which a child sits and that is designed to protect a child in case of a motor-vehicle collision. It must fit the child, and the child must be properly strapped into the seat for it to be effective.

chronic disease: a long-lasting or recurrent illness that may be underlying the acute problem that prompted need for emergency care. Signs and symptoms between the chronic disease and trauma may need to be distinguished.

closed-ended questions: questions that can be answered with a "yes" or "no." This is often the best approach with patients under the influence of alcohol or drugs due to their limited ability to concentrate.

closed fracture: a break in a bone in which there is no break in the continuity of the overlying skin.

compartment syndrome: a condition in which increased tissue pressure in a confined space causes decreased blood flow, leading to hypoxia and possible muscle, nerve, and vessel impairment, which may be permanent if the cells die.

compensate: the body's natural ability to adapt to a range of conditions. In the elderly patient there may be a decrease in the ability, or even an absence of the ability, to compensate for shock or other conditions.

consent: the permission that must be obtained before emergency care may be provided. In the case of an injured child, the granting of permission to treat the child. It is usually given by the parents or legal guardian but is not required in an emergency situation if neither are present.

contracoup: an injury to the brain on the opposite side of the original impact.

COPD: short for chronic obstructive pulmonary disease.

coup: an injury to the brain in the area of original impact.

crepitation: the sound or feel of broken fragments of bone grinding against each other.

Cushing's reflex: a reflex whereby the body reacts to increased intracerebral pressure by raising the blood pressure. Also called Cushing's response.

D

DCAP-BLS: short for deformities, contusions, abrasions, penetrations, burns, lacerations, and swelling.

domestic violence: physical abuse in the home. Through the second and third trimester of pregnancy, it is estimated that 1 in 10 pregnant women experiences physical abuse.

drug-assisted intubation (DAI): a technique to improve the likelihood of intubating a difficult patient by administering a sedative and paralytic agent. Previously called rapid sequence intubation or rapid sequence induction.

E

ECG: short for electrocardiogram.

electrical injury: an injury from the passage of electrical current through the body. The injuries can be from heat generated in tissue from electrical current passing through the body, cardiac dysrhythmia from current passing through the heart, and thermal burns from ignition of clothing.

emergency rescue: the immediate removal, without use of spinal motion restriction, of a patient from an immediately life-threatening situation.

essential equipment: equipment that is worn or carried when the responders approach the trauma patient. It includes personal protective equipment, long backboard and strapping, rigid cervical extrication collar, oxygen and airway equipment, and trauma box.

evisceration: the protruding of intestinal organs through a wound.

external laryngeal manipulation (ELM): a maneuver to improve visualization of the vocal cords during endotracheal intubation.

F

flail chest: the fracture of two or more adjacent ribs in two or more places, causing instability of the chest wall and paradoxical movement of the "flail segment" in a spontaneously breathing patient.

flow-restricted oxygen-powered ventilation device (FROPVD): an artificial ventilation device that provides 100% oxygen at a flow rate of 40 liters per minute at a maximum pressure of 50 + 5 cm water.

fluid resuscitation: the replacement of intravascular volume in a hypovolemic patient by infusing a crystalloid solution.

focused exam: an exam used when there is a focused (localized) mechanism of injury or an isolated injury. The exam is limited to the area of injury.

foreign body airway obstruction (FBAO): any foreign body (vomitus, blood, food, etc.) that obstructs the airway.

G

GCS: short for Glasgow Coma Scale; a method used to measure the severity of a head injury.

H

heat-inhalation injury: thermal burns of the upper airway caused by inhaling flame or hot gases. The lower airways are usually not affected because of efficient cooling by moist mucous membranes.

hemorrhagic shock: a type of shock caused by insufficient blood within the vascular system.

hemostatic agents: chemical or physical agents that help stop hemorrhage by facilitating clotting of the blood at the bleeding site.

hepatitis B virus (HBV): an infectious virus usually spread by exposure to infected blood. It is the major cause of acute and chronic hepatitis, cirrhosis, and liver cancer. An effective vaccine to prevent infection is available.

hepatitis C virus (HCV): an infectious virus primarily spread by exposure to infected blood, though it is no longer spread by blood transfusions. There is no current vaccine.

high-energy event: a mechanism of injury in which it is likely that there was a large release of uncontrolled kinetic energy transmitted to the patient, thus increasing the chances for serious injury.

human immunodeficiency virus (HIV): a virus that weakens the immune system, predisposing a patient to a wide range of unusual infections.

hypoventilation: the movement of air in and out of the lungs is unable to maintain the carbon dioxide level below 45 mm Hg.

hypovolemic shock: a type of shock caused by insufficient volume (blood or fluid) within the vascular system.

I

impaled object: an injury in which an object is embedded in the body tissue.

initial assessment: a rapid assessment of airway, breathing, and circulation to prioritize the patient and identify immediately life-threatening conditions; part of the ITLS Primary Survey.

interactive style: the speech and body language used by an EMS responder during interaction with a patient. A positive, nonjudgmental style facilitates assessment and interventions while decreasing scene time.

intracranial pressure (ICP): the pressure of the brain and contents within the skull.

intrathoracic abdomen: that part of the abdomen enclosed by the lower ribs; contains the liver, gallbladder, spleen, stomach, and transverse colon.

ITLS Ongoing Exam: an abbreviated exam to determine changes in the patient's condition.

ITLS Primary Survey: a brief exam to find immediately life-threatening conditions. It is made up of the scene size-up, initial assessment, and either the rapid trauma survey or the focused exam.

ITLS Secondary Survey: a comprehensive heat-to-toe exam to find additional injuries that may have been missed in the ITLS Primary Survey.

J

joint dislocation: a complete disruption of a joint with total loss of contact between the joint's articular surfaces.

JVD: short for jugular vein distention.

K

kyphotic deformity: a condition caused by narrowing of the vertebral discs and gradual collapse of the osteoporotic thoracic vertebral bodies often seen in the elderly who present in a stooped posture with an "S" shape to the spine.

L

length-based tape: a method of estimating the appropriate size equipment and doses of medications for children. The method is based on the fact that a child's weight is proportional to his length.

lightning injury: an injury by the multiple effects of very short duration, very high voltage direct current on the body. The most serious effect is cardiac and respiratory arrest.

LOC: short for level of consciousness.

lung compliance: the "give" or elasticity of the lungs.

M

massive hemothorax: the presence of at least 1,500 cc of blood loss into the pleural space of the thoracic cavity.

MCI: short for multi-casualty incident.

mean arterial blood pressure (MAP): the sum of the diastolic blood pressure plus one-third (systolic blood pressure minus the diastolic blood pressure).

mechanical shock: a type of shock produced by conditions that affect the ability of the heart to pump blood; caused by a damaged heart (myocardial contusion) or by conditions preventing the filling of the heart (pericardial tamponade, tension pneumothorax).

mechanism of injury: the means by which the patient was injured, such as fall, motor-vehicle collision, or explosion.

mediastinum: the anatomic region within the thorax, located between the lungs, that contains the heart and great vessels, trachea, major bronchi, and the esophagus.

minute volume: the volume of air breathed in and out in one minute; varies from 5 to 12 liters per minute.

MMAP: a technique for predicting when a patient will be difficult to intubate; the letters MMAP stand for Mallampati, measurement 3-3-1, atlanto-occipital extension, and pathology.

N

neurogenic shock: a type of shock caused by spinal injury in which the spinal connections to the adrenal glands are interrupted and the vasoconstrictors, epinephrine and norepinephrine, are not produced. Without the vasoconstrictors the blood vessels dilate and redistribute blood flow to a larger vascular volume causing a relative hypovolemia.

neurovascular injury: an injury that involves nerves and blood vessels. Also called neurovascular compromise.

neutral alignment: aligning the patient according to the baseline physiologic spinal position.

no-reflow phenomenon: the inability of restoring oxygenation and blood pressure to restore perfusion to the cortex after an anoxic episode of 4 to 6 minutes or more. It is caused by irreversible spasm of the arterioles.

normal ventilation: the movement of air into and out of the lungs that maintains the carbon dioxide level between 35 and 45 mm Hg.

O

occupant restraint systems: systems built into a vehicle to prevent the driver and passengers from being thrown about the interior of the vehicle or from being ejected from the vehicle in the event of a collision.

open fracture: a broken bone in which a piece of the bone is protruding or has protruded through the overlying skin.

open pneumothorax: the accumulation of air in the pleural space secondary to penetrating injury, presenting as an open or sucking chest wound (> 3 cm in diameter).

open-book pelvic fracture: a severe pelvic fracture in which the symphysis is torn apart and the anterior pelvis is "opened" like a book; frequently associated with disruption of both sacroiliac joints.

OPIM: short for other potentially infectious material to which a rescuer may be exposed (other than blood).

osteoporosis: a condition frequently seen in the elderly in which there is gradual loss of calcium from the bones with a decrease in bone mass and density, causing the bones to be more easily fractured.

P

paradoxical pulse: a clinical sign of cardiac tamponade. It is an exaggeration of the normal variation of the strength of the pulse during the inspiratory phase of respiration, in which the blood pressure decreases as one inhales and increases as one exhales. The paradox is that, in the case of a pericardial tamponade with decreased cardiac output, the palpated radial pulse disappears during inspiration. Also called *pulsus paradoxus*.

paresthesia: an abnormal sensation; a "tingling" or "burning" sensation.

Parkland formula: a formula to calculate initial fluid resuscitation of the burn patient. The formula is: fluid needs for first 24 hours equal 4 cc of Ringer's lactate or normal saline multiplied times the % of burn area multiplied times the body weight in kilograms.

patent airway: an open airway.

pathophysiology of aging: the process of aging that consists of the gradual decline in the normal function of many body systems, which in part may be responsible for greater risk of injury in the elderly population.

patient assessment: the process by which the EMS responder evaluates a trauma patient to determine injuries sustained and the patient's physiologic status; made up of the ITLS Primary Survey, ITLS Ongoing Exam, and ITLS Secondary Survey.

patient restraint: limiting the patient's motion and mobility to prevent him from becoming a danger to himself or others.

pericardial tamponade: the rapid collection of blood between the heart and pericardium from a cardiac injury. The accumulating blood compresses the ventricles of the heart, preventing the ventricles from filling between contractions and causing cardiac output to fall.

peritoneum: a thin serous membrane that lines the abdominal cavity and encloses the organs of the intrathoracic and true abdomen.

personal protective equipment (PPE): the equipment that an EMS rescuer dons for protection from various dangers that may be present at a trauma scene. At a minimum that entails wearing protective gloves. At a maximum the rescuer may require a chemical suit and self-contained breathing apparatus.

physiological changes of pregnancy: the normal changes that occur to the body of a woman as she progresses through her pregnancy. They affect blood volume, vital signs, and even response to hypovolemia.

pleural space: the potential space between the visceral and parietal pleura within the thorax. In disease or injury states this space can accumulate air, fluid, or blood.

PMS: short for pulses, motor function, and sensation.

postexposure prophylaxis (PEP): the administration of medications to prevent infection from the agent to which the person was exposed.

PPE: short for personal protective equipment.

primary brain injury: the immediate damage to the brain tissue that is the direct result of an injury force.

primary spinal-cord injury: injury to the spinal cord that occurs at the time of the trauma itself. This injury results from the cord being cut, torn, or crushed, or by its blood supply being cut off.

pulse oximeter: a noninvasive device for measuring the oxygen saturation of the blood.

pulse pressure: the pressure driving blood through the vascular system; calculated by subtracting the diastolic from the systolic blood pressure.

R

radiation injury: an injury to the skin and tissues from the effect of ionizing radiation; caused by radiation breaking molecular bonds within the cell. This type of injury cannot be differentiated from thermal burns by appearance alone.

rapid extrication: the rapid removal of a patient from a dangerous position or situation using modified spinal motion restriction.

rapid sequence intubation (RSI): a technique to improve the likelihood of intubating a difficult patient by administering a sedative and paralytic agent. Also called rapid sequence induction or drug-assisted intubation.

rapid trauma survey: a brief exam from head to toe performed to identify life-threatening injuries.

Reeves sleeve: a dual-purpose motion-restriction device that is effective for both spinal motion restriction and patient restraint.

respiration: the exchange of oxygen between the alveoli and the red blood cells.

retroperitoneal abdomen: that part of the abdomen behind the thoracic and true portions of the abdomen separated from the other abdominal regions by the thin retroperitoneal membrane; includes the kidneys, ureters, pancreas, posterior duodenum, ascending and descending colon, abdominal aorta, and the inferior vena cava.

rhabdomyolysis: the disintegration (lysis) or dissolution of muscle. This releases large amounts of myoglobin into the blood, which can precipitate in the kidneys, causing renal failure.

rule of nines: a method of estimating the body surface area burned by a division of the body into regions, each of which represents approximately 9% of the total surface area, plus 1% for the genital area.

S

SAMPLE history: the minimum amount of information needed for a trauma patient; the letters in SAMPLE stand for symptoms, allergies, medications, past medical history, and last oral intake.

scene size-up: observations made and actions taken at a trauma scene before actually approaching the patient. It is the initial step in the ITLS Primary Survey.

seat-belt sign: a bruise or abrasion across the abdomen from an improperly positioned lap belt. It can be a clue to blunt intra-abdominal injury.

secondary brain injury: an injury to the brain that is the result of hypoxia or decreased perfusion of brain tissue after a primary injury.

secondary spinal-cord injury: an injury to the spinal cord that occurs from hypotension, generalized hypoxia, injury to blood vessels, swelling, compression of the cord from surrounding hemorrhage, or injury to the cord from movement of a damaged and unstable spinal column.

Sellick maneuver: a maneuver (posterior pressure on the cricoid cartilage) to close the esophagus and prevent gastric insufflation and vomiting.

smoke-inhalation injury: an injury to the lungs or other body organs from inhalation of toxic gases found in smoke.

spinal column: the 33 vertebrae that house and protect the spinal cord.

spinal cord: an electrical conduit composed of specific bundles of nerve tracts. It connects the brain to the muscles and organs of the body.

spinal motion restriction (SMR): techniques and equipment used to minimize movement of the spine and attempt to prevent further spinal column or cord injury.

sprain: a sudden twist of a joint with stretching or tearing of ligaments.

standard precautions: procedures used to prevent contamination by a patient's body fluids. This always entails wearing gloves, frequently requires a face shield, and occasionally requires a protective gown or suit; includes treating each patient and the rescuer himself as if they were infectious.

strain: a stretching or partial tearing of a muscle or musculotendinous unit.

supine hypotension syndrome: the drop in blood pressure seen when a woman who is greater than 20 weeks pregnant is in the supine position. The hypotension is caused by the weight of the pregnant uterus pressing on the inferior vena cava and decreasing the return of blood to the heart by up to 30%.

T

tension pneumothorax: a condition in which air continuously leaks out of the lung into the pleural space. The air continues to accumulate there without means of exit, resulting in increasing intrathoracic pressure on the affected side and eventual collapse of the superior and inferior vena cava as well as the lung.

thermal injury: an injury to the skin caused by heat from flame, hot liquids, hot gases, or hot solids.

TIC: short for tenderness, instability, and crepitus.

tidal volume: the amount of air that is inspired and expired during one respiratory cycle.

traumatic cardiopulmonary arrest (TCPA): a grouping of conditions defined by the common precipitating factor of trauma being the origin for the cardiac arrest.

true abdomen: that part of the abdomen from the lower ribs and including the pelvis but anterior to the retroperitoneum; contains the large and small intestines, a portion of the liver, and the bladder. In a female, the uterus, fallopian tubes, and ovaries are also part of the true abdomen.

U

uncooperative patient: a patient who behaves inappropriately and does not respond to reasonable requests and limits placed on him for his own safety and that of caregivers. Based on jurisdiction, a range of options are available for restraining patients against their will when warranted for patient safety, assessment, and care.

unsalvageable patient: one who does not have a reasonable expectation for resuscitation and survival based on defined clinical indicators and parameters. It is acceptable to withhold resuscitation under those conditions.

V

vasoconstriction: the constriction (narrowing) of the arteries to maintain the blood pressure and perfusion of vital organs.

ventilation: the movement of air or gases in and out of the lungs.

W

withholding or terminating resuscitation: based on research and published guidelines, an attempt to resuscitate the patient in cardiac arrest is not initiated or is stopped in certain instances.

Index

Q

R

S

T